Hematopathology

Renu Saxena • Hara Prasad Pati
Editors

Hematopathology

Advances in Understanding

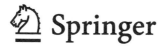 Springer

Editors
Renu Saxena
Department of Hematology
All India Institute of Medical Sciences
New Delhi
India

Hara Prasad Pati
Department of Hematology
All India Institute of Medical Sciences
New Delhi
India

ISBN 978-981-13-7715-0   ISBN 978-981-13-7713-6   (eBook)
https://doi.org/10.1007/978-981-13-7713-6

This Springer imprint is published by the registered company Springer Nature Singapore Pte Ltd.
The registered company address is: 152 Beach Road, #21-01/04 Gateway East, Singapore 189721, Singapore

Contents

About the Editors

Hara Prasad Pati received his MD pathology from All India Institute of Medical Sciences (AIIMS), New Delhi and subsequently worked as a senior resident/senior research officer at the Department of Pathology at the same institute. He is currently working as the Professor of Hematology at AIIMS. His research areas include acute leukemia, chronic leukemia (CML), MDS, drug trials (deferiprone), hemostasis, functional platelet disorders, venous thrombosis particularly splanchnic venous thrombosis, red cell enzymology, hematopoietic cell colony culture, electron microscopy, angiogenesis, immunohistochemistry, and flow cytometry.

Dr Pati has published more than 200 papers in national and international journals and 30 book chapters and has co-edited six hematology books. Presently, he is the Editor-in-Chief of the Indian Journal of Hematology and Blood Transfusion. Dr Pati is a fellow of the International Medical Sciences Academy, Indian College of Pathologists, and Indian Society of Hematology, and a member of the American Society of Hematology and British Society of Hematology.

Renu Saxena is the Professor and Head of the Department of Hematology, All India Institutes of Medical Sciences (AIIMS), New Delhi. Her main interests are in the diagnosis and molecular genetics of hemostasis, thrombosis, thalassemia, hemoglobinopathies, hemolytic disorders, and acute and chronic leukemias. DNA analysis for hemophilia A linkage studies, intron 22 and 1 inversion, von Willebrand disease characterization, F V Leiden, prothrombin 20210, and MTHFR gene mutations are some of the areas in which she has been actively involved. Dr Saxena has published more than 350 papers in national and international journals and is a fellow of the National Academy of Medical Sciences (FNAMS) and International Medical Sciences Academy.

In addition, Dr Saxena serves on the editorial boards of numerous national and international journals and on subject expert committees for national scientific bodies like the Indian Council for Medical Research (ICMR), Department of Science and Technology (DST), Council of Scientific and Industrial Research (CSIR), and Department of Biotechnology (DBT). She has been the principal investigator for 26 funded research projects and has received 17 prestigious national and international awards for her contributions in hematology, including the BC Roy Award from the Medical Council of India.

Part I

Red Cell Disorders

Newer CBC Parameters of Clinical Significance

Shanaz Khodaiji

As technology advances, recently developed automated hematology analyzers (HA) determine routine CBC parameters with better accuracy. In addition, they yield novel parameters also called Advanced Clinical Parameters (ACP) whose clinical utility is being assessed by several researchers in the field of laboratory hematology. Many of these ACP have been found to enhance clinical information and are now integrated into the routine Complete Blood Count (CBC) report.

ACPs can be obtained on the following analyzers:

- Sysmex XE and now XN-series
- Abbot Diagnostics Cell Dyn Sapphire
- Beckman Coulter LH750 and UniCel DxH 800
- Horiba Medical Pentra
- Mindray BC 6800
- Siemens Advia

Evolution of CBC parameters from basic to advanced is shown in Table 1.1.

ACP are a result of constant improvement in hardware and software technology along with use of newer improved reagents and fluorescent dyes.

S. Khodaiji (✉)
P.D. Hinduja Hospital and Medical Research Centre, Mumbai, India
e-mail: dr_skhodaiji@hindujahospital.com

Table 1.1 Evolution of CBC analyzers over the years

1960	1970/1980	1990
WBC	5 part differential	Immature grans (IG)
RBC	Reticulocytes and fractions	RET-HE & RBC-HE
Hb		NRBC and frag RBC
Hct	Platelet (I) impedance	Platelet (O) optical/(F) fluorescence
MCV	MPV	Hematopoietic progenitor cells (HPC)
MCH	RDW	

1.1 Reticulocyte Parameters

These parameters are obtained from the reticulocyte channel of the Sysmex XE and XN HAs.

1.1.1 Reticulocyte Count and Reticulocyte Fractions

The reticulocyte count is a very useful hematological parameter but highly under-utilized in clinical practice because manual reticulocyte counting is tedious to perform and prone to inter-observer variation resulting in unreliable counts with very high CVs.

The RET channel available on many newer hematology analyzers performs reticulocyte measurements automatically with no preprepapation of sample required.

R. Saxena, H. P. Pati (eds.), *Hematopathology*, https://doi.org/10.1007/978-981-13-7713-6_1

1.1.2 Principle

This is based on the principle of fluorescence flow cytometry using the nucleic acid dye oxazine 750 which stains the RNA of the cell. RBCs do not contain RNA and hence do not take up the dye, whereas reticulocytes fluoresce brightly and can thus be counted. The forward-scattered light (FSC) and the fluorescence signal (FSL), separate reticulocytes from mature RBCs (Fig. 1.1).

According to their stage of maturity, reticulocytes have varying fluorescence intensity, and based on this they are fractionated into three subtypes as follows:

- Those that fluorescence dimly are low fluorescence reticulocytes or **LFR**
- Those showing medium fluorescence, the medium fluorescence reticulocytes or **MFR**
- Those with high fluorescence called **HFR**

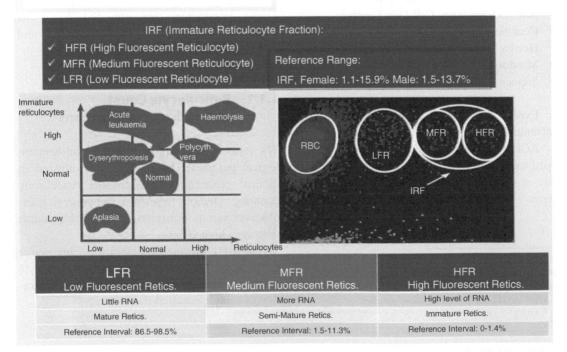

Fig. 1.1 Utility of reticulocyte count and reticulocyte fractions in hematological diagnosis. Alongside is a normal RET scattergram showing reticulocyte fractions on Sysmex analyser

The immature reticulocyte fraction (IRF) is the percentage of immature reticulocytes, calculated from the sum of MFR and HFR. IRF is a reflection of erythropoietic activity and is increased in bone marrow engraftment following transplant. It is an earlier indication of regenerating marrow than absolute neutrophil count (ANC).

1.2 Reticulocyte Production Index (RPI)

The RPI, is a correction of the reticulocyte count, and is useful in the diagnosis of anemia because the percent reticulocyte count can be misleading in anemia (Table 1.2)

Table 1.2 Calculation of RPI on automated HA

Reticulocyte Production Index is calculated as follows:
1. $\text{ReticIndex} = \text{ReticCount} * \dfrac{\text{Hematocrit}}{\text{Normal Hematocrit}}$
A value of 45 is usually used as a normal hematocrit
2. The next step is to correct for the longer life span of prematurely released reticulocytes in the blood—a phenomenon of increased red blood cell production
This relies on a table:

Hematocrit (%)	Retic survival(days) = maturation correction
36–45	1.0
26–35	1.5
16–25	2.0
15 and below	2.5

So, in a person whose reticulocyte count is 5%, hemoglobin 7.5 g/dL, hematocrit 25%, the RPI would be:

$$\text{RPI} = \frac{\text{ReticIndex}}{\text{MaturationCorrection}} \rightarrow \textbf{RPI} = \frac{5 * \dfrac{25}{45}}{2} = 1.4$$

- RPI is used for evaluation only in anemic patients
- RPI < 2 with anemia is seen when production of reticulocytes (and RBC) is reduced
- RPI > 2 with anemia is suggestive of loss of RBC as in hemolysis or hemorrhage and this is accompanied by increased compensatory production of reticulocytes
- **RPI is difficult to calculate manually and is available only on automated HAs**

Availability of the reticulocyte fractions has improved the classification of anemias as demonstrated in Fig. 1.2. The reticulocyte count is plotted against the reticulocyte fraction and cause of anemia can be ascertained from this plot (Table 1.3).

The normal ranges of reticulocyte parameters as determined in our lab are:

Reticulocyte count	0.20–2.50%
RPI	0.1 in normal individuals. In anemic adults, RPI >2 indicates increased erythropoiesis and <2 suppressed erythropoiesis at BM level
IRF	2.0–16.20%

1.3 RET-HE (Reticulocyte Hemoglobin Equivalent)

The RET-HE is a measure of the hemoglobin (Hb) content of reticulocytes and is available on the Sysmex analyzers. This parameter is called CHr (reticulocyte Hb content) on the Bayer

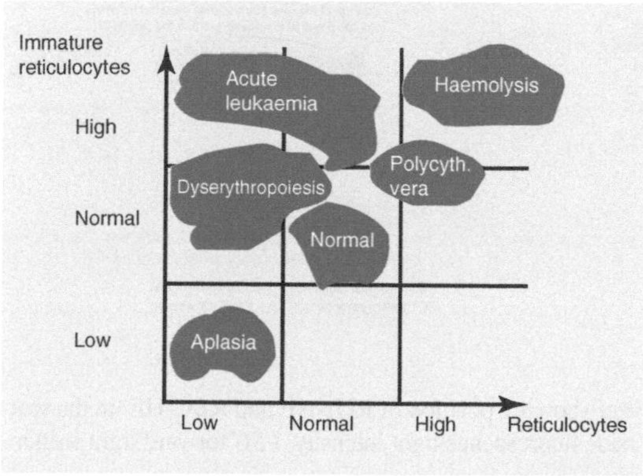

Clinical Condition	Reticulocyte Count	IRF
Dyserythropoiesis (e.g. acute myeloid leukemia or myelodysplastic syndromes, megaloblastic anemia)	N or ↓	↑
Reduced erythropoiesis (e.g. iron deficiency, anemia of chronic disease	↓	N
Increased erythropoiesis (e.g. acquired hemolytic anemia, blood loss)	↑	↑

Fig. 1.2 Reticulocyte count vs. reticulocyte fractions. (*Taken from d'Onofrio et al. 1996; Briggs 2009*)

ADVIA analyzer. Brugnara et al. found good correlation between these two parameters.

Since RBCs have a 120-day life span, changes in Hb of RBC (RBC-HE) are detected relatively late by routine parameters such as Hb, Mean Corpuscular Volume (MCV), Mean Corpuscular Hemoglobin (MCH), or hypochromic red blood cells (HYPO-HE). On the other hand, since reticulocytes mature over 2–4 days, RET-HE is a real-time snap shot of current Hb content of developing RBCs. Changes in iron status are instantly reflected in the RET-HE value and is useful in diagnosis and monitoring of iron deficiency anemia (IDA). The published reference range is 28.2–36.6 pg.

1.3.1 Principle

The RET-HE and RBC-HE are determined in the reticulocyte channel by flow cytometry. The mean FSC estimates the cell volume and simulta-

Table 1.3 Reticulocyte count vs. reticulocyte fractions

Clinical condition	Reticulocyte count	IRF
Dyserythropoiesis (e.g., acute myeloid leukemia or myelodysplastic syndromes, megaloblastic anemia)	N or ↓	↑
Reduced erythropoiesis (e.g., iron deficiency, anemia of chronic disease)	↓	N
Increased erythropoiesis (e.g., acquired hemolytic anemia, blood loss)	↑	↑

neously measures the Hb content of RBCs and reticulocytes. These parameters were initially called RBC-Y and Ret-Y, but subsequently, were transformed into the Hb equivalents (He) by application of certain algorithms (Fig. 1.3).

1.4 DELTA-He

DELTA-He is a calculated value of the difference between RET-HE and RBC-HE. A value higher than the normal range is an indication of improved erythropoietic activity, whereas consistently low values over a period of time, may indicate suppressed erythropoiesis.

Why is RET-HE a more effective marker?
- Inability to release iron from the bone marrow stores rapidly enough to keep pace with erythropoiesis, even in the presence of adequate iron stores, leads to a state of functional iron deficiency (FID). RET-HE is an indicator of adequacy of iron available for erythropoiesis. It is thus useful in the diagnosis of iron deficiency and monitoring response to treatment.
- Traditional biochemical tests for assessing iron status, such as serum iron, transferrin or ferritin, are also acute phase reactants and hence not reliable in our setting. For example, a normal or elevated serum ferritin as seen in anemia of chronic disease, does not predict the bioavailability of the iron correctly because in spite of a raised ferritin level FID can exist in these

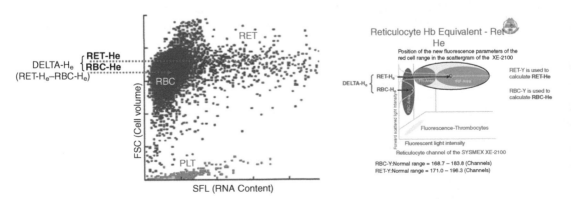

Fig. 1.3 Reticulocyte channel of the Sysmex Hematology analyzer showing position of RET-HE and RBC-HE in the scattergram *(Provided by Sysmex Europe, Hamburg, Germany)*. *SFL* side fluorescence light intensity, *FSC* forward light scatter

patients. Therefore, RET-HE has the potential to be the most sensitive index for immediate availability of iron for erythropoiesis

- It appears earlier and is more accurate than biochemical parameters for diagnosis of FID.
- It is fast, inexpensive, and easy to perform. Results are obtained along with CBC report.

Uses of RET-HE

- Reduced RET-HE and ferritin values are suggestive of classical iron deficiency. In patients with CKD, a RET-HE less than 25 pg suggests iron deficiency.
- A patient will not respond to iron therapy if the RET-HE is above the normal range.
- A combination of high/normal ferritin and low RET-HE value is suggestive of FID provided infection is ruled out as the cause of raised ferritin.
- A RET-HE value below 27.2 pg is able to predict iron deficiency with a sensitivity of 93.3%, and a specificity of 83.2%.
- It is useful to determine **iron status in patients on EPO therapy**. If it is low, then parenteral iron needs to be administered to the patient along with EPO. The best response to IV EPO in dialysis patients is seen with a RET-HE less than 30.6 pg. The RET-HE rises post-EPO therapy, indicating a response to treatment.
- The National Kidney Foundation guidelines have included RET-HE as a parameter for assessing the initial iron status. It also assesses need of IV iron replacement of hemodialysis patients. According to The Clinical Practice Guidelines and Clinical Practice Recommendations for anemia in chronic kidney disease in adults, initial assessment of anemia should include a CBC, absolute reticulocyte count, serum ferritin to assess iron stores, and **serum transferrin saturation (TSAT) or RET-HE/CHr to assess adequacy of iron for erythropoiesis.**
- European Best Practice Guidelines for **management of anemia in chronic renal failure** recommends that functional iron available for erythropoiesis can be assessed by any one parameter; % hypochromic RBC, TSAT, or **RET-HE.**
- It is particularly helpful in **pediatric patients** as diagnosis is quick and an extra blood collection can be avoided in children.

- No other test provides similar information.

In a study carried out at Hinduja Hospital, ROC analysis of RET-HE showed an **AUC of 0.999** with a cut-off value of **28 pg** below which IDA could be diagnosed with a **sensitivity of 100% and a specificity of 97.92%.** The ROC analysis of RBC-HE showed that with a cut-off value of **24.8 pg (AUC of 1)** IDA could be diagnosed with **sensitivity of 98.46% and specificity of 100%.**

The normal ranges as determined in our lab are:

RET-HE in females	27.70–33.40 pg
RET-HE in males	28.70–34.10 pg

1.4.1   Thomas Plot

Thomas et al. introduced a diagnostic model using RET-HE/CHr in combination with the soluble transferrin receptor/log ferritin ratio (sTfR-F index) for monitoring progression of iron deficiency, regardless of acute phase response (Fig. 1.4). The Thomas plot can be used in the differentiating FID from classical iron deficiency.

A case to demonstrate usefulness of RET-HE

- A 25-year-old, female came with fatigue and mild dyspnea.
- On day 0: Hb–10.6 g/dL (11.5–16.5), MCV–70.5 pg (76–96) retic count–0.58% (0.2–2.5), serum iron–10 μg/dL (65–175), TIBC–504 μg/dL (235–400) and TSAT–2% (20–40). RET-HE–20 pg.
- She was diagnosed as having IDA and treated with Orofer tablet OD. CBC + retic was repeated on day 5.
- Day 5: Hb, MCV, serum iron, TIBC, and Tsat remained constant. However, the RET-HE (27) and retic count (1.18) rose significantly demonstrating response to treatment.
- Day 30: All values had come within their reference ranges.
- Hence, we conclude that RET-HE is a useful indicator of gauging response to iron therapy

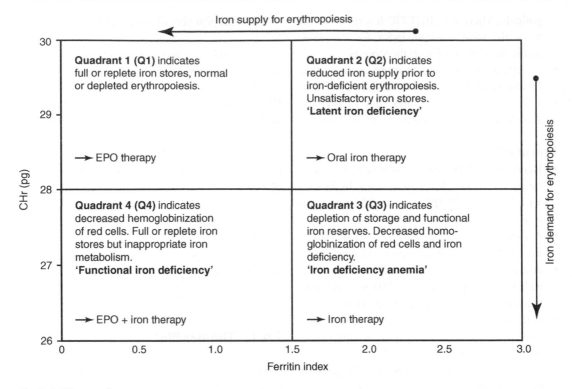

Fig. 1.4 Thomas plot

when performed on day 5 of starting iron therapy. Treatment should be continued till all parameters are normal including serum ferritin.

1.5 Newer RBC Parameters

Four novel RBC extended parameters are available on Sysmex XE analyzers, but on the XE instruments, these are research parameters only. They are:

- **% HYPO-HE**, the percentage of hypochromic RBCs with Hb content equivalent to less than 17 pg.
- **% HYPER-HE**, the percentage of hyperchromic RBCs with Hb content equivalent to more than 49 pg.
- **% MICRO-R**, the percentage of microcytic RBCs with a volume less than 60 fL.
- **% MACRO-R**, the percentage of macrocytic RBCs with a volume greater than 120 fL. These

correspond to a subpopulation of mature red cells with insufficient iron content.

On XN-Class analyzers, the MICRO-R and MACRO-R, are new diagnostic reportable parameters and are part of the CBC.

1.5.1 Principle for Measurement of HYPO-HE

The RBC-HE is calculated on the high-angle FSC in the retic channel (Fig. 1.5). HYPO-HE and HYPER-HE are derived from RBC-HE using a proprietary algorithm. RBC-HE is analogous to the MCH. HYPO-HE is the percentage of RBC with cellular Hb content lower than 17 pg, whereas HYPER-HE is the percentage of RBC with cellular Hb content higher than 49 pg.

The x-axis represents the fluorescence intensity. The high-angle forward-scattered light signal, which reflects cell size and internal structure is on the y-axis (Fig. 1.5). The left scattergram

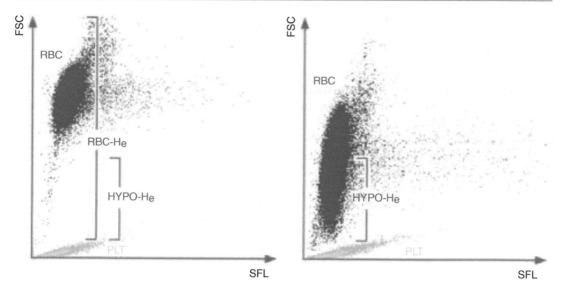

Fig. 1.5 RET scattergram showing HYPO-HE

(Fig. 1.5) shows a normal sample with HYPO-HE less than 1% whereas the right scattergram shows a sample with 60% HYPO-HE.

1.5.2 Principle of Measurement of MICRO-R and MACRO-R on Sysmex XN Analyzers

MICRO-R and MACRO-R values are obtained from both ends of the RBC histogram. With microcytes in the sample, the RBC histogram is shifted to the left and often a shoulder can be seen. Conversely, macrocytic RBC generate histograms with a longer slope on the right. With the help of two distinct discriminators at either end, a microcytic and a macrocytic population of RBC can be derived. The MICRO-R and MACRO-R are expressed as a percentage of all RBCs (Fig. 1.6).

Clinical utility
- CKD patients on EPO can have either iron-deficient or iron-sufficient erythropoiesis and this can be determined by %HYPO.
- Urrechaga et al. devised a mathematical formula using %MICRO-R and %HYPO-HE, which could discriminate β-thalassemia from IDA with a sensitivity of 97.4% and specificity of 97.1%.

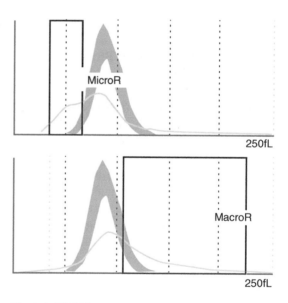

Fig. 1.6 RBC histogram showing Micro-R (upper panel) and Macro-R (lower panel)

- RET-HE and RET-HE/RBC-HE ratio are decreased (<29.5 pg and <1.02, respectively) in patients with a combination of β-thalassemia and IDA.
- Additionally, in this group of patients, also a combination of %HYPO-HE and M-H index seems to be promising. A markedly increased %HYPO-HE (>20) is seen along with a decreased M-H index (<11.5) (*personal*

communication). Further investigation is required.

- The %HYPO-HE and %MICRO-R RBCs is increased in iron-deficient erythropoiesis. These parameters can pick up small changes in the number of RBC with inadequate hemoglobinization.
- The European Best Practice Guidelines (EBPG), National Kidney Foundation Kidney Disease Outcome Quality Initiative (NKF KDOQI) guidelines recommend the use of HYPO-HE as well as MICRO-R.
- A normal MCV along with an increased MICRO-R or MACRO-R is observed in myelodysplastic syndrome patients.

Thus, MICRO-R and MACRO-R are helpful in narrowing down the possible causes of anemia.

1.6 Fragmented Red Blood Cells (FRC)

Fragmented red blood cells (FRC% and FRC#) is a research parameter on the Sysmex analyzers. It is based on the principle of fluorescence flow cytometry and measured in the reticulocyte channel. FRC is present in an area below the RBC population in the RET scattergram. FRC displays extremely low SFL signal (due to the absence of nucleic acids in RBC) and a high-angle FSC which is lower than that of normal RBC (Fig. 1.7).

SFL intensity of each cell is on *x*-axis and the high-angle FSC on *y*-axis. The cells are characterized on basis of cell size and cellular content. FRC are visible in the RET scattergram below the RBC population.

FRCs appear as "helmets" (cells with two tapered and horn-like projections on either end) and other odd shapes on the peripheral smear.

1.7 The New WNR Channel

The New WNR Channel on the Sysmex XN analyzers has made NRBC assessment possible with every CBC. Parameters reported in this channel

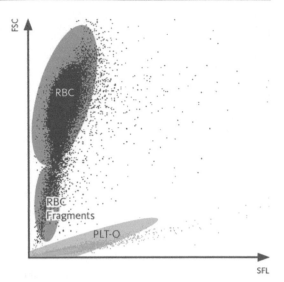

Fig. 1.7 Scattergram of RET channel showing position of FRC

are WBC count, BASO# (absolute count), BASO%, NRBC#, and NRBC%.

1.8 Nucleated Red Blood Cell (NRBC)

Nucleated red blood cells can be mistaken for lymphocytes by hematology analyzers, thereby resulting in an erroneous WBC and lymphocyte count. NRBC is absent in healthy adults. When a sample contains NRBC, the Sysmex XE analyzers generate a flag and the slide has to be reviewed. NRBCs in the blood film are counted manually and a mathematical calculation is applied to give a corrected total WBC count. This is subjective and inaccurate. If a sample containing NRBC is not flagged, an erroneously high WBC and lymphocyte count may be reported. Automated NRBC detection has great clinical utility and goes far beyond correction of WBC count.

1.8.1 Principle

In the WNR channel of the Sysmex XN analyzer, a polymethine dye for nucleic acids and cell-specific lyse are used specifically for NRBC

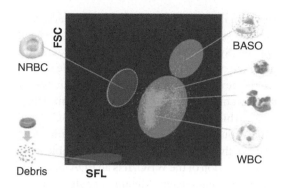

Fig. 1.8 Scattergram of NRBC channel showing position of NRBC cluster

detection. Here, the cells are actually counted and this is not a mere estimation. NRBCs are identified in the same channel as WBCs. The SFL reflects the nucleic acid content and FSC the cell size (Fig. 1.8).

Advantages of automated NRBC count
- The NRBC count is included with every CBC on Sysmex XN analyzers. It is quick and there is no added cost involved. On other X-Class analyzers such as XE, only a flag is generated to indicate the presence of NRBC.
- NRBC are reported as a percentage (%/100 WBC) as well as absolute counts (#—per μL).
- No extra sample preparation or mathematical correction is required.
- There is no impact of interference from lipids or lyse-resistant RBCs.
- Sysmex XN provides an NRBC count that is accurate for both high and low counts. This accuracy is needed because:
  - In neonates and in blood samples with high NRBC counts, a correction has to be made to the WBC count.
  - In adults, even very low NRBC counts are clinically significant.

Clinical value of NRBC counts
- NRBCs are raised in conditions of increased erythropoiesis as seen in acute hemolysis, severe hypoxia, and in thalassemia syndromes.
- They can be seen in hematological malignancies, bone marrow metastases of solid

tumors, and extramedullary hematopoiesis (leucoerythroblastosis).
- They can also appear in conditions of hematopoietic stress such as sepsis, or massive hemorrhage. In these situations, their presence correlates with severity of disease.
- Studies have shown that persistence of NRBCs in peripheral blood is associated with a poorer prognosis in hematological and non-hematological conditions and in ICU patients, they indicate increased mortality.
- It is extremely useful in neonatology and pediatric practice. NRBC counts can be physiologically raised in new-borns and young infants to up to 100 NRBC/100 WBC and automated counts are superior and quicker than manual counts in giving accurate and reliable WBC counts.
- Patients of thalassemia or sickle cell disease needing transfusion usually have high NRBC counts and can benefit greatly from NRBC monitoring.

Thus, automated NRBC count is extremely useful to exclude a spurious rise in WBC count, which is crucial in neonatal patients with sepsis and low WBC counts. Therefore, an NRBC count should be routinely performed for all pediatric and neonatal patients and also in adult patients if clinically warranted.

1.9 The New WDF Channel

On the new Sysmex XN analyzer, Immature Granulocytes (IG) value is standard with every WBC Diff count. The new WDF channel improves reporting accuracy and precision for samples with very low WBC counts (<500 cells) because it includes a **Low WBC mode**, which triples the number of cells counted, giving a differential on every low WBC count. Thus, the WDF channel increases the number of reportable WBC and differential results by giving fewer vote-outs. Sysmex has improved the sensitivity and specificity of the six-part diff by developing a new method for discriminating monocytes, lymphocytes, atypical lymphocytes, and blasts.

Sysmex Adaptive Flagging Algorithm based **on Shape-recognition (SAFLAS)** allows linear discrimination of cell clusters in the WDF scattergram using shape and positioning of different mononuclear cell populations (Fig. 1.9). The parameters reported in this channel are NEUT%, NEUT#, LYMPH%, LYMPH#, MONO%, MONO#, EO%, EO# and IG%, IG# (Fig. 1.10).

Targeting lymphocytes and monocytes, SAFLAS recognizes not only the numbers of cells but also the shape of each cluster's position, angle, size, length, etc.

1.10 Immature Granulocyte (IG) Count

Immature granulocytes are manually counted on the peripheral smear as part of the differential count (DC). They may be missed when present in

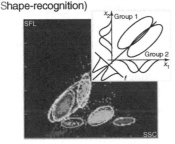

SAFLAS method
(Sysmex Adaptive FLagging Algorithm based on Shape-recognition)

Detects abnormal cells - (with high sensitivity)
LDA (Linear Discriminant Analysis)

Fig. 1.9 SAFLAS in WDF channel

very small numbers, especially in leucopenic samples, because the manual count is imprecise On the Sysmex XE hematology analyzers, the presence of IG is flagged, requiring a slide review. On the newer Sysmex XN hematology analyzers, the IG counts (# and %) are a direct measurement, which is part of the CBC and WBC differential counts. It becomes available with every CBC within minutes, making it a valuable sixth subpopulation of the WBC. It is an FDA-approved reportable parameter. Metamyelocytes, myelocytes, and promyelocytes are counted as IGs. Band cells are not included in the IG count.

1.10.1 Principle

IGs are measured by fluorescence flow cytometry in the WDF channel.

The cell membrane is lysed by the unique lyse reagent while the intracellular DNA and RNA are labelled with a fluorescent dye. The strongest fluorescence signals are displayed by cells having high RNA content such as immature and activated cells. In the scattergram, the cells are differentiated according to their fluorescence and internal structure. These form separate populations which can be measured (Fig. 1.11).

An example of the scattergrams with the presence and absence of IGs is shown below (Fig. 1.12).

IGs in the peripheral blood are early indicators of infection, inflammation, or other bone marrow conditions. Quick and reliable detection of IGs enables early diagnosis of these diseases.

Fig. 1.10 Shows separation of different cell populations, particularly monocytes and lymphocytes, using population density readings and SSC vs. FSL analysis

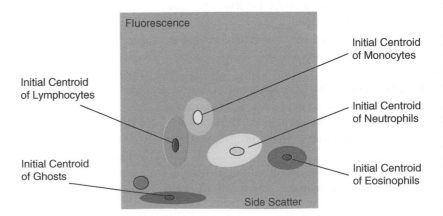

Fluorescence

Initial Centroid of Monocytes

Initial Centroid of Lymphocytes

Initial Centroid of Neutrophils

Initial Centroid of Ghosts

Initial Centroid of Eosinophils

Side Scatter

Benefits and utility of IG count

- Automated IG counts are early indicators of sepsis and infections and enable implementation of immediate action.
- For patients with unknown history/diagnosis, who have an increased IG count, a slide review is recommended. However, in **known patients on follow-up**, a daily manual review need not be done if IG count is available. It thus reduces the slide review rate and improves TAT.

- The IG count is physiologically raised in neonates and pregnant women.

1.10.2 Hypo- and Hyper-Granulated Neutrophils on the New Sysmex XN Hematology Analyzer

It has been observed that the values of hematological parameters differ between the new XN and the older XE analyzers because reagents and algorithms have been optimized in the newer XN analyzers. Hence, new reference ranges need to be validated for these parameters. An example is the **Neutrophil-Granularity-Intensity or NEUT-GI** on the XN-series and **NEUT-X** on the XE-series which are an important tool to detect hypo-granulated neutrophils seen in myelodysplasia or hyper-granulated neutrophils seen in inflammation.

Neutrophil Activation is measured by Neutrophil Reactivity Intensity (**NEUT-RI**) and Neutrophil-Granularity-Intensity (**NEUT-GI**)

Why measure neutrophil activation?

- It is now recognized that in inflammation, neutrophils do not merely play a passive role by simply responding to external signals, but acti-

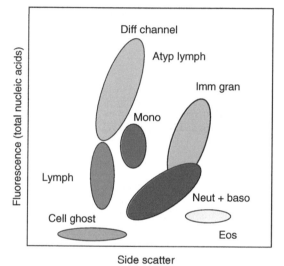

Fig. 1.11 Position of the IGs in the WBC + Diff scattergram

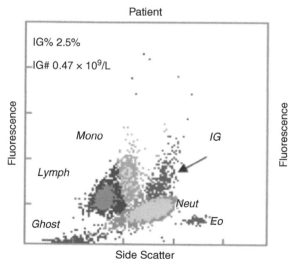

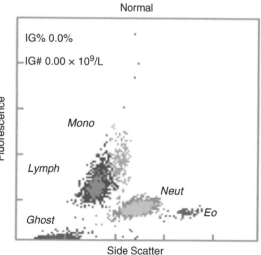

Fig. 1.12 Diff scattergram: IG-positive and IG-negative cases

vated neutrophils can perform most of the functions of macrophages. They are known to secrete a variety of pro-inflammatory cytokines and surface molecules (MHCII) which enable antigen presentation, and activation of T cells.

- Both, NEUT-GI and NEUT-RI, will be increased in conditions showing early innate immune response due to neutrophil activation.
- These parameters of inflammation allow an early diagnosis of sepsis so that targeted therapy can be instituted/modified immediately in order to avoid unnecessary use of antibiotics.
- The activation markers, NEUT-GI and NEUT-RI on neutrophils and RE-LYMP, AS-LYMP on lymphocytes are available on Sysmex XN HAs as "Extended Inflammation Parameters" package.

NEUT-RI and NEUT-GI measurement in the Sysmex XN analyzers

- Activated cells have altered membrane lipid composition and show greater cytoplasmic activity due to cytokine production leading to higher intensity of the FSL than resting cells. NEUT-RI is a parameter, which reflects neutrophil reactivity intensity, as per the metabolic activity of the cell.
- The 90° side scatter signal (SSC) reflects the inner complexity/granularity of the cell. Therefore, in toxic granulation or vacuolization, the position of the neutrophil cloud in the scattergram is shifted from it is normal location. Thus NEUT-GI, which is an indicator of scatter intensity, (expressed in SI units) changes accordingly (Fig. 1.13).

Neutrophil population with SSC on the x-axis, (granularity and internal structure) and fluorescence intensity, on the y-axis (RNA/DNA content of cell) (Fig. 1.13).

1.10.3 Neutrophil Granulation (NEUT-SSC)

Neutrophils and eosinophils have the highest SSC of all WBCs because they have more

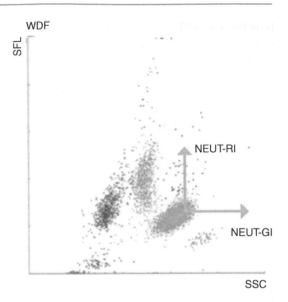

Fig. 1.13 Scattergram from Sysmex XN showing position of NEUT-GI and NEUT-RI in WDF channel

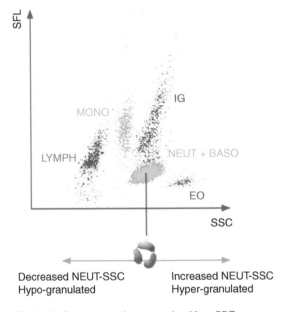

Fig. 1.14 Scattergram demonstrating Neut-SSC

granules than any other leucocyte (Fig. 1.14). Hypo-granular neutrophils have a low NEUT-SSC which is a feature of dysplastic neutrophil, as seen in myelodysplastic syndromes (MDS). High NEUT-SSC is associated with hypergranularity. The NEUT-SSC is a research parameter found in the WDF channel on

XN-Series analyzers. In the XE analyzers, it is called NEUT-X.

The SSC signal of the neutrophil population, which is plotted on the x-axis of the scattergram, is an indication of the granularity and internal structure of the cells. Fluorescence intensity, which corresponds to RNA/DNA cell content, is plotted on the y-axis (Fig. 1.14).

1.10.4 Lymphocyte Activation

1.10.4.1 RE-LYMP and AS-LYMP

Reactive Lymphocytes (RE-LYMP) and Antibody-Synthesizing activated B lymphocytes (plasma cells) (AS-LYMP) are new diagnostic parameters which can measure activated lymphocytes on all XN-Series instruments. They provides additional information about the cell-mediated response of the innate and adaptive immune processes. Both parameters are expressed as absolute counts and percentages.

RE-LYMP has a higher FSL than normal lymphocytes The **AS-LYMP** has the highest FSL. The AS-LYMP cells are always included in the RE-LYMP count (Fig. 1.15).

The values depend on the nature and severity of the inflammatory stimulus.

These parameters can differentiate between a cell-mediated or humoral immune-response to pathogens, thus making it possible to distinguish between

- Infectious vs. non-infectious cause of inflammation where they help in diagnosis, treatment, and monitoring
- Viral or bacterial infections
- Acute or subsiding infections

These parameters are early indicators of infection and have great potential in dedicated infection wards and ICUs.

RE-LYMP and AS-LYMP are part of the "Extended Inflammation Parameters" package available from a routine blood count, together with the CBC and DIFF.

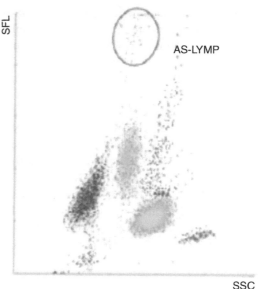

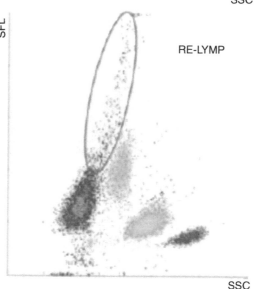

Fig. 1.15 WDF channel scattergrams showing position of AS-LYMP and RE-LYMP. Top position shows AS-LYMP, bottom position shows RE-LYMP

1.11 Platelet Parameters

1.11.1 Optical and Fluorescent Platelet Counts (PLT-O and PLT-F)

The impedance platelet count (PLT-I) is the primary method for platelet counting in all hematology analyzers. When particles of similar size as platelets are present in the sample, accuracy of PLT-I is compromised and the count is flagged. These interfering factors are large platelets, small RBCs, or WBC fragments (Fig. 1.16). To overcome this, provision was made on the Sysmex XE analyzers for optical counting of platelets (PLT-O) in the reticulocyte channel using a polymethine dye. Now a new fluorescent channel dedicated for counting platelets is available on Sysmex XN, the PLT-F channel. The PLT-O/F counts are more accurate and show excellent correlation with platelet counts by flow cytometry (CD41/61) which is the International Reference Method (IRM) for counting platelets.

False increases	False decreases
RBC fragments	Aggregates
WBC fragments	Giant platelets
Microcytes	Platelet satellitism
Bacteria	
Cryoglobulin Immune complexes Chylomicrons	

Fig. 1.16 Factors interfering with PLT-I count

1.11.2 Principle

Platelets are separated from RBC due to their higher fluorescence signal in the reticulocyte channel of the Sysmex XE analyzer (Fig. 1.17). A switching algorithm in the software allows the more reliable platelet result to be reported between PLT-I AND PLT-O, and this is indicated by the symbol "&". On the XN analyzer, in the PLT-F channel, platelets are identified and counted using a platelet-specific, fluorescent dye, Oxazine, which stains the rough surface endoplasmic reticulum and mitochondria (Fig. 1.17). PLT-F is considered more accurate than the PLT-I and is reported as the default platelet count.

A study conducted by Dadu T, Khodaiji S et al., compared accuracy of platelet counting by impedance and optical methods and showed that out of a total of 118 blood samples with platelet count <50,000/μL, Sysmex-R (reported count) had the least bias with 95% linear agreement and thus correlated best with IRM. In five cases, the PLT-R values were based on the PLT-I values. In all these cases, the IRM correlated best with PLT-I value (Table 1.4).

Table 1.4 Comparison of PLT-I and PLT-F and Sysmex reported count by Pearson correlation

Method	Pearson correlation (r)
Sysmex reported	0.9537
Sysmex impedance	0.9138
Sysmex optical	0.9483

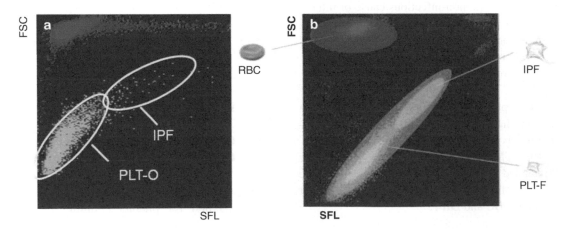

Fig. 1.17 Scattergrams of PLT-O and PLT-F channels. (**a**) Plt-O channel on Sysmex XE. (**b**) Plt-F on Sysmex XN

Patients with low platelet counts have a higher risk of bleeding and may require platelet transfusions. According to various recommendations, a stable patient is transfused if the platelet count falls below 10,000/µL. However, in case of co-existing risk factors such as splenomegaly, coagulation factor deficiencies, or severe bleeding the threshold used is 20,000/µL.

The PLT-F is of great value in these situations as it is the most accurate method of counting platelets and can be relied upon as a transfusion trigger in severely bleeding patients with very low platelet counts.

Evolution of platelet counting technologies (Table 1.5 and Fig. 1.18) on newer hematology analyzers has vastly improved the accuracy of platelet counts.

Table 1.5 Evolving platelet counting techniques

PLT-I	PLT-O	PLT-F
Hydrodynamic focusing DC (direct current) method using size discriminators to separate platelet from other blood cells	Fluorescence FC method based on staining of the remnant RNA in platelets by **polymethine fluorescent retic dye**	Fluorescence FC method based on the staining of remnant RNA in platelets by **Oxazine fluorescent platelet dye**

1.12 Immature Platelet Fraction (IPF)

On the newer hematology analyzers, optical and fluorescence platelet measurements are done flow cytometrically by using fluorescent intensity (SFL) and forward scatter (FSC) to separate out the platelets from the RBC and reticulocyte populations.

Young platelets, which have a higher FSC and SFL are measured as the immature platelet fraction with the Sysmex XE (Fig. 1.19) and XN (Fig. 1.18) instruments, and as the "reticulated platelet fraction" with the Abbott Cell Dyn Sapphire instrument. Just as the reticulocyte count reflects the bone marrow production of the RBCs, the IPF reflects bone marrow platelet production. The IPF is a direct cellular measurement of thrombopoiesis that measures young and more reactive platelets in peripheral blood. It can be used with other available clinical information to help determine the pathophysiological mechanism of thrombocytopenia.

The IPF is an FDA approved parameter and can be reported as the absolute count (IPF#) and/or the percentage (IPF%). The sample is run in the RETIC mode on Sysmex XE and PLT-F and IPF mode on Sysmex XN analyzers.

IPF is an improvement over the mean platelet volume, (MPV) which is not very reliable as

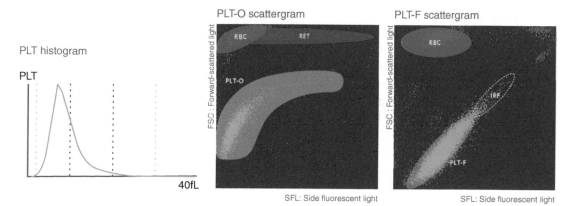

Fig. 1.18 Impedance, optical, and fluorescence methods of platelet counting

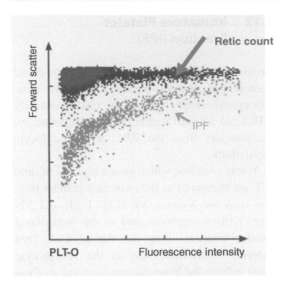

Fig. 1.19 Scattergram of Sysmex XE showing position of IPF

observed by biases between different hematology analyzers.

Utility of IPF in clinical practice
- IPF is an indicator of bone marrow activity and is raised when there is excess destruction of platelets in peripheral blood. Thus, it supports the diagnosis of autoimmune thrombocytopenic purpura, (ITP) thrombotic thrombocytopenic purpura (TTP), and is useful in distinguishing these from bone marrow suppression or failure, where the IPF value is low.
- As IPF rises before the platelet counts recover, it can be used as a predictor of platelet recovery after BMT or chemotherapy.
- Immature platelets are more reactive and have a raised prothrombotic potential. They are also more resistant to inhibition by aspirin and P2Y12 receptor antagonists. Many studies have shown that the absolute count of IPF reflects residual platelet reactivity. Thus, IPF can be used to predict the efficacy of antiplatelet therapy and to assess the risk of cardiovascular thrombotic events.
- **Use in Thrombocytosis:** IPF cannot differentiate between reactive thrombocytosis and clonal proliferation such as essential thrombo-

cythemia (ET), with certainty, although some data shows that platelet distribution width (PDW) is increased in the latter compared with the former. Also, IPF was found to be greatly increased in patients with ET compared with control subjects.

The published normal values are: NR: 1.1–6.1%. Normal mean IPF = 3.1% *(Briggs et al. 2004)*.

The normal range as determined in our lab is:

IPF	0.70–4.30%
PLT-F	150–400 × 10^9/L

Benefits of IPF are:
- A bone marrow procedure can be avoided for uncomplicated thrombocytopenia evaluation.
- IPF is a better parameter than mean platelet volume (MPV) to differentiate between the causes of thrombocytopenia because younger platelets are not necessarily larger.
- Can be reliable even when platelet count is very low.
- It is a useful indicator in effective risk assessment and therapy monitoring of coronary artery diseases.

A word of caution
- Newer platelet parameters display time-dependent variations in their values. Thus, strict control for time of collection, transportation, and performance of the assay needs to be observed.
- Scattergrams from HA should be compared with the results of the microscopic examination of the blood smear, before relying on a multiple quantitative indices from the analyzers.

1.13   Body Fluid Analysis (BF)

Currently, body fluid counts are performed manually in Fuchs-Rosenthal or Neubauer counting chamber (hemacytometer) which is considered the gold standard method.

Cell differentiation is done on smears made by cytocentrifugation, sedimentation, or filtration and staining of the film with MGG or Wright staining. These methods are time consuming and inaccurate.

Sysmex launched its fully automated HA, the XE-2100 in 1999. A few years later, it was FDA approved for measuring most body fluids (BF) except CSF because of its high background count; the Limit of Quantification (LoQ) for WBC is 50×10^6/L.

In 2007, the XE-5000 was introduced which had unique software for BF analysis called the **body fluid mode**. It could analyze all fluids without any pre-treatment and counted three times more cells, thereby improving the precision and accuracy of the cell counts. The limit of quantification (LoQ) of WBC is 10×10^6/L.

Sysmex's latest HA the XN-Series contains a BF mode which measures a variety of BFs and counts two times more cells than the XE-5000 to increase precision. The limit of detection (LOD) of WBC is 1 cell/μL and LoQ of WBC is 5 cells/μL (Fleming et al.).

It is FDA approved for CSF and can perform 38 samples per hour.

Features such as an extra rinse, and stringent background checks are incorporated to improve the precision and accuracy.

1.13.1 Principle

A combination of fluorescent flow cytometry and impedance techniques are used to characterize cells based on their size, volume, granularity, surface area, and fluorescence signal. Parameters reported are the total nucleated cell count (TNC), RBC count, WBC count, MN, count, PMN count, and high fluorescent (HF-BF) cells such as macrophages, malignant, and mesothelial cells. The HF-BF cells are located just above the MN cluster and are not included in the WBC differential count, but are included in the TNC (Fig. 1.20).

Reportable Parameters are (Fig. 1.21) WBC-BF, MN (#/%), PMN (#/%), TC-BF, RBC-BF (RBC Channel) (Fig. 1.21).

Research Parameters are HF-BF (#/%), NE-BF (#/%), LY-BF (#/%), EO-BF (#/%), MO-BF (#/%).

1.14 Hematopoietic Progenitor Cells (HPC)

There is a high individual variability in peripheral blood stem cell (PBSC) mobilization as compared to bone marrow transplantation (BMT) because it is more difficult to predict the time to harvest the stem cells for transplantation.

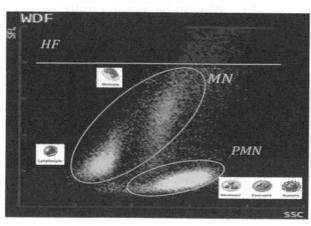
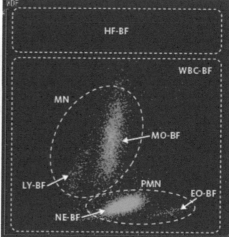

Fig. 1.20 Scattergram of body fluid channel

Fig. 1.21 Screenshot of body fluid report on Sysmex XN

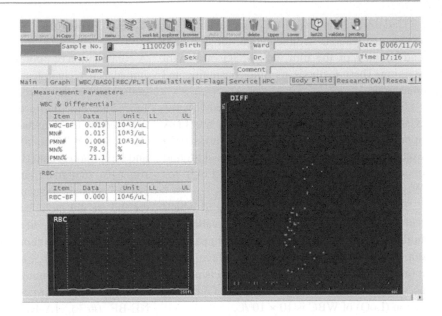

1.14.1 Measuring Stem Cells

The earlier, in vitro cell culture method is impractical for routine use as it requires over 2 weeks for the colonies to grow and hence has been abandoned. The flow cytometric measurement of CD34 cells is the gold standard for CD34 counts in PBSC and bone marrow harvests. However, this is costly and takes at least 2 h for the result.

An option is now available on the XN-Series in the WPC measurement channel called "**XN Stem Cells**" which measures HPC.

Advantage of HPC Counts

- As compared to flow cytometry, it is simple, fast, and reliable
- It is available within a few minutes because no intervention is required like sample preparation or gating, etc.
- Excellent correlation has been reported with the CD34 counting by flow cytometry.
- It is useful in predicting the optimal time to collect stem cell from mobilized donors.
- Additionally, stem cell enumeration can be done during the apheresis procedure to monitor stem cell yield and optimize collection.
- This optimization of the process can help to lower the cost.

1.14.2 Principle

Stem cell counting is done in the WPC channel. Membrane lipids of immature cells are different from that of mature cells or abnormal blasts. Stem cell membranes are relatively resistant to damage by the WPC reagent. Stem cells are detected based on abnormal membrane composition and nuclear content. Stem cells are medium in size (medium FSC), have a low granularity (low SSC) and relatively low SFL (Fig. 1.22).

1.15 ACP on Beckman Coulter Hematology Analyzers

The Beckman Coulter analyzers offer **Cellular Morphometric Parameters (CMP)**, which provide a powerful way to gain new insights into red and white blood cell morphology. CMP include extended 3D scatterplots and numerical values assigned to cell subpopulations with characteristic shapes.

The proprietary **Automated Intelligent Morphology (AIM) technology** and unique design of Beckman Coulter's DxH series of hematology analyzers has made it possible to offer 70 additional parameters that correspond to cell shape in three dimensions. It offers

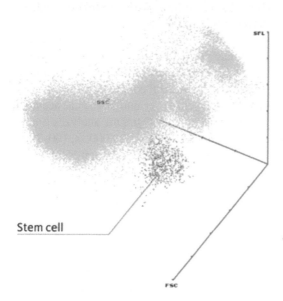

Fig. 1.22 XN Stem cells cluster (purple) in the 3D model of the WPC channel

- More detailed morphological information with higher resolution
- Proprietary data synthesis to yield deeper insights into cellular behavior

Many researchers around the globe have used the CMP to better understand cellular morphological changes in various disease states.

1.16 White Blood Cells

With CMP, researchers can analyze the four major WBC types to detect aberrant cells. The AIM technology records 14 numerical values of parameters that can help pinpoint abnormal cells. Some parameters include:

- Mean neutrophil/monocyte/lymphocyte volume
- Neutrophil/monocyte/lymphocyte width

These parameters are also called **Cell Population Data (CPD)** and can be used for early detection of sepsis and in differentiating

bacterial from viral infections. They are very useful in pediatric practice.

1.17 Red Blood Cells

These are for research use only (RUO) and provide useful information about cell morphology, enhancing the ability to detect altered cells.

These parameters are,

- Red blood cell size factor, which characterizes size of the cell across the full age continuum of circulating cells
- Un-ghosted cells, which indicate the presence of red blood cell abnormalities, such as inclusions, target cells, and abnormal hemoglobin

1.18 Platelets

Platelet researchers uses advanced data synthesis to provide unique insights into platelet morphology, including:

- Platelet distribution, which calculates variation in platelet size
- Plateletcrit, which computes the volume of platelet packed cells

1.19 Reticulocytes

Reticulocyte parameters use the DxH 800's unique hardware design to allow deeper insights into cell morphology, including:

- Reticulocyte distribution width by standard deviation/coefficient of variation. Together, these parameters can indicate the cell population's size dispersion
- Immature reticulocyte fraction calculations, which compare the percentage of high light scatter reticulocytes to the total count to detect immature cells

1.20 Hematoflow Technology with CytoDiff[1]

HematoFlow is Beckman Coulter's exclusive technology that links hematology and flow cytometry with a multi-color monoclonal antibody solution. It provides automated, accurate, and detailed differential information. With HematoFlow, WBC differentials go beyond traditional cellular analysis while producing results more quickly with a reduced need for manual review. The system also offers enhanced differential results and standardization across the laboratory, providing additional clinical information and improving patient management.

1.20.1 How CytoDiff Implementation Can Reduce Your Manual Review Rate to 5%

CytoDiff software applies proprietary algorithms to automatically separate and detail cell populations using a reagent cocktail composed of six monoclonal antibodies in five colors. The result is an automated 10-part cytometric WBC differential—the five-part traditional WBC differential with additional immunologic subpopulations of B and T/NK lymphocytes, as well as abnormal populations of immature granulocytes and blasts (Fig. 1.23).

_____
[1]Not Available in the USA

How HematoFlow with CytoDiff Delivers Better Reviews Faster

- Enhanced clinical utility: The automated 10-part differential provides far greater insights than those available from a traditional complete blood cell count.
- Improved sensitivity and statistical accuracy: HematoFlow with CytoDiff analyzes a much larger number of cells—20,000 vs. 100–200 in a manual slide review, making it ideal for low WBC populations.
- Improved standardization: Increased precision eliminates subjective variability within the laboratory and enables reproducible charts and graphs.
- Significantly reduced manual review rates: Laboratories can reduce the need for manual review by up to eight times, thereby eliminating unnecessary slide making, staining, drying, and microscopic examination.
- Easy to learn, easy to use: HematoFlow with CytoDiff analysis can be learned in 2–3 days, vs. the years of practice required for effective microscopic review.

1.21 Malaria Parasite Detection

Since a complete blood count (CBC) is an essential investigation for fever, there is growing interest to utilize the automated HA to provide an early and sensitive indication for malaria detection.

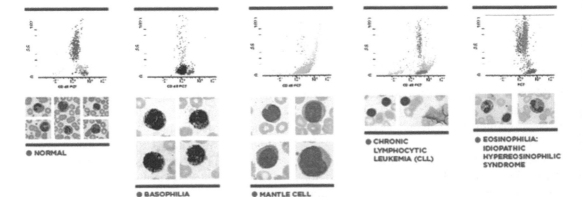

Fig. 1.23 Selected examples of CytoDiff data compared to cell images

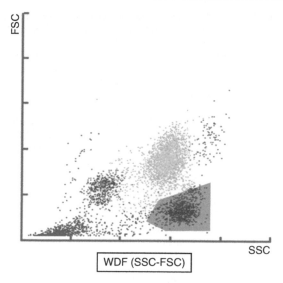

Fig. 1.24 Scattergram of P.vivax malaria positive sample on XN (IR 2.0%) showing cluster of infected RBCs (purple area)

Studies done so far show that the HAs can detect malarial infection by several different principles, such as (1) detection of malaria pigment, hemozoin, in monocytes, (2) analysis of depolarized laser light (DLL), and (3) detection of increased activated monocytes. Up until now, hematology analyzers have utilized surrogate parameters for malaria detection. These provide subtle clues in the form of abnormalities in the scattergram, but need further validation for making an accurate diagnosis.

In the Sysmex XN and XN-L hematology analyzers, malaria-infected RBCs can be picked up while performing a CBC. Malaria is detected in the WDF channel on a scattergram with SSC on the *x*-axis and SFL on the *y*-axis. It is seen as an additional cluster made up of infected RBC (Fig. 1.24) and a flag is generated when these clusters exceed a preset threshold, prompting the user to do a slide review for malaria.

Contrary to earlier surrogate modes of detection, **this method gives a specific indication of the presence of parasite in the RBC.**

1.22 Conclusion

Technological advances incorporated in HA over several years have made the CBC report more accurate and meaningful. The TAT is improved by reducing false-positive flagging for fragmented RBCs, abnormal WBCs, and platelet clumps, thus reducing the need for unnecessary slide reviews. Accurate detection and enumeration of abnormal/atypical cells is now possible along with measurement of novel parameters of potential clinical relevance.

Clinical utility of the newer parameters sometimes remains poorly documented. External quality control is not always possible due to lack of sufficient participants, and even internal quality control may not be available. The reproducibility is better validated for the well-established parameters, such as cell counts, though it is not so robust for volume-based parameters such as Mean Neutrophil Volume.

There are marked differences in measurement principles, calibration, and algorithms of different analyzers with the result some parameters give widely varying results across analyzers. The most conspicuous example of this is the MPV, whose clinical significance is uncertain in spite of being available for years.

Another drawback is that parameters obtained on a specific instrument from one manufacturer cannot be used by other laboratories that do not use that instrument.

In order to derive maximum benefit from the newer parameters, it is required for every laboratory to validate these before using them for clinical reporting.

Bibliography

1. Bartels PC, Schoorl M, Schoorl M. Hemoglobinization and functional availability of iron for erythropoiesis in case of thalassemia and iron deficiency anemia. Clin Lab. 2006;52(3–4):107–14.
2. Briggs C, Hart D, Kunka S, Oguni S, Machin SJ. Immature platelet fraction measurement: a future guide to platelet transfusion requirement after haematopoietic

stem cell transplantation. Transfus Med. 2006;16: 101–9. https://doi.org/10.1111/j.1365-3148.2006.00654.x.

3. Briggs C, Costa AD, Freeman L, Aucamp I, Ngubeni B, Machin SJ. Development of an automated malaria discriminant factor using VCS technology. Am J Clin Pathol. 2006;126:691–8. https://doi.org/10.1309/0PL 3C674M39D6GEN.

4. Brugnara C, Mohandas N. Red cell indices in classification and treatment of anemias: from M.M. Wintrobes's original 1934 classification to the third millennium. Curr Opin Hematol. 2013;20:222–30.

5. Brugnara C, Schiller B, Moran J. Reticulocyte hemoglobin equivalent (ret He) and assessment of iron-deficient states. Clin Lab Haematol. 2006;28(5):303–8. https://doi.org/10.1111/j.1365-2257.2006.00812.x.

6. Buttarello M, Pajola R, Novello E, Rebeschini M, Cantaro S, Oliosi F, Naso A, Plebani M. Diagnosis of iron deficiency in patients undergoing hemodialysis. Am J Clin Pathol. 2010;133:949–54.

7. Campuzano-Zuluaga G, Hänscheid T, Grobusch MP. Automated haematology analysis to diagnose malaria. Malar J. 2010;9:346. https://doi.org/10.1186/1475-2875-9-346.

8. Canals C, Remacha AF, Sarda MP, Piazuelo JM, Royo MT, Romero MA. Clinical utility of the new Sysmex XE2100 parameter—reticulocyte hemoglobin equivalent—in the diagnosis of anemia. Hematologica. 2005;90:1133–4.

9. Brugnara C. Reticulocyte cellular indices: a new approach in the diagnosis of anemias and monitoring of erythropoietic function. Crit Rev Clin Lab Sci. 2008;37(2):93–130. https://doi.org/10.1080/10408360091174196.

10. Miguel A, Orero M, Simon R, Collado R, Perez PL, Pacios A, Iglesias R, Martinez A, Carbonell F. Automated neutrophil morphology and its utility in the assessment of neutrophil dysplasia. Lab Hematol. 2007;13:98–102.

11. Cornbleet PJ, Novak RW. Classifying segmented and band neutrophils. CAP Today. 1994;8:37–41.

12. Tina D, Kunal S, Anjum S, Shanaz K. Comparison of platelet counts by Sysmex XE 2100 and LH-750 with the international flow reference method in thrombocytopenic patients. Indian J Pathol Microbiol. 2013;56(2):114–9.

13. Fleming CKA. From manual microscopy to automated cell counters for first line screening of body fluids: but not without a special body fluid mode. Ned Tijdschr Klin Chem Labgeneesk. 2016;41(3):229–34.. hdl.handle.net/1765/80130

14. Principle for automated leukocyte differentiation with XE Family analysers, making use of bioimaging technology. The Cell Analysis Center—Scientific Bulletin Part 4. Sysmex Corporation 1-5-1, Wakinohama-Kaigandori, Chuo-ku, Kobe 651-0073, Japan. www.sysmex.co.jp & www.sysmex-europe.com.

15. Fujimoto K. Principles of measurement in hematology analyzers manufactured by Sysmex corporation. Sysmex J Int. 1999;9(1):31–44.

16. D'onofrio G, Zini G, Brugnara C. Clinical applications of automated reticulocyte indices. Hematology. 2016;3(2):165–76. https://doi.org/10.1080/10245332.1998.11746388.

17. Herklotz R, et al. Precision and accuracy of the leukocyte differential on the Sysmex XE-2100. Sysmex J Int. 2001;11(1):8–21. https://www.beckmancoulter.com/wsrportal/.../hematology/...parameters/index.htm; https://www.sysmex.at/fileadmin/media/f103/Scientific.../ScientificBulletin_Part4.pdf Sysmex J Int 1999;9(1):21–30.

18. Leers MP, Keuren JF, Oosterhuis WP. The value of the Thomas-plot in the diagnostic work up of anemic patients referred by general practitioners. Int J Lab Hematol. 2010;32:572–81. https://doi.org/10.1111/j.1751-553X.2010.01221.x.

19. Miwa N, Akiba T, Kimata N, Hamaguchi Y, Arakawa Y, Tamura T, Nitta K, Tsuchiya K. Usefulness of measuring reticulocyte hemoglobin equivalent in the management of haemodialysis patients with iron deficiency. Int J Lab Hematol. 2010;32:248–55. https://doi.org/10.1111/j.1751-553X.2009.01179.x.

20. Tessitore N, Solero GP, Lippi G, Bassi A, Faccini GB, Bedogna V, Gammaro L, Brocco G, Restivo G, Bernich P, Lupo A, Maschio G. The role of iron status markers in predicting response to intravenous iron in haemodialysis patients on maintenance erythropoietin. Nephrol Dial Transplant. 2001;16(7):1416–23. https://doi.org/10.1093/ndt/16.7.1416.

21. NKF-K/DOQI. NKF-K/DOQI clinical practice guidelines for hemodialysis adequacy, peritoneal dialysis adequacy, vascular access, and anemia of chronic kidney disease: update 2000. Am J Kidney Dis. 2001;37:S7–S238.

22. d'Onofrio G, Chirillo R, Zini G, Caenaro G, Tommasi M, Micciulli G. Simultaneous measurement of reticulocyte and red blood cell indices in healthy subjects and patients with microcytic and macrocytic anemia. Blood. 1995;85:818–23.

23. Letestu R, Marzac C, Audat F, Belhocine R, Tondeur S, Baccini V, Garçon L, Cortivo LD, Perrot J-Y, Lefrère F, Valensi F, Ajchenbaum-Cymbalista F. Use of hematopoietic progenitor cell count on the Sysmex XE-2100 for peripheral blood stem cell harvest monitoring. Leuk Lymphoma. 2009;48(1):89–96. https://doi.org/10.1080/10428190600886149.

24. Schoorl M, Schoorl M, van Pelt J, Bartels PCM. Application of innovative hemocytometric parameters and algorithms for improvement of microcytic anemia discrimination. Hematol Rep. 2015;7(2):5843. https://doi.org/10.4081/hr.2015.5843.

25. Thomas C, Thomas L. Biochemical markers and hematologic indices in the diagnosis of functional iron deficiency. Clin Chem. 2002;48:1066–76.

26. Thomas DW, Hinchliffe RF, Briggs C, Macdougall IC, Littlewood T, Cavill I, British Committee for Standards in Haematology. Guideline for the laboratory diagnosis of functional iron deficiency. Br J Haematol. 2013;161(5):639–48. https://doi.org/10.1111/bjh.12311. Epub 2013 Apr 10.

27. Lecompte TP, Bernimoulin MP. Novel parameters in blood cell counters. Clin Lab Med. 2015;35(1):209–24, Copyright © 2015 Elsevier Inc.

28. Torino ABB, Gilberti Mde FP, da Costa E, de Lima GAF, Grotto HZW. Evaluation of red cell and reticulocyte parameters as indicative of iron deficiency in patients with anemia of chronic disease. Rev Bras Hematol Hemoter. 2014;36(6):424–9. https://doi.org/10.1016/j.bjhh.2014.09.004.

29. Urrechaga E, Borque L, Escanero F. The role of automated measurement of RBC subpopulations in differential diagnosis of microcytic anemia and β-thalassemia. Am J Clin Pathol. 2011;135:374–9.

30. Zucker ML, Murphy CA, Rachel JM, Martinez GA, Abhyankar S, McGuirk JP, Reid KJ, Plapp FV. Immature platelet fraction as a predictor of platelet recovery following hematopoietic progenitor cell transplantation. Lab Hematol. 2006;12(3):125–3.. PMID:16950671

Iron Metabolism and Iron Deficiency Anemia

2

Meera Sikka and Harresh B. Kumar

2.1 Introduction

Iron is an essential micronutrient which plays an important role in several reactions in the human body. With its ability to easily exchange electrons, associate with proteins and bind oxygen, it is indispensable in fundamental biochemical activities. Iron is incorporated into proteins including hemoglobin, myoglobin and cytochromes, iron-sulfur clusters such as respiratory complexes and other functional groups. These iron containing proteins are essential for vital functions including oxygen transport, mitochondrial respiration, nucleic acid replication, and repair. Iron also serves an important role in various enzymes such as peroxidases, ribonucleotide reductase, and P450 class of detoxifying cytochromes [1].

2.2 Iron Metabolism

2.2.1 Total Body Iron and its Distribution

The total body iron content of an adult is 3–5 g, i.e., 35 mg/kg in females and 4–5 g or 50 mg/kg in males. Iron is distributed in two compartments: functional and storage compartments. Majority

(65%) of functional iron is incorporated in hemoglobin of circulating red cells and serves to transport oxygen. Rest of the functional iron is present in myoglobin, cytochromes, and other enzymes which use iron in electron transfer including enzymes containing iron-sulfur clusters (15%).

About 20% of the total iron is stored as ferritin and hemosiderin in macrophages. A tiny fraction (0.1%) is in the plasma bound to the iron carrier protein transferrin [2] (Fig. 2.1).

2.2.2 Dietary Iron

Dietary iron is present in two forms: **heme iron** and **non-heme iron**.

Heme iron which is found in foods of animal origin accounts for only 10% of the dietary iron with even lesser amounts in developing countries like India. Despite its low concentration, it represents a highly bioavailable form of iron and accounts for almost 40% of total absorbed iron. Its absorption is significantly more efficient than that of non-heme iron being unaffected by other constituents of the diet.

Non-heme iron is present in foods of plant origin and accounts for about 90% of the total iron present in food. The absorption of non-heme iron is affected by constituents of the diet and is reduced by phytates (cereals), oxalates, bran, other fibers, phosphates, tannins (tea, coffee), and calcium. Ascorbic acid, dietary protein, heme iron, and low gastric pH increase iron absorption.

M. Sikka (✉) · H. B. Kumar
Department of Pathology, UCMS and GTB Hospital, Delhi, India

© Springer Nature Singapore Pte Ltd. 2019
R. Saxena, H. P. Pati (eds.), *Hematopathology*, https://doi.org/10.1007/978-981-13-7713-6_2

Fig. 2.1 Distribution of body iron

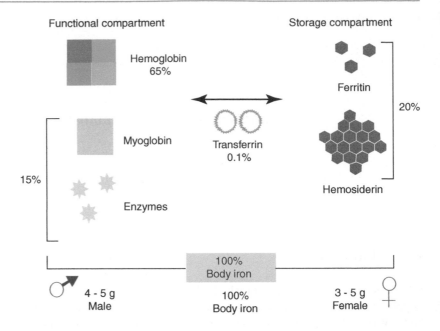

Depending on the combination of enhancers and inhibitors of absorption, non-heme iron assimilation varies several fold. Only 10% of dietary iron is absorbed [3, 4].

2.2.3 Recommended Iron Intake

The recommended daily intake of iron for children aged 0–5 and 5–12 years is 2 mg/kg and 30 mg, respectively. Adult men require an intake of 8 mg while premenopausal women and pregnant women (PW) need 18 mg and 27 mg, respectively [5].

2.3 Absorption of Iron

Iron absorption occurs in the **duodenum and upper jejunum** where enterocytes absorb ferrous iron via their apical membrane.

Absorption of heme iron. On exposure to gastric acid and proteases, heme is freed from the apoprotein and enters the mucosal cell intact. It is absorbed by the enterocytes using heme carrier protein 1 (HCP1), a transport protein which is expressed at high levels in the duodenum and is regulated by Iron regulatory proteins (IRPs).

Within the cell, iron is released from the protoporphyrin ring by heme oxygenase and enters the cytosolic iron pool [6].

Absorption of non-heme iron. Non-heme iron is in ferric form and must be reduced to ferrous iron to be absorbed. This reduction is mediated by the brush border, duodenal cytochrome b reductase (Dcytb) expressed on the apical surface of the enterocyte. The gene for Dcytb is located on chromosome 2, and its expression is induced in response to stimuli that increase iron absorption. Ferrous iron is transported across the cell membrane into the cytoplasm by divalent metal ion transporter 1 (DMT 1) expressed on the apical membrane of the enterocytes. It also transports other divalent ions and acts as a proton symporter, i.e., protons accompany metal ions into the cell. The gastric fluid provides the required protons for transport of iron [6].

Due to lack of a regulated mechanism for iron excretion, body iron balance is maintained by controlling iron absorption. The amount of iron lost is replaced by uptake of an equal amount from the diet. The intestinal mucosa responds to changes in body iron stores and alters the absorption accordingly. While the absorption can increase 3–5 times in iron-deficient states, it decreases in situations of iron overload [3].

2.3.1 Intracellular Iron Transport

Once iron enters the mucosal cell, it can either be incorporated as ferritin or is transported into the circulation across the basolateral membrane within minutes to hours. Iron which is retained as mucosal ferritin is not absorbed and is lost to the body when the cell is exfoliated at the end of its life span (2–4 days). Exfoliation of intestinal epithelial cells represents a pathway of regulated iron excretion. The amount of iron which moves into the plasma and that which remains in the cell as ferritin is regulated. Transport of iron across the cytoplasm of the enterocyte is possible because of its association with proteins which act as iron chaperones [6].

2.3.2 Basolateral Transport of Iron

Iron which is not stored in the enterocytes is transferred across the basolateral membrane into the plasma by ferroportin, a multi-transmembrane segment protein, and the only known iron exporter.

Ferroportin (Fpn) is present in all tissues that export iron into plasma which includes duodenal enterocytes, macrophages of spleen and liver, and hepatocytes. Fpn is also required for transfer of iron from the mother to fetus early in gestation. It plays a role in the export of iron from macrophages which recycle iron from senescent erythrocytes. Ferroportin is known to be expressed in the lung, renal tubules, and marrow erythroid precursors where its function is not known. Mutations in the ferroportin gene result in disturbances in iron homeostasis, elevated serum ferritin, and a hemochromatosis like state.

The basolateral export of iron requires change of its redox state from the ferrous to ferric form which is mediated by **hephaestin** [3] (Fig. 2.2).

2.3.3 Factors Influencing Iron Absorption

The total body iron content is maintained by regulating absorption. There are two factors which determine the rate of absorption of iron: **iron stores and rate of erythropoiesis.**

If iron stores are depleted as occurs in IDA, more iron is transferred to the plasma and less remains within the enterocytes as ferritin. The reverse happens when iron stores are normal and this is referred to as the stores regulator.

Rate of erythropoiesis irrespective of whether it is effective or ineffective also determines absorption. When the rate of production of red cells is increased, there is an increase in the absorption of iron from the intestine (erythroid regulator). In conditions associated with ineffective erythropoiesis such as beta thalassemia major, the increased iron absorbed deposits in various organs [3].

2.3.4 Iron Transport in Plasma

Iron is transported in the plasma bound to the protein **transferrin** which is synthesized in the liver. It is a glycoprotein with a MW of about 80 kDa which is initially synthesized as a preprotein and modified to produce the mature protein. The rate of transferrin synthesis shows an inverse relationship with iron stores.

Transferrin has two homologous iron binding domains each of which can bind an atom of ferric iron. As the iron atoms are incorporated one at a time, iron loaded transferrin can exist in monoferric or diferric forms. At any point of time, only one-third of transferrin binding sites are occupied with iron.

When iron binds to transferrin, one mole of anion (bicarbonate usually) is taken up and three moles of hydrogen ions are released. The binding of bicarbonate and its interaction with iron give transferrin its characteristic pink color with an absorption peak at a wavelength of 465 nm. Patients with congenital atransferrinemia develop a severe microcytic hypochromic anemia. The iron transport compartment is dynamic and changes approximately ten times during the day. Binding of iron to transferrin provides solubility, reduces reactivity, and thus ensures a safe and controlled delivery of iron to all cells [7]. In the laboratory, transferrin can be measured directly

Fig. 2.2 Absorption of
heme and non-heme iron

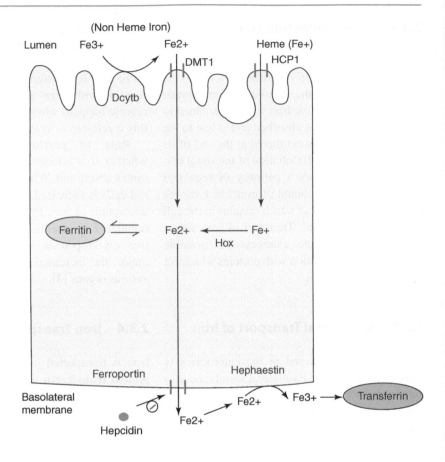

Dcytb- Duodenal cytochrome b
DMT1- Divalent metal transporter 1
Hox-Heme oxygenase
HCP1-heme carrier protein 1

(normal levels 2–3 g/L) or quantified as total iron binding capacity, i.e., in terms of the amount of iron it can bind.

2.3.5 Uptake of Iron by Tissues

Transferrin delivers the bound iron to developing erythroid cells as also other cells by binding to cell surface receptors, transferrin receptors (TfR). The TfR-transferrin iron complex is internalized via an endocytic vesicle. Once within the cell, iron dissociates from the complex and remains in the cytosol while the TfR-transferrin complex is recycled back to the cell surface. Both transferrin

and TfR participate in multiple rounds of iron delivery (Fig. 2.3).

Transferrin receptor is a transmembrane protein with two polypeptide chains each of which weighs 95 kD. Both the chains are identical and mediate the delivery of iron to erythroblasts. The receptor has a membrane spanning segment and a cytoplasmic segment. Each TfR can bind two transferrin molecules. The diferric form of transferrin is bound with a higher affinity.

TfRs are present on all cells with the majority (80%) being in the erythroid marrow. Their number is modulated during erythroid development. Very few receptors are identified on CFU-E and BFU-E, with numbers increasing in basophilic

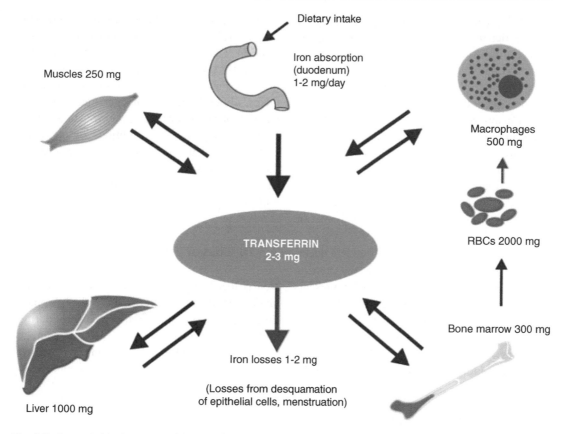

Fig. 2.3 Systemic iron homeostasis

normoblasts. The numbers peak at the stage of polychromatic normoblast and decrease as reticulocytes mature. The number of transferrin receptors on the cell surface reflects its iron requirement. Mature red cells shed all the receptors which are found in the plasma (a truncated form of the tissue receptor) and their number correlates with the rate of erythropoiesis [1].

TfR 2 shares 45% homology with TfR in its extracellular domain. The receptor which binds transferrin with lesser affinity is highly expressed in the liver and erythroid precursors. Mutation in the gene for TfR2 leads to an iron overload disorder suggesting that the receptor plays a role in iron homeostasis [8].

In iron-deficient states, there is a prompt induction of receptor synthesis. sTfR levels reflect the degree of depletion of the functional iron compartment well before IDA develops and are a reliable index of early tissue iron deficiency.

2.3.6   Iron Utilization in Normoblasts

Once inside the cell, iron moves to the mitochondria and is incorporated into protoporphyrin and used for heme synthesis. Almost 80–90% of the iron which enters the erythroid precursors is incorporated into heme. Iron which is not used is stored as ferritin and hemosiderin and can be identified in erythroid precursors as blue granules on Perl's staining [1].

2.3.7   Storage Iron

Iron is stored in two forms: ferritin and hemosiderin.

Ferritin is comprised of an apoferritin with iron incorporated in the central core. The protein shell is constructed of two distinct ferritin subunits:

H and L which are structurally homologous. Ferritins rich in H chains acquire iron more rapidly while L chain-rich ferritins are more stable. The ratio of H and L chains varies depending on the tissue subtype. Several isoforms of ferritin have been described. Each molecule of ferritin can hold 4500 iron atoms when fully saturated. Iron stored in ferritin is utilized in iron-deficient states.

Ferritin is also found in the plasma in small amounts and the level correlates with iron stores. Its estimation is used as a non-invasive indicator of iron deficiency with 1 µg/L of plasma ferritin concentration corresponding to 8–10 mg of tissue iron stores.

Hemosiderin is formed by incomplete degradation of ferritin. It is less soluble than ferritin and has a higher iron to protein ratio. It represents a more stable and less available form of storage iron and the size of the compartment changes only after prolonged mobilization of iron. In conditions associated with iron overload, hemosiderin is the predominant iron storage protein [6].

2.3.8 Systemic Iron Homeostasis

Systemic iron homeostasis regulates intestinal iron absorption and its entry and mobilization from stores to meet demands of erythropoiesis. It also ensures a stable milieu wherein each cell regulates its iron uptake according to needs (Fig. 2.3).

2.3.9 Recycling of Macrophage Iron

Iron recycling accounts for most of the iron homeostasis in humans. Iron is liberated from phagocytosis of effete red cells in the macrophages of liver and spleen. A significant proportion of the released iron is stored within macrophages as ferritin and is rapidly mobilized when the demand for iron is more. The remaining iron is released in two phases: an early phase which occurs within a few hours of erythrophagocytosis and a later phase which takes place over days. Mobilization in the later phase occurs in response to demand of iron and is a critical

determinant of the availability of iron for erythropoiesis. This release of iron is mediated by ferroportin. The recycling of erythrocytes generates about 20–25 mg iron/day and is essential to meet iron requirements of erythropoiesis. In adult males, about 1 mg of iron is stored in macrophages, the amount being less in women of reproductive age group. In conditions of increased erythropoiesis, the amount of iron which leaves the macrophages exceeds that which enters it. The reverse happens in conditions associated with increased destruction of red cells [2].

2.3.10 Loss of Iron

Iron is lost from the body when intestinal cells and epithelial cells of the skin are shed. Women during their reproductive life lose iron during menstruation and pregnancy. The total average loss in normal adult males and non-menstruating females is about 1–2 mg/day. This amount is balanced by intestinal absorption [3].

2.3.11 Iron Homeostasis: Role of Hepcidin

Hepcidin, initially characterized as an antimicrobial peptide, is a 25 amino acid peptide hormone synthesized by the liver. The human hepcidin gene codes for the formation of a 84 amino acid preprohepcidin which is then processed to the active form. The structure of the 25 amino acid molecule resembles a hairpin with 8 cysteines that form 4 disulfide bonds in a ladder-like configuration. Hepcidin that readily passes through the glomerular membrane is taken up and degraded in the proximal tubules. A small proportion of the filtered hepcidin passes into the urine intact. Hence, it can be detected both in plasma and urine. Urine also contains 20 and 22 amino acid forms. The expression of hepcidin is mediated by bone morphogenetic protein (BMP) and JAK2/STAT 3 signaling pathway [9, 10].

Hepcidin acts by binding to the iron transporter ferroportin. The binding induces a conformational change in ferroportin and triggers its endocytosis and consequent lysosomal degradation. This reduces dietary iron absorption and inhibits release of recycled iron from macrophages and hepatocytes.

Several factors regulate the production of hepcidin. Important among these are **body iron content and rate of erythropoiesis.** In iron-deficient states, the synthesis of hepcidin is inhibited allowing more iron to enter the plasma; the reverse occurs when iron is adequate. Proteins such as hemojuvelin, TfR2, and receptor for BMP are involved in this. When erythropoiesis is increased, hepcidin production is suppressed, making more iron available for Hb synthesis and this is mediated by growth differentiation factor-15 (GDF-15). The suppression of hepcidin is particularly prominent in conditions with ineffective erythropoiesis such as β-thalassemia major [7].

Inflammation and infections increase hepcidin synthesis. This is mediated by IL-6 which activates the BMP6 receptor complex followed by activation of the SMAD pathway and over-expression of hepcidin. The increased hepcidin causes hypoferremia which develops early in infections. It limits availability of iron for erythropoiesis and contributes to anemia associated with infection.

Hypoxia stimulates the marrow to produce more erythrocytes leading to decrease in hepcidin. **Anemia** modulates hepcidin levels through multiple effects: hypoxia, increased erythropoietic activity, decreased tissue iron [10].

In order to coordinate the apical absorption of iron by DMT 1 with the basolateral transfer into plasma by ferroportin, the effect of hepcidin on ferroportin is communicated to the apical iron absorption mechanism so that iron uptake is reduced. This is mediated by iron regulatory proteins 1 and 2 (IRP-1, IRP-2) [11].

2.3.12 Iron Regulatory Proteins Regulate Cellular Iron

Iron is present in many cells each of which has specific functions related to iron metabolism. Cellular iron homeostasis is post-transcriptionally regulated by IRP1 and IRP2. IRPs are cytosolic RNA binding proteins which bind to iron-responsive element (IRE) located in the untranslated regions of genes as also mRNA encoding proteins involved in uptake of iron, its storage, utilization, and export. The binding inhibits initiation of translation. When cellular iron is reduced, IRPs do not bind to IREs allowing an increased rate of mRNA translation. High iron levels suppress these changes. Hence, IRP and IREs are both involved in regulating the synthesis and suppression of multiple proteins involved in iron metabolism [12].

2.3.13 Iron Deficiency Anemia (IDA)

Iron deficiency (ID) is a condition in which iron availability is insufficient to meet the body's needs. It can be present with or without anemia.

2.3.14 Prevalence

Iron deficiency is the most common nutritional deficiency in the world. It is estimated that over 30% of the world's population is anemic largely due to deficiency of iron. Besides its high prevalence in developing countries, it is the only micronutrient deficiency which is significantly prevalent in developed nations also. It is estimated that 60–80% of the world's population suffers from deficiency of iron. However, 40% of the global burden of ID is reported to occur in SE Asia.

Pregnant women and children are particularly susceptible to the occurrence of IDA. With anemia as an indirect indicator of ID, up to 88% of Indian pregnant women (PW) are affected. The prevalence among preschool children is similar to that in PW with nearly 79% children below the age of 3 years being anemic. In nonpregnant women of reproductive age group, the prevalence of anemia is reported to be 52% [13]. In a study which compiled global data from several large studies, it was estimated that 50% of anemia in women and children is attributable to deficiency of iron [14]. These prevalence rates are not different from those in 1970s indicating that the anemia epidemic is persisting in India.

Based on the prevalence of anemia of which the most common cause is iron deficiency, there are no countries where ID is not a mild public health problem. For PW, more than 80% countries have a moderate-to-severe public health problem. In India, it is a **severe public health problem** for preschool children, PW, and non-pregnant women [15].

2.3.15 Etiology of IDA

The etiology of IDA is multifaceted. It generally results from inadequate intake of iron due to poor quantity/quality of diet, impaired absorption, or increased demand for iron. Chronic blood loss from any site is an important cause of IDA. Bleeding from GIT (ulcers, parasites, malignancies) as also from any other site causes IDA (Table 2.1).

2.3.16 Stages of ID

Iron deficiency and IDA result from a prolonged period of negative iron balance leading to a compromised supply of iron to the tissues. The first stage of prelatent iron deficiency is characterized by the absence of measurable iron stores. Iron-deficient erythropoiesis shows evidence of restricted iron supply but no anemia. Finally, IDA occurs with reduction in Hb concentration [3] (Table 2.2).

2.3.17 Clinical Features

Low plasma concentration of iron limits hemoglobin synthesis leading to **anemia**. The clinical features depend on the severity of anemia, its duration and speed of onset. Some patients may be asymptomatic while others present with pallor, weakness, easy fatiguability, exertional dyspnea which progresses to dyspnea at rest as anemia becomes severe, irritability, dizziness, and palpitations. ID even without anemia also results in fatigue [4]. Dryness and roughness of skin and hair, alopecia, glossitis, and restless leg syndrome are other clinical manifestations.

2.3.18 Adverse Consequences of IDA

It is now well recognized that iron deficiency even without anemia is associated with several adverse consequences.

Table 2.2 Stages in the development of iron deficiency

Parameter	Prelatent	Latent	IDA
Bone marrow iron	Reduced	Absent	Absent
Serum ferritin (μg/L)	<16	<16	<16
FEP	N	Increased	Increased
sTfR	N	Increased	Increased
TS (%)	N	<16	<16
CHr	N	Decreased	Decreased
Hb	N	N	Decreased

Table 2.1 Etiology of IDA

Decreased intake	Impaired absorption	Increased loss	Increased demand
Diets low in iron	Achlorhydria Gastrectomy/gastric bypass surgery	Chronic blood loss from any site:GIT, hematuria, epistaxis	Pregnancy
Low quantity of bioavailable iron	Celiac disease H.pylori infection	Gynecological loss	Lactation
Less food intake	Phytates, tannins, other inhibitors	Drugs:aspirin NSAIDs	Infancy
	Drugs:NSAIDs, aspirin, H_2 blockers Proton pump inhibitors	Parasites:hookworm	

2.3.19 Developmental and Neurophysiological Deficits in Infants and Children

Several neurologic and non-neurologic sequelae of ID have been reported, some of which are not reversed completely with iron supplementation.

2.3.20 Cognitive Development

Iron plays a key role in brain function and is present, often in large quantities in several areas of the brain. A significant correlation has been found between IDA and cognition. ID even without anemia has an effect on cognitive and motor scores with lower scores observed when IDA sets in. Reduced mental, motor, social, and neurophysiological functioning has been observed in these patients. Iron-deficient children were found to achieve lower scores on IQ testing and other cognitive performance activities.

Infants are particularly vulnerable during 6–23 months of age as iron is essential for developing cognitive functions at this stage of life. Anemic infants have trouble with motor functions specially those involving balance and coordination. Even after receiving iron therapy for 3 months with correction of anemia, previously anemic infants continue to have lower mental and motor development. Delayed psychomotor development has also been shown in iron-deficient infants. On reaching school going age, they have impaired performance in tests of language skills as also motor skills and coordination. Impaired scholastic performance has also been reported [3, 16].

Children with IDA show **behavioral disturbances.** These children are disruptive, irritable with short attention span and lack of interest in their surroundings. Children, adolescents, and women show increased attention and concentration with iron supplementation [17].

2.3.21 Evoked Response Potentials (ERP)

Studies using ERP, both auditory and visual, in iron-deficient children show prolonged latencies and reduced amplitudes of waves responses possibly due to impaired myelination which remain uncorrected with iron supplementation. The changes persisted in children when repeat testing was done at 4 years of age supporting the role of iron as an essential element for myelination in early infancy [16].

2.3.22 Other Consequences

ID results in **impaired growth.** The high iron requirement in infancy cannot be met by diet alone especially in developing countries. Maternal iron reserves are depleted after 4–6 months of feeding and if these infants are not supplemented, their growth is impaired. Iron supplementation improves growth [18].

Immune abnormalities such as defects in cellular immunity, reduction in number of both helper and suppressor T cells and impaired killing of microorganisms by phagocytes are observed in IDA which **impairs resistance to infection.** Supplementation with iron reduces morbidity from infectious diseases [3].

A higher risk of **maternal mortality** is observed with decreasing Hb levels. About 18% of maternal mortality in low- and middle income countries is attributable to deficiency of iron [19]. Maternal IDA has a negative correlation with the length of gestation. **Prematurity, low birth weight,** and other pregnancy-related complications are observed in IDA [20].

2.3.23 Economic Consequences of IDA

2.3.23.1 Work Capacity and Productivity

Skeletal muscle contains 10–15% of the body's iron mainly in oxidative fibers which appear red because of the iron in myoglobin. Skeletal muscle oxidative capacity and oxygen consumption both determine exercise performance. Lack of iron affects physical performance especially in women. A linear relationship has been reported between ID and aerobic work capacity. Anemia is known to impair work performance, endurance, and productivity all of which improve with supplementation. For every increase in Hb of 1 g/dL, there is an improvement in production efficiency of 14% [21].

Iron deficiency **impairs national socioeconomic development**. The estimation of disability adjusted life years (DALYs) provides an estimate of the magnitude of economic losses to a population. The impact of ID on maternal mortality, growth, and cognitive function in children and adults results in 19.7 million DALYs [19]. It has been estimated that anemia accounts for 68 million years of living with disability, almost 9% of the total for all conditions [22].

2.3.24 Laboratory Diagnosis of IDA

Several tests are available for the laboratory diagnosis of IDA. The results of the tests must be interpreted in the clinical context. A combination of tests can be used for diagnosis.

2.3.24.1 Complete Blood Counts

Hemoglobin (Hb) and Hematocrit (Hct). Patients with IDA have mild-moderate reduction in Hb concentration and Hct. Hb < 13 g/dL in males and <12 g/dL in females defines the last stage of iron deficiency which is IDA. In pregnancy, this cutoff is 11 g/dL [14]. Hb provides a quantitative measure of the severity of ID once anemia has developed but lacks sensitivity and specificity. As anemia can occur in several conditions, Hb concentration alone cannot be used to diagnose IDA.

Red cell count and indices. Total RBC count, MCV, and MCH are reduced while MCHC is reduced in long-standing/severe disease. The reduction is proportional to the severity and duration of anemia. MCV and MCH are inexpensive and widely available parameters but become abnormal in late stages of ID. The values may be normal in co-existent deficiency of B_{12}/folate and are reduced in other disorders also.

The **total leucocyte count** is usually normal. **Thrombocytosis** is observed in these patients with counts being 1.5–2 times normal.

Red cell distribution width (RDW). This is a measure of an isocytosis of red cells and is elevated early in IDA. It can be measured as coefficient of variation (RDW-CV) or standard deviation (RDW-SD). RDW can be used to distinguish between IDA and β-thalassemia trait (normal RDW).

Reticulocyte Hb content (CHr). CHr provides a measure of the iron available to recently produced red cells. It is a strong predictor of ID as it provides a more real-time view of bone marrow iron status. In the early phase of ID, there is fluctuation in the iron supply to the marrow resulting in reticulocytes with less Hb and decrease in CHr before the development of anemia. CHr less than 29 pg is diagnostic of IDA. It needs no additional blood sample, is reported as part of the reticulocyte count in the analyzer, and has been recommended as a screening test for the early detection of ID. Unlike biochemical tests of iron status, it does not show biological variability and is not affected by inflammation. It is also used to monitor iron therapy as it rises early after iron supplementation and to diagnose functional ID during r-Hu EPO therapy. Its limitations are that it is available on only few automated analyzers. In patients with co-existent deficiency of B_{12}/folate, the value may be elevated. It is also low in other disorders associated with impaired iron availability [20, 23].

Reticulocyte Hb equivalent. This is available on some automated hematology analyzers and is a reliable, sensitive, and specific parameter to identify iron-deficient states [24].

Percentage of hypochromic red cells. This is a measure of the concentration of Hb in red cells and takes into account the absolute amount of Hb as also the size of the red cell. As the size of the red cell changes with storage, it does not give reliable results on stored samples necessitating the need for a fresh sample. This limits its application even though it is comparable to CHr in terms of its utility. The parameter is independent of erythropoietic activity and is useful in monitoring hemodialysis patients on r-Hu EPO [25].

2.3.25 Examination of a Stained Peripheral Blood Film (PBF)

The blood smear shows microcytes with an increase in central pallor. The number of erythrocytes affected and the degree of hypochromia are related to the severity of anemia. In severe disease, most of the red cells appear as rings. Poikilocytes in the form of elongated cells may be seen (Fig. 2.4).

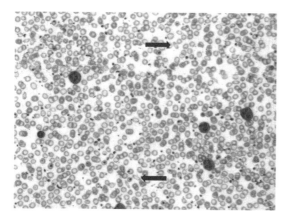

Fig. 2.4 PBF of patient with IDA showing microcytic hypochromic red cells. Few elongated cells (arrow) are also seen (Leishman stain ×400)

2.3.26 Biochemical Tests of Iron Status

2.3.26.1 Serum Iron (SI), Total Iron Binding Capacity (TIBC), and Percent Transferrin Saturation (%TS)

These tests are widely used for assessment of iron status. SI is reduced and TIBC elevated in IDA resulting in a substantial reduction in %TS with levels <16% being diagnostic of IDA [15].

SI shows diurnal variation with higher concentrations seen later in the day. Patients on iron-rich diet or those on iron supplements have falsely elevated levels. As the results are affected by lipemia, testing is done on a fasting state. There is a variation in the level of SI based on the assay methodology and the presence of hemolysis. The level is low in anemia of chronic disease and must not be used on its own to diagnose ID. Elevated TIBC is specific for ID but has a low sensitivity. %TS also has acute phase reactivity and shows diurnal variation. However, it is a more useful indicator of iron status than SI or TIBC alone. These iron markers are considerably altered by inflammation. If IDA co-exists with inflammation, the interpretation of results is difficult thus limiting their applicability [26].

2.3.26.2 Serum Ferritin (SF)

SF concentration correlates well with total body iron stores. It is extensively used to diagnose ID and is especially useful in populations where the prevalence of infections is low. The test is not invasive, widely available, specific, and frequently used to diagnose ID. A low SF is a reliable index of ID and levels <16 μg/L are diagnostic of ID [27].

Ferritin is an acute phase reactant and rises in the presence of co-existing infection/inflammation/malignancy making interpretation of SF levels in these situations problematic. The problem can be overcome by simultaneous measurement of markers of inflammation such as CRP which will help in identification of co-existing inflammation. Another approach is to raise the cut-off value of SF which defines iron deficiency when it co-exists with infection with the best predictor being SF < 100 µg/L. If serum ferritin is between 100 and 300 µg/L, %TS is recommended to confirm ID [28].

2.3.26.3 Zinc Protoporphyrin (ZPP)/Free Erythrocyte Protoporphyrin (FEP)

Protoporphyrin is normally produced during the synthesis of Hb and remains in the RBC for its entire life span. FEP is elevated in IDA as less iron is available for Hb synthesis. It detects stage II iron deficiency, i.e., iron-deficient erythropoiesis being normal in Stage I. The level reflects the events of the preceding 2–3 months. Changes in FEP levels occur relatively slowly. It can be measured as ZPP which reflects aberrant incorporation of zinc into protoporphyrin instead of iron when iron is not available.

FEP is measured in a hematofluorometer which requires only a drop of blood and can be performed within minutes along with CBC. It has been used as a screening test in field surveys. It is simple, cheap but not specific as it is also elevated in infection, lead poisoning, and hemolysis. Studies indicate that in patients with microcytic hypochromic anemias, FEP done as an initial test is helpful in the differential diagnosis. While an elevated level is sufficient for a presumptive diagnosis of IDA, a normal level rules out disorders of heme synthesis. Additional tests such as %TS, SF may then be done as required. Some studies recommend simultaneous measurement of FEP, SF, and Hb in assessing iron deficiency [29].

2.3.26.4 Serum TfR

Receptor levels are increased in IDA. Measurement of sTfR is especially useful in the differentiation of IDA from anemia of chronic disease as its concentration is unaffected by the acute phase response. sTfR has shown to be a promising tool for the diagnosis of ID. The levels are also raised in conditions associated with increased erythropoietic activity such as hemolytic anemia.

sTfR is measured using commercially available ELISA assays. A major advantage of sTfR measurement over SF is that it is more specific to changes in iron status and erythropoiesis. The clinical interpretation of sTfR result is simpler if confounding factors such as hemolysis are excluded. Its day-to-day variation is more acceptable than the conventional indices of functional iron status such as %TS and provides an alternative to these tests. As almost 30% of susceptible population such as pregnant women can have ID without anemia, sTfR levels can detect tissue ID before the onset of anemia and help prevent its deleterious effects. Limitations of the assay include lack of standardized reference material and nonavailability of standardized cutoffs which has made the test underutilized [23].

2.3.26.5 sTfR/Log Ferritin (sTfR-F Index)

This ratio provides a better indicator of iron depletion than either of the tests alone. Ferritin reflects storage iron and sTfR the functional iron compartment, combining the two values provides a ratio which is reciprocally regulated. It takes advantage of the increase in TfR and decrease in SF in ID. Both the variables in the ratio are influenced by iron stores, availability of iron for erythropoiesis, and the total erythroid marrow mass.

The ratio has a high sensitivity and specificity and can distinguish between iron replete and iron deplete anemic subjects effectively. It has been found to be useful in accurately classifying anemia especially when it accompanies diseases with active inflammation. A low index indicates anemia of chronic disease while a high index suggests ID. Although thresholds are not well defined, ratio > 2–3 can be used to diagnose IDA [30]. However, its utility in diagnosing non anemic ID is not established. The ratio has also been used for assessment of supplementation induced changes [31].

2.3.26.6 Serum Hepcidin

Assays have been developed to measure hepcidin. These include ELISA using anti-hepcidin antibodies and mass spectrometry with a close correlation existing between both techniques. While ELISA measures low levels more accurately, mass spectrometry measures the active form (25 amino acid) of hepcidin accurately.

Hepcidin can be measured in serum and urine with the former being preferred. Urinary estimation requires measurement of creatinine to correct for the difference in the concentrating ability of the kidney. Hepcidin levels are reduced in IDA.

The levels show a diurnal variation with lower levels seen in the morning and are lower in women as compared to men. Use of hepcidin as a routine diagnostic test of ID is still limited due to lack of studies on large number of subjects and of international standardization thresholds [32].

Other uses of hepcidin estimation. Results from a pilot study suggest that hepcidin levels can be used to determine which patients will respond to oral iron [33]. In regions with high infection burden, estimation of hepcidin can help decide the appropriateness of oral iron therapy. This is necessary as supplementation with iron to children with infections is associated with serious adverse outcomes including high mortality attributed to increased vulnerability to malaria and other microbial agents [34].

2.3.27 Examination of Bone Marrow Aspirate for Iron

Examination of stained bone marrow aspirates for hemosiderin is a specific test for ID and is still considered the gold standard for evaluation of iron stores (Fig. 2.5). On staining with Prussian blue,

Table 2.3 Laboratory tests of IDA

Parameter	Reference range	Change in IDA
Hemoglobin (g/dL)	Females 13.5 ± 1.5 Males 15.0 ± 2.0	Reduced Males < 13, Females < 12 PW < 11
MCV (fL) MCH (pg)	MCV 80–100 MCH 29.5 ± 2.5	MCV < 80 MCH < 27
MCHC (g/dL)	33.0 ± 1.5	Reduced in severe disease
RDW (%)	12.8 ± 1.2	Increased >14%
CHr (pg)		Reduced <29
%Hypochromic cells	<5	Increased
Serum iron (µg/dL)	60–180	Reduced
TIBC (µg/dL)	250–450	Elevated
%TS		<16
SF (µg/L)	20–200	Reduced <16
sTfR	Lab to establish	Elevated
ZPP/FEP (µmol/mol heme)	<40	Elevated
BM iron	1+ to 3+	Absent
Serum hepcidin	Lab to establish	Reduced

iron granules can be identified in erythroid precursors and macrophages. The positivity is graded on the basis of intensity of staining from 1 to 6.

Normoblasts which show siderotic blue granules are called sideroblasts. In normal individuals, about half of the normoblasts are sideroblasts, each of which contains less than five small granules. If the granules form a ring; complete or partial around the nucleus of the normoblast, the cell is a ring sideroblast which is seen under pathological conditions.

The disadvantages of this method are that it is invasive, causes discomfort to the patient, and hence is not suitable for screening [3].

The reference range and the abnormality of tests used for diagnosis of IDA is shown in Table 2.3.

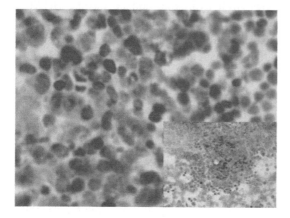

Fig. 2.5 Perl's stain of BM aspirate (×400) showing absent iron stores in a patient with IDA. Inset shows normal iron stores (×400)

2.3.28 Treatment of IDA

IDA is treated with iron supplementation which can be given orally or through intravenous route.

The treatment aims to correct the Hb concentration and also replenish iron stores.

Oral iron therapy is inexpensive, convenient, effective, easy to obtain, and the first choice of treatment in most cases. The common oral preparations used are ferrous sulfate, ferrous fumarate, and ferrous gluconate of which ferrous sulfate is most commonly used. Oral iron is usually indicated when Hb concentration is less than 12 g/dL and more than 8 g/dL. The recommended daily dose for adults with ID is 100–200 mg of elemental iron and that for children is 3–6 mg/kg body weight of a liquid preparation. Though it is preferable to take iron on an empty stomach, various side effects including nausea, vomiting, epigastric discomfort, constipation, diarrhea, metallic taste, and dark colored stools are reported. The patient can then be advised to take the supplement with meals though it reduces absorption. As the side effects are dose related, they can also be reduced by starting therapy with a small dose and gradually increasing it.

Sustained release preparations are also available for oral administration. They are better tolerated but are more expensive and are not absorbed as efficiently as other oral drugs [23].

Duration of therapy. Oral iron therapy is given till the Hb concentration reaches normal. It should be further continued for 3–6 months to replenish stores [32].

Failure to respond to oral iron results from lack of adherence to therapy, low tolerance, true refractoriness, continued loss of blood as also impaired absorption or an incorrect diagnosis [23].

Estimation of serum hepcidin can identify patients who will probably respond to oral iron (hepcidin low) and those who will not (normal/elevated hepcidin) [33]. However, these assays are not available routinely.

Parenteral iron is indicated when oral therapy is poorly tolerated, the patient does not respond to oral iron and in patients with malabsorption. Patients with chronic blood loss in whom bleeding cannot be adequately controlled also need parenteral iron.

The preparations commonly in use are ferric carboxymaltose (FCM), iron dextran, and iron sucrose. These compounds comprise of a core which contains the iron salt and is surrounded by a carbohydrate shell. In the RES, iron is released from the complex and used. The kinetics of iron release varies with the compound used. The speed of release determines how much iron can be given as a single dose.

Intravenous iron can be given as a **single dose or in multiple doses**. Single dose preparations are low molecular weight iron dextran, ferumoxytol, ferric carboxymaltose, and iron isomaltoside. These preparations can be given in high doses of 500–1000 mg in a single infusion resulting in replacement of the total deficit in one or two infusions. The advantage is that a single dose can be given in 1–2 sessions [5]. Multiple dose preparations are iron sucrose and ferrous gluconate. Even though they can be used as single dose, multiple doses are used for better delivery rate and replacement. Ferric carboxymaltose (FCM) has been successfully used to treat ID of varied etiology in children and adults. The preparation is reported to be safe and extremely effective and is recommended when oral iron therapy fails, a quick increase in hemoglobin or replacement of the total iron deficit at a single or few settings is required [35, 36].

Ferumoxytol is a newer compound approved in the USA and Europe which is as effective as other iron compounds. It is a iron oxide nanoparticle with a polyglucose sorbitol carboxymethyl ether coating. This minimizes sensitivity and larger doses can be given rapidly. **Iron nanoparticles** (iron hydroxide adipate tartrate [IHAT]) mimicking the ferritin molecule which have high bioavailability are under trial [29, 32]. The indications for parenteral iron are given in Table 2.4.

As formulae calculating the total iron deficit are not reliable, a 1000 mg replacement dose is used. This may not be sufficient for patients with severe IDA and so SF should be measured after 2–4 weeks of the infusion. If SF is <50 µg/L, another dose is given.

The chief **advantage** of parenteral iron is that it replenishes iron stores more effectively and reliably and increases Hb more quickly as compared to oral iron. For the new formulations, a single dose is sufficient thus reducing hospital visits. These preparations have an extremely low

Table 2.4 Indications of parenteral iron

1. Hb ≤8 g/dL
2. Intolerance/not responsive to oral iron
3. Rapid correction of anemia required
4. Selected cases of anemia of chronic disease
5. Chronic heart failure
6. Iron malabsorption
7. Ongoing blood loss
8. Use of erythropoietin and erythropoietin stimulating agents in CKD
9. Inflammatory bowel disease
10. IRIDA
11. Substitute for blood transfusion (religious reasons, post-surgery transfusion sparing)

Table 2.5 Strategies in preventing IDA

• Removing poverty
• Awareness and education regarding diet
• Food fortification
• Biofortification
• Iron supplementation to susceptible populations
• Delayed cord clamping
• Prevention and treatment of infection
• Screening for ID in vulnerable population

risk of serious adverse effects, do not require a test dose, and can be given over a short period of time.

Side effects include abdominal pain, nausea, headache flushing, myalgia, arthralgia. and diarrhea. Infusion reactions including serious anaphylactic reactions have been reported especially with high MW iron dextran [32].

2.3.29 Monitoring Response to Iron Supplementation

The response to iron can be monitored by reticulocyte count which begins to rise after 3–4 days, peaks at 5–7 days and then returns to normal. The count is inversely related to Hb concentration which begins to increase by the second week of therapy and normalizes by 2 months of initiation of therapy. An increase of 2 g/dL of Hb concentration is an appropriate response to iron therapy. The red cell indices remain abnormal for some time after Hb returns to normal [37].

2.3.30 Follow-Up After Iron Supplementation

After normalization of Hb, CBC and parameters of iron status must be measured each month for 3 months and then once every 3 months for a year [37]. Long-term follow-up is needed for patients with severe IDA and those receiving intravenous iron. Ferritin should be checked every 3–4 months and if it falls below 50 µg/L, another dose of

intravenous iron is given. Recently, measurement of Hb concentration at day 14 has been proposed to decide if the patient needs to be shifted from oral to intravenous iron therapy [38].

Caution. In malaria endemic areas, iron supplementation may increase parasitemia and have negative effects on other types of infections like diarrhea and acute respiratory illness. There is hence a need for caution [28]. Estimation of serum hepcidin helps determine the best time to provide children in these regions with iron supplementation [34].

2.3.31 Prevention of IDA

Preventive measures are especially required for populations at risk of IDA such as PW, infants, and children (Table 2.5).

Preventive measures include

• Nations must provide information about and promote access to foods rich in iron such as foods of animal origin, legumes, green leafy vegetables, kidney beans, and lentils. Adding enhancers and reducing inhibitors of absorption will increase iron bioavailability. Ferritin is used by plants and animals for storage of iron and this phytoferritin has high potential as a food fortificant. As this is not available commercially, consumption of foods naturally rich in this protein such as pulses and lentils will help increase iron intake.
• Fortification is addition of iron supplements to the most widely consumed food of a particular population at the point of manufacture without changing the property of the food item. Rice, bread, wheat flour, and salt are some of the foods which have been fortified. The choice of

these ingredients is influenced by the characteristics of the product such as taste and color and may be constrained by cost. Fortification gives access to all socioeconomic groups. Products must contain at least 15% of the relevant Nutrient Reference Value (NRV) per measure of product to have claim of being fortified with iron. The limitation is that the iron compounds used are insoluble/poorly soluble and strongly chelated making them less bioavailable. Iron can react with other components in the food affecting the shelf life.

- Biofortification is targeted breeding of crops rich in micronutrients. Iron biofortification is applicable to wheat, rice, millets, beans, peas, and lentils. These foods have higher concentrations of iron [29, 39].
- Iron supplementation is given as part of prevention to populations susceptible to ID (PW, women in the reproductive age group, adolescents, and preschool children). WHO recommends that governments of low income countries with high prevalence of ID should implement universal iron supplementation for young children and PW. However, the approach has low levels of implementation and the risk of side effects [40].
- As children need additional iron after 6 months of breast feeding, they may be given multiple micronutrient powders. WHO recommends micronutrient powders which contain lipid encapsulated iron with other micronutrients in the form of sachets for children 6–23 month which can be added to prepared food. This is easier for children to take as they have problem in swallowing tablets [40].
- As worm infestation is a common cause of IDA in tropical countries, deworming at regular intervals may help increase the Hb concentration.
- Cord clamping 1–3 min after delivery improves infant iron stores at 6 months of age. Delayed cord clamping is recommended for all uncomplicated deliveries by WHO [29].

- Screening for IDA should be done at regular intervals in children, adolescents, pregnant women, and women in the reproductive age group [v29, 39].

2.4 Functional Iron Deficiency

Functional iron deficiency (FID) is defined as a state where there is insufficient incorporation of iron into erythroid precursors despite adequate iron stores as identified by the presence of stainable iron in the marrow together with normal or elevated serum ferritin [3]. FID is characteristically seen in anemia of chronic disease (ACD) which is associated with chronic diseases of varied etiology including chronic kidney disease (CKD). Disorders associated with ACD have in common the ability to induce the production of cytokines such as IL-6, TNF, and IL-1. These cytokines induce the transcription of hepcidin which downregulates ferroportin expression to inhibit the absorption of dietary iron. Hypoferremia diminishes the amount of iron available for Hb synthesis and erythrocyte production. Because of the inflammatory state, the RE storage iron gets locked up thus restricting the supply of iron to the erythroid marrow [28].

FID is frequently seen in patients of chronic kidney disease (CKD) on dialysis. Anemia is present in 80% of these patients and is multifactorial in etiology. Both absolute and functional ID are present in 25–38% patients of CKD. Recombinant erythropoietin is the treatment of choice for anemia in CKD. Therapy with erythropoiesis stimulating agents (ESA) stimulates the erythroid marrow leading to an increased iron requirement which outstrips the ability of circulating iron to provide adequate substrate for Hb synthesis. A high prevalence of iron deficiency is observed in CKD patients on HD. ID in CKD is a combination of absolute and functional ID and is a major factor which limits response to ESA. It is recommended that CKD patients

Table 2.6 Uses and limitations of laboratory parameters of FID

Parameter	Use	Limitation
Red cell indices MCV and MCH	Must be determined at diagnosis as baseline parameters to assess the change over a time period	– They are mean values over a period of 20–120 days – Are slow to change – Do not reflect any acute change in iron lack – Confounded by co-existing deficiency of folate/B12 and thalassemias
% hypochromic red cells	Direct indicator of FID Reliable Sensitive Specific ≥10% consistent with absolute ID/FID	– Available on only few analyzers – Each analyzer has defined the cutoff – Influenced by the time between sampling and analysis
Reticulocyte count	Used to assess response to ESA (increase ≥40 × 10^9/L from baseline by 4 weeks)	By itself does not provide information on iron status
CHr	Predicts response to intravenous iron Levels of <29 pg indicate iron restricted erythropoiesis in patients with FID and those on ESA	– Available on only few analyzers – Each analyzer has defined the cutoff
Reticulocyte Hb content	Helps distinguish absolute ID (<25 pg) from ACD (>25 pg) Best predictive value for response to intravenous iron in patients of CKD on HD (<30.6 pg)	– Available on only few analyzers
SI, TIBC, %TS	%TS < 20 indicates the need for parenteral iron therapy in patients on ESA	– SI and TIBC do not identify FID – %TS must be used together with sTfR to identify patients who will respond to ESA
SF	Essential as a baseline parameter <100 μg/L:CKD not on dialysis and <200 μg/L >CKD-HD indicates FID	– No consensus on upper limit above which iron not to be given – Suggested target values have limitations – Not helpful in predicting responsiveness to ESA
sTfR, TfR index	Useful in the diagnosis of ID with ACD Used in predicting response to intravenous iron in patients on ESA (superior to SF)	– Expensive – Not widely available – Can be used with SF when automated measures are not available

should be monitored for FID and be given intravenous iron supplementation along with ESA to prevent iron restricted erythropoiesis. Oral iron agents are not helpful as the increased hepcidin inhibits its absorption [41].

- The **laboratory diagnosis** of FID is challenging as the conventional parameters used for the diagnosis of absolute ID are not applicable due to their alteration by the acute phase response.
- The parameters which can be used for diagnosis are briefly discussed below (Table 2.6).
- **% hypochromic red cells** is the best parameter for the diagnosis of FID. At a cutoff ≥6%, it was found to be superior to SF, TIBC, ZPP, and sTfR in the diagnosis of iron-deficient and iron-sufficient CKD patients.

- **ZPP** is a reliable indicator of FID. It can be used as an alternative to CHr or Ret-Hb. However, the test lacks specificity in the diagnosis of FID.
- **SF** being an acute phase reactant is elevated in these patients. Hence, a normal value does not exclude FID. SF values <100 µg/L in CKD patients not on dialysis and <200 µg/L in CKD patients on dialysis are suggestive of FID which can be treated with intravenous iron therapy. There is no consensus on the upper limit of SF above which intravenous iron is not recommended. If the level is >800 µg/L, iron supplementation must not be given. However, levels up to 1200 µg/L do not preclude IRE.
- **SI, TIBC, %TS** SI and TIBC fail to identify FID. %TS less than 20% indicates the need for parenteral iron therapy in patients on ESA. It has poor sensitivity and specificity in identifying patients who will respond to ESA and/or iron in CKD. %TS can be used in combination with sTfR to identify FID as an alternative to CHr and Ret-He. In anemic patients with CKD, if there is laboratory evidence of IRE (% hypochromic red cells > 6%, Ret-He < 30.6 pg) SF must be estimated. If it is <200 µg/L/<100 µg/L in patients on HD/not on HD, respectively, it indicates absolute ID. If SF > 200 µg/L/>100 µg/L in patients on HD/not on HD but <800 µg/L, a diagnosis of FID can be considered. In both situations, iron therapy is warranted [42, 43].

Treatment

- Functional iron deficiency is treated by modifying dosage of recombinant human erythropoietin or ESA along with intravenous iron [42].

Iron deficiency anemia and thalassemia traits

- Beta thalassemia trait (BTT) is an important cause of microcytic hypochromic anemia and often co-exist with IDA [44]. After a detailed clinical history and examination, a CBC should be assessed along with examination of a stained PBF. BTT is characterized by mild anemia, with a disproportianate decrease in MCV and MCH, relative erythrocytosis, and a normal RDW. Co-existent ID reduces the Hb concentration to a greater degree. Mean MCV and MCH have been reported to be significantly lower in traits with ID as compared to those without ID. Discriminant functions like Mentzer index, Shine & Lal index, and England & Fraser index can be applied though none of them are 100% sensitive or specific [45, 46]. Peripheral smear shows the presence of microcytic hypochromic red cells, target cells, and basophilic stippling in BTT. Serum ferritin and iron studies should be undertaken to identify IDA. The parameters are normal in BTT uncomplicated by iron deficiency while the SF is reduced in IDA. If the SF is normal, quantitation of HbA_2 is done. Elevated HbA_2 (3.5–7%) which is measured by cellulose acetate electrophoresis/HPLC/other method quantitation is diagnostic of BTT [47]. As red cell indices are altered by co-existing disorders, screening for BTT should be considered in any patient with unexplained microcytosis even if the red cell indices are not typical of BTT [48]. HbA_2 may be reduced in BTT patients with co-existent iron deficiency. However, studies from India have shown that the presence of ID did not preclude the detection of BTT. If the RBC indices are suggestive of thalassemia trait and the HbA_2 is normal, the level may be repeated after correction of iron deficiency [49]. In cases with low RBC indices, normal iron parameters and HbA_2 levels, it is appropriate to examine for HbH inclusions using brilliant cresyl blue. Their absence does not exclude α-thalassemia trait but their presence indicates that family studies and DNA assay are required [50] (Fig. 2.6).

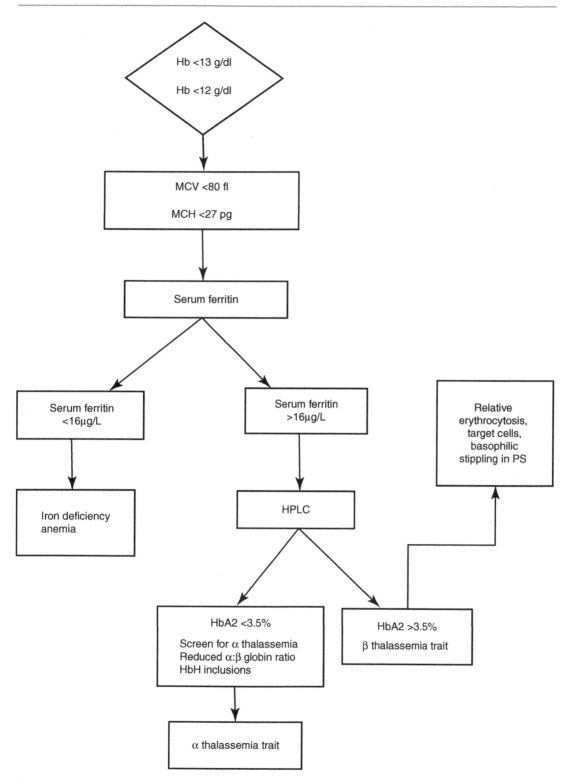

Fig. 2.6 Approach to diagnosis of iron deficiency anemia co-existing with thalassemia trait

References

1. Winter WE, Bazydlo LA, Harris NS. The molecular biology of human iron metabolism. Medicine. 2014;45:92–102.
2. Barragan-Ibanez G, Santoyo-Sanchez A, Ramos-Penafiel CO. Iron deficiency anemia. Rev Med Hosp Gen Mex. 2016;79:41–114. https://doi.org/10.1016/j.hgmx.2015.06.008.
3. Andrews NC. Iron deficiency and related disorders. In: Greer JP, Foerster J, Rodgers GM, Paraskevas F, Glader B, Arber DA, Means RT, editors. Wintrobe's clinical hematology. 12th ed. Philadelphia: Lippincott Williams and Wilkins; 2009. p. 810–34.
4. Lopez A, Cacoub P, Macdougall IC, Peyrin-Biroulet L. Iron deficiency anaemia. Lancet. 2016;387(10021):907–16.
5. DeLoughery TG. Iron deficiency anemia. Med Clin North Am. 2017;101:319–32.
6. Tandara L, Salamunic I. Iron metabolism: current facts and future directions. Biochem Med. 2012;22:311–28.
7. Wang J, Pantopoulos K. Regulation of cellular iron metabolism. Biochem J. 2011;434:365–81.
8. Punnonen K, Rajamaki A. Serum transferrin receptor and it's ratio to serum ferritin in the diagnosis of iron deficiency. Blood. 1997;89:1052–7.
9. Silva B, Faustino P. An overview of molecular basis of iron metabolism regulation and the associated pathologies. Biochim Biophys Acta. 2015;1852:1347–59.
10. Zhao N, Zhang A, Enns CA. Iron regulation by hepcidin. J Clin Invest. 2013;123:2337–43.
11. Ganz T, Nemeth E. Hepcidin and iron homeostasis. Biochim Biophys Acta. 2012;1823:1434–43.
12. Muckenthaler MU, Rivella S, Hentze MW, Galy B. A red carpet for iron metabolism. Cell. 2017;168:344–58.
13. De Benoist B, McLean E, Egil I, Cogswell M. Worldwide prevalence of anaemia 1993–2005. WHO global database on anaemia. Geneva: WHO; 2008.
14. DeMaeyer EM, AdielsTegman M. The prevalence of anemia in the world. World Health Stat Q. 1985;38:302–16.
15. WHO. Iron deficiency anemia assessment, prevention and control: a guide for programme managers. Geneva: World Health Organization; 2001.
16. Madan N, Rusia U, Sikka M, Sharma S, Shankar N. Developmental and neurophysiologic deficits in iron deficiency in children. Indian J Pediatr. 2011;78:58–64.
17. Falkingham M, Abdelhamid A, Curtis P, Fairweather-Tait S, Dye L, Hooper L. The effects of oral iron supplementation on cognition in older children and adults: a systematic review and meta-analysis. Nutr J. 2010;9:4–10.
18. Stoltzfus RM, Mullany L, Black RE. Iron deficiency anaemia. In: Ezzati M, Lopez AD, Rodgers A, Murray CJL, editors. Comparative quantification of health risks: global and regional burden of disease attributable to selected major risk factors, vol. 1. Geneva: World Health Organization; 2005. p. 163–209.
19. WHO. Global health risks: mortality and burden of disease attributable to selected major risks. Geneva: World Health Organization; 2009.
20. Charles CV. Iron deficiency anemia: a public health problem of global proportions. In: Maddock J, editor. Public health—methodology, environmental and systems issues. Rijeka: InTech; 2012. ISBN: 978-953-51-0641.
21. Buratti P, Gammella E, Rybinska I, Cairo G, Recalcati S. Recent advances in iron metabolism: relevance for health, exercise and performance. Med Sci Sports Exerc. 2015;47:1–8.
22. Kassebaum NJ, Jasrasaria R, Naghavi M. A systematic analysis of global anemia burden from 1990-2010. Blood. 2013;123:615–24.
23. Auerbach M, Adamson JW. How we diagnose and treat iron deficiency anemia. Am J Hematol. 2016;91:31–8.
24. Brugnara C, Schiller B, Moran J. Reticulocyte hemoglobin equivalent (Ret-He) and assessment of iron deficient states. Clin Lab Haematol. 2006;28:303–8.
25. Bovy C, Gothot A, Krzesinski JM, Beguin Y, Sart-Tilman CHU. Mature erythrocyte indices: new markers of iron availability. Hematologica. 2005;90:549–51.
26. Cappellini DM, Comin-Colet J, de Francisco A, Dignass A, Doehner W, Lam CSP, et al. Iron deficiency across chronic inflammatory conditions: international expert opinion on definition, diagnosis, and management on behalf of the IRON CORE Group. Am J Hematol. 2017;92:1068–78.
27. Hallberg L, Bengtsson C, lapidus L, Lindstedt G, Hulten L. Screening for iron deficiency: an analysis based on bone marrow examinations and serum ferritin determinations in a population sample of women. Br J Haematol. 1993;85:787–98.
28. Camaschella C. Iron deficiency anemia. N Engl J Med. 2015;372:1832–43.
29. Pasricha SR, Drakesmith H. Iron deficiency anemia. Problems in diagnosis and prevention at the population level. Hematol Oncol Clin North Am. 2016;30:309–25.
30. Skikne BS, Punnonen K, Caldron PH, Bennett MT, Rehu M, Gasior GH, Chamberlin JS, Sullivan LA, Bray KR, Southwick PC. Improved differential diagnosis of anemia of chronic disease and iron deficiency anemia: a prospective multicenter evaluation of soluble transferrin receptor and the sTfR/log ferritin index. Am J Hematol. 2011;86:923–7.
31. Suominen P, Punnonen K, Rajamaki A, Irjala K. Serum transferrin receptor and transferrin receptor-ferritin index identify healthy subjects with subclinical iron deficits. Blood. 1998;8:2934–9.
32. Franceschi LD, Iolascon A, Taher A, Cappellini MD. Clinical management of iron deficiency anemia in adults: systematic review on advances in diagno-

sis and treatment. Eur J Intern Med. 2017;42:16–23. https://doi.org/10.1016/j.ejim.2017.04.018.

33. Bregman DB, Goodnough LT. Experience with intravenous ferric carboxymaltose in patients with iron deficiency anemia. Ther Adv Hematol. 2014;5:48–60.

34. Pasricha SR, Atkinson SH, Armitage AE, Khandwala S, Veenemans J, Cox SE, et al. Expression of the iron hormone hepcidin distinguishes different types of anemia in African children. Sci Transl Med. 2014;6:235re3.

35. Mantadakis E, Roganovic J. Safety and efficacy of ferric carboxymaltose in children and adolescents with iron deficiency anemia. J Pediatr. 2017; 184:241.

36. Powers JM, Shamoun M, McCavit TL, Adix L, Buchanan GR. Intravenous ferric carboxymaltose in children with iron deficiency anemia who respond poorly to oral iron. J Pediatr. 2016;108: 221–6.

37. Goddard AF, James MW, McIntyre AS, Scott BB, The British Society of Gastroenterology. Guidelines for the management of iron deficiency anaemia. Gut. 2011;60:1309–16.

38. Okam MM, Koch TA, Tran MH. Iron deficiency anemia treatment response to oral iron therapy: a pooled analysis of five randomized controlled trials. Haematologica. 2016;101:e6–7.

39. Prentice AM, Mendoza YA, Pereira D, Cerami C, Wegmuller R, Constable A, Spieldenner J. Dietary strategies for improving iron status: balancing safety and efficacy. Nutr Rev. 2016;75:49–60.

40. WHO. Recommendations on wheat and maize flour fortification meeting report: interim. Geneva: World Health Organization; 2009.

41. Wish JB. Assessing iron status: beyond serum ferritin and transferrin saturation. Clin J Am Soc Nephrol. 2006;1:S4–8.

42. Archer NM, Brugnara C. Diagnosis of iron-deficient states. Crit Rev Clin Lab Sci. 2015;52(5):256–72.

43. Wayne Thomas D, Hinchliffe RF, Briggs C, Macdougall IC, Littlewood T, Cavill I. Guideline for the laboratory diagnosis of functional iron deficiency. Br J Haematol. 2013;161:639–48.

44. Madan N, Sikka M, Sharma S, Rusia U. Serum ferritin levels in carriers of beta thalassemia trait. Acta Haematol. 1996;96:267.

45. Bain BJ. The α, β, δ, and γ thalassaemias and related conditions. In: Bain BJ, editor. Hemoglobinopathy diagnosis. 2nd ed. Malden: Blackwell; 2006. p. 63–138.

46. Batebi APA, Esmailian R. Discrimination of beta-thalassemia minor and iron deficiency anemia by screening test for red blood cell indices. Turk J Med Sci. 2012;42(2):275–80.

47. Rao S, Kar R, Gupta SK, Chopra A, Saxena R. Spectrum of hemoglobinopathies diagnosed by cation exchange-HPLC and modulating effects of nutritional deficiency anemias from North India. Indian J Med Res. 2010;132:513–9.

48. Ryan K, Bain BJ, Worthington D, James J, Plews D, Mason A, Roper D, Rees DC, de la Salle B, Streetly A, British Committee for Standards in Haematology. Significant haemoglobinopathies: guidelines for screening and diagnosis. Br J Haematol. 2010;149(1):35–49.

49. Madan N, Sikka M, Sharma S, Rusia U. Phenotypic expression of HbA$_2$ in beta thalassemia trait with iron deficiency. Ann Hematol. 1998;77:93–6.

50. Higgs DR. The pathophysiology and clinical features of α thalassaemia. In: Steinberg MH, Forget BG, Higgs DR, Weatherall DJ, editors. Disorders of hemoglobin: genetics, pathophysiology, and clinical management. 2nd ed. New York: Cambridge University Press; 2009. p. 266–95.

Megaloblastic Anemia and Dual Nutritional Deficiency Anemia

3

K. V. Karthika and Hara Prasad Pati

3.1 Megaloblastic Anemia

3.1.1 Definition

Megaloblastic anemia is a general term used to describe a group of anemias caused by impaired DNA synthesis and characterized by macro-ovalocytes in peripheral blood smear and mega-loblastic erythroid hyperplasia in the bone marrow.

3.1.2 Pathophysiology of Megaloblast Morphology

Megaloblasts, the hallmark of these anemias, are caused by asynchronous maturation between the nucleus and the cytoplasm due to impairment of DNA synthesis. When DNA synthesis is impaired, the cell cannot proceed from the G2 growth stage to the mitosis (M) stage. Hence, the DNA synthesis is retarded, whereas the RNA and protein synthesis of the cell occurs at a normal pace. This leads to continuing cell growth without division, resulting in a mature cytoplasm with an immature nucleus.

3.1.3 History

1849—Addison described this condition as anemia, general languor, and debility

1877—Osler and Gardner found its association with neuropathy

1880—Ehrlich first described megaloblasts

1926—Minot and Murphy identified that this condition could be reversed by ingestion of large quantities of liver

1929—Castle established that gastric acid contains an "intrinsic factor" (IF) that combines with an "extrinsic factor" to allow the latter to be absorbed

1934—Dorothy Hodgkin described the structure of vitamin B_{12} for which she received the Nobel Prize

1948—Herbert discovered the structure of folic acid and its association with megaloblastic anemia

3.2 Folic Acid Metabolism

The synthetic form of folate is more commonly known as folic acid. The metabolically active form of folic acid is known as tetrahydrofolic acid. The main dietary sources include green leafy vegetables, lemons, oranges, banana, cereals, fish, liver, kidneys, etc. Folate in food can be lost on prolonged storage or overcooking. The daily requirement varies from 50 to 100 µg; however,

K. V. Karthika (✉) · H. P. Pati (✉)
Department of Hematology, All India Institute of Medical Sciences, New Delhi, India

© Springer Nature Singapore Pte Ltd. 2019
R. Saxena, H. P. Pati (eds.), *Hematopathology*, https://doi.org/10.1007/978-981-13-7713-6_3

recommended daily allowances are kept at a higher level of around 400 μg. This is because the bioavailability depends on the conversion of the polyglutamated form in the diet into monoglutamated form for absorption [1]. The body stores are found in the liver. They range from 3 to 5 mg and last for about 3–5 months [2].

3.2.1 Folate Absorption

Folate is absorbed in the small intestine, primarily the duodenum and the upper part of jejunum. Natural folates are absorbed faster than folic acid. The polyglutamated folates are converted to the monoglutamated form by the enzymes carboxypeptidase or polyglutamate hydrolase (also known as intestinal conjugase). The monoglutamated form is then absorbed either passively along the concentration gradient or actively by binding to the transporters RFT-1, RFT-2, and folate-binding protein (FBP). Once within the enterocyte, they are further converted to dihydro- and tetrahydro-folate by a reductase enzyme and further converted to methyltetrahydrofolate which then passes into the systemic circulation freely or bound to albumin. This form (5-MTHF) then enters the target cell membrane through the reduced folate carrier and is demethylated (Fig. 3.1).

Physiological function of THF: The most important role of THF is in the synthesis of thymidylate (a pyrimidine base of DNA). In the absence of thymidylate, uracil is incorporated which results in deranged DNA function [4]. Folic acid deficiency in pregnant women may cause neural tube defects in the fetus, underlining its role in neural development of fetus.

3.2.2 Causes of Folic Acid Deficiency [5]

Deficiency of folic acid is usually due to low folate in food or imbalance between demand and intake.

Causes of Reduced Availability
- Dietary deficiency can occur in generalized malnutrition states, elderly and in association with alcohol intake.
- Impaired absorption usually occurs in primary gastrointestinal conditions such as tropical sprue, celiac disease, Crohn's disease, extensive small bowel resection, infiltrative disorders, Whipple's disease, scleroderma, amyloidosis, and diabetes mellitus.
- Genetic defects of enzymes involved in their uptake such as intestinal conjugase deficiency, resulting in malabsorption, dihydrofolate reductase, methylenetetrahydrofolate, and glutamate formiminotransferase deficiencies.
- Drugs can also reduce absorption by several mechanisms:
  (a) Trimethoprim, pyrimethamine, methotrexate—inhibit dihydrofolate reductase
  (b) Phenytoin and valproic acid—reduce absorption and also affect its metabolism

Fig. 3.1 Absorption of folate in the intestine [3]

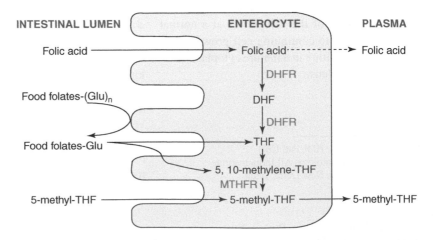

Causes of Increased Demand

- Increased requirements can occur in physiological and pathological states such as pregnancy, breastfeeding, chronic hemolytic anemia, and chronic exfoliative dermatitis.

Chronic hemolytic anemias cause rapid depletion of the folate reserves due to the associated erythroid hyperplasia. This can further result in megaloblastic crisis in the presence of exacerbating factors such as fever and illness, which can impede oral intake. Hence, prophylactic folic acid should be given to patients with hemolytic anemias such as hereditary spherocytosis and sickle cell anemia.

3.3 Vitamin B_{12} Metabolism

The chemical name of vitamin B_{12} is cyanocobalamin. There are also other forms depending upon the radical to which they are bound such as adenosylcobalamin and methylcobalamin. The source of vitamin B_{12} includes animal foods such as fish, liver, and dairy products. Plant foods do not contain vitamin B_{12}. The RDA of vitamin B_{12} is around 2 μg though requirements may increase in pregnant and breastfeeding women. Similar to folic acid, vitamin B_{12} is stored in the liver, the storage lasting for about 3–5 months.

3.3.1 Absorption of Vitamin B_{12}

When vitamin B_{12} is ingested in diet, it is normally found bound to proteins. These proteins are degraded by the enzyme pepsin released by the parietal cells of the stomach. The free vitamin B_{12} binds to R-binder (also known as haptocorrin or transcobalamin I [TC-I]) which protects the molecule and carries it till the second part of duodenum. The R-binder is secreted by the salivary glands of the oropharynx and is also found in neutrophils and monocytes. Here, the proteases in the pancreatic juice (trypsin, chymotrypsin, elastase) degrade TC-I and release vitamin B_{12} from the complex [6].

The free vitamin B_{12} now binds to IF which is also released from the parietal cells in the fundus and cardia of the stomach. The IF-B_{12} complex finally reaches the ileum. The ileal enterocytes possess the IF receptor (also known as cubilin-amnionless complex). The complex binds to this receptor and is internalized. Once within the enterocyte, the IF is degraded and cobalamin released. It then binds to transcobalamin II (TC-II) which carries vitamin B_{12} in the systemic circulation. The target cells take up this bound cobalamin by the virtue of TC-II receptors on their surface [6] (Fig. 3.2).

Physiological function of vitamin B_{12}: It acts as a coenzyme in the synthesis of methionine and tetrahydrofolate from methyltetrahydrofolate and homocysteine. This process is known as "folate trapping" since folate needs to be demethylated to remain in the cell, failing which they escape the cell without being used. This demethylation is brought about by the above reaction. Thus, it is hypothesized that manifestations of cobalamin deficiency is primarily due to folate deficiency. Cobalamin also acts as a coenzyme in the conversion of methylmalonic acid (MMA) to succinic acid, the latter being an important substrate in the Krebs cycle [6].

3.3.2 Causes of Cobalamin Deficiency [5, 8]

Vitamin B_{12} deficiency is most commonly due to impaired absorption rather than due to reduced uptake. Reduced uptake occurs mostly in strict vegetarians, due to dietary deficiency. Impaired absorption can be caused by the following disorders:

- Gastric disorders—pernicious anemia, gastritis, old age, atrophic gastritis, use of proton pump inhibitors or H2 antagonists, *Helicobacter pylori* infection, total or partial gastrectomy, Zollinger–Ellison syndrome
- Intestinal disorders—extensive ileal resection, ileitis, leukemic/lymphomatous infiltration, tuberculosis, Crohn's disease, postradiation ileitis, tropical sprue or celiac disease, scleroderma, amyloidosis, blind loop syndrome with bacterial overgrowth, parasitic infections such as *Diphyllobothrium latum*, *Giardia lamblia*, and *Strongyloides stercoralis*.

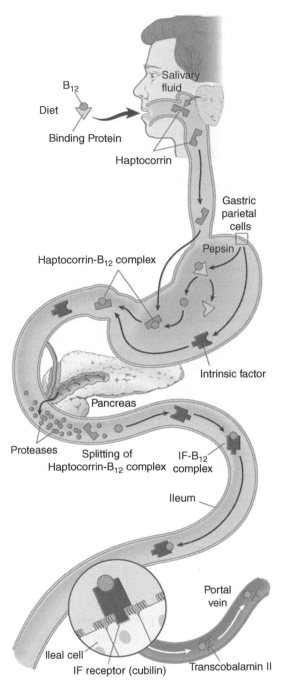

Fig. 3.2 Schematic illustration of vitamin B_{12} absorption [7]

- Pancreatic disorders—hereditary chronic pancreatitis, Imerslund–Gräsbeck disease (inherited cubilin deficiency)
- Genetic defects—TC-II deficiency, functional impairment of TC-II, haptocorrin or TC-I defi-

ciency, homocystinuria, methylmalonicacidemia, methylenetetrahydrofolate deficiency collectively known as congenital megaloblastic anemias
- Drugs—cholestyramine, metformin, colchicine

3.4 Pernicious Anemia

Pernicious anemia is caused due to impaired IF secretion by the gastric parietal cells, resulting in impaired vitamin B_{12} absorption. It can be inherited or acquired. The inherited form is a rare autosomal recessive disorder causing deficient secretion of IF in the absence of gastric atrophy and is seen in children below 2 years of age. The acquired form is more common and occurs in adults. It is an autoimmune disorder with genetic predisposition and is associated with HLA A2, A3, B7, patients with type A blood group and other autoimmune disorders. Patients with pernicious anemia have a higher risk of irreversible gastric atrophy, achlorhydria with concomitant iron deficiency, and gastric carcinoma.

The antibodies in pernicious anemia are of two types: anti-parietal cell and anti-IF antibodies. Anti-parietal cell antibodies are the most common and present in 90% of patients with pernicious anemia but in only 5% of healthy adults. Similarly, antibodies to IF are also found in most patients with pernicious anemia. IF antibodies, type 1 and type 2, are present in 50% of patients with pernicious anemia and are highly specific. Therefore, they can be used as a confirmatory test. Treatment requires parenteral administration of vitamin B_{12} to circumvent the impaired absorption of oral vitamin B_{12}.

3.5 Congenital Megaloblastic Anemia

Congenital megaloblastic anemia is due to deficiency or altered activity of the enzymes, carrier proteins, or receptors involved in the metabolism (absorption, transport, and conversion to active form) of vitamin B_{12} or folate, resulting in impaired utilization of these nutrients. This group has been explored in detail in the context of vitamin B_{12} deficiency. These disorders need to be suspected when clinical manifestations of cobalamin deficiency are observed in infancy or childhood. Three disorders where absorption and transport of cobalamin are affected have been identified, and another seven alter cellular use and coenzyme production. The disorders of absorption and transport are TC-II deficiency, IF deficiency (also known as inherited pernicious anemia), and IF receptor deficiency (Imerslund–Gräsbeck syndrome). These defects cause developmental delay and megaloblastic anemia since birth, which can be treated with pharmacologic doses of parenteral cobalamin. Serum cobalamin values are reduced in the IF defects and normal in TC-II deficiency.

The defects of cellular use, commonly denoted by letters CblA to G, can be detected by the presence or absence of methylmalonic aciduria and homocystinuria. The presence of only methylmalonic aciduria indicates a block in conversion of methylmalonic CoA to succinyl-CoA and results due to defect in the methylmalonyl-CoA mutase enzyme that catalyzes the reaction or a defect in the synthesis of its cobalamin coenzyme (cobalamin A and cobalamin B deficiency).

The presence of only homocystinuria can result either from poor binding of cobalamin to methionine synthase due to cobalamin E deficiency or defect in producing methylcobalamin from cobalamin and S-adenosylmethionine due to cobalamin G deficiency. This results in a reduction in methionine synthesis, with accumulation of the enzyme substrates causing homocystinemia and consequent homocystinuria.

Methylmalonic aciduria and homocystinuria occur when the metabolic defect impairs conversion of cobalamin III to cobalamin II (cobalamin C, cobalamin D, and cobalamin F deficiency). This reaction is common for the formation of both MMA and homocystinuria. Early detection of these disorders is important because most patients respond favorably to supra-pharmacological doses of cobalamin, thereby preventing the neurological abnormalities associated with them.

3.6 Imerslund–Gräsbeck Syndrome

This is an autosomal recessive disorder caused due to biallelic mutations in the IF receptor also known as cubilin-amnionless receptor. This receptor is essential not only for intestinal vitamin B_{12} absorption but also for renal reabsorption of proteins. The deficiency of this receptor (either cubilin or amnionless) therefore results in selective vitamin B_{12} malabsorption and proteinuria. The diagnosis of this disorder is suspected by a decreased excretion of cobalamin-IF complex in urine and is confirmed by mutation study of the involved genes. The treatment involves lifelong administration of parenteral vitamin B_{12}.

3.7 Pathophysiology of Megaloblastic Anemia

The pathophysiology of megaloblastic anemia is due to ineffective erythropoiesis resulting from intramedullary apoptosis of hematopoietic precursors (rapidly dividing cells). This apoptosis is not solely due to deficiency of thymidylate. In the absence of thymidylate, it is replaced by uracil which activates the DNA repair pathways resulting in p53-mediated apoptosis. To some extent, RNA and protein synthesis is also affected. This results in asynchronous maturation of the nucleus and cytoplasm. The nucleus devoid of DNA does not mature, whereas the cytoplasm matures at a normal rate due to normal RNA and hemoglobin synthesis, thus resulting in megaloblastosis [5]. It is also important to keep in mind that DNA synthesis can also be impaired directly in HIV and myelodysplastic syndromes in the absence of vitamin B_{12} and folate deficiency.

3.8 Pathophysiology of Neurological Changes

Neurological symptoms are confined to cobalamin deficiency. Two factors contribute to these symptoms. The first factor is the impaired synthesis of the amino acid methionine which is essential for myelin synthesis. The second factor is the accumulation of MMA, a neurotoxic intermediate. These factors together cause degeneration of myelin fibers of the posterior and lateral grey horn of the spinal cord, resulting in subacute combined degeneration [5]. Increased levels of cytokines such as TGF-α and EGF have also been identified in these patients, which may also contribute to the pathogenesis of neurodegeneration [9].

3.9 Clinical Features

When patients present with the symptoms of chronic anemia, there may be mild jaundice due to the associated intramedullary hemolysis. The combination of pallor and jaundice gives the skin a lemon yellow color, characteristic of megaloblastic anemia. There may also be glossitis (beefy tongue), nail pigmentation, change of hair color (due to increased melanin synthesis), etc. The neurological symptoms of cobalamin deficiency include loss of joint position sense, loss of vibration sense in toes and fingers, paresthesia, hypoesthesia, tingling, gait abnormalities, loss of coordination, muscle weakness, spasticity, optic neuropathy, urinary and fecal incontinence, erectile dysfunction, dementia, and memory loss. Neuropathy is symmetric and mainly affects the lower extremities (stock and glove distribution). Clinically, patients with subacute combined degeneration have a positive Romberg's test. Patients with pernicious anemia have symptoms of other associated autoimmune disorders such as type 1 diabetes, thyroid disorders, and Addison's disease.

3.10 Laboratory Findings

3.10.1 Hemogram and Peripheral Smear

The characteristic peripheral smear finding is macrocytic anemia (increased mean corpuscular volume) with macro-ovalocytes and reticulocytopenia. There may also be leukopenia and thrombocytope-

nia in severe cases. Hypersegmented neutrophils are another characteristic finding in megaloblastic anemia. Hypersegmented neutrophils refer to the presence of >5% of neutrophils with five segments, or >1% with six segments. Macrocytosis is defined as increased mean corpuscular volume, which may be masked in patients with iron deficiency. However, hypersegmented neutrophils persist in iron deficiency and aid in the diagnosis of megaloblastic anemia. Other findings include anisocytosis, basophilic stippling, Howell–Jolly bodies, Cabot rings (remnants of mitotic spindle), etc. Increased bilirubin and LDH reflect ongoing intramedullary hemolysis.

3.10.2 Bone Marrow Examination

Bone marrow aspiration is usually done to rule out myelodysplastic syndromes and to assess iron stores. There is panmyelosis with megaloblastic changes in the erythroid and myeloid series. There is erythroid hyperplasia with increase in orthochromatic erythroid precursors showing megaloblastic change. The cells are enlarged with immature nucleus and a sieve like chromatin, whereas the cytoplasm is mature and adequately hemoglobinized (Fig. 3.3). In the myeloid series, there are giant metamyelocytes and band forms. A less common finding is the presence of hyperlobated and hyperdiploid megakaryocytes and giant platelets. Lymphocytes and plasma cells are spared from the cellular gigantism and cytoplasmic asynchrony observed in other cell lineages. Bone marrow megaloblastosis is reversed within 24 h of vitamin B_{12}/folate therapy and returns to normal in 2–3 days [5, 10].

3.11 Primary Tests for B_{12} and Folate Deficiencies [10]

3.11.1 Serum B_{12} (Cobalamin)

Reference range: 200–900 pg/mL

Anemia and neuropathy can be seen at levels of <180 mg/L; however, levels <150 mg/L are diagnostic of B_{12} deficiency. The serum cobalamin

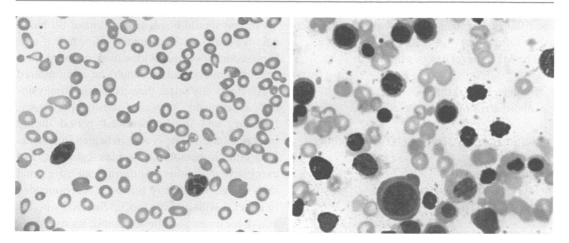

Fig. 3.3 Peripheral smear showing macro-ovalocytes and hypersegmented neutrophils and occasional polychromato-phils (left) and bone marrow aspirate smear showing megaloblasts with erythroid hyperplasia (right)

level can however be within normal range in the following circumstances:

- TC-II deficiency
- Acute cobalamin deficiency due to nitrous oxide (prevalent in older times)

Serum cobalamin levels may be physiologically low in pregnancy, intake of oral contraceptives, severe folic acid deficiency, and patients taking large doses of ascorbic acid.

3.11.2 Serum Folate

Reference range: 2.5–20 ng/mL

A diagnosis of folate deficiency can be made when the folate levels are less than 2.5 ng/mL. However, in some cases of folate deficiency, there can be an overlap with the normal range (2.5–5 ng/mL).

The following precautions need to be considered when assessing serum folate values:

- A single dose of folate either by medication or meal may falsely elevate serum folate levels to normal. Hence, blood sample should be drawn prior to any intervention (transfusions, meals, and therapy) to achieve accurate results.
- Hemolysis can cause false results due to release of red cell folate.

3.11.3 RBC Folate

Reference range: >140 ng/mL

- Not affected by diet and reflects tissue stores since folate content is established early in RBCs.
- Red cell folate levels may be affected by hemolysis.
- Low in severe B_{12} deficiency.
- Test is complex and expensive.

Serum for folate and cobalamin should be collected prior to meals or therapy, frozen and then stored if the tests cannot be performed immediately.

3.12 Lab Tests to Confirm and Distinguish Vitamin B_{12} and Folate Deficiencies

Serum homocysteine and MMA levels together are helpful to distinguish between cobalamin and folate deficiencies. Both are increased in cobalamine deficiency. Homocysteine is increased in folate deficiency; however, MMA is normal in these cases. These should be used if the clinical presentation and serum vitamin B_{12} and folate levels do not correlate. However, homocysteine and vitamin B_{12} levels may be altered in conditions other than megaloblastic anemia such as the following:

The MMA level can be elevated in

- End-stage renal disease
- Inborn error of MMA metabolism

Serum homocysteine can be increased in

- Homocystinuria
- Hyperhomocysteinemia
- Certain MTHFR polymorphisms

3.13 Testing for Parietal Cell/IF Antibodies

Antibodies against both IF and gastric parietal cells can be demonstrated in patients with pernicious anemia. The former is seen in 50% of cases and is specific. The latter though seen in 90% of patients is not specific as it can be positive in other autoimmune and thyroid disorders.

3.14 Diagnostic Therapeutic Trial

In under-resourced laboratories where serum studies are unavailable, a therapeutic trial of vitamin B_{12}/folate can be given and the reticulocyte response can be assessed after 72 h. However, a trial of folate therapy alone is contraindicated since this may exacerbate neurological symptoms in patients with coexisting cobalamin deficiency. Therapeutic trial may also be useful in elderly patients with subclinical deficiency in whom laboratory tests are within normal limits.

3.15 Treatment

3.15.1 Folic Acid Deficiency

Folic acid therapy in a patient with coexisting cobalamin deficiency may alleviate symptoms of anemia; however, neurological symptoms worsen. Hence, they need to be given together. Folic acid is given at a dosage of 1–5 mg/day for 3–4 months along with cyanocobalamin.

Treatment should be ideally continued till blood counts normalize. Treat underlying cause if any. If no secondary cause is identified, continue therapy indefinitely. Folate should be administered prophylactically when there is increased physiological demand such as during pregnancy, lactation, and in the perinatal period during breastfeeding. Folate is also indicated in patients with chronic hemolytic anemias, psoriasis, and exfoliative dermatitis and during extensive renal dialysis. Folate therapy has been recommended in patients with hyperhomocysteinemia, who are at risk for thromboembolic complications [11].

3.15.2 Cobalamin Deficiency

Cyanocobalamin is given at a dosage of 1000 µg intramuscularly daily for 2 weeks, followed by weekly once until blood count normalizes, then continued monthly once for life. Prophylaxis for life is especially important in strict vegetarians, elderly, and patients with prior gastric surgery. Oral route is usually preferred in patients with contraindications to intramuscular injections such as hemophilias. Patients with genetic causes such as TC-II deficiency may require higher doses.

3.16 Monitoring of Therapy

- 1–2 days: Reduction of serum iron, indirect bilirubin, and lactate dehydrogenase
- 3–4 days: Reticulocytosis
- 10 days: Hemoglobin starts to increase, reduction of MCV
- 14 days: Hypersegmented neutrophils start to disappear though they may persist for longer
- 2 months: Resolution of anemia
- 3–12 months: Resolution of neurological symptoms

3.17 Dual Nutritional Deficiency Anemia

Megaloblastic anemia may sometimes be masked by coexistent iron deficiency. Thus, the macrocytic anemia may be masked by the microcytic hypochromic anemia of iron deficiency. This clinical picture is known as dimorphic anemia or dual nutritional deficiency anemia. According to NHANES III data, dual nutritional deficiency anemia constitutes for about 10% of nutritional anemias [12]. This is commonly seen in elderly patients, pregnancy, extensive bowel resection, pernicious anemia, malnutrition, etc. Iron deficiency may also be precipitated by the treatment of megaloblastic anemia (associated with accelerated erythropoiesis). Combined deficiency may also be suspected in patients who do not show appropriate response to iron/vitamin B_{12}/folate monotherapy. Peripheral smear characteristically shows two distinct red cell populations. There is one population of hypochromic, microcytic cells and another of macrocytic cells with reticulocytopenia. There may also be hypochromic macroovalocytes. The MCV may be normal though the RDW is increased. In dimorphic anemia, all three types of erythropoiesis can usually be detected—hypochromic, megaloblastic, and normoblastic—the latter, however, usually predominating. Variability in red blood cell morphologic characteristics in this setting reflects the relative degree of deficiency of each of these substrates. The diagnosis relies upon a high degree of suspicion along with proper clinical examination and specific investigations. A bone marrow examination may be done to assess iron stores. Serum ferritin levels may not truly reflect the degree of iron deficiency in patients with coexisting megaloblastic anemia. Treatment is by administration of iron and vitamin B_{12}/folate either orally or parenterally depending on the cause of deficiency. Clinical course may be monitored by the reticulocyte response.

References

1. Pitkin RM, Allen LB, Bailey LB, et al. Dietary reference intakes for thiamin, riboflavin, niacin, vitamin B6, folate, vitamin B12, pantothenic acid, biotin and choline. Washington: National Academies Press; 1998.
2. Butler CC, Vidal-Alaball J, Cannings-John R, et al. Oral vitamin B12 versus intramuscular vitamin B12 for vitamin B12 deficiency: a systematic review of randomized controlled trials. Fam Pract. 2006;23:279–85.
3. Pietrzik K, Bailey L, Shane B. Folic acid and L-5-methyltetrahydrofolate: comparison of clinical pharmacokinetics and pharmacodynamics. Clin Pharmacokinet. 2010;49:535–48.
4. Verhoef H, Veenemans J, Mwangi M, Prentice AM. Safety and benefits of interventions to increase folate status in malaria-endemic areas. Br J Haematol. 2017;177(6):905–18.
5. Carmel R, Green R, Rosenblatt DS, et al. Update on cobalamin, folate, and homocysteine. Hematology Am Soc Hematol Educ Program. 2003;62:81.
6. Lieberman M, Marks AD. Tetrahydrofolate, vitamin B12, and S-adenosylmethionine. Mark's basic medical biochemistry: a clinical approach. 3rd ed. Philadelphia: Wolters Kluwer/Lippincott Williams &Wilkins; 2009.
7. Kumar V, Abbas AK, Aster JC. Robbins and Cotran. Pathologic basis of disease. 9th ed. Philadelphia: Elsevier Saunders; 2015.
8. Truswell AS. Vitamin B12. Nutr Diet. 2007;64: S120–5.
9. Hemmer B, Glocker FX, Schumacher M, et al. Subacute combined degeneration: clinical, electrophysiological, and magnetic resonance imaging findings. J Neurol Neurosurg Psychiatry. 1998;65:822–7.
10. Green R, Kinsella LJ. Current concepts in the diagnosis of cobalamin deficiency. Neurology. 1995;45:1435–40.
11. Andres E, Fothergill H, Mecili M. Efficacy of oral cobalamin (vitamin B12) therapy. Expert Opin Pharmacother. 2010;11(2):249–56.
12. Patel KV. Epidemiology of anemia in older adults. Semin Hematol. 2008;45(4):210–7.

References

Pathogenesis and Investigations in Hereditary Red Blood Cell Membrane Disorders

4

Monica Sharma

4.1 Pathogenesis of Red Blood Cell Membrane Disorders

Red blood cell (RBC) membrane disorders are chiefly inherited conditions caused by mutations in the genes encoding for cytoskeletal proteins or transmembrane transporters, leading to decreased red cell deformability and permeability leading to premature removal of the erythrocytes from the circulation. RBC membrane disorders can be categorized into two main subgroups:

1. **Structural defects**: Hereditary spherocytosis (HS), Hereditary elliptocytosis (HE), Hereditary pyropoikilocytosis (HPP), and Southeast Asian ovalocytosis (SAO).
2. **Altered permeability of the RBC membrane**: Dehydrated hereditary stomatocytosis (DHS), Overhydrated hereditary stomatocytosis (OHS), Familial pseudohyperkalemia (FP), and Cryohydrocytosis (CHC).

M. Sharma (✉)
Department of Hematology, Safdarjung Hospital and Vardhman Mahavir Medical College,
New Delhi, India
e-mail: drmsharma@vmmc-sjh.nic.in

4.1.1 Structure of Red Cell Membrane

The lipid bilayer interspersed with several transmembrane proteins is made up of equal amounts of cholesterol and asymmetrically distributed phospholipids, with phosphatidylcholine and sphingomyelin placed in the outer leaflet of the bilayer while phosphatidylethanolamine, phosphatidylserine, and phosphoinositides are localized in the inner leaflet [1]. The asymmetry of phospholipids helps in anchoring the skeletal network and also protects from phagocytosis of red cells by the macrophages.

4.1.2 Membrane Proteins (Fig. 4.1)

Skeletal proteins made of α/β-spectrin, actin, and protein 4.1/4.1 R are like a laminate on the inner surface of the lipid bilayer, which maintains the biconcave shape. Linkage proteins maintain cohesion between bilayer and membrane skeleton. Vertical linkage, made of band 3-RhAG-protein 4.2-ankyrin and β-spectrin, provides cohesion between phospholipid bilayer and the membrane skeleton. Horizontal linkage, made of spectrin self-association sites and spectrin–actin–protein 4.1R junctional complex, confers elasticity and deformability.

Both membrane cohesion and mechanical stability are critical to maintain the excess surface

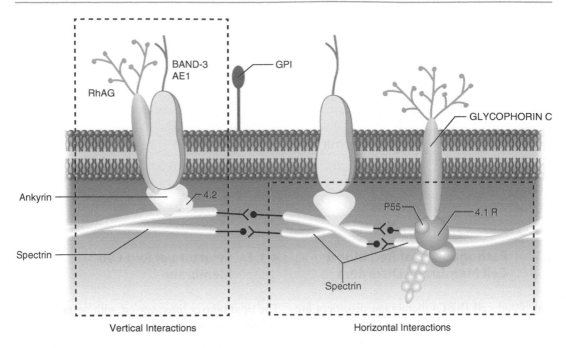

Fig. 4.1 Schematic representation of red cell membrane

area that allows deformability of the RBC. Loss of linkages results in lipid loss in the form of vesiculations and decreased membrane surface area, which compromises the red cell deformability in the circulation [2, 3].

Transmembrane proteins, acting as anion-cation transporters, form the bulk of membrane protein, chief of which is the anion exchanger band 3, which is the core of the "band 3 complex" (ankyrin-1, protein 4.2, and glycophorin A). The "Rh complex" (the Rh-associated glycoprotein (RhAG), the CD47, glycophorin B, and the Landsteiner–Wiener glycoprotein) is also associated with "band 3 complex." The transmembrane proteins regulate cell volume homeostasis as passive transporters they are Na+-K+-Cl− co-transporter, Na+-Cl− co-transporter, Band 3 anion exchanger and Na+-K+ co-transporter; the active ATP-dependent Na+-K+ ATPase, and Ca2+ ATPase. The calcium-activated potassium channel, the Gardos channel and AQP1, the water channel also contribute to the red cell volume regulation.

4.1.3 Significance of the RBC Membrane Structure

The passage of the RBC for 120 days in the blood stream is possible only because of three distinct factors in the red cell membrane:

1. Cell surface area-to-volume ratio
2. Cell volume homeostasis
3. Membrane deformability

Cell surface area-to-volume ratio: The normal biconcave human RBC with about 90 fL volume and surface area of about 140/m^2 possesses an excess of surface area to undergo extensive cellular deformations. Decreased cell surface area-to-volume ratio leading to a spherical cell is the defining feature in HS, HE, and OHS. Sphericity in HS and HE is the result of loss of cell surface area while that in the OHS results from increased cell volume.

Cell volume homeostasis: The cell volume homeostasis is maintained by intracellular concentration of Na+ and K+ and the consequent water content. A volume of 90 fL with cell hemoglobin content of 30 pg enables the red cell to maintain the intracellular hemoglobin concentration at 33 g/dL and a cytoplasmic viscosity, which is only six times higher than that of water. Cell volume homeostasis is required to maintain the surface area-to-volume ratio enabling red cellular deformations, and the low intracellular viscosity minimizes any viscous dissipation during red cell deformation. Red cell dehydration and hence increased cytoplasmic viscosity is a feature of DHS.

Membrane deformability: Unfolding and refolding of the spectrin repeats is central to the elasticity of the normal red cell membrane. Decreased membrane deformability is a distinct feature of red cells in SAO.

Knowledge of biogenesis of the membrane cytoskeleton during erythropoiesis is essential to understand the role of each gene or protein in the pathogenesis of the spherocyte. The synthesis of erythroid membrane proteins starts early and is asynchronous. The synthesis of spectrins and ankyrin is initiated earlier than that of band 3, and the synthesis of α-spectrin is about 3–4 times more than that of β-spectrin. Thus, homozygous or double heterozygous defects of α-spectrin can cause HS, whereas due to its limited amount (with respect to α-spectrin), the deficiency of β-spectrin can cause HS even in the heterozygous state [4, 5].

Decreased membrane cohesion, or mechanical stability causing loss of surface area, or increased cell volume due to defective ion transporters, each can compromise the deformability of the cell leading to its premature removal from circulation.

4.1.4 Investigations of Red Cell Membrane Disorders

4.1.4.1 Red Cell Morphology
Presence of spherocytes, pincered erythrocytes (band 3) or spherocytic acanthocytes (β-spectrin), elliptocytes (HE), poikilocytes, pyknocytes, and microspherocytes (HPP) on a freshly made peripheral blood smear are all a clue to the presence of a membrane defect. Their number though

is variable from few to numerous; however, the elliptocytes should definitely be more than 20% to be significant. Stomatocytes are seen as cup-shaped red cells characterized by a central hemoglobin-free area [6, 7].

4.1.4.2 Red Cell Indices
Various hematological analyzers provide erythrocyte indicators, which may aid in screening for membrane defects. But most of these parameters are research parameters not commonly used by the laboratories.

1. Automated MCHC: In moderate and severe cases, MCHC is increased, but may be normal in mild cases. MCHC >35 g/dL and RDW >14% are reported to have a sensitivity of 50% and a specificity of 100% for the identification of HS [8].
2. Hyper-dense cell percentage (% Hyper): Advia 2120 analyzer (Siemens Medical Solutions Diagnostics, NY, USA)—% Hyper cut-off point of 6.4% showed an excellent sensitivity (92.3%) and specificity (90.7%) to detect HS [9].
3. Mean sphered corpuscular volume (MSCV): Beckmann Coulter Inc., Fullerton, CA, USA—an artificial volume measurement during the reticulocyte count. A delta (MCV-MSCV) value >9.6 fL is a good indicator for HS (90.6% specificity and 100% sensitivity) when there is a negative DAT result [10].
4. Hyperchromic RBC (% HPR)—CELL-DYN Sapphire (Abbott Diagnostics, Santa Clara, CA, USA)—erythrocytes with hemoglobin >41 g/dL [11, 12].
5. Percent Hyper-He-Sysmex XE-5000 (Sysmex, Kobe, Japan)—indicates the percentage of hyperchromic red cells with an Hb content >49 pg [13, 14].

4.1.4.3 Reticulocyte Count
Automated reticulocyte indices are particularly very useful to differentiate hereditary from acquired spherocytosis. Since membrane remodeling begins at the reticulocyte stage in HS, a reduced reticulocyte volume less than 100 fL is seen, except in the neonates.

Table 4.1 Application of screening tests in the differential diagnosis of various RBC membrane defects

Diagnosis	OFT	AGLT	Ektacytometry	Cryohemolysis	EMA binding
HS	↑	<900 s	DImax ↓ Omin ↑ Hydration ↓	↑	↓
HE, HPP	↑	N, ↓	Trapezoidal shape	↑	↓ and ↓↓↓
OHSt	↑	No data	DImax N Omin ↑ Hydration ↑	No data	↑
DHSt	↓	>900 s	DImax N Omin ↓ Hydration ↓	No data	↑
CHC	No data	No data	No data	No data	↓
SAO	No data	No data	Not deformable	↑	↓
CDA	↑	No data	No data	N/↑	N/↓
AIHA	↑	>900 s	HS like	No data	N/↑

The reticulocyte indices using a (Ret/IRF) ratio higher than 7.7 have a high predictive value to identify spherocyte population. This ratio is generally high (>19) in mild or subclinical HS. Moderate and severe HS is identified based on an increased MicroR/Hypo-He ratio (MicroR—microcytic cells representing the formed microparticles and Hypo-He—hypochromic erythrocytes) [14, 15].

Specific biochemical tests are available with variable sensitivities and specificities to characterize the membrane defects. Table 4.1 describes the utility of the various tests in the differential diagnosis.

4.1.4.4 Osmotic Fragility Test (OFT) [16]

The test has traditionally been considered as the gold standard for the laboratory diagnosis of HS.

Principle: OFT measures the in vitro lysis of red cells suspended in solutions of decreasing osmolarity. Due to the loss of membrane surface area relative to intracellular volume, HS red cells are unable to withstand the entry of water that occurs when they are placed in increasingly hypotonic saline solutions; hence, they hemolyze more readily than normal red cells at any saline concentration. The red cells conditioned by the spleen form a tail that disappears after splenectomy. Post incubation at 37 °C for 24 h, the RBCs become metabolically depleted, which accelerates the loss of membrane surface area and the spheroid shape, thus making it more sensitive.

Results: Hemolysis is determined colorimetrically measuring the amount of hemoglobin released from red cells into the extracellular fluid. The absorbance is measured at 540 nm for fresh blood and after 24 h incubation, and a graph of % hemolysis versus NaCl concentration is plotted.

Interpretation: The shift of OF curve reflects the red cell response to hypotonic medium due to reduced cell volume and surface area. The shift to right of the curve is suggestive of spherocytes. Osmotic fragility is within reference range in HE, but is increased in spherocytic HE and HPP [17].

Limitations

- It is labor-intensive and time-consuming procedure and requires ≥2 mL of whole blood, thus making it unsuitable for use in newborn babies or as a population screening test.
- It has low sensitivity and specificity.
- OFT may be normal in 10–20% of HS cases because it cannot detect atypical and mild cases, also the test may be normal in the presence of iron deficiency, obstructive jaundice and during the recovery phase of an aplastic crisis, affected by elevated reticulocyte counts.
- It does not differentiate spherocytosis seen in other conditions, like AIHA, recent blood transfusion, enzymopathies, and unstable hemoglobin variants.

4.1.4.5 Sensitivity

HS cases: 68% on fresh; 81% on incubated blood (incubated OFT).

Compensated HS cases: 53% on fresh, 64% with incubated OFT.

4.1.4.6 Flow Cytometry-Based Fragility Tests

There are two flow cytometry-based tests to measure erythrocyte fragility:

1. Flow cytometric osmotic fragility test (FCM OFT)
2. Eosin-5′-maleimide (EMA) binding test

4.1.4.7 Flow Cytometric Osmotic Fragility [18–21]

Principle: The red cells are susceptible to lysis when exposed to deionized water (DW), a hemolysis-inducing agent. A red cell suspension in isotonic normal saline undergoes hemolysis when exposed to DW, subsequently red cell count is measured in real time by FCM before and after DW spiking.

Results: The degree of osmotic hemolysis is expressed as "% residual red cells."

$$\% \; Residual\, red\, cells = \frac{Mean\; event\; count\; of\; last\; two\; regions \left(residual\; cells\right)}{Event\; count\; of\; first\; region \left(cells\; present\; initially\right) \times dilution\; factor} \times 100$$

Interpretation: Increased osmotic fragility is indicated by a low percentage of residual red cells.

Advantages

- Time and labor-saving
- Quantitative and objective
- Cost-effective
- Pre-incubation of blood samples not required
- High test efficiency rates
- Can indicate clinical severity in HS patients

Sensitivity and specificity: 85.7% and 97.2%, respectively.

4.1.4.8 Eosin-5-Maleimide (EMA) Binding Test [20]

Principle: The dye eosin-5-maleimide on the intact labeled red cells binds with Lys-430 on the first extracellular loop of band 3 protein and the Rh-related proteins of the RBC membrane, then the relative fluorescence intensity is measured by flow cytometry. Reduced band 3 and related membrane proteins lead to a decreased fluorescence intensity, characteristically to <65% of normal.

Advantages

- It is time-efficient (results within 2–3 h), labor-saving, quantitative, and objective.
- The results are not influenced by storage for up to 6 days, allowing shipping of samples.
- Requirement of only 5 μL of peripheral blood makes it easy to perform in neonates.
- The test can detect HS red cells as well as SAO, cryohydrocytosis, and some cases of CDA type II, even HPP red cells.
- The test can be used alone when adequate clinical and laboratory information on the patient are available.

Limitations

1. EMA dye is expensive and its working solution is unstable to light.
2. Nonavailability of universal reference ranges for normal controls and HS.
3. HS cases associated with ankyrin defects cannot be picked up and is equivocal for other RBC membrane disorders such as elliptocytosis, pyropoikilocytosis, stomatocytosis, and SAO.

4.1.5 Results

$$Mean\; channel\; fluorescence\% \left(MCF\right) = \frac{\left(mean\; normal\; fluorescence\; controls - fluorescence\; test\right) \times 100}{mean\; normal\; fluorescence\; controls}$$

The test is positive for HS when the percentage of fluorescence reduction is >21%, negative when <16%, and equivocal if the percentage is between 16 and 21% [22].

Hereditary pyropoikilocytosis (HPP, MCV < 60 fL) and HE can be differentiated from HS, based on the graded reduction in fluorescence intensity for HPP (the lowest) < HS < HE ≤ normal controls [20, 23]. Fluorescence readings of some rare red cell disorders—CDAII, SAO, and cryohydrocytosis which are similar can be distinguished from HS based on their clinical features.

4.1.5.1 Interpretation of Results

Low MCF indicates defect in band 3 or protein 4.2, hence it is specific for though can also be positive in HPP.

Sensitivity and Specificity: 92.7% and 99.1%; positive predictive value of 97.8% and a negative predictive value of 96.9%.

4.1.5.2 Glycerol Lysis-Time Test/ Acidified Glycerol Lysis-Time Test [24, 25]

Principle: Glycerol in a hypotonic buffered saline solution slows the rate of entry of water molecules into the red cells, so that the time taken for lysis can be very conveniently measured. GLT 50 is a one-tube test, to measure the time taken for 50% lysis of a blood sample after addition of glycerol. The original method although had more sensitivity in the osmotic-resistant range, but could identify most patients with HS by a shorter GLT50.

Zanella et al. modified the original test by lowering the pH of the buffered solutions to 6.85, which improved the sensitivity and specificity for HS. As a result, the lysis of normal red cells can be measured at a more manageable time of >900 s.

4.1.6 Results

AGLT50 Normal blood (normal adults, newborn infants and cord samples): >30 min (1800 s).

AGLT50 in Hereditary Spherocytosis: Between 25 and 150 s.

This AGLT is also seen in acquired spherocytosis, such as AIHA, in some pregnant women, chronic renal failure, and myelodysplastic syndrome.

Sensitivity for β-thalassemia 95% and specificity 97%, for iron deficiency 53% and for HS, only 36%, so PPV of a positive result is practically nil for HS.

4.1.6.1 Significance of the AGLT

Sensitivity of the AGLT is high in compensated HS and with an undetected biochemical defect cases.

4.1.6.2 The Pink Test [26]

Principle: The pink test is a modification of the acidified glycerol lysis test in which red cells in a drop of peripheral blood are added to a solution of acidic hypotonic glycerol (pH 6.66) and evaluated for final hemolysis.

4.1.7 Results

Healthy controls: 4.1 and 21.7% of hemolysis. **HS**: Above 41.3%.

It is also positive in some cases of renal failure, AIHA, normal pregnant women and negative in other microcytic anemias (β-thalassemia, iron deficiency anemia).

Sensitivity is 100% in hereditary spherocytosis; it clearly discriminates them from healthy subjects.

4.1.7.1 Cryohemolysis Test [27]

Principle: The red cells when cooled from 37° to 0 °C, while suspended in hypertonic medium, rupture; because of the cell shrinkage, their membrane cannot undergo mechanical accommodation. The amount of hemoglobin released is then measured spectrophotometrically. The strain imposed on the skeleton during the temperature changes exposes not only changes in the surface area-to-volume ratio but also defects in the proteins of the vertical linkages.

Advantages

- This test is reported to identify all patients with HS, including asymptomatic carriers.
- SAO has also increased cryohemolysis.
- The test can be carried out on EDTA blood up to 1 day old.

4.1.8 Results

$$\%\text{hemolysis} = \frac{\text{Absorbance at } 540\,(\text{test})}{\text{Absorbance } 540\,\text{of } 100\%\ \text{cell lysate}} \times 100\%$$

4.1.9 Interpretation

Range of cryohemolysis in normal subjects is 3–15%; in hereditary spherocytosis, it is >20% [27].

However, it is recommended that individual laboratories establish their own reference values for the method.

Sensitivity is 100% and specificity is 90% in relation to the general population of hospitalized patients and 87% in relation to AIHA.

4.1.9.1 Ektacytometry [28]

Principle: Blood sample is subjected to a defined value of shear stress which induces change of red cell shape from circular at rest to elliptical at a high shear stress, this is projected as a laser diffraction pattern. It is a measure of the average RBC deformability, and a deformability index for the red cells is derived.

Advantages

- Amount of blood required to perform the test is small (100 μL); hence, it can be used for neonates.
- Distinct osmotic deformability profiles generated can help diagnosis of not only HS but the other RBC membrane disorders such as elliptocytosis, HPP, stomatocytosis, and SAO.

Limitations

- The instrument is complex and not readily available.
- There is a need for specialized staff members in order to process the samples and analyze the data.
- The test can be done only after 3 months post-transfusion.
- Analysis should be done within 48 h of blood sampling.

A new generation ektacytometer Osmoscan LoRRca MaxSis has been engineered by Mechatronics Instruments BV® (Zwaag, The Netherlands). It is a unique instrument, with research and clinical applications, which enables simultaneous analysis of three major RBC properties, RBC cell geometry, viscosity, and deformability. Even though it diagnoses most of the membrane defects, ektacytometry has not even been evaluated in the 2011 guidelines.

4.1.10 Results

In both systems, a measure of cellular deformability defined as the deformability index (DI) is generated.

- HS. DImax↓; Omin↑: osmotic fragility↑; O'↓: cell hydration↓
- HE and HPP. DImax↓; in both instances the curve has a trapezoidal shape
- DHS. DImax normal; Omin↓: osmotic fragility↓; O'↓: cell hydration ↓
- OHS. DImax normal; Omin↑: osmotic fragility↑; O'↑: cell hydration↑

4.1.10.1 Sodium Dodecyl Sulfate Polyacrylamide Gel Electrophoresis (SDS-PAGE) [29]

Identifying a protein defect red cell membrane confirms the diagnosis. SDS-PAGE is used on red cell membrane ghosts not only for identification of the protein defect (e.g., CDAII band 3 and spectrin variants in HE/HPP) but also the quantitation of protein (decreased proteins in both HS and HE, or increased spectrin dimer in HE/HPP). It can detect protein 4.1 defect in HE. Although not mandatory for diagnosis of HS, it is useful where the proband has a clinical condition inconsistent with that of the affected parent(s) and siblings.

Limitation: The facility is largely unavailable and the sample has to be processed rapidly within

24 h. The test also lacks sensitivity for very mild or asymptomatic "carrier" HS.

4.1.10.2 Molecular Genetics [30]

Several mutations have been identified, the testing provides no extra information nor is it required for treatment decision-making for a patient of HS or HE with a positive family history. NGS (next generation sequencing) to identify the protein gene mutation in the proband, and less expensive molecular techniques (namely PCR and sequencing) to test the other family members (e.g., parents and affected relatives).

Table 4.1 summarizes the laboratory features of RBC membrane defects.

4.2 Hereditary Spherocytosis

HS is a group of inherited disorders characterized by the presence of spherical shaped erythrocytes in a peripheral blood smear. Approximately 1 in 2000 Caucasians has HS. It has also been found in other ethnic groups (in Africa, Algeria, Tunisia, Egypt, Japan, North India, and Brazil) [31].

4.2.1 Pathobiology of Hereditary Spherocytosis (HS) [32]

The weakened vertical linkages due to deficiency of one of the membrane proteins destabilize the lipid bilayer, leading to loss of membrane in the form of microvesicles. This reduces the surface area of the cell and leads to spherocyte formation. Red cells with a deficiency of spectrin or ankyrin produce microvesicles containing band 3, whereas a reduced amount of band 3 or protein 4.1R gives rise to band 3-free microvesicles. Consequent to the decreased deformability, the spherocytes get trapped in the spleen where the membrane is further damaged by splenic conditioning and ultimately lyse. The membrane lipid loss is symmetrical, i.e., the relative proportions of cholesterol and phospholipids are normal and the asymmetrical distribution of phospholipids is maintained. Secondary to the underlying membrane defect, the increased cation permeability leads to a loss of monovalent cations accompanied by the loss of water leaving the spherocytes dehydrated.

4.2.2 Red Cell Membrane Protein Defects

Membrane loss in hereditary spherocytosis is as a result of deficiency or dysfunction of one or combined membrane proteins [2, 33, 34] based on which the disease can be divided into subsets.

- Deficiency of spectrin
- Combined deficiency of spectrin and ankyrin
- Deficiency of band 3 protein
- Deficiency of protein 4.2
- Deficiency of Rh complex
- Undefined protein abnormalities

Different molecular mechanisms can generate similar membrane protein deficiency in HS. Most of the protein gene mutations in HS are "private" or sporadic occurrences, i.e., they are specific to one family or found in a few families from different countries.

4.2.3 Hereditary Spherocytosis in the Neonate

The disease very often presents as jaundice in the first few days of life which has to be managed by phototherapy or sometimes exchange transfusions. Co-inheritance of Gilbert's syndrome as detected by homozygosity for a TATA box polymorphism in the uridine-diphosphate glucuronyl-transferase 1A1 gene (UGT1A1) increases both the frequency and severity of hyperbilirubinemia [35] in neonates with HS. The hemoglobin at birth is within the normal range, which decreases sharply during the first 3 weeks of life, leading to a transient, severe anemia requiring blood transfusions. The severity of hemolysis in the neonatal period has been related to the presence of fetal hemoglobin, which does not bind to 2,3-diphosphoglycerate

(2,3-DPG). The resulting elevated free 2,3-DPG levels destabilize the spectrin–protein 4.1 interaction, thereby augmenting the skeletal defect. The erythropoiesis at this age is slow and most infants outgrow the need for transfusion by the end of their first year of life.

Close follow-up of infants with HS is necessary; in the first 6 months hemoglobin and reticulocyte counts should be monitored every month to detect and treat late anemia. After 6 months every 6–8 weeks, and thereafter to 3–4 months in the second year of life. Up till the age of 5 years, hemoglobin, bilirubin levels and reticulocyte counts should be checked every 6–12 months, and every year thereafter. Annual screening for parvovirus B19 serology should be done until a positive result for IgG is obtained.

The diagnosis of hereditary spherocytosis is more difficult in the neonatal period than later in life. Splenomegaly is infrequent; reticulocytosis is usually not severe, i.e., not >10%, and spherocytes are commonly seen in neonatal blood films even in the absence of disease. The neonatal red cells are osmotically resistant compared to that of the adult cells, hence the osmotic fragility test is also less reliable. For these reasons, investigations should be postponed until at least 6 months of age and age appropriate osmotic fragility curves should be used.

4.3 Complications in HS

4.3.1 Gallbladder Disease

The formation of bilirubinate gallstones is the most common complication of hereditary spherocytosis arising between 10 and 30 years of age. The co-inheritance of Gilbert's syndrome (as detected by homozygosity for a TATA box polymorphism in the uridine-diphosphate glucuronyl-transferase 1A1 gene (UGT1A1)) increases the risk by 4–5 folds. An abdominal ultrasound is recommended every third to fifth year in patients with HS, every year in those with both HS and Gilbert's syndrome, and before splenectomy.

4.3.2 Hemolytic, Aplastic, and Megaloblastic Crises

Hemolytic crises are usually associated with viral illnesses and typically occur in childhood. They are mild and characterized by jaundice, splenomegaly, anemia, and reticulocytosis. Medical intervention is seldom necessary.

Aplastic crises following viral infections (most common being parvovirus B19) are uncommon but marrow suppression may be profound anemia requiring hospitalization and transfusion with serious complications, including congestive heart failure or even death. The aplastic crises usually last for 10–14 days. The diagnosis can be confirmed by documenting raised parvovirus IgM titers in the acute illness. The family members should be warned of the risk of catching this contagious viral infection.

Megaloblastic crises are seen in HS patients during periods of increased folate demands, such as growth spurt in pediatric age and pregnancy.

4.3.3 Other Complications

Leg ulcers, chronic dermatitis in the legs and gout are rare manifestations of HS, which usually heal rapidly after splenectomy. In severe cases, skeletal abnormalities resulting from expansion of the marrow can occur. Extramedullary hematopoiesis can lead to tumors, particularly along the thoracic and lumbar spine or in the kidney hila, in nonsplenectomized patients with mild to moderate HS. Postsplenectomy, the masses involute and undergo fatty metamorphosis. Thrombosis has been reported in several HS patients, usually postsplenectomy.

4.3.4 Diagnostic Value of the Various Lab Tests

The laboratory diagnosis is based upon a combination of clinical history, family history, physical examination (splenomegaly, jaundice), and laboratory data (full blood count, morphology, and reticulocyte count) [36]. Additional, specialized tests utilizing the surface area-to-volume ratio are needed to confirm the diagnosis, including the red cell osmotic fragility test (OFT), Glycerol Lysis (GLT), Acidified Glycerol Lysis (AGLT), and Pink test. However, these tests may miss the mild HS cases and do not differentiate HS from secondary spherocytosis as in AIHA. The cryohemolysis test and the flow cytometric EMA-binding test are the recommended methods of lab diagnosis of HS [35]. The latter in particular has been proven to be a sensitive and specific diagnostic tool for HS.

EMA-binding shows 98% specificity and 93% sensitivity which is independent of the type and amount of molecular defect and the clinical phenotype. A comparable sensitivity has been shown by the AGLT (95%) and Pink test (91%). The sensitivity of NaCl osmotic fragility tests, traditionally considered the gold standard for diagnosis, is only 68% on fresh and 81% on incubated blood, which is further reduced in compensated cases (53% and 64%) [37]. EMA test has comparable specificity and sensitivity to the acidified glycerol lysis test and ektacytometry [38] and is better than OFT [39].

Differentiation between HS and CDA II is a challenge, the latter mimics HS both in terms of clinical presentation and increased red cell osmotic fragility, and can only be distinguished by detection of hypoglycosylation of band 3. Patients with dominantly inherited HS and relatives with clinical heterogeneity should also be assessed for another co-existing RBC defect (thalassemic trait, sickle hemoglobin, or pyruvate kinase or glucose-6-phosphate dehydrogenase deficiency) or for low-expression alleles occurring in trans to the hereditary spherocytosis allele using SDS-PAGE of membrane proteins.

Thus molecular diagnosis is useful in patients with atypical features, severe disease, unclear or recessive inheritance, de novo mutations or undiagnosed hemolytic anemia and also aids in identification of silent carriers and prenatal diagnosis.

Although none of the currently available methods have 100% sensitivity, British Committee for Standards in Haematology guidelines (BCSH) 2011 recommends the use of the EMA test or cryohemolysis for the diagnosis [40].

4.3.5 Treatment

Splenectomy cures almost all patients with this disorder, eliminating the anemia and hyperbilirubinemia and near-normalization of reticulocyte count. Spherocytes and altered osmotic fragility persist even after splenectomy; however, the tail of the osmotic fragility curve disappears. Splenectomy in infancy and early childhood even in severely transfusion dependent cases should not be done before 3 years of age and is best delayed until 6–9 years of age. Delay after 10 years increases the risk of cholelithiasis.

4.4 Hereditary Elliptocytosis (HE)/Hereditary Pyropoikilocytosis (HPP)

HE characterized by the presence of elliptical or oval erythrocytes on the blood films is estimated to be 1 in 2000–4000 individuals and is inherited as an autosomal dominant disorder [41].

4.4.1 Etiology and Pathogenesis

HE/HPP is due to defects in the horizontal interactions of the cytoskeletal network involving the spectrin dimer–dimer interaction or the spectrin–actin–protein 4.1R junctional complex and glycophorin C(GPC), which weakens the skeleton and compromises its deformability during circulatory shear stress [41]. HE reticulocytes have a normal shape when released into the circulation but become progressively more elliptical as they age and ultimately the abnormal shape becomes permanent [41]. As the severity of the defect increases, the cells become prone to fragmentation. HPP patients exhibit a combination of horizontal (impaired spectrin tetramer formation) and vertical (spectrin deficiency) defects, with the latter causing microspherocytes and exacerbating the hemolytic anemia [42].

4.4.2 Red Cell Membrane Protein Defects

Spectrin: Commonly mutations that affect spectrin heterodimer self-associations are found in HE. There is increase in spectrin dimers and decrease in spectrin tetramers, which weakens the membrane skeleton and facilitates the formation of elliptocytes under circulatory shear stress [42, 43].

Protein 4.1R: Mutated red cells are mechanically unstable and fragment at moderate shear stress but provide protection from *P. falciparum* [43]. An acquired deficit in 4.1R is reported in myelodysplastic syndromes [44].

Glycophorin C(GPC): Heterozygous carriers of this defect are asymptomatic, with normal red cell morphology, whereas homozygous subjects present with mild HE and exhibit elliptocytes on the blood film [45].

4.4.3 Clinical Features

The clinical presentation of HE is heterogeneous, from asymptomatic carriers to patients with severe, life-threatening anemia. Majority of patients are asymptomatic, found incidentally or are carriers who possess the same molecular defect as an affected HE relative. The erythrocyte life span is normal, and the patients are not anemic and have normal blood films. HE patients with chronic hemolysis experience moderate to severe hemolytic anemia with elliptocytes and poikilocytes on the blood film and may develop complications of chronic hemolysis, such as gallstones. The clinical expression of HE may vary within the same family despite all the affected individuals carrying the same causative mutation. This is a result of the inheritance of modifier alleles or co-inheritance of other molecular defects which modify the clinical expression. The hemolytic anemia can also be exacerbated by acquired conditions, which alter microcirculatory stress on the red cells. HPP is typically picked up in patients with family history of HE.

4.4.4 Hereditary Elliptocytosis in Infants

Clinical symptoms of elliptocytosis are uncommon in the neonatal period. Only severe forms of HE/HPP are present in the neonatal period with severe, hemolytic anemia with marked poikilocytosis and jaundice requiring red cell transfusion, phototherapy, or exchange transfusion. The clinical severity of HE can be affected by the weak binding of DPG to fetal hemoglobin leading to an increased free DPG, which further destabilizes the spectrin–actin–protein 4.1 interaction [46]. The hemolysis abates usually between 9 and 12 months of age, and the patient progresses to typical HE with mild anemia. The typical elliptocytes begin to appear on the blood film at 4–6 months of age.

4.4.5 Laboratory Features

The hallmark of HE is the presence of classically normochromic, normocytic elliptical cells varying from the short stick shape (4.1 deficiency) to more oblong on the blood smears from few to 100% in number although the number does not correlate with severity of hemolysis.

In HPP along with elliptocytes, extreme poikilocytosis in form of bizarre cells fragmented or budding and microspherocytes are seen with low MCV from 50 to 70 fL. Some of the fragmented red cells are counted as platelets by the hematology analyzer and overestimate the platelets counts. The reticulocyte count generally is <5%, but may be higher when hemolysis is severe, along with increased serum bilirubin, increased urinary urobilinogen, and decreased serum haptoglobin.

Osmotic fragility is abnormal in severe HE and in HPP patients. The ektacytometry curve exhibits a trapezoidal form with a decrease in the red cell deformability. SDS-PAGE electrophoresis and analysis of spectrin tetramer–dimer ratios using non-denaturing gels help in detection. Molecular biological studies to determine the underlying mutation are not necessary for diagnosis.

4.4.6　Treatment and Prognosis

Treatment is rarely needed in patients with HE. Occasional, red blood cell transfusions may be required. In severe cases of HE and HPP, splenectomy has been palliative.

4.5　Southeast Asian Ovalocytosis (SAO)

SAO is characterized by the presence of large oval red cells which contain one or two transverse ridges or a longitudinal slit. It is a very common autosomal dominant condition in the aboriginals from Papua New Guinea, Indonesia, Malaysia, the Philippines, and southern Thailand, in areas where malaria is endemic, with prevalence varying between 5 and 25% providing protection against all forms of malaria [47, 48].

The defect results due to a mutation in the SLC4A1 gene encoding band 3. The erythrocytes are rigid and hyperstable and show a slight loss of monovalent cations when exposed to low temperatures, with a reduction of anion flux. In SAO, band 3 binds tightly to ankyrin, forming oligomers, which exhibit restricted lateral and rotational mobility and inability to transport anions. Interestingly, this rigidity does not affect red cell survival in vivo, and the affected adult individuals are completely asymptomatic [49, 50].

4.5.1　Lab Diagnosis

The diagnosis is usually made coincidentally on examination of blood smears with at least 20% of oval shaped red cells and absence of clinical and laboratory evidence of hemolysis. Few may present as hemolytic anemia in the neonates requiring phototherapy. Deformability of SAO red cells is quantitated by ektacytometry [51].

4.6　Red Cell Membrane Transport Defects: Hereditary Stomatocytosis

The hereditary stomatocytoses described as the "channelopathies" of the red cell are dominantly inherited diseases where abnormal transport of Na+ and K+ is the key to the pathophysiology [52]. A "pump" forces Na+ out of the cell and K+ in, and this action is balanced by a process called "the passive leak." In the hereditary stomatocytoses, the passive leak is increased and the red cell becomes overwhelmed with salt and water resulting in hemolysis. The main types are overhydrated (OHSt), dehydrated (DHSt/xerocytosis), cryohydrocytosis (CHC), and familial pseudohyperkalemia (FP). Recently discovered genes, the clinical course, and treatment have been summarized in Table 4.2.

4.6.1　Acquired Red Cell Membrane Defects

Normal individuals may show up to 3% stomatocytes on blood films. Acquired *stomatocytosis* is common in alcoholics, particularly acute alcoholism. Vinca alkaloids used for chemotherapy may induce hemolysis with increased sodium permeability [60].

Transient stomatocytosis is seen in long distance runners immediately after a race. *Spherocytes* are hallmark of AIHA, where RBCs coated with autoantibodies are either entirely or partly phagocytosed in the cords of spleen. Micro- and macrospherocytes are also seen in chronic hepatitis C virus infection treated with protease inhibitors (telaprevir and boceprevir) which induce oxidative stress, thus destabilizing the membrane-cytoskeletal structure by reducing α- and β-spectrins. *Spiculated/spur cells* can occur transiently in several conditions, such as after transfusion with stored blood, ingestion of alcohol and certain drugs, exposure to ionizing radiation or certain venoms and hemodialysis, in patients with functional or actual splenectomy,

Table 4.2 Salient features of various red cell membrane transport defects

	Overhydrated HSt (OHSt)	Dehydrated HSt (DHSt)	Cryohydrocytosis (CHC) [57]	Familial psuedohyperkalemia (FP) [59] coles
Prevalence	1/1,000,000	1/10,000 [54]	Rare	Rare
Inheritance	ADD	ADD		
Mutation	RhAG protein [53, 54]	*PIEZO1* mechanoreceptor protein *KCNN4* gene (Gardos channel) [55, 56]	*SLC4A1* gene [58]	*ABCB6* gene
Morphology	Macrocytes, stomatocytes	Stomatocytes, target cells	Stomatocytes	Normal
Hb	8–10 g/dL	12–15 g/dL	10–12 g/dL	Normal
MCV	120–140 fL	98–120 g/dL	Normal	Normal/high
MCHC	24–28 g/dL	35–37 g/dL [53]	Normal	Normal
Reticulocyte count	10–15%	10%	08%	Normal
Haptoglobin	Undetectable	Undetectable	Undetectable	Present
Intracellular cation	40× normal Na$^+$/ K$^+$ transport rate	Abnormal	K$^+$ leak at low temperature and 4 °C	High plasma K$^+$ in blood sample on long standing at RT
OFT Ektacytometry deformability	Increased STR	Decreased STL		
Course	Mild anemia	Significant anemia, monitor for cholelithiasis, parvovirus Iron overload		
Treatment	Folate Splenectomy contraindicated	Folates Splenectomy ± in severe cases		

severe liver disease, severe uremia, abetalipoproteinemia, certain inherited neurologic disorders and abnormalities of the Kell blood group. *Acanthocytes and/or echinocytes* may be present in patients with glycolytic enzyme defects, myelodysplasia, hypothyroidism, anorexia nervosa, and vitamin E deficiency; in premature infants; and in individuals with suppressed expression of Lu a and Lu b (Lutheran blood group system). The altered phospholipid distribution as in abetalipoproteinemia or increased cholesterol content (liver diseases) on the outer leaflets causes increased surface area-to-volume ratio, which in turn modifies band 3 causing irregular cell surface which becomes more pronounced after passage through spleen. In acanthocytes, it is the altered intramembrane proteins, which disrupts the band 3 and its cytoskeletal interactions causing membrane protrusions.

4.6.2 Summary

Using peripheral blood smear along with specific lab tests red cell membrane defects, inherited or acquired, can be diagnosed. In hereditary spherocytosis, spherocytes seen on PBF have a good positive predictive value in a patient with a family history and compatible red cell indices but in the absence of a family history, both DAT and a screening test for HS should be performed. All the screening tests described can detect typical HS. When in doubt, two screening tests can be used. When the screening tests give negative or equivocal results, molecular testing should be resorted to especially when the family members are hematologically normal [61]. For hereditary elliptocytosis in the absence of a family history of HE or only a few elliptocytes on the PBF, it is advised to confirm the

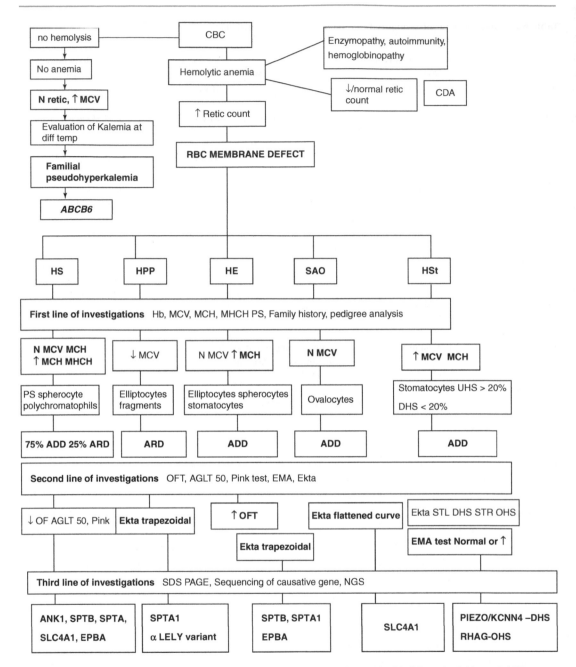

Fig. 4.2 Algorithm for the differential diagnosis of RBC membrane defects. Modified from Andolfo et al. [62]

diagnosis using SDS-PAGE for quantitation of protein 4.1 and spectrin analysis (spectrin dimer content and spectrin variant), or use ektacytometry to obtain characteristic DI profile [61]. It is important to identify disordered membrane permeability defects as splenectomy is of no benefit to a patient with dehydrated HSt and overhydrated HSt; in fact, they are more prone to severe postsplenectomy thrombotic complications. Apart from the increased or decreased red cell volume, the confirmation requires ion flux measurement, ektacytometry, or DNA sequencing for specific genes [61] (Fig. 4.2).

References

1. Zwaal RFA, Schroit AJ. Pathophysiologic implications of membrane phospholipid asymmetry in blood cells. Blood. 1997;89(4):1121–32.
2. Mohandas N, Gallagher PG. Red cell membrane: past, present, and future. Blood. 2008;112(10): 3939–48.
3. Perrotta S, Gallagher PG, Mohandas N. Hereditary spherocytosis. Lancet. 2008;372(9647):1411–26.
4. Chen K, Liu J, Heck S, Chasis JA, An X, Mohandas N. Resolving the distinct stages in erythroid differentiation based on dynamic changes in membrane protein expression during erythropoiesis. Proc Natl Acad Sci U S A. 2009;106(41):17413–8.
5. Lazarides E, Woods C. Biogenesis of the red blood cell membrane-skeleton and the control of erythroid morphogenesis. Annu Rev Cell Biol. 1989;5: 427–52.
6. Mariani M, Barcellini W, Vercellati C, et al. Clinical and hematologic features of 300 patients affected by hereditary spherocytosis grouped according to the type of the membrane protein defect. Haematologica. 2008;93(9):1310–7.
7. Grace RF, Lux SE. Disorders of red cell membrane. In: Orkin SH, Nathan DG, Ginsburg D, Fisher DE, Lux SE, editors. Hematology of infancy and childhood. Philadelphia: Saunders; 2009. p. 659–838.
8. Michaels LA, Cohen AR, Zaho H, et al. Screening for hereditary spherocytosis by use of automated erythrocyte indexes. J Pediatr. 1997;130(6):957–60.
9. Farias MG, Freitas PA. Percentage of hyperdense cells: automated parameter to hereditary spherocytosis screening. Clin Biochem. 2015;48(18): 1341–3.
10. Broséus J, Visomblain B, Guy J, Maynadié M, Girodon F. Evaluation of mean sphered corpuscular volume for predicting hereditary spherocytosis. Int J Lab Hematol. 2010;32(5):519–23.
11. Urrechaga E, Borque L, Escanero JF. Biomarkers of hypochromia: the contemporary assessment of iron status and erythropoiesis. Biomed Res Int. 2013;2013:603786.
12. Rooney S, Hoffmann JJ, Cormack OM, McMahon C. Screening and confirmation of hereditary spherocytosis in children using a CELL-DYN sapphire haematology analyser. Int J Lab Hematol. 2015;37(1):98–104.
13. Urrechaga E, Borque L, Escanero JF. Potential utility of the new Sysmex XE 5000 red blood cell extended parameters in the study of disorders of iron metabolism. Clin Chem Lab Med. 2009;47(11):1411–6.
14. Mullier F, Lainey E, Fenneteau O, Da Costa L, Schillinger F, Bailly N, et al. Additional erythrocytic and reticulocytic parameters helpful for diagnosis of hereditary spherocytosis: results of a multicentre study. Ann Hematol. 2011;90(7):759–68.
15. Lazarova E, Pradier O, Cotton F, Gulbis B. Automated reticulocyte parameters for hereditary spherocytosis screening. Ann Hematol. 2014;93:1809–18.
16. Parpart AK, Lorenz PB, Parpart ER, Gregg JR, Chase AM. The osmotic resistance (fragility) of human red cells. J Clin Invest. 1947;26(4):636–40.
17. King MJ, Zanella A. Hereditary red cell membrane disorders and laboratory diagnostic testing. Int J Lab Hematol. 2013;35(3):237–43.
18. Stoya G, Gruhn B, Vogelsang H, Baumann E, Linss W. Flow cytometry as a diagnostic tool for hereditary spherocytosis. Acta Haematol. 2006;116(3): 186–91.
19. Warang P, Gupta M, Kedar P, Ghosh K, Colah R. Flow cytometric osmotic fragility—an effective screening approach for red cell membranopathies. Cytometry B Clin Cytom. 2011;80(3):186–90.
20. King MJ, Behrens J, Rogers C, Flynn C, Greenwood D, Chambers K. Rapid flow cytometry test for the diagnosis of membrane cytoskeleton-associated haemolytic anaemia. Br J Haematol. 2000;111(3): 924–33.
21. Yamamoto A, Saito N, Yamauchi Y, Takeda M, Ueki S, Itoga M, et al. Flow cytometric analysis of red blood cell osmotic fragility. J Lab Autom. 2014;19(5):483–7.
22. King MJ, Telfer P, MacKinnon H, Langabeer L, McMahon C, Darbyshire P, et al. Using the eosin-5-maleimide binding test in the differential diagnosis of hereditary spherocytosis and hereditary pyropoikilocytosis. Cytometry B Clin Cytom. 2008;74(4): 244–50.
23. King MJ, Chapman L, Mackinnon H, Mills W, Psiachou-Leonnard E, Murrin R. Examination of flow cytometric histograms of eosin-5-maleimide labelled red cells can assist in differential diagnosis of membranopathy. Br J Haematol. 2003;121(Suppl 1):75.
24. Gottfried EL, Robertson NA. Glycerol lysis time of incubated erythrocytes in the diagnosis of hereditary spherocytosis. J Lab Clin Med. 1974;84(5): 746–51.
25. Zanella A, Milani S, Fagnani G, Mariani M, Sirchia G. Diagnostic value of the glycerol lysis test. J Lab Clin Med. 1983;102(5):743–50.
26. Vettore L, Zanella A, Molaro GL, De Matteis MC, Pavesi M, Mariani M. A new test for laboratory diagnosis of spherocytosis. Acta Haematol. 1984;72(4):258–63.
27. Streichman S, Gescheidt Y. Cryohemolysis for the detection of hereditary spherocytosis: correlation studies with osmotic fragility and autohemolysis. Am J Hematol. 1998;58(3):206–12.
28. Clark MR, Mohandas N, Shohet SB. Osmotic gradient ektacytometry: comprehensive characterization of the red cell volume and surface maintenance. Blood. 1983;61(5):899–910.
29. Iolascon A, Avvisati RA. Genotype/phenotype correlation in hereditary spherocytosis. Haematologica. 2008;93(9):1283–8.
30. Delaunay J. The molecular basis of hereditary red cell membrane disorders. Blood Rev. 2007;21(1):1–20.
31. Eber SW, Pekrun A, Neufeldt A, Schröter W. Prevalence of increased osmotic fragility of

erythrocytes in German blood donors: screening using a modified glycerol lysis test. Ann Hematol. 1992;64(2):88–92.

32. Gallagher PG, Jarolim P. Red cell membrane disorders. In: Hoffman R, Benz Jr EJ, Shattil SJ, et al., editors. Hematology: basic principles and practice. 4th ed. Philadelphia: WB Saunders; 2005.

33. Delaunay J, Alloisio N, Morle L, Baklouti F, Dalla Venezia N, et al. Molecular genetics of hereditary elliptocytosis and hereditary spherocytosis. Ann Genet. 1996;39(4):209–21.

34. Tse WT, Lux SE. Red blood cell membrane disorders. Br J Haematol. 1999;104(1):2–13.

35. Rocha S, Costa E, Ferreira F, Cleto E, Barbot J, Rocha-Pereira P, et al. Hereditary spherocytosis and the (TA)nTAA polymorphism of UGTA1A1 gene promoter region—a comparison of the bilirubin plasmatic levels in the different clinical forms. Blood Cells Mol Dis. 2010;44(2):117–9.

36. Bolton-Maggs PH, Stevens RF, Dodd NJ, Lamont G, Tittensor P, King MJ, General Haematology Task Force of the British Committee for Standards in Haematology. Guidelines for the diagnosis and management of hereditary spherocytosis. Br J Haematol. 2004;126(4):455–74.

37. Bianchi P, Fermo E, Vercellati C, Marcello AP, Porretti L, Cortelezzi A, et al. Diagnostic power of laboratory tests for hereditary spherocytosis: a comparison study in 150 patients grouped according to molecular and clinical characteristics. Haematologica. 2012;97(4):516–23.

38. Girodon F, Garçon L, Bergoin E, Largier M, Delaunay J, Fénéant-Thibault M, et al. Usefulness of the eosin-5′-maleimide cytometric method as a first-line screening test for the diagnosis of hereditary spherocytosis: comparison with ektacytometry and protein electrophoresis. Br J Haematol. 2008;140(4):468–70.

39. Kar R, Mishra P, Pati HP. Evaluation of eosin-5-maleimide flow cytometric test in diagnosis of hereditary spherocytosis. Int J Lab Hematol. 2010;32(1 pt 2):8–16.

40. Bolton-Maggs PH, Langer JC, Iolascon A, Tittensor P, King MJ, General Haematology Task Force of the British Committee for Standards in Haematology. Guidelines for the diagnosis and management of hereditary spherocytosis—2011 update. Br J Haematol. 2012;156(1):37–49.

41. Gallagher PG. Hereditary elliptocytosis: spectrin and protein 4.1R. Semin Hematol. 2004;41(2):142–64.

42. Coetzer T, Palek J, Lawler J, et al. Structural and functional heterogeneity of α spectrin mutations involving the spectrin heterodimer self-association site: relationships to hematologic expression of homozygous hereditary elliptocytosis and hereditary pyropoikilocytosis. Blood. 1990;75(11):2235–44.

43. Coetzer T, Lawler J, Prchal JT, Palek J. Molecular determinants of clinical expression of hereditary elliptocytosis and pyropoikilocytosis. Blood. 1987;70(3):766–72.

44. Takakuwa Y, Tchernia G, Rossi M, Benabadji M, Mohandas N. Restoration of normal membrane stability to unstable protein 4.1-deficient erythrocyte membranes by incorporation of purified protein 4.1. J Clin Invest. 1986;78(1):80–5.

45. Winardi R, Reid M, Conboy J, Mohandas N. Molecular analysis of glycophorin C deficiency in human erythrocytes. Blood. 1993;81(10):2799–803.

46. Mentzer WC Jr, Iarocci TA, Mohandas N, Lane PA, Smith B, Lazerson J, et al. Modulation of erythrocyte membrane mechanical stability by 2,3-diphosphoglycerate in the neonatal poikilocytosis/elliptocytosis syndrome. J Clin Invest. 1987;79(3):943–9.

47. Iolascon A, Perrotta S, Stewart GW. Red blood cell membrane defects. Rev Clin Exp Hematol. 2003;7(1):22–56.

48. Mohandas N, An X. Malaria and human red blood cells. Med Microbiol Immunol. 2012;20(14):593–8.

49. Liu SC, Zhai S, Palek J, Golan DE, Amato D, Hassan K, et al. Molecular defect of the band 3 protein in southeast Asian ovalocytosis. N Engl J Med. 1990;323(22):1530–8.

50. Mohandas N, Winardi R, Knowles D, Leung A, Parra M, George E, et al. Molecular basis for membrane rigidity of hereditary ovalocytosis. J Clin Invest. 1992;89(2):686–92.

51. Mohandas N. Molecular basis for red cell membrane viscoelastic properties. Biochem Soc Trans. 1992;20(4):776–82.

52. Stewart GW. Hemolytic disease due to membrane ion channel disorders. Curr Opin Hematol. 2004;11(4):244–50.

53. Bruce LJ. Hereditary stomatocytosis and cation-leaky red cells-recent developments. Blood Cells Mol Dis. 2009;42(3):216–22.

54. Bruce LJ, Burton NM, Gabillat N, Gabillat N, Poole J, Flatt JF, et al. The monovalent cation leak in overhydrated stomatocytic red blood cells results from amino acid substitutions in the Rh-associated glycoprotein. Blood. 2009;113(6):1350–7.

55. Andolfo I, Alper SL, De Franceschi L, Auriemma C, Russo R, De Falco L, et al. Multiple clinical forms of dehydrated hereditary stomatocytosis arise from mutations in PIEZO1. Blood. 2013;121(19):3925–35.

56. Zarychanski R, Schulz VP, Houston BL, Maksimova Y, Houston DS, Smith B, et al. Mutations in the mechanotransduction protein PIEZO1 are associated with hereditary xerocytosis. Blood. 2012;20(9):1908–15.

57. Bogdanova A, Goede JS, Weiss E, Bogdanov N, Bennekou P, Bernhardt I, et al. Cryohydrocytosis: increased activity of cation carriers in red cells from a patient with a band 3 mutation. Haematologica. 2010;95(2):189–98.

58. Guizouarn H, Martial S, Gabillat N, Borgese F. Point mutations involved in red cell stomatocytosis convert

the electroneutral anion exchanger 1 to a nonselective cation conductance. Blood. 2007;110(6):2158–65.

59. Coles SE, Ho MM, Chetty M, Nicolaou A, Stewart GW. A variant of hereditary stomatocytosis with marked pseudohyperkalaemia. Br J Haematol. 1999;104(2):275–83.

60. Neville AJ, Rand CA, Barr RD, Mohan Pai KR. Drug-induced stomatocytosis and anemia during consolidation chemotherapy of childhood acute leukemia. Am J Med Sci. 1984;287(1):3–7.

61. King MJ, Garcon L, Hoyer JD, Iolason A, Picard V, Stewart G, et al; International Council for Standardization in Haematology. ICSH guidelines for the laboratory diagnosis of nonimmune hereditary red cell membrane disorders. Int J Lab Hematol. 2015;37(3):304–25.

62. Andolfo I, Russo R, Gambale A, Iolascon A. New insights on hereditary erythrocyte membrane defects. Haematologica. 2016;101(11): 1284–94.

Molecular Genetics of Inherited Red Cell Membrane Disorders

5

Anu Aggarwal, Manu Jamwal, and Reena Das

Inherited red cell membrane disorders constitute a diverse group of disorders which are characterized by wide clinical and molecular heterogeneity. They are nonimmune hereditary hemolytic anemia, and patients present with variable degrees of pallor, episodic jaundice, splenomegaly, and elevated lactate dehydrogenase (LDH) levels. The underlying cause is the defects either in the organization of membrane structure or membrane transport function arising because of mutations in genes encoding erythrocyte membrane proteins essential for stable structure and function. The commonest disorder is hereditary spherocytosis (HS) followed by relatively uncommon conditions such as hereditary elliptocytosis (HE) and hereditary pyropoikilocytosis (HPP). Disorders of alterations of hydration include hereditary stomatocytosis (HSt) where cation permeability in the red cell membrane is disturbed, leading to overhydrated HSt and hereditary xerocytosis/dehydrated HSt. Extensive biochemical, biophysical, and genetic studies of the red cell membrane in the decades have provided detailed molecular insights into the structural basis for normal red cell membrane function

and for altered function in various inherited red cell membrane disorders [1–5].

5.1 Laboratory Diagnosis of Red Cell Membrane Disorders

Laboratory diagnosis of a patient suspected to have red cell membrane disorder is done by hierarchal testing based on automated red cell indices, the morphology of RBCs, and reticulocytosis in the context of an appropriate clinical presentation. Different diagnostic tests are performed to find the cause of the underlying hemolysis in a systematic manner as shown in Fig. 5.1.

Glucose-6-phosphate dehydrogenase (G6PD) deficiency, thalassemia syndromes, and other hemoglobinopathies like sickle cell disorders and hemoglobin E syndromes, unstable hemoglobins, autoimmune hemolytic anemia (AIHA), pyruvate kinase (PK) deficiency, and sometimes congenital dyserythropoietic anemia (CDA) type II need to be appropriately excluded. Diagnosis for patients with classic HS is straightforward, based on a positive family history especially when the inheritance is autosomal dominant, the presence of spherocytes on peripheral blood film, increased reticulocyte count, increased incubated osmotic fragility test (iOFT), and decreased mean channel fluorescence for eosin 5′ maleimide (EMA) dye by flow cytometry. Similarly, other disorders like HE, HPP, or HSt could be diagnosed by the morphology of red

A. Aggarwal · M. Jamwal · R. Das (✉)
Department of Hematology, Post Graduate Institute of Medical Education and Research,
Chandigarh, India
e-mail: das.reena@pgimer.edu.in

© Springer Nature Singapore Pte Ltd. 2019
R. Saxena, H. P. Pati (eds.), *Hematopathology*, https://doi.org/10.1007/978-981-13-7713-6_5

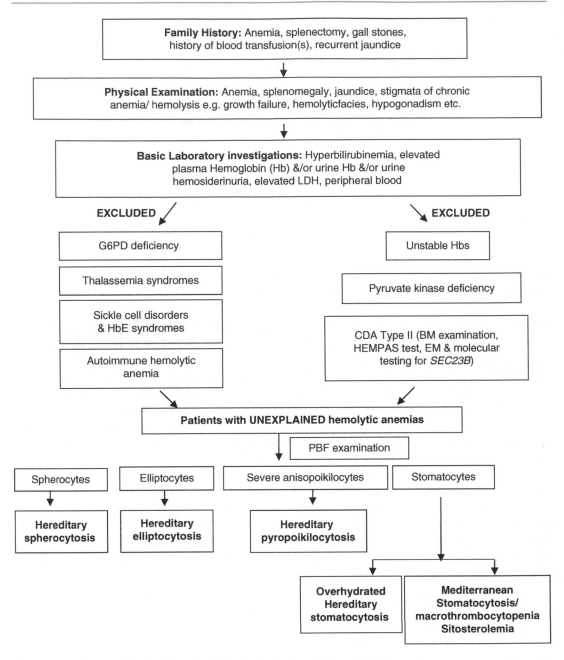

Fig. 5.1 Algorithm used in the diagnosis of inherited red cell membrane disorders

blood cells on peripheral smear. However, the difficulty lies when there is overlapping clinical features, protean manifestations, post-blood transfusion samples, and co-inheritance of other disorders. Traditional diagnostic testing approaches fail to identify the cause in such cases, and therefore, genetic testing to identify the underlying defect could be implemented. Sanger sequencing for the region of interest is the first approach to proceed to find the defect. However, the number and complexity of the genes involved make it cumbersome and time-consuming. Next-generation sequencing (NGS)/targeted re-sequencing of the panel of implicated genes provides a rapid and cost-effective approach to the molecular diagnosis of hemolytic anemias [6].

5.2 Hereditary Spherocytosis (HS)

HS is a heterogeneous disease characterized by the presence of microspherocytes in the peripheral blood smear (PBS) with increased osmotic fragility which was first described in 1871. Spherocytes show reduction of normal surface area and increased rigidity. During circulation, the abnormal erythrocytes get trapped in the spleen where they encounter in a metabolically unfavorable environment in the splenic pulp and are phagocytosed. The hemolysis in the spleen results directly in varying degrees of anemia and hyperbilirubinemia, which in turn results in pallor, fatigue, and jaundice in the patient. The loss of surface area results from increased membrane fragility due to defects in the erythrocyte membrane proteins, like ankyrin, band 3, beta spectrin, alpha spectrin, and protein 4 [3, 7].

5.2.1 Geographical Distribution

HS occurs universally in all populations and happens to be the commonest cause of inherited chronic hemolytic anemias among people of North European descent, affecting approximately one case in 2000 people. It is also prevalent in Japan and less frequently in the Southeast Asian and African-American populations; however, comprehensive data is not available for them [7]. In India, HS has been reported chiefly from the northern states (Punjab, Delhi, Uttar Pradesh, and Maharashtra) as well as sporadically from eastern and southern states like Andhra Pradesh and West Bengal [8–10].

Although precise incidence data is unavailable, anecdotal evidence suggests that it is a relatively frequently encountered membrane disorder.

5.2.2 Genetics of HS

Majority of the cases (~70%) of HS is autosomal dominant (AD) in inheritance, and others show autosomal recessive (AR) inheritance or *de novo* mutations [11–13]. Homozygosity for dominantly inherited HS gene has not been known, suggestive of the incompatibility of the homozygous state with life. Dominant HS is predominantly associated with null phenotypes due to nonsense or frameshift mutations resulting from insertions or deletions, whereas recessive HS is caused by promoter or missense mutations, which are probably *de novo* mutations [14–17]. Mutations causing HS are in genes like ankyrin, β-spectrin, band 3, α-spectrin, and protein 4.2 that act as transmembrane proteins, membrane skeletal proteins, and mediating proteins helping in the attachment of the transmembrane proteins to the skeletal proteins of erythrocyte membrane respectively as shown in Table 5.1.

HS may be subclassified depending upon the genes implicated as given in Table 5.2.

Table 5.2 Classification of HS depending upon the implicated genes

Type	MIM ID #	Gene implicated
HS type 1 (SPH 1)	# 182900	*ANK1*
HS type 2 (SPH 2)	# 182870	*SPTB*
HS type 3 (SPH 3)	# 270970	*SPTA1*
HS type 4 (SPH 4)	# 612653	*EPB3/SLC4A1*
HS type 5 (SPH 5)	# 612690	*EPB42/ELB42*

Compiled from OMIM [19]

Table 5.1 Main features of the genes involved in hereditary spherocytosis

Gene symbol	Chromosome location	Gene size (kb)	No. of exons	AA
SPTA1/EL2	1q23.1	80	53	2429
SPTB/EL3	14q23.3	100	38	2137
ANK1	8p11.21	160	49	1880
EPB3/SLC4A1	17q21.31	18	21	911
EPB42/ELB42	15q15.2	20	16	691

Iolascon et al. [18]; Online Mendelian Inheritance in Man, OMIM [19]

Table 5.3 Clinical classification of HS

	Mild	Moderate	Moderately severe	Severe
Percent of cases	10–15	60–70	10–15	5–15
Hb; mean (range) in g/dL	11–15	8–12	6–8	<6
Reticulocyte count (%)	10–15	20–30	15–25	15–25
Bilirubin level (mg/dL)	1–2	2	2–3	3
Blood transfusions	No	0–3	1–4	3–8
Transmission pattern	AD or *De novo*	*De novo* and AD	*De novo* and AD	AR

5.2.3 Clinical Manifestations

Clinical manifestations of HS are quite variable among the patients and are marked by

1. Hemolysis with or without anemia
2. Elevated absolute reticulocyte count
3. Splenomegaly
4. Jaundice
5. Presence of gallstones
6. Increased mean corpuscular hemoglobin concentration (MCHC)
7. Presence of spherocytes on PBS
8. Increased osmotic fragility test
9. Family history of anemia, jaundice, and gallstones

The clinical presentation is extremely variable among the patients, and many patients may not be identified until later in life when an infection or other process aggravates hemolysis. The degree of hemolysis varies considerably from asymptomatic to severely transfusion-dependent patients. The anemia seen in HS is usually mild to moderate, but may be worsened with fatigue, cold exposure, pregnancy, deficiencies of iron, vitamin B12, folate in addition to co-inheritance of β-thalassemia, PK deficiency, G6PD deficiency or due to viral infection likely parvovirus B19. Jaundice in anemic patients is due to increased red cell destruction leading to hyperbilirubinemia. Some patients also develop pigment (calcium bilirubinate) gallstones due to chronic hemolysis. The disease worsens with the co-inheritance of Gilbert syndrome or G6PD deficiency especially in the neonatal period. HS is clinically subclassified based on the severity of disease as mild, moderate, moderately severe, and severe phenotypes which is shown in the Table 5.3 based on the classification given by Perrotta et al. (2008) [7]. The classification is modified according to Indian population (unpublished).

5.2.4 Laboratory Diagnosis of HS

The diagnosis of HS is based on clinical findings and various laboratory tests. Clinical features like variable degree of anemia, jaundice, and splenomegaly are suggestive in the patient. In laboratory diagnosis, the most important is PBS showing spherocytes, mushroom red cells, poikilocytosis, acanthocytes, or ovalostomatocytes with abnormal red blood cell indices (increased MCHC and increased RDW) and high reticulocyte count. Various laboratory tests including OFT (incubated and fresh), acidified glycerol lysis test (AGLT), and Pink test may be used as the first line of screening test for the diagnosis. These tests vary in their specificity and sensitivity in patients. Figure 5.2 shows the increased reticulocytes, presence of spherocytes and acanthocytes in PBS, and increased iOFT.

The sensitivity of these tests is low, and a rapid flow cytometric analysis by eosin-5-maleimide (EMA) binding dye for erythrocytes has been considered as a sensitive and specific screening test for the diagnosis of HS [20]. The maleimide moiety of EMA dye predominantly binds to band 3 protein at the Lys-430 (in the first extracellular loop). In addition, it also binds to sulfhydryl groups expressed by Rh, RhAg, and CD47. In HS, absent or decreased expression of

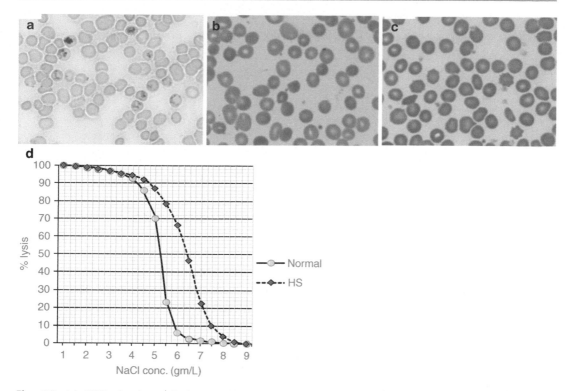

Fig. 5.2 (**a**) PBS showing reticulocytes (Azure B, 1000×); (**b**) PBS showing spherocytes and occasional stomatocytes (Leishman, 1000×); (**c**) PBS showing acantho-cytes and spherocytes (Leishman, 1000×); (**d**) HS patient showing increased susceptibility to lysis using iOFT

red blood cell membrane proteins causes reduced binding of EMA to band 3 and thus shows decreased fluorescence emission. The sensitivity of the tests varies from 90 to 95%, whereas its specificity ranges from 95 to 99%.

5.2.5 Status of EMA Flow Cytometry Test in India

Studies are available from three different centers of India. In the study by Kedar et al., patients with HS and HE showed significant reduced MCF values ($P < 0.001$) than the control group and the other patient group of hemolytic anemia [21]. Another study by Kar et al. enrolled 114 subjects belonging to different categories of hemolytic anemias and showed the decreased MCF values of erythrocytes labeled with EMA dye in HS than other hemolytic and non-hemolytic anemias ($P < 0.01$). False-positive values were obtained in AIHA and CDA patients. Therefore, the sensitivity and specificity determined were 96.4% and 94.2%, respectively [22]. Joshi et al. established the cutoff value for MCF ratio of 0.79 and percent decrease of MCF as 17% in HS patients. Figure 5.3 describes the gating strategy and histograms depicting control and HS case. In their study, they proved the efficiency of EMA dye fluorescence test to capably diagnose the splenectomized cases of HS when hematological parameters improved considerably [23].

$$\text{MCF ratio} = \frac{\text{MCF of patient}}{\text{Mean MCF of normal controls}}$$
$$= <0.8 \text{ is consistent with the diagnosis of HS.}$$

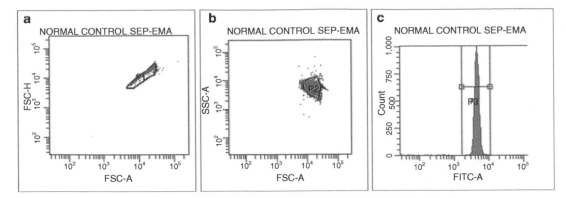

Fig. 5.3 (**a**) Gating strategy for RBCs; (**b**) Normal control subject showing population of RBC, stained with EMA; (**c**) Confirmed case of HS with reduced MCF and decreased CV

In few atypical cases where diagnosis cannot be made or in transfused patients, the underlying molecular diagnosis of HS may be detected using freshly prepared red cell ghosts on 4–12% gradient polyacrylamide gels. It can act as the third line of investigation in many subjects for analysis of erythrocyte membrane proteins but still in many cases it may not be helpful [3]. SDS-PAGE is useful to distinguish CDA type II from HS as gel electrophoresis of erythrocyte membrane proteins demonstrate the characteristic compact band 3 in CDA type II patients in comparison with HS patients [24].

5.2.6 Molecular Spectrum of HS

Various types of mutations (point mutations, splice site mutations, small deletions, duplications, and insertions) occur throughout the lengths of *ANK1*, *SPTB*, *SPTA1*, *EBP3/SLC4A1*, and *EPB42/ELB42* genes. Protein-truncating mutations (frameshift and nonsense) are more frequently observed as compared to missense mutations, in these genes. Mutations in the ankyrin 1 (50%), β-spectrin (20%), and band 3 (15–20%) are most frequently found in autosomal dominant pattern of inheritance. In few cases, ankyrin defects can also cause autosomal recessive inheritance of HS. The production of α-spectrin is three- to fourfold greater than that of

β-spectrin in normal erythroid cells; therefore, only homozygous/compound heterozygous defects of α-spectrin can cause HS. The mutations in protein 4.2 are rare and are mostly present in the Japanese patients in autosomal recessive pattern.

5.2.7 Co-inheritance of G6PD Deficiency, Gilbert Syndrome, or Thalassemia with HS

There is heterogeneity in the phenotypes of HS, and even within the same family, the clinical characteristics are varied due to other genetic conditions that can modify disease phenotype in hemolytic anemias. Concomitant genetic modifiers such as red cell enzymopathies, thalassemia syndrome, and Gilbert syndrome can attribute to this intra-familial heterogeneity. Several reports state that the presence of other simultaneous disorders may worsen [25, 26] or ameliorate [27] HS phenotype.

G6PD deficiency is the most common enzyme deficiency in erythrocytes present in India and marks the initial point of molecular testing [28]. There are reports showing HS occurring concomitantly with G6PD deficiency [25]. G6PD deficiency needs to be ruled out as this could lead to inappropriate therapeutic interventions.

HS with Gilbert syndrome [26, 29, 30] has also been described previously. In Gilbert syndrome, hyperbilirubinemia is the prime clinical feature which is associated with decreased activity of the UGT1A1 enzyme. Co-inheritance of Gilbert syndrome with HS can aggravate the symptoms in patients and is reported to have a greater tendency to form gallstones in these patients [26, 31]. Gilbert syndrome is caused by the insertion of [TA] repeat in the promoter region of *UGT1A1* gene (Fig. 5.4) where the reference sequence consists of six TA repeats [A(TA)6TAA].

Co-inheritance of Gilbert syndrome and G6PD deficiency with HS was also seen in the relatively severe phenotypes. Thalassemia is also seen in concurrence with HS [27, 32, 33]. One of the patients with HS carried the single gene alpha 4.2 deletion with G6PD deficiency and Gilbert syndrome and was less symptomatic [32].

Clinical observations and correct analysis of laboratory tests are required to diagnose such complex conditions.

5.3 Hereditary Elliptocytosis (HE)

HE is characterized by the presence of elliptocytes on the blood film with a variable degree of anemia, ranging from asymptomatic to severe. They may have reticulocytosis depending on the degree of hemolysis, but mostly HE patients are asymptomatic who rarely require therapy and are diagnosed incidentally. HE is caused by abnormalities in the membrane skeleton proteins like α-spectrin, β-spectrin, protein 4.1, and glycophorin C. Figure 5.5 shows a case of hereditary elliptocytosis and reticulocytosis.

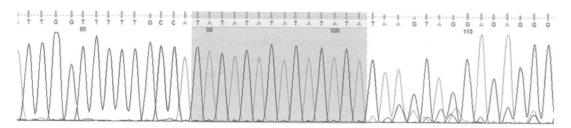

Fig. 5.4 Chromatogram showing homozygosity for TA (7/7) repeats in promoter of *UGT1A1* gene

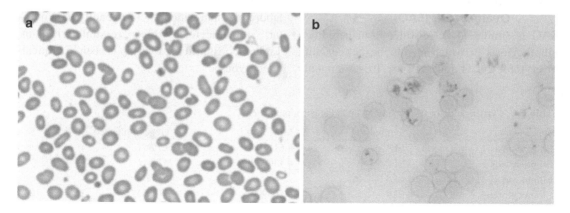

Fig. 5.5 (**a**) PBS showing elliptocytes; (**b**) Increased reticulocytes

5.3.1 Geographical Distribution

The incidence of HE is estimated as 1:2000–4000 globally, but is observed upto 1:100 in parts of Africa. As most of the patients are asymptomatic, the actual incidence of the disease remains unknown. It has been postulated that elliptocytes confer resistance to malaria.

5.3.2 Molecular Spectrum of HE

HE is usually an autosomal dominant disorder, and the leading causes are the mutations in genes coding for membrane skeleton, namely *EPB41*, *SPTA1*, and *SPTB* which disrupts self-association regions of spectrin dimers/tetramers (Table 5.4) [34, 35].

5.3.2.1 Hereditary Pyropoikilocytosis (HPP)

HPP is classified as a subtype of HE and its related disorders which characteristically shows poikilocytosis, fragmented erythrocytes, and microspherocytes. There is severe anemia with reticulocytosis and other hemolytic features. HPP is an autosomal recessive disease caused by compound heterozygous or homozygous mutations in *SPTA1* gene often inherited from asymptomatic HE parents. Severe poikilocytosis results in low MCV (50–60 fL).

5.3.2.2 Southeast Asian Ovalocytosis (SAO)

SAO is similar to but distinct from hereditary elliptocytosis in which membrane permeability of erythrocytes is affected [36]. It is commonly found in Thailand, Malaysia, Philippines, Brunei, Cambodia, Indonesia, Papua, and New Guinea. Cases are diagnosed incidentally as majority remain asymptomatic. Rarely patients are reported to have mild hemolysis and jaundice [37]. It is an autosomal dominant condition and is caused by heterozygous deletion of 27 nucleotides in *SLC4A1* gene. SAO is known to provide resistance against malaria [38]. Only one case of homozygosity for the 27 bp is known, and the phenotype is severe with the requirement of intrauterine transfusions [39].

5.4 Hemolytic Anemias Caused by Defects in Red Cell Cation Permeability and Transport

Red cell membrane disorders arising because of the defects in genes encoding red cell membrane channels or transport proteins primarily have defective cation permeability or transport mechanism across the membrane. The distinct feature is the presence of stomatocytes in the peripheral blood film. Stomatocytosis could be the manifestation of underlying genetic defect or can occur in association with several acquired conditions. Stomatocytes can be artifacts, so multiple evaluations are required. There is wide heterogeneity in the clinical and laboratory manifestations in the stomatocytic syndromes ranging from compensated hemolysis to severe anemia. There is a varied degree of clinical, laboratory, and genetic heterogeneity in hereditary stomatocytosis which are summarized in Table 5.5. Significant overlap is seen in clinical phenotypes.

Table 5.4 Classification of HE depending upon the gene implicated

Type	Symbol	MIM ID #	Gene implicated
Elliptocytosis-1	EL1	# 611804	*EPB41*
Elliptocytosis-2	EL2	# 130600	*SPTA1*
Elliptocytosis-3	EL3	–	*SPTB*
Elliptocytosis-4	EL4	# 166900	*SLC4A1*

Compiled from OMIM [19]

Table 5.5 Classification of defects in red cell cation permeability and transport

Type	MIM ID #	Inheritance	Gene
Overhydrated hereditary stomatocytosis(OHS)	# 185000	AD	*RHAG*
Cryohydrocytosis/stomatocytosis, cold-sensitive (CHC)	# 185020	AD	*SLC4A1*
Stomatin-deficient cryohydrocytosis with neurologic defects	# 608885	AD	*SLC2A1*
Pseudohyperkalemia, familial, 2, due to red cell leak PSHK2	# 609153	AD	*ABCB6*
Dehydrated hereditary stomatocytosis with or without pseudohyperkalemia and/or perinatal edema (DHS1)	# 194380	AD	*PIEZO1*
Dehydrated hereditary stomatocytosis 2 (DHS2)	# 616689	AD	*KCNN4*
Sitosterolemia Mediterranean stomatocytosis/macrothrombocytopenia	# 210250	AR	*ABCG5/ABCG8*

Compiled from OMIM [19]

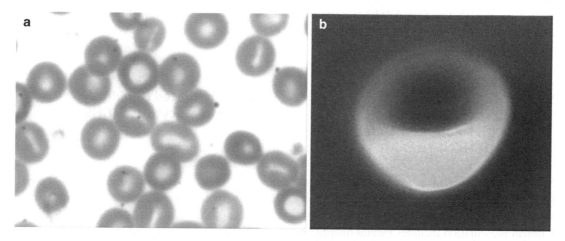

Fig. 5.6 (**a**) Blood film showing stomatocytes (Leishman stain, 1000×); (**b**) Scanning electron microscopy showing stomatocyte

5.5 Overhydrated Hereditary Stomatocytosis (OHS)

OHS is characterized by the presence of stomatocytes (Fig. 5.6), and clinically most patients present with compensated hemolysis to mild macrocytic anemia, osmotic fragile red cells, splenomegaly, and unconjugated hyperbilirubinemia.

OHS is caused by heterozygous mutations in the *RHAG* (Rh-associated glycoprotein) gene. It is also caused by heterozygous mutations in the membrane channel protein-coding genes *SLC4A1* and *SLC2A1* [40]. It is relatively rare and mostly underdiagnosed condition with approximately 20 cases reported worldwide so far [3].

De novo mutations are very frequent in this disorder. Only two studies from India describe the phenotype of hereditary stomatocytosis [41, 42]. The SDS-PAGE analysis shows OHS to be stomatin (EPB72) deficient; however, no mutation in the *EPB72* gene is reported so far.

Correct diagnosis of OHS is however critical since postsplenectomy thrombotic complications have been documented in affected individuals and have been fatal in a few. Splenectomy has been shown to have limited therapeutic benefit in hereditary stomatocytosis and should be performed after careful consideration [43]. Iron overload is usually seen in patients of OHS despite being transfusion-independent.

5.6 Cryohydrocytosis/ Stomatocytosis, Cold-Sensitive (CHC)

CHC is an extremely rare form of stomatocytosis and is characterized by the presence of stomatocytes (overhydrated erythrocytes) that have defective activity at lower temperatures [44]. Major laboratory finding is mild anemia and pseudohyperkalemia. This is an autosomal dominant disorder and occurs due to heterozygous mutations in the *SLC4A1* gene. The same gene is known to cause HS type 4 and SAO. Splenomegaly can be present, but splenectomy is known to have no therapeutic benefits to the patients.

5.7 Stomatin-Deficient Cryohydrocytosis with Neurologic Defects (SDCHCN)

SDCHCN is also known as GLUT1 deficiency syndrome with pseudohyperkalemia and hemolysis and is an asyndromic form of stomatocytosis. Clinical presentation includes mental retardation, movement disorders, seizures, cataracts, and massive hepatosplenomegaly. Hemolytic anemia is characterized by the presence of stomatocytes on blood film and pseudohyperkalemia resulting from defects in the red blood cell membrane. The cause is found to be heterozygous mutations in the *SLC2A1* gene. The disorder combines the neurologic features of GLUT1 deficiency syndrome-1 resulting from impaired glucose transport at the blood–brain barrier.

5.8 Dehydrated Hereditary Stomatocytosis (DHS)/ Hereditary Xerocytosis

5.8.1 DHS With or Without Pseudohyperkalemia and/or Perinatal Edema (DHS 1)

DHS1 also known as hereditary xerocytosis or hereditary desiccytosis is caused by a heterozy-

gous mutation in the *PIEZO1* gene with an autosomal dominant inheritance. Clinical features include jaundice and hepatosplenomegaly. It is characterized by primary erythrocyte dehydration (dessicytes cells with their hemoglobin puddled at the periphery). The red cell indices show a very high MCHC and decreased red cell osmotic fragility. Stomatocytes are rarely seen [45]. Macrocytosis is observed with mild to moderate compensated hemolytic anemia. Some patients may also have perinatal edema or pseudohyperkalemia. Like OHS, iron overload may be present without the history of blood transfusion and may require chelation [40, 46].

5.8.2 Dehydrated Hereditary Stomatocytosis 2 (DHS2)

In DHS2 clinical and laboratory features are similar to *PIEZO1*-associated DHS. However, no mutation was detected in the *PIEZO1* gene. Recently with the advent of whole exome sequencing, a novel gene, *KCNN4*, was identified as causative and a second form of DHS was found [47–49]. Rapetti-Mauss et al. (2015) studied French and Polish families with same heterozygous mutation R352H and noted the varying degree of anemia between the two families. Variation in the clinical phenotypes carrying the same mutation could be explained by the differences in *PIEZO1* polymorphisms carried by those individuals. Splenectomy offered no therapeutic benefits as it did not improve the symptoms; however, no thrombotic complications were observed [47].

5.8.3 Pseudohyperkalemia, Familial, 2, Due to Red Cell Leak (PSHK2)

This disorder is clinically benign, a non-hemolytic variant of DHS1. Red blood cells show a "passive leak" of K+ cations into the plasma upon storage at room temperature (or below). It is an asymptomatic autosomal dominant disorder caused by heterozygous mutations in *ABCB6* gene [50]. Peripheral blood smear usually does not show features of hemolytic anemia including stomatocytes.

5.8.4 Sitosterolemia/ Phytosterolemia

Sitosterolemia is an autosomal recessive metabolic condition caused by homozygous or compound heterozygous mutation in *ABCG8* or *ABCG5* gene. It results from an excess of plasma phytosterols arising as a consequence of unrestricted intestinal sterol absorption. Plant sterols in the patient plasma are markedly elevated, and clinically tendon and tuberous xanthomas with accelerated atherosclerosis and premature coronary artery disease are noted. Mediterranean stomatocytosis/macrothrombocytopenia was recognized as the hematologic presentation of sitosterolemia by Rees et al. in 2005 [51]. It is characterized by chronic hemolysis, stomatocytic red cells, macrothrombocytopenia, and varied systemic manifestations (Fig. 5.7). Recently, three siblings affected in the same family with *ABCG5* [c.727C>T (p.Arg243Ter), rs119479066] mutation with autosomal recessive inheritance were reported for the first time from India [52].

5.9 Recent Advances in Diagnosis of Red Cell Membrane Disorders

Diagnosis of red cell membrane disorders is usually based on laboratory testing followed by morphological screening as described in Fig. 5.1. Genetic diagnosis becomes important where

- Traditional testing has failed.
- Family history is lacking.
- Clinical phenotype is unexplained.
- Patient has required multiple transfusions, confounding the results of laboratory tests.

Establishing a molecular diagnosis offers insight into the pathophysiology and etiology of the disease and is crucial for patient management. Sanger sequencing is a method of choice when finding the molecular defect. Since the number of causative conditions are numerous and includes many and large genes, gene-by-gene approach is not helpful. Recently, targeted resequencing is becoming a popular approach for providing rapid and accurate diagnosis, as the limited panel of genes facilitates the data interpretation [6, 53–55].

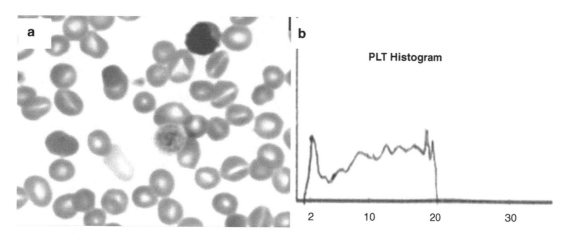

Fig. 5.7 (**a**) PBF showing stomatocytes, spherocytes, and giant platelet (May Grunwald-Giemsa, 1000×); (**b**) Platelet histogram showing the presence of giant platelets

Different laboratories have utilized different customized hemolytic anemia panels of next-generation sequencing to provide a rapid and sensitive assay [6, 54]. Hence, due to the genetic heterogeneity and complexity of the genes involved, red cell membrane disorders are perfect candidates for next-generation sequencing/targeted resequencing. Targeted resequencing is efficient to detect mutations causing hemolytic anemia, including novel variants and is ready for application in clinical laboratories.

References

1. Lux SE, Wolfe LC. Inherited disorders of the red cell membrane skeleton. Pediatr Clin North Am. 1980;27:463–86.
2. Bruce LJ, Guizouarn H, Burton NM, Gabillat N, Poole J, Flatt JF, et al. The monovalent cation leak in overhydrated stomatocytic red blood cells results from amino acid substitutions in the Rh-associated glycoprotein. Blood. 2009;113:1350–7. http://www.ncbi.nlm.nih.gov/pubmed/18931342.
3. Andolfo I, Russo R, Gambale A, Iolascon A. New insights on hereditary erythrocyte membrane defects. Haematologica. 2016;101:1284–94.
4. Narla J, Mohandas N. Red cell membrane disorders. Int J Lab Hematol. 2017;39:47–52.
5. Delaunay J, Stewart G, Iolascon A. Hereditary dehydrated and overhydrated stomatocytosis: recent advances. Curr Opin Hematol. 1999;6:110–4. http://www.ncbi.nlm.nih.gov/pubmed/10088641.
6. Agarwal AM, Nussenzveig RH, Reading NS, Patel JL, Sangle N, Salama ME, et al. Clinical utility of next-generation sequencing in the diagnosis of hereditary haemolytic anaemias. Br J Haematol. 2016;174:806–14. https://doi.org/10.1111/bjh.14131.
7. Perrotta S, Gallagher PG, Mohandas N. Hereditary spherocytosis. Lancet. 2008;372:1411–26. https://doi.org/10.1016/S0140-6736(08)61588-3.
8. Kedar P. Red cell membrane pathology in hereditary spherocytosis in India. Indian J Hematol Blood Transfus. 2013;29(4):245–6.
9. Karan AS, Saxena R, Choudhry VP. Autosomal non-dominant hereditary spherocytosis: does it occur in India? Am J Hematol. 2002;70:266–7.
10. Das A, Bansal D, Das R, Trehan A, Marwaha RK. Hereditary spherocytosis in children: profile and post-splenectomy outcome. Indian Pediatr. 2014;51:139–41.
11. Tse WT, Lux SE. Red blood cell membrane disorders. Br J Haematol. 1999;104:2–13.
12. Eber SW, Gonzalez JM, Lux ML, Scarpa AL, Tse WT, Dornwell M, et al. Ankyrin–1 mutations are a major cause of dominant and recessive hereditary spherocytosis. Nat Genet. 1996;13:214–8. http://www.ncbi.nlm.nih.gov/pubmed/8640229.
13. Del Giudice EM, Nobili B, Francese M, D'Urso L, Iolascon A, Eber S, et al. Clinical and molecular evaluation of non-dominant hereditary spherocytosis. Br J Haematol. 2001;112:42–7.
14. del Giudice EM, Hayette S, Bozon M, Perrotta S, Alloisio N, Vallier A, et al. Ankyrin Napoli: a de novo deletional frameshift mutation in exon 16 of ankyrin gene (ANK1) associated with spherocytosis. Br J Haematol. 1996;93:828–34. http://www.ncbi.nlm.nih.gov/pubmed/8703812.
15. Morlé L, Bozon M, Alloisio N, Vallier A, Hayette S, Pascal O, et al. Ankyrin Bugey: a de novo deletional frameshift variant in exon 6 of the ankyrin gene associated with spherocytosis. Am J Hematol. 1997;54:242–8. http://www.ncbi.nlm.nih.gov/pubmed/9067504.
16. Hayette S, Carré G, Bozon M, Alloisio N, Maillet P, Wilmotte R, et al. Two distinct truncated variants of ankyrin associated with hereditary spherocytosis. Am J Hematol. 1998;58:36–41. http://www.ncbi.nlm.nih.gov/pubmed/9590147.
17. Random J, Miraglia Del Giudice E, Bozon M, Perrotta S, De Vivo M, Iolascon A, et al. Frequent de novo mutations of the ANK1 gene mimic a recessive mode of transmission in hereditary spherocytosis: three new ANK1 variants: Ankyrins Bari, Napoli II and Anzio. Br J Haematol. 1997;96:500–6.
18. Iolascon A, Miraglia del Giudice E, Perrotta S, Alloisio N, Morlé L, Delaunay J. Hereditary spherocytosis: from clinical to molecular defects. Haematologica. 1998;83:240–57. http://www.ncbi.nlm.nih.gov/pubmed/9573679.
19. Hamosh A, Scott AF, Amberger J, Valle D, McKusick VA. Online Mendelian inheritance in man (OMIM). Hum Mutat. 2000;15:57–61.
20. Bianchi P, Fermo E, Vercellati C, Marcello AP, Porretti L, Cortelezzi A, et al. Diagnostic power of laboratory tests for hereditary spherocytosis: a comparison study in 150 patients grouped according to molecular and clinical characteristics. Haematologica. 2012;97:516–23. http://www.ncbi.nlm.nih.gov/pubmed/22058213.
21. Kedar PS, Colah RB, Kulkarni S, Ghosh K, Mohanty D. Experience with eosin-5′-maleimide as a diagnostic tool for red cell membrane cytoskeleton disorders. Clin Lab Haematol. 2003;25:373–6.
22. Kar R, Mishra P, Pati HP. Evaluation of eosin-5-maleimide flow cytometric test in diagnosis of hereditary spherocytosis. Int J Lab Hematol. 2010;32:8–16.
23. Joshi P, Aggarwal A, Jamwal M, Sachdeva MUS, Bansal D, Malhotra P, et al. A comparative evaluation of Eosin-5′-maleimide flow cytometry reveals a high diagnostic efficacy for hereditary spherocytosis. Int J Lab Hematol. 2016;38:520–6.
24. Bolton-Maggs PHB, Langer JC, Iolascon A, Tittensor P, King M-J. Guidelines for the diagnosis and man-

agement of hereditary spherocytosis - 2011 update. Br J Haematol [Internet]. 2012;156:37–49. https:// doi.org/10.1111/j.1365-2141.2011.08921.x.

25. Alfinito F, Calabro V, Cappellini MD, Fiorelli G, Filosa S, Iolascon A, et al. Glucose 6-phosphate dehydrogenase deficiency and red cell membrane defects: additive or synergistic interaction in producing chronic haemolytic anaemia. Br J Haematol. 1994;87:148–52.

26. del Giudice EM, Perrotta S, Nobili B, Specchia C, d'Urzo G, Iolascon A. Coinheritance of Gilbert syndrome increases the risk for developing gallstones in patients with hereditary spherocytosis. Blood. 1999;94:2259–62.

27. Li CK, Heung-Ling Ng M, Cheung KL, Lam TK, Ming-Kong SM. Interaction of hereditary spherocytosis and alpha thalassaemia: a family study. Acta Haematol. 1994;91:201–5.

28. Sukumar S, Mukherjee MB, Colah RB, Mohanty D. Molecular basis of G6PD deficiency in India. Blood Cells Mol Dis. 2004;33:141–5.

29. Lee HJ, Moon HS, Lee ES, Kim SH, Sung JK, Lee BS, et al. A case of concomitant Gilbert's syndrome and hereditary spherocytosis. Korean J Hepatol. 2010;16:321–4. https://doi.org/10.3350/ kjhep.2010.16.3.321.

30. Iijima S, Ohzeki T, Maruo Y. Hereditary spherocytosis coexisting with UDP-glucuronosyltransferase deficiency highly suggestive of Crigler-Najjar syndrome type II. Yonsei Med J. 2011;52:369–72.

31. Rivet C, Caron N, Lachaux A, Morel B, Pracros JP, Francina A, et al. Association of a glucose-6-phosphate deficiency and a Gilbert syndrome as risk factors for a severe choledocholithiasis in a 2-month-old male infant. Pediatr Blood Cancer. 2012;58:316.

32. Jamwal M, Aggarwal A, Kumar V, Sharma P, Sachdeva MUS, Bansal D, et al. Disease-modifying influences of coexistent G6PD-deficiency, Gilbert syndrome and deletional alpha thalassemia in hereditary spherocytosis: a report of three cases. Clin Chim Acta. 2016;458:51–4. http://linkinghub.elsevier.com/ retrieve/pii/S0009898116301450.

33. Heaton DC, Fellowes AP, George PM. Concurrence of hereditary spherocytosis and alpha thalassaemia. Aust NZ J Med. 1991;21:485–6.

34. Gallagher PG. Hereditary elliptocytosis: spectrin and protein 4.1R. Semin Hematol. 2004;41:142–64.

35. Zhang Z, Weed SA, Gallagher PG, Morrow JS. Dynamic molecular modeling of pathogenic mutations in the spectrin self-association domain. Blood. 2001;98:1645–53.

36. Wrong O, Bruce LJ, Unwin RJ, Toye AM, Tanner MJA. Band 3 mutations, distal renal tubular acidosis, and Southeast Asian ovalocytosis. Kidney Int. 2002;62:10–9.

37. Reardon DM, Seymour CA, Cox TM, Pinder JC, Schofield AE, Tanner MJA. Hereditary ovalocytosis with compensated haemolysis. Br J Haematol. 1993;85:197–9.

38. Jarolim P, Palek J, Amato D, Hassan K, Sapak P, Nurse GT, et al. Deletion in erythrocyte band 3 gene in malaria-resistant Southeast Asian ovalocytosis. Proc Natl Acad Sci U S A. 1991;88:11022–6. http:// www.pubmedcentral.nih.gov/articlerender.fcgi?artid =53065&tool=pmcentrez&rendertype=abstract.

39. Picard V, Proust A, Eveillard M, Flatt JF, Couec ML, Caillaux G, et al. Homozygous Southeast Asian ovalocytosis is a severe dyserythropoietic anemia associated with distal renal tubular acidosis. Blood. 2014;123:1963–5.

40. Glogowska E, Gallagher PG. Disorders of erythrocyte volume homeostasis. Int J Lab Hematol. 2015;37:85–91.

41. Manzoor F, Bhat S, Bashir N, Geelani S, Rasool J. Hereditary stomatocytosis: first case report from Valley of Kashmir. Med J Dr DY Patil Univ. 2015;8:347. http://www.mjdrdypu.org/text. asp?2015/8/3/347/157083.

42. Jamwal M, Aggarwal A, Sachdeva MUS, Sharma P, Malhotra P, Maitra A, et al. Overhydrated stomatocytosis associated with a complex RHAG genotype including a novel de novo mutation. J Clin Pathol. 2018;71:648–52. https://doi.org/10.1136/ jclinpath-2018-205018.

43. Stewart GW, Amess JA, Eber SW, Kingswood C, Lane PA, Smith BD, et al. Thrombo-embolic disease after splenectomy for hereditary stomatocytosis. Br J Haematol. 1996;93:303–10.

44. Bruce LJ. Hereditary stomatocytosis and cation leaky red cells—recent developments. Blood Cells Mol Dis. 2009;42:216–22.

45. Houston BL, Zelinski T, Israels SJ, Coghlan G, Chodirker BN, Gallagher PG, et al. Refinement of the hereditary xerocytosis locus on chromosome 16q in a large Canadian kindred. Blood Cells Mol Dis. 2011;47:226–31.

46. Grootenboer S, Schischmanoff PO, Laurendeau I, Cynober T, Tchernia G, Dommergues JP, et al. Pleiotropic syndrome of dehydrated hereditary stomatocytosis, pseudohyperkalemia, and perinatal edema maps to 16q23-q24. Blood. 2000;96:2599–605. http://www.ncbi.nlm.nih.gov/pubmed/11001917.

47. Andolfo I, Russo R, Manna F, Shmukler BE, Gambale A, Vitiello G, et al. Novel Gardos channel mutations linked to dehydrated hereditary stomatocytosis (xerocytosis). Am J Hematol. 2015;90:921–6.

48. Rapetti-Mauss R, Lacoste C, Picard V, Guitton C, Lombard E, Loosveld M, et al. A mutation in the Gardos channel is associated with hereditary xerocytosis. Blood. 2015;126:1273–80.

49. Glogowska E, Lezon-Geyda K, Maksimova Y, Schulz VP, Gallagher PG. Mutations in the Gardos channel (KCNN4) are associated with hereditary xerocytosis. Blood. 2015;126:1281–4.

50. Andolfo I, Alper SL, Delaunay J, Auriemma C, Russo R, Asci R, et al. Missense mutations in the ABCB6 transporter cause dominant familialpseudohyperkalemia. Am J Hematol. 2013;88:66–72.

51. Rees DC, Iolascon A, Carella M, O'Marcaigh AS, Kendra JR, Jowitt SN, et al. Stomatocytic haemolysis and macrothrombocytopenia (Mediterranean stomatocytosis/macrothrombocytopenia) is the haematological presentation of phytosterolaemia. Br J Haematol. 2005;130:297–309.

52. Jamwal M, Aggarwal A, Maitra A, Sharma P, Bansal D, Trehan A, et al. First report of Mediterranean stomatocytosis/macrothrombocytopenia in an Indian family: a diagnostic dilemma. Pathology. 2017; 49:811.

53. Sun Y, Ruivenkamp CAL, Hoffer MJV, Vrijenhoek T, Kriek M, van Asperen CJ, et al. Next-generation diagnostics: gene panel, exome, or whole genome? Hum Mutat. 2015;36:648–55.

54. Roy NBA, Wilson EA, Henderson S, Wray K, Babbs C, Okoli S, et al. A novel 33-gene targeted resequencing panel provides accurate, clinical-grade diagnosis and improves patient management for rare inherited anaemias. Br J Haematol. 2016;175:318–30.

55. Del Orbe BR, Arrizabalaga B, De la Hoz AB, García-Orad A, Tejada MI, Garcia-Ruiz JC, et al. Detection of new pathogenic mutations in patients with congenital haemolytic anaemia using next-generation sequencing. Int J Lab Hematol. 2016;38: 629–38.

Historical Investigations and Advances in Flow Cytometry-Based Tests in Paroxysmal Nocturnal Hemoglobinuria

Khaliqur Rahman and Dinesh Chandra

6.1 Introduction

Paroxysmal nocturnal hemoglobinuria (PNH) is a nonmalignant, clonal hematopoietic stem cell disorder, which is characterized by features of hemolysis, thrombosis, and bone marrow (BM) failure. The genetic mechanism behind PNH is a somatic mutation in a gene known as phosphatidylinositol glycan class A (PIGA), present on chromosome "X." PIGA gene is required for the synthesis of glycosylphosphatidylinositol (GPI), the anchor through which many proteins are attached to the cell membrane. These proteins are collectively known as GPI-anchored proteins (GPI-APs) [1, 2]. Among these GPI-APs are CD55 and CD59, the two important complement regulatory proteins. Absence of these leads to complement-mediated red blood cell lysis, one of the characteristic features of PNH [3, 4]. The term "PNH," however, appears imprecise as only a fraction of patients presents with hemoglobinuria, which is also not always nocturnal.

It is a well-known fact that BM failure syndrome, especially aplastic anemia (AA), has a frequent association of PNH. A fair proportion of AA patients, as high as 70%, have been found to harbor a PNH clone, depending upon the sensitivity of the screening method used [5]. The clone size in these patients is usually much smaller as compared to those seen in classic PNH patients [6, 7]. However, a proportion of these patients may exhibit the clonal expansion and can progress to clinical hemolytic PNH. Hence, a careful screening to detect the presence of PNH clone in these cases is of utmost importance. The drug eculizumab, a humanized monoclonal antibody which inhibits the action of complement C5, has been a boon for PNH patient. Before its advent, a fair proportion of patients (~35%) used to die within 5 years of diagnosis even with the administration of the best available treatment option [8]. This drug significantly reduces the symptoms associated with PNH and the transfusion requirement of these patients. It has been shown to improve the life expectancy as well as the quality of life of PNH patient. Eculizumab (Soliris, Alexion Pharmaceuticals) is one of the costliest drugs of the world, and this fact again underscores the utility of an accurate clone size estimation [PNH clone in MDS and other diseases need to be also included here].

Presence of PNH clones in myelodysplastic syndrome is also a well-established fact. With a stringent flow cytometry-based screening, about 35% of refractory anemia can show the presence of PNH clone, and there can be a clonal expansion of PNH in the cases with MDS. It has now been well established that PNH is more

K. Rahman (✉) · D. Chandra
Department of Hematology, Sanjay Gandhi Post Graduate Institute of Medical Sciences, Lucknow, Uttar Pradesh, India
e-mail: khaliq@sgpgi.ac.in

© Springer Nature Singapore Pte Ltd. 2019
R. Saxena, H. P. Pati (eds.), *Hematopathology*, https://doi.org/10.1007/978-981-13-7713-6_6

frequently noted in MDS patients who present with BM failure. These patients with an associated PNH clone are less likely to transform into leukemia and have a better prognosis [9–11].

There are also reports of finding a PNH clone in JAK2-mutated myeloproliferative neoplasm [12]. However, their exact significance as well as follow-up of the clone sizes is largely unknown.

6.2   Historical Perspective of PNH

Some of the landmark developments related to PNH are summarized as follows:

1882: Paul Strubing from Germany first identified PNH as an entity, separate from paroxysmal cold hemoglobinuria (PCH) and march hemoglobinuria. He concluded that sleep played an important role in hemolysis. Accumulation of lactic acid and carbon dioxide because of slowing of the circulation during sleep was reasoned for this phenomenon. According to him, normal RBCs were resistant to acidic conditions; while, the defective RBCs were sensitive and got lysed [13].

Early twentieth Century: Marchiafava and Micheli got interested in this disease, and PNH got its eponym as Marchiafava–Micheli disease [14].

1911: Dutch physician Hijmans van den Berg first suggested the role of a plasma factor, now known as complement, in hemolysis of PNH patients. It was shown that when the RBCs from PNH patients were suspended in serum of normal subjects or patients' own serum, they got lysed because of the presence of complements in the serum [15].

1928: Dutch physician Ennekin first used the term "paroxysmal nocturnal hemoglobinuria" [16].

1937: Thomas Hale Ham reported that treatment of PNH patients with sodium bicarbonate reduces hemoglobinemia and hemoglobinuria. He performed some in vitro tests by acidifying the plasma with CO_2 or lactic acid and putting the patients' RBCs in it. This test remained one of the most common and useful tests for screening of PNH. He observed that there was rapid hemolysis when the serum or plasma was acidified. This hemolysis could be inhibited by adding sodium bicarbonate. An important additional information was that the red cells from blood group "O" volunteers did not hemolyze when resuspended in patients' serum or plasma. He thus concluded that the main defect lied in the red cells of these patients, whereas the factor for the lysis is present in plasma of all individuals. He also noted that the lysis was not noted when the acidified serum was heated at 60 degrees and thus concluded that a thermolabile factor (complement) was responsible for the hemolysis [17, 18].

1939: Ham and Dingle published a landmark paper titled "Certain immunological aspects of the hemolytic mechanisms with special reference to serum complement" that had repercussion on the PNH research for next five decades [19].

1954: Pillemer identified the properdin system (the alternative complement pathway system) which was later confirmed to be involved in PNH pathogenesis [20].

1963: Dacie identified the phenotypic mosaicism in PNH RBC [21].

1966: Rosse developed an assay to test the complement sensitivity of PNH RBCs, better known as complement lysis sensitivity assay. Based on this test, he concluded that PNH mostly has a mosaic of two abnormal populations of RBC, which were later known as type II and type III cells [22].

1969: Aster and Enright demonstrated that platelets and neutrophils from PNH patients are abnormally sensitive to complement-mediated lysis [23]. Hoffmann showed the presence of factors that inhibited complement-mediated hemolysis in human RBC stroma [24, 25].

1970: Studies by Oni and colleagues indicated the monoclonal nature of the complement-sensitive erythrocytes [26].

1974: Hoffmann used the name decay accelerating factor (DAF) describing the functional property of the substance that enhanced the decay rate of classic pathway C3 convertase. This is now commonly known as CD55 [27].

1979: Stern and Rosse demonstrated the mosaic nature of granulocytes, similar to RBCs [28].

1983: Pangburn et al. demonstrated functional as well as immunochemical evidence of DAF deficiency in PNH [29].

1986: It was first hypothesized that on the hematopoietic cells of PNH, all the deficient proteins are GPI anchored, and all the GPI-APs are deficient in case of PNH [30].

1987: The complex structure of the GPI anchor was fully elucidated. It was suggested that the expression of the GPI-AP on cell surface would require multiple enzymes and cofactors.

1989: Holguin and colleagues reported the isolation membrane inhibitor of reactive lysis from the cell surface of normal human RBCs. This substance is now commonly known as CD59 [31].

1993: Kinoshita and colleagues suggested the defect in a common gene in the complementation class A. This gene was named as phosphatidylinositol glycan A (PIGA). Due to a defect in this gene, PNH cells fail to synthesize N-acetylglucosamine phosphatidylinositol [32].

Early 1990s: Flow cytometric detection of cells lacking the expression of GPI AP.

2000: Use of fluorescent aerolysin (FLAER) for better sensitive detection of PNH clones using flow cytometry [33].

2008: Two hit concept in PNH, first hit leading to PIGA mutation, the second hit usually an epigenetic phenomenon giving survival advantage for the proliferation of PNH clones [34].

2010: ICCS guideline for flow cytometry-based detection of PNH clones [35].

2012: Practical guidelines for high sensitivity analysis and monitoring of PNH clones by flow cytometry was published [36].

6.3 Diagnostic Modalities for PNH

6.3.1 In Vitro Methods Demonstrating Complement-Mediated Hemolysis

Introduction of these tests started with the discovery that the lysis of RBC in PNH is dependent on a thermolabile serum factor (now known as a complement). Increased susceptibility of RBC lysis with activated complement could be demonstrated by a variety of tests like acidified serum [18], thrombin [37], cold antibody lysis [38],

sucrose [39], cobra venom [40], and inulin [41]. Acidified serum, cobra venom, and inulin activate the complement via the alternative pathway; whereas cold antibody test and thrombin test activate the complement via the classic pathway. In sucrose lysis tests, the low ionic strength leads to nonspecific binding of IgG to the cell surface and subsequent activation of complement via classic as well as an alternate pathway. Among the abovementioned tests, the Hams acidified serum lysis and sucrose lysis tests were most commonly used. But these have now become obsolete owing to their cumbersome nature, low sensitivity, specificity, and not being quantitative. The classic Hams test is negative if <5% type III PNH cells are present. Additionally, it may give false positivity in CDA type II (HEMPAS). Similarly, false positivity of sucrose lysis test can be seen in megaloblastic anemia, autoimmune hemolytic anemia, etc. The complement lysis tests developed by Rosse and colleagues could give an idea of the quantity and type of hemolytic RBCs [42, 43]. They showed that PNH was a heterogeneous disease with three populations of red cells. These were cells with normal sensitivity (type I), cells of medium sensitivity (type II, which are 3–5 times more sensitive), and very sensitive cells (which are 10–15 times more sensitive than the normal cells, type III).

6.3.2 Methods Utilizing Hemagglutinition and Gel Card System

This method was utilized in the 1980s when antibodies against CD55 (DAF) and CD59 (MIRL) were used to see the RBC agglutinition in the microcolumns of the gel card. Normal RBCs would agglutinate, while the RBCs deficient in CD55/CD59 would not agglutinate [44]. The commercially available kits have micro typing cards containing sephacryl and anti-mouse antibody from rabbit within a gel matrix. Erythrocyte suspension in low ionic strength buffer is added to three microtubes; followed by anti-CD55 antibody, anti-CD59 antibody, and a negative control in these three tubes and labeling them, respectively. The card is centrifuged for 10 min. PNH cells lacking CD55 or CD59 epitopes settle down at the bottom, whereas normal cells expressing CD55 and CD59 clump on top of the sephacryl gel. This test is easier to perform compared with complement-based tests. However, certain limitations include its poor sensitivity, which has been reported as 2–10% of type III RBCs, and not being quantitative [45].

6.3.3 Flow Cytometry-Based Methods

Flow cytometric methods have been in vogue for PNH clone detection since the late 1980s and early 1990s. Classically, they utilize fluorescently tagged antibodies against the GPI-APs. Numerous GPI-APs have been identified in different cell lineages that can be targeted for this purpose (Fig. 6.1). Absent expression of these antigens (GPI-AP) suggests a diagnosis of PNH. More recently, FLAER has been used, which directly binds to the GPI anchor. Use of FLAER has markedly increased the sensitivity of flow-based assay [46].

6.4 Flow Cytometry-Based PNH Testing

Flow cytometric detection of differential expression of DAF (CD55) on the normal and PNH RBCs can be traced back to 1985 [47]. The flow cytometric methods for the detection of GPI-linked antibody have now become the method of choice. Since the clinical manifestation of PNH predominantly involved complement-mediated hemolysis, all the initial research studies were focused on finding the proteins involved it. CD55 (DAF) was identified first, which was named after the functional property of this material to enhance the rate at which the activity of a classic pathway C3 convertase diminished [25]. Subsequently, it

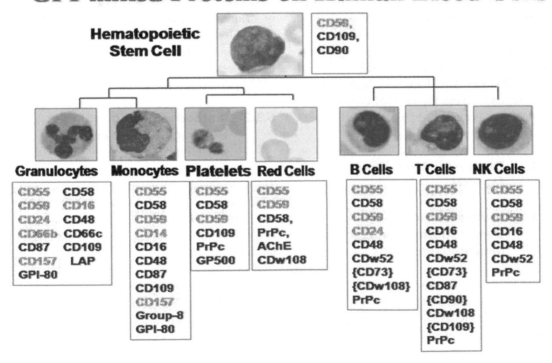

Fig. 6.1 GPI-linked protein in different blood cells. Commonly used markers in flow cytometry analysis are highlighted in blue

was realized that DAF cannot be the sole mechanism responsible for all the abnormalities of the membrane attack complex (MAC). Hence, search for substances which regulated the MAC led to the identification of a protein from the surface of normal erythrocytes that inhibited reactive lysis of PNH erythrocytes [31]. As soon as the deficiencies of CD55 and CD59 in PNH were confirmed, their absence found using flow cytometry techniques was being used to define a PNH clone. Sooner it was noted that a few patients in spite of being deficient for CD55 or CD59 did not have any manifestation of PNH. It was subsequently realized that these were some familial cases of isolated CD55 or CD59 deficiency. Hence, it was recommended to use both CD55 and CD59. True PNH cases used to be deficient for both these antibodies, in contrast to familial cases where RBC was deficient for either CD55 or CD59. The simple flow cytometric assays using CD55- and CD59-based approaches, however, are neither sensitive nor accurate, rendering them inadequate to detect small clone size which is frequently seen in AA and MDS. Hence, development and validation of standardized methodologies using other robust GPI-linked reagents were required.

6.4.1 Specimen Consideration

The preferred and widely accepted sample for the flow cytometric testing of PNH is ethylene-diamine-tetra-acetic acid (EDTA) anticoagulated peripheral blood. However, other anticoagulants like heparin and acid citrate dextrose (ACD) can also be used. BM is not preferred owing to variable expression of antibodies used for screening in different stages of RBC and WBC development. However, some of the newer antibodies used like FLAER and CD157 do not have a much variable expression on different stages of cells.

The sample should be processed preferably within 48 h. However, inevitable delay in the RBC analysis can be overcome by storing the sample in the refrigerator at 4 °C for a period of 7 days. Long-term storage of RBC can be done by freezing the sample in 25% dextrose. For WBC screening, sample storage may lead to

change in scatter properties, ultimately leading to difficulty in gating the polymorphs and monocytes. Hence, it is recommended to complete the analysis within 48 h.

6.4.2 Cell Lineages to be Screened for PNH

Screening of PNH clone and accurate estimation of the clone size in red cells is of utmost importance, as the clone size directly correlates with hemolysis and thrombosis, the main clinical manifestation of this disease. However, isolated testing of RBCs is never recommended because of underestimation of exact clone size owing to an ongoing hemolysis and subsequent transfusion. Hence, WBC (granulocytes and monocytes) screening is recommended with RBC screening and a comparison of RBC and WBC clone sizes provides useful clinical information. It may be a frequent observation to have a PNH clone in WBCs without PNH RBC clone. But, the vice versa is almost never seen. In our own experience of FLAER-based PNH screening in leukocytes, almost all the cases with a PNH clone size of less than 2% in WBC did not show any PNH RBC clone [7]. Screening of lymphocytes is not recommended owing to their long life as well as variable expression of the GPI-linked antigens on lymphoid cells.

6.4.3 Analysis of RBC

CD59 is expressed at a more abundant level as compared to CD55. Additionally, CD55 does not provide a good separation of type II cell population. Hence, for the single reagent analysis, CD59 is preferred over CD55.

One of the important considerations in RBC analysis is frequent aggregate formation on the addition of antibodies. Hence extra wash steps and frequent vortexing/racking are required to disaggregate the RBC clumps. It is also recommended to dilute the antibodies to an extent which gives sufficient positive signals without producing much of RBC clumps. The use of IgM antibody is to be avoided. Strategies which include both CD55 and CD59 should be carried out after a careful titration of antibodies. Antibodies should be diluted, and the lowest concentration that gives acceptable positive signals should be used.

CD235a (glycophorin A) which is used to gate the RBCs in a high sensitivity analysis causes significant aggregation of RBC, owing to its very high surface density. Aggregation is typically higher with the PE conjugates as compared to FITC. In general, a much higher dilution of this antibody is required for PNH RBC analysis, as compared to those used for BM leukemia immunophenotyping. In our practice, the CD235a-FITC reagent from BD Biosciences (San Jose, CA, USA) is diluted 1:200 times before adding 10 microliters of the diluted form for gating RBC. It is thus stressed that each laboratory should carefully evaluate the optimal dilution of antibodies, so that acceptable signals are noted with very limited aggregation (Fig. 6.2).

Gating and Analysis: RBCs can be identified in a log-scaled FSC vs. SSC scatterplot. When no lysis is used, almost all the cells seen in the scatterplot are RBCs. The tube should be vortexed vigorously before acquisition, in order to disaggregate the RBC clumps. Voltage and threshold should be adjusted so that the RBCs are seen in the center of the scatterplot. For high sensitivity analysis, it is recommended to use a gating marker (CD235a—glycophorin A). This is done to get a pure population of RBCs and exclude the platelet clumps, which could falsely get included in FSC vs. SSC gate. As mentioned above, adding CD235 may significantly increase the aggregation of RBCs and hence optimum dilution is required. Gated RBCs are displayed on the single parameter histogram of CD55 or CD59. A negative control consisting of CD235a-stained RBC is only used to identify the expected position of type III RBCs. Normal RBCs represent the type I cells, while type II cells are represented in area between type I and type III cells. Dots plots provide better representation of small PNH clones, which are usually not very well seen with one dimensional histogram. RBCs are the easiest targets for a high sensitivity analysis, especially in cases of AA, where getting 2.5 lakh leukocytes may be difficult.

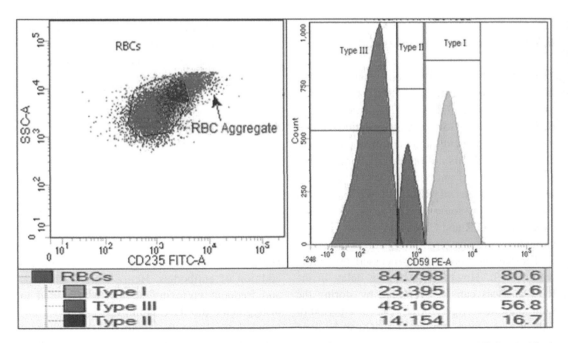

Fig. 6.2 Gating of RBCs using CD235. The RBC aggregates are seen as projection of scatter dots at 45° diagonal line. On one dimensional histogram of CD59 PE, the RBCs exhibit three populations of RBCs

6.4.4 Leukocyte Assay

Analyses of neutrophils and monocytes are widely used for accessing the clone size. However, there are instances where a sufficient number of monocytes or neutrophils are difficult to acquire. Lymphocytes are not used for screening purpose owing to their long life as well as variable expression of the GPI-linked antigens on their surface.

For dealing with leukocytes, getting rid of RBCs by lysing them is an important step in cell processing. Mostly, the stain-lyse-wash method is preferred, where lysis can be performed by any commercially available or in-house method that does not compromise the scatter properties. For screening of leukocytes in cases of pancytopenia (AA or myelodysplastic syndrome), it may be necessary to prelyse the red cells taking more samples. In these situations, especially for high sensitivity PNH screening, a bulk lysis with 500 μL of the sample using formalin-free ammonium chloride-based lysing agent is preferred.

Since the leukocyte screening grew out of the experience from RBC staining, earlier CD59 and CD55 were the commonly used markers. Slowly, the knowledge about other GPI-linked leukocyte surface antigens grew, and these were explored for PNH testing using flow cytometry. CD66b, CD24, and CD16 were commonly used for granulocytes, while CD14 was commonly used as a monocytic marker. CD48 and CD157 were some of the other used markers, but their experience was limited.

6.5 FLAER as Marker for Both Granulocyte and Monocyte

Discovery of FLAER had a great impact on leukocyte screening for PNH. It was noted that the binding of aerolysin, a channel-forming toxin from bacterium *Aeromonas hydrophila*, is determined by the presence of GPI anchors of membrane glycoproteins. Hence, PNH cells which were deficient in GPI anchor were not lysed by this bacterium. Aerolysin is secreted as an inactive form, pro-aerolysin, activation of which

requires a proteolytic cleavage of the C-terminal peptide [48, 49]. FLAER is a mutant form of pro-aerolysin, labeled with a fluorophore Alexa Fluor 488. It has the binding property but lacks the channel-forming property of active aerolysin. Peripheral blood nucleated cells are able to bind to FLAER because they are able to convert pro-aerolysin to aerolysin by using proteases like furin present on their cell surface. RBCs lack these proteases and hence are unable to bind [33, 49]. FLAER is manufactured by Pinewood Scientific (Vancouver, BC, Canada). For some years after its discovery, its wide use was limited owing to its lyophilized preparation, which was inconvenient to use as well as unstable. Later, more stable reagents were available. Nowadays the liquid form of this reagent is available, that has better stability and storage requirement comparable to commonly used antibodies. However, there are still some countries where this reagent is not available. Screening of PNH clone in leukocytes using FLAER is currently the gold standard for flow cytometry-based screening (Fig. 6.3).

6.5.1 CD157 as Marker for Both Granulocyte and Monocyte

CD157 has been identified as one of the promising reagents which is expressed on both polymorphs and monocytes [50]. CD157 is also known as bone marrow stromal cell antigen 1 (BST 1). It is a single-chain GPI-AP which is helpful in pre-B cell growth. It is expressed on B cell progenitors, T progenitors, granulocytes, monocytes, and some other cells as well. It is structurally and functionally similar to CD38.

Sutherland et al. reported the use of CD157 as a common PNH marker and demonstrated its utility in a two-tube four-color as well as single-tube five-color combinations in FLAER-based PNH screening [51]. It has been found as a sensitive marker with a low background rate in normal sample [52]. CD157-based PNH screening was found to be very precise with minimal inter-assay and intra-assay variations [52, 53]. It provided a better separation between the PNH-negative and

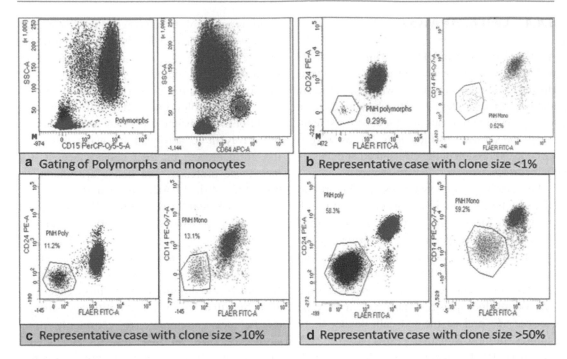

Fig. 6.3 Screening of PNH clones in leukocytes using flow cytometry. (**a**) Gating strategy. (**b–d**) representative scatterplots showing detectable PNH clone of variable size

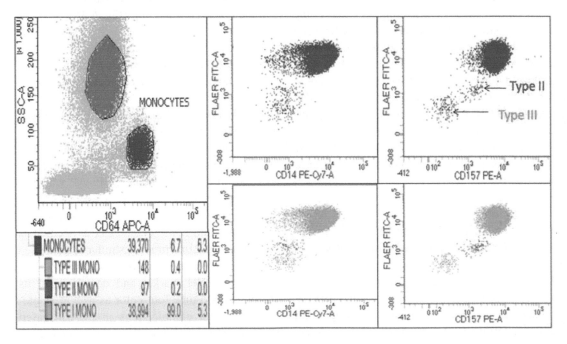

Fig. 6.4 Advantage of CD157 in better distinction of type II and type III clones

PNH-positive populations. Additionally, there was a better identification of type II PNH clones compared to CD24/CD14-based assay (Fig. 6.4). It can be used in a single-tube five-color combi-nation and can replace the two-tube four-color assay, thus leading to reduction in both reagent and technical time cost. Replacing the single-tube six-color assay will not reduce the cost of

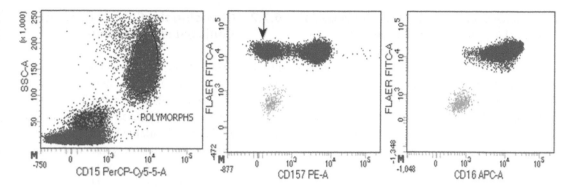

Fig. 6.5 A proportion of gated polymorphs (shown by arrow) showing loss of CD157 expression, but are positive for FLAER, indicating them to be normal cells. These cells are seen to co-express FLAER and CD16 (another PNH marker) at normal level. The true PNH clone is negative for FLAER, CD157, as well as CD16 (shown in blue)

technical time, but will definitely reduce the reagent (antibody) cost.

Some of the papers as well as verbal communication with some of the researchers have shown that there are cases which show a subset of granulocytes and monocytes population to be negative for CD157 but express FLAER. Hence, these were not considered as the true PNH clones. The exact reason for this phenomenon has not yet been established. But, the phenotypic polymorphism has been suggested as one of the probable reason. In our own experience, we had one such case out of some 200 odd cases that were screened using FLAER/CD157 in a single-tube five-color combination (Fig. 6.5). Recently, one of the papers has highlighted the importance of CD157 in a non-FLAER-based screening [54]. They confirmed a good performance characteristic and agreement between the FLAER- and non-FLAER-based approaches, using CD157. They highlighted its importance in a cost-effective analysis especially in those areas of the world where FLAER is not available. However, taking in view the selective absence of CD157 in a proportion of cases, replacement of FLAER does not seem to be a wise step at this point of time.

Gating and Analysis: For routine sensitivity analysis, FSC vs. SSC or CD45 vs. SSC analysis is sufficient for gating granulocytes and monocytes. However, in cases of MDS where the scatter properties are altered, gating the granulocytes and separating them from monocytes may be difficult. Getting a pure population based on CD45

vs. SSC plot may be difficult for monocytes as well, especially if they are in low number. Hence, for better delineation and for high sensitivity analysis, use of gating markers like CD15 for granulocytes and CD33/CD64 for monocytes is recommended. CD64 has been found to be a better marker as compared to CD33 to get a purer population of monocytes [7]. For routine analysis, acquisition of 5000–10,000 gated population is sufficient, but for high sensitivity analysis, 2.5 lakh events are recommended. This may be difficult for monocytes especially in cases with pancytopenia, and hence a lower number of monocytes is acceptable.

6.6 Routine Sensitivity Versus High Sensitivity Analysis

A routine sensitivity analysis is one which is sufficient enough for detecting PNH clones at 1% level, while high sensitivity analysis should be able to detect the clone sizes of 0.01%. For classic PNH patients, who present with features of hemolysis or thrombosis, a routine analysis may be sufficient enough to detect the presence of PNH clone. However, in patients with AA and MDS who usually do not have the clinical features of hemolysis, the clone size is small and in a majority of patients less than 1%. In these cases, a routine sensitivity analysis will miss the PNH clone detection in a majority of cases. Identifying these minor clones are important as ~25% of these patients may show expansion of clone size and may later present with clinical PNH.

For routine analysis, RBCs are gated on log-scaled FSC vs. SSC plot. The use of CD235a as a gating marker is optional and not mandatory. But for high sensitivity analysis, use of CD235a as a gating marker for RBCs is mandatory. For gating the leukocytes, CD45 vs. side scatter may be sufficient to gate the granulocytes as well as monocytes in a routine sensitivity analysis. However, for high sensitivity analysis, it is desirable to use a gating marker (CD15 for granulocytes and CD33/CD64 for monocytes); to get a pure population, FLAER plus one other informative reagent is mandatory for identifying a PNH clone. About 5000–10,000 gated events may be sufficient for routine sensitivity analysis, but for high sensitivity analysis, 2.5 lakhs of gated population is recommended [35].

6.7 Quality Assurance for High Sensitivity Analysis

6.7.1 Instrument Setup

As with any other high sensitivity analysis of rare events, an optimum instrument setup is required. The PMT voltage setup, scatter properties, and optimal fluorescence compensation are required. PMT voltage is set using unstained cells and making them lie on the scale in the negative area. It is cross-checked using the bright antibody-fluorochrome conjugate, usually CD3, ensuring that CD3-positive T cells do not go off scale and CD3-negative B cells are properly on the scale in the negative region and not crushed against the axis. If required, the PMT voltage is lowered down to bring the positive signal on the scale. Fluorochrome compensations can be set using the beads or the cells. If antibody capture beads are used, these are stained with the same antibody-fluorochrome conjugate which is to be used in the panel, except for FLAER, which can be replaced by CD3-AF488. Using cells, the compensation can be set up, staining the lymphocytes in different tubes with CD3 in different fluorochromes. The compensation can be cross-checked by staining the cells using antibody cocktails.

6.7.2 Choosing the Correct Reagent Conjugates and Clones

FLAER and CD24/CD157 are the most commonly used combination for the screening of granulocytes, while FLAER and CD14/CD157 are the most commonly used combination for monocytes [36, 51]. Available literature has some recommendations for the reagents and fluorochrome conjugates, which can be used in 4, 5, or 6 color combinations [35, 55]. These reagents and clones have extensively been checked to be preferred over other clone and conjugate combination. These are mentioned in Tables 6.1, 6.2, 6.3, 6.4, and 6.5 [55]. If some laboratory wants to use its own combination, it should be thoroughly checked for the proper functioning of these reagents.

6.7.3 Frequency of PNH-Positive Cells in Normal Samples

At least 10–20 peripheral blood samples from healthy volunteers should be subjected to PNH testing to determine the background level of PNH-positive cells. Studies have shown an average of 0.0004% PNH-type RBCs, 0.0013% PNH-type granulocytes, and 0.0033% PNH-type monocytes in normal individuals [36]. If the assay is fully optimized, the laboratory cutoff can be determined using mean value + 4 standard deviation from these normal samples.

Table 6.1 Recommended red blood cell antibodies and clones: Beckman Coulter and Becton Dickinson instruments

Antibody conjugate	Purpose	Clone (source)
CD235a-FITC	Gating the RBCs	YTH89.1 (Cedarlane Laboratories) 10F7MN (eBiosciences / Thermo Fisher Scientific) KC16 (Beckman Coulter) JC159 (DAKO, Agilent Technologies)
CD59 PE	GPI linked for RBCs	OV9A2 (eBiosciences) MEM43 (Invitrogen) MEM43 (ExBio)

Table 6.2 Recommended white blood cell antibodies and clones: Beckman Coulter

Antibody conjugate	Purpose	Clone (source)
FLAER	GPI linked (granulocytes and monocytes)	NA (Cedarlane Lab, Ontario, Canada)
CD24 PE	GPI linked (granulocytes)	SN3 (eBiosciences, Thermo Fisher Scientific) ALB9 (Beckman Coulter)
CD24 APC	GPI linked (granulocytes)	SN3 (eBiosciences)
CD14 PE	GPI linked (monocytes)	61D3 (eBiosciences) RMO52 (Beckman Coulter) Tuk4 (Invitrogen)
CD14 APC700	GPI linked (monocytes)	RMO52 (BC)
CD157 PE	GPI linked (granulocytes and monocytes)	SY11B5 (eBiosciences)
CD64 PC5	Gating (monocytes)	22 (Beckman Coulter)
CD64 ECD	Gating (monocytes)	22 (Beckman Coulter)
CD64 PC7	Gating (monocytes)	22 (Beckman Coulter)
CD15 PC5	Gating (granulocytes)	80H5 (Beckman Coulter)
CD15 PerCP eF710	Gating (granulocytes)	MMA (eBiosciences)
CD45 PC7	Leukocyte gating, pattern recognition, and debris exclusion	J33 (Beckman Coulter)
CD45 KO	Leukocyte gating, pattern recognition, and debris exclusion	J33 (Beckman Coulter)
CD45 eF450	Leukocyte gating, pattern recognition, and debris exclusion	2D1 (eBio)

Table 6.4 Recommended white blood cell antibodies and clone for Becton Dickinson

Antibody conjugate	Purpose	Clone (source)
FLAER	GPI linked (granulocytes and monocytes)	NA (Cedarlane Lab, Ontario, Canada)
CD24 PE	GPI linked (granulocytes)	SN3 (eBiosciences, Thermo Fisher Scientific) ML5 (Becton Dickinson)
CD24 APC	GPI linked (granulocytes)	SN3 (eBiosciences)
CD14 PE	GPI linked (monocytes)	61D3 (eBiosciences) MOP9 (Becton Dickinson) Tuk4 (Invitrogen)
CD14 APC	GPI linked (monocytes)	MOP9 (Becton Dickinson)
CD157 PE	GPI linked (granulocytes and monocytes)	SY11B5 (eBiosciences)
CD64 APC	Gating (monocytes)	10.1 (Becton Dickinson) 10.1 (eBiosciences)
CD64 PC7	Gating (monocytes)	10.1 (Becton Dickinson)
CD15 APC	Gating (granulocytes)	HI98 (Becton Dickinson)
CD15 PerCP eF710	Gating (granulocytes)	MMA (eBiosciences)
CD15 eF450	Gating (granulocytes)	MMA (eBiosciences)
CD45 PerCP	Leukocyte gating, pattern recognition, and debris exclusion	2D1 (eBiosciences)
CD45 APCH7	Leukocyte gating, pattern recognition, and debris exclusion	2D1 (Becton Dickinson)
CD45 eF450	Leukocyte gating, pattern recognition, and debris exclusion	2D1 (eBiosciences)

Table 6.3 Recommended white blood cell panel: Beckman Coulter cytometers

	AF488	PE	ECD	PC5	eF710	PC7	APC	APCA 700	KrO	eF450
4 C Gran	FLAER	CD24	–	CD15	–	CD45	–	–	–	–
4 C Mono	FLAER	CD14	–	CD64	–	CD45	–	–	–	–
5 C (Gran + Mono)	FLAER	CD157	CD64	CD15	–	CD45	–	–	–	–
6 C (Gran + Mono)	FLAER	CD24	–	CD15	–	CD64	–	CD14	CD45	–
6 C (Gran + Mono)	FLAER	CD157	–	–	CD15	CD64	CD24	–	–	CD45

Table 6.5 Recommended white blood cells panel: Becton Dickinson cytometers

	AF488	PE	PerCP	PCPeF710	PC7	APC	APCH7	eF450
4 C Gran	FLAER	CD24	CD45	–	–	CD15	–	–
4 C Mono	FLAER	CD14	CD45	–	–	CD64	–	–
5 C (Gran + Mono)	FLAER	CD157	CD45	–	–	CD64	–	CD15
5 C (Gran + Mono)	FLAER	CD157	–	CD15		CD64	CD45	
6 C (Gran + Mono)	FLAER	CD24	CD45	–	CD64	CD14	–	CD15
6 C (Gran + Mono)	FLAER	CD24	–	CD15	CD64	CD14	CD45	
6 C (Gran + Mono)	FLAER	CD157	–	CD15	CD64	CD24		CD45

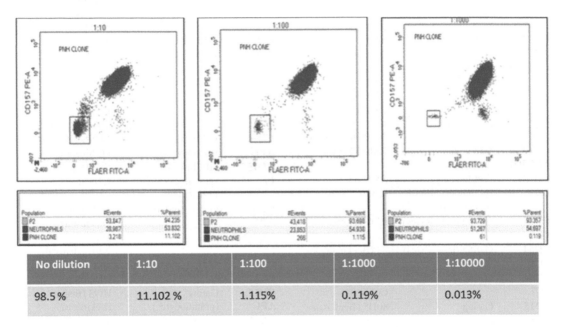

No dilution	1:10	1:100	1:1000	1:10000
98.5%	11.102%	1.115%	0.119%	0.013%

Fig. 6.6 Spiking experiment done during validation of CD157. A linear relation was noted between the dilution and proportion of PNH-positive cells

6.7.4 Sensitivity of the Assay Using Dilution/Spiking Experiments

Fresh PNH-positive sample can be diluted in a normal peripheral blood sample. A serial tenfold dilution yielding 1:10, 1:100, 1:1000, and 1:10,000 should be tested for the linearity of dilution and size of PNH clone. It is desirable to get 100 PNH (FLAER-negative CD14/CD24 or CD157-negative) events. However, for higher dilutions, 30–50 clustered events or one million total gated leukocytes may be acceptable (Fig. 6.6).

6.7.5 Inter-Assay and Intra-Assay Variability

This can be tested by running the same stained tube multiple times (minimum three times) for intra-assay variability testing or staining the same sample multiple times in separate tubes and analyzing each tube individually. This should be done with samples having a wide range of PNH clone size. A higher variation may be observed in cases with lower clone sizes as compared to those having a higher clone size. Any variation of less than 10% is acceptable.

6.7.6 External Quality Assurance Program

College of American Pathologists in North America and the United Kingdom National External Quality Assessment Service in Europe provide the external quality assurance program. The former provides EQA for RBC analysis only while the latter is for leukocyte immunophenotyping. It has been demonstrated that stabilized whole blood sample is suitable for the currently recommended high sensitivity analysis. It has also been highlighted that using the carefully selected conjugates and standardized protocol can lead to reduced variation around the median even for experienced laboratories [56]. A recent study has demonstrated that using same standardized four-color assay on fresh samples had good precision and reproducibility performance. It also had a good correlation and agreement between centers (both novice and experienced) for all target PNH clone sizes [57]. Whatever be the approach, it is important to have continuing education for standardized testing and reporting of PNH. Exchange of samples between the laboratories is also recommended as one of the important steps for standardizing the testing of this rare condition.

6.8 Data Interpretation and Reporting

Clinical PNH cases, who present with hemolysis, usually have large PNH clone sizes. The PNH clone size in AA is usually significantly lower in comparison with classic PNH group. Routinely, these cases have a clone size of less than 10%, with most of them showing a minor clone of less than 1%. The clinical significance of this small size clone is controversial. But it is important to detect PNH clones in AA because of three important reasons. (1) Some studies, but not all, have shown that AA with the presence of PNH clone had a better response to immunosuppressive therapy [58–60]. (2) Finding a PNH clone virtually rules out other causes of inherited BM failure syndrome. Studies have shown that none of the cases of AA with PNH clone exhibit increased chromosome breakage [7, 46]. (3) A fair proportion of these patients may show an increase in clone size and progression of these subclinical PNH cases to frank clinical hemolytic PNH. Use of immunosuppressive therapy in the form of ATG may also lead to an increase in clone size [61].

Some of the cases of AA may have a large clone size of more than 50% [7, 46, 61]. Interestingly, even in the presence of a large clone size, many of these patients do not show clinical or laboratory evidence of hemolysis. The probable reason for this would be a reduced absolute mass of newly formed RBCs/reticulocytes (as a result of marrow hypoplasia in AA), which are the most sensitive cells to complement-mediated lysis. In contrast, classic PNH cases have more of these neocytes (as a result of compensatory erythropoiesis) and thus more features of hemolysis.

The PNH clone size of leukocytes is usually greater than that of RBCs. This can be explained by two mechanisms: one being the complement-mediated lysis of RBC and the other being the dilution of the PNH-positive RBCs following transfusion. However, RBC analysis is useful as RBC clone size directly correlates with the clinical features. Additionally, RBC staining is better in demonstrating the partial antigen deficiency as compared to the granulocytes. There is no specific cutoff, but cases with more than 20% type III RBCs are likely to be symptomatic. Cases with large type II and absence of significant type III populations show reticulocytosis with elevated LDH levels but less hemolysis [35]. Monitoring RBC clone is also important in cases with eculizumab therapy, as the drug prevents the complement-mediated hemolysis and hence the size of RBC clone increases with ongoing therapy.

Among the leukocytes, the reliability of neutrophils in assessing the clone sizes is better than monocytes, owing to the relatively lower number of monocytes that could be acquired and analyzed. But, for the cases where a sufficient number of monocytes could be analyzed, the clone size of monocytes is usually found to be greater than neutrophils [7, 36, 46]. There have been reports by some authors documenting that the analysis of monocytes and reticulocytes gives the best estimation of clone sizes in patients with small PNH clone [62].

It is of utmost importance to avoid the term negative or positive in the reports to avoid confusion (the cells "Positive" for GPI markers are actually "negative" for PNH and vice versa). Hence it is better to use the term "PNH clones detected" and "no PNH clones detected." The total proportion of abnormal cells (type II + type III) should be mentioned for each lineage of cells analyzed. For RBCs, it is important to give information about the type II clone sizes. The importance of type II clone size for leukocytes is not well understood. Repeat testing is recommended for cases of AA. However, there is no requirement of repeat testing for the patient with unexplained thrombosis or hemolysis, where no PNH clone is detected. The small clone size should include a language in the report that should make clear that this is not the same as a diagnosis of hemolytic PNH. A mention of the antibody cocktail used along with the sensitivity of the assay should also be incorporated in the report.

For PNH detection using high sensitivity analysis, where small clones are detected, it is important to follow the rule of two. PNH clone should be detected in two lineages (RBCs, granulocyte or monocytes) using two gating markers for leukocytes (including CD45 and one other, usually CD15 for granulocyte and CD33/CD64 for monocytes) and two PNH markers (including FLAER and one other, usually CD24 for granulocyte and CD14 for monocytes). For RBCs, CD235 is the only gating marker and CD59 is the only PNH marker. When using separate tubes for granulocytes, monocytes, and RBCs, it is recommended that a high sensitivity screening for RBC and granulocytes should be done first, followed by a high sensitivity monocyte assay for all cases which contain PNH RBCs or granulocyte [36]. Since we perform a common five-color/six-color assays for granulocyte and monocyte, our strategy is to perform high sensitivity screening for leukocytes first. This is followed by high sensitivity screening of RBC for the cases which demonstrate PNH granulocytes or monocytes.

6.9 Conclusion

PNH is a clonal, non-neoplastic stem cell disorder with varied clinical manifestation. Its association with AA and MDS has been well established. The diagnosis can be established through various techniques, but flow cytometry is the preferred one owing to its sensitivity, specificity, and ability to accurately provide the clone size. Discovery of FLAER has been a major breakthrough, and currently, FLAER-based flow cytometric analysis is the "gold standard" diagnostic modality for PNH. CD157 also seems to be a promising reagent that can target both granulocyte and monocytes. Recent guidelines have been established for the diagnosis and monitoring of PNH using flow cytometry by International Clinical Cytometry Society (ICCS). It was followed by practical guidelines for high sensitivity analysis of PNH clones, where specific reagent cocktails and analytical strategies were directly addressed. Following these guidelines will lead to standardized comparable results across various laboratories. These guidelines do not prevent the laboratories from making the modification, but these should be extensively validated. Given the rarity of this disease and presence of small size clones in BM failure (AA and MDS) cases, it is important to address all the quality assurance steps for improving the detection of PNH clones. Data interpretation should be diligently done, with the generation of simple but informative reports, avoiding the terms that can create confusion.

References

1. Nagarajan S, Brodsky RA, Young NS, Medof ME. Genetic defects underlying paroxysmal nocturnal hemoglobinuria that arises out of aplastic anemia. Blood. 1995;86:4656–61.
2. Takahashi M, Takeda J, Hirose S, Hyman R, Inoue N, Miyata T, et al. Deficient biosynthesis of N-acetylglucosaminyl-phosphatidylinositol, the first

intermediate of glycosyl phosphatidylinositol anchor biosynthesis, in cell lines established from patients with paroxysmal nocturnal hemoglobinuria. J Exp Med. 1993;177:517–21.

3. Medof ME, Kinoshita T, Nussenzweig V. Inhibition of complement activation on the surface of cells after incorporation of decay-accelerating factor (DAF) into their membranes. J Exp Med. 1984;160: 1558–78.

4. Rollins SA, Sims PJ. The complement-inhibitory activity of CD59 resides in its capacity to block incorporation of C9 into membrane C5b-9. J Immunol. 1990;144:3478–83.

5. Mukhina GL, Buckley TJ, Barber JP, Jones RJ, Brodsky RA. Multilineage glycophosphatidylinositol anchor deficient haematopoeisis in untreated aplastic anemia. Br J Haematol. 2001;115:476–82.

6. Sachdeva MUS, Varma N, Chandra D, Bose P, Malhotra P, Varma S. Multiparameter FLAER-based flow cytometry for screening of paroxysmal nocturnal hemoglobluniera enhances detection rate in patients with aplastic anemia. Ann Hematol. 2015;94(5):721–8.

7. Rahman K, Gupta R, Yadav G, Hussein N, Singh MK, Nityanand S. Fluorescent Aerolysin (FLAER)-based paroxysmal nocturnal hemoglobinuria (PNH) screening: a single center experience from India. Int J Lab Hematol. 2017;39(3):261–71.

8. Hillmen P, Lewis SM, Bessler M, et al. Natural history of paroxysmal nocturnal hemoglobinuria. N Engl J Med. 1995;333(19):1253–8.

9. Wang SA, Pozdnyakova O, Jorgensen JL, Medeiros LJ, Stachurski D, Anderson M, et al. Detection of paroxysmal nocturnal hemoglobinuria clones in patients with myelodysplastic syndromes and related bone marrow diseases, with emphasis on diagnostic pitfalls and caveats. Haematologica. 2009;94:29–36.

10. Iwanaga M, Furukawa K, Amenomori T, Mori H, Nakamura H, Fuchigami K, et al. Paroxysmal nocturnal hemoglobinuria clones in patients with myelodysplastic syndromes. Br J Haematol. 1998;102:465–74.

11. Young NS. Paroxysmal nocturnal hemoglobinuria and myelodysplastic sydromes: clonal expansion of PIG-A-mutant hematopoietic cells in bone marrow failure. Haematologica. 2009;94(1):3–7.

12. Sugimori C, Padron E, Caceres G, Shain K, Sokol L, Zhang L, et al. Paroxysmal nocturnal hemoglobinuria and concurrent JAK2V617F mutation. Blood Cancer J. 2012;2(3):e63.

13. Strubing P. Paroxysmale Ha¨moglobinurie. Deutsch Medicinische Wochenschrift. 1882;8:17–21.

14. Marchiafava E, Nazari A. Nuovo conttributo allo studiodegli itteri cronici emolitici. Il Policlinico. Sezion Med. 1911;18:241–8.

15. van den Bergh HAA. Ictére hémolytique avec crise-shé moglobinuriques. Fragilité globulaire. Rev Med. 1911;31:63–9.

16. Crosby WH. Paroxysmal nocturnal hemoglobinuria. A classic description by Paul Strübing in 1882 and a bibliography of the disease. Blood. 1951;6: 270–84.

17. Ham TH. Chronic hemolytic anemia with paroxysmal nocturnal hemoglobinuria. A study of the mechanism of hemolysis in relation to acid-base equilibrium. N Engl J Med. 1937;217:915–7.

18. Ham TH. Studies on destruction of red blood cells. Chronic hemolytic anemia with paroxysmal nocturnal hemoglobinuria: an investigation of the mechanism of hemolysis, with observations of five cases. Arch Intern Med. 1939;64:1271–305.

19. Ham TH, Dingle JH. Studies on destruction of red blood cells. II. Chronic hemolytic anemia and paroxysmal nocturnal hemoglobinuria: certain immunological aspects of the hemolytic mechanism with special reference to serum complement. J Clin Investig. 1939;18:657–72.

20. Pillemer L, Blum L, Lepow IH, Ross OA, Todd EW, Wardlaw AC. The properdin system and immunity. Demonstration and isolation of a new serum protein, properdin, and its role in immune phenomena. Science. 1954;120:279–85.

21. Dacie JV. Paroxysmal nocturnal haemoglobinuria. Proc R Soc Med U S A. 1963;56:587–96.

22. Rosse WF, Dacie JV. Immune lysis of normal human and paroxysmal nocturnal hemoglobinuria (PNH) redcells. The sensitivity of PNH red cells to lysis by complement and specific antibody. J Clin Investig. 1966;45:736–48.

23. Aster RH, Enright SE. A platelet and granulocyte membrane defect in paroxysmal nocturnal hemoglobinuria: usefulness for the detection of platelet antibodies. J Clin Investig. 1969;48:1199–210.

24. Hoffmann EM. Inhibition of complement by a substrate isolated from human erythrocytes. Extraction from human erythrocyte stomata. Immunochemistry. 1969;6:391–403.

25. Hoffmann EM. Inhibition of complement by a substrate isolated from human erythrocytes. Studies on the site and mechanism of action. Immunochemistry. 1969;6:405–19.

26. Oni SB, Osunkoya BO, Luzzatto L. Paroxysmalnocturnal hemoglobinuria: evidence for monoclonal origin of abnormal red cells. Blood. 1970;36:145–52.

27. Hoffmann E, Cheng W, Tomeu E, Renk C. Resistance of sheep erythrocytes to immune lysis by treatment of the cells with a human erythrocyte extract: studies on the site of inhibition. J Immunol. 1974;113:1501–9.

28. Stern M, Rosse WF. Two populations of granulocytes in paroxysmal nocturnal hemoglobinuria. Blood. 1979;53:928–34.

29. Pangburn MK, Schreiber RD, Müller-Eberhard HJ. Deficiency of an erythrocyte membrane protein with complement regulatory activity in paroxysmal nocturnal hemoglobinuria. Proc Natl Acad Sci U S A. 1983;80:5430–4.

30. Davitz MA, Low MG, Nussenzweig V. Release of decay accelerating factor from the cell membrane by phosphatidylinositol-specific phospholipase C. J Exp Med. 1986;163:1150–61.

31. Holguin MH, Fredrick LR, Bernshaw NJ, Parker CJ. Isolation and characterization of a protein from

normal erythrocytes that inhibits reactive lysis of the erythrocytes of paroxysmal nocturnal hemoglobinuria. J Clin Investig. 1989;84:7–17.

32. Miyata T, Takeda J, Iida J, Yamada N, Inoue N, Takahashi M, et al. The cloning of PIG-A, a component in the early step in GPI-anchor synthesis. Science. 1993;259:1318–20.

33. Brodsky RA, Mukhina G, Li S, Nelson KL, Chiurrazi PL, Buckley T, et al. Improved detection and characterization of paroxysmal nocturnal hemoglobinuria using florescent aerolysin. Am J Clin Pathol. 2000;114:459–66.

34. Bessler M, Hiken J. The pathophysiology of disease in patients with paroxysmal nocturnal hemoglobinuria. Hematology Am Soc Hematol Educ Program. 2008;2008:104–8.

35. Borowitz MJ, Craig FE, DiGuiseppe JA. On behalf of the Clinical Cytometry Society et al Guidelines for the diagnosis andmonitoring of paroxysmal nocturnal hemoglobinuria and related disorders by flow cytometry. Cytometry B Clin Cytom. 2010; 78:211–30.

36. Sutherland DR, Keeney M, Illingworth A. Practical guidelines for high sensitivity detection and monitoring of paroxysmal nocturnal hemoglobinuria clones by flow cytometry. Cytometry B. 2012;82B:195–208.

37. Crosby WH. Paroxysmal nocturnal hemoglobinuria. A specific test for the disease based ability of thrombin to activate the hemolytic factor. Blood. 1950;5: 843–6.

38. Dacie JV, Lewis SM, Tills D. Comparative sensitivity of erythrocytes in paroxysmal nocturnal hemoglobinuria to hemolysis by normal serum and by high titre cold antibody. Br J Hematol. 1960;6:362–71.

39. Hartman RC, Jenkins DE Jr, Arnold AB. Diagnostic specificity of sucrose hemolysis tests for paroxysmal nocturnal hemoglobinuria. Blood. 1970;35:462–75.

40. Kabaksi T, Rosse WF, Logue GL. The lysis of paroxysmal nocturnal hemoglobinuria red cells by serum and cobra factor. Br J Haematol. 1972;23:693–705.

41. Brubaker LH, Schaberg DR, Jefferson DH, Mengel CE. A potential rapid screening test for paroxysmal nocturnal hemoglobinuria. N Engl J Med. 1973;288:1059–60.

42. Rosse WF, Dacie JV. The role of complement in the sensitivity of the paroxysmal nocturnal hemoglobinuria red cell to immune lysis. Bibl Haematol. 1965;23:11–8.

43. Rosse WF. Variations in the red cells in paroxysmal nocturnal haemoglobinuria. Br J Haematol. 1973;24:327–42.

44. Navenot JM, Bernard D, Petit-Frioux Y, Loirat MJ, Guimbretière J, Muller JY, Blanchard D. Rapid diagnosis of paroxysmal nocturnal hemoglobinuria by gel test agglutination. Rev Fr Transfus Hemobiol. 1993;36(2):135–47.

45. Gupta R, Pandey P, Choudhry R, Kashyap R, MehrotraM NS, Nityanand S. A prospective comparison of four techniques for diagnosis of paroxys-

mal nocturnal haemoglobinuria. Int J Lab Hematol. 2007;29:119–26.

46. Sachdeva MU, Varma N, Chandra D, Bose P, Malhotra P, Varma S. Multiparameter FLAER-based flow cytometry for screening of paroxysmal nocturnal hemoglobinuria enhances detection rates in patients with aplastic anemia. Ann Hematol. 2015;94:721–8.

47. Kinoshita T, Medof ME, Silber R, Nussenzweig V. Distributionof decay-accelerating factor in the peripheral blood of normal individuals and patients with paroxysmal nocturnal hemoglobinuria. J Exp Med. 1985;162:75–92.

48. Diep DB, Nelson KL, Raja SM, Pleshak EN, Buckley TJ. Glycosylphosphatidylinositol anchors of membrane glycoproteins are binding determinants for the channel-forming toxin aerolysin. J Biol Chem. 1998;273:2355–60.

49. Sutherland DR, Kuek N, Davidson J, et al. Diagnosing PNH with FLAER and multiparameter flow cytometry. Cytometry B Clin Cytom. 2007;72:167–77.

50. Hernandez-Campo PM, Almeida J, Sanchez ML, Malvezzi M, Orfao A. Normal patterns of expression of glycosylphosphatidylinositol anchored proteins on different subsets of peripheral blood cells: a frame of reference for the diagnosis of paroxysmal nocturnal hemoglobinuria. Cytometry B. 2006;70B:71–81.

51. Sutherland DR, Acton E, Keeney M, Davis BH, Illingworth A. Use of CD157 in FLAER based assay for high sensitivity PNH granulocyte and PNH monocyte detection. Cytometry Part B. 2014;86B:44–55.

52. Rahman K, Gupta R, Harankhedkar S, Gupta T, Sarkar MK, Nityanand S. Utility of CD157 as a common leukocytes marker for paroxysmal nocturnal hemoglobinuria screening in a single tube five color combination. Indian J Hematol Blood Transfus. 2018;34(2):304–9. https://doi.org/10.1007/s12288-017-0867-z.

53. Marinov I, Kohutova M, Tkakova V, Pesek A, Cermak J, Cetkovsky P. Clinical relevance of CD157 for rapid and cost effective simultaneous evaluation of PNH granulocyte and monocytes by low cytometry. Int J Lab Hematol. 2015;37:231–7.

54. Marinov I, Illingworth AJ, Benko M, Sutherland DR. Performance characteristics of a non-fluorescent aerolysin-based paroxysmal nocturnal hemoglobinuria (PNH) assay for simultaneous evaluation of PNH neutrophils and PNH monocytes by flow cytometry, following published PNH guidelines. Cytometry B Clin Cytom. 2018;94(2):257–63. https://doi.org/10.1002/cyto.b.21389.

55. Keeney M, Illingworth A, Sutherland DR. Paroxysmal nocturnal hemoglobinuria assessment by flow cytometric analysis. Clin Lab Med. 2017;37(4):855–67. https://doi.org/10.1016/j.cll.2017.07.007.

56. Fletcher M, Sutherland DR, Whitby L, et al. Standardizing leucocyte PNH clonedetection: an international study. Cytometry B Clin Cytom. 2014;86(5):311–8.

57. Marinov I, Kohoutova M, Tkacova V, et al. Intra- and interlaboratory variability of paroxysmal nocturnal hemoglobinuria testing by flow cytometry following

the2012 practical guidelines for high-sensitivity paroxysmal nocturnal hemoglobinuria testing. Cytometry B Clin Cytom. 2013;84(4):229–36.

58. Scienberg P, Wu CO, Numez O, Young NS. Predictive response of immunosuppressive therapy and survival in severe aplastic anemia. Br J Hematol. 2009;144:206–16.

59. Sugimori C, Chuhjo T, Feng X, Yamazaki H, Takami A, Teramura M, Mizoguchi H, Omine M, Nakao S. Minor population of CD55-CD59-blood cells predicts response to immunosuppressive therapy and prognosis in patients with aplastic anemia. Blood. 2006;107:1308–14.

60. Yoshida N, Yagasaki H, Takahashi Y, Yamamoto T, Liang J, Wang Y, Tanaka M, Hama A, Nishio N, Kobayashi R, Hotta N, Asami K, Kikuta A, Fukushima T, Hirano N, Kojima S. Clinical impact of HLA-DR15, a minor population of paroxysmal nocturnal haemoglobinuria-type cells, and an aplastic anaemia-associated autoantibody in children with acquired aplastic anaemia. Br J Haematol. 2008;142:427–35.

61. Scheinberg P, Marte M, Nunez O, Young NS. Paroxysmal nocturnal hemoglobinuria clones in severe aplastic anemia patients treated with horse anti-thymocyte globulin plus cyclosporine. Haematologica. 2010;95:1075–80.

62. Hochsmann B, Rojewski M, Schrezenmeier H. Paroxysmal nocturnal hemoglobinuria (PNH): higher sensitivity and validity in diagnosis and serial monitoring by flow cytometric analysis of reticulocytes. Ann Hematol. 2011;90:887–9.

Laboratory Diagnosis of Microangiopathic Hemolytic Anemia Including TTP, DIC, and HUS

Aakanksha Singh and Mrinalini Kotru

Microangiopathic hemolytic anemia (MAHA) is a type of hemolytic anemia characterized by non-immune intravascular destruction of red cells secondary to the presence of microthrombi in the circulation or abnormal vascular surfaces. It is often accompanied by thrombocytopenia. This syndrome of hemolytic anemia and thrombocytopenia occurring secondary to the formation of microthrombi is also called thrombotic microangiopathy (TMA) or red cell fragmentation syndrome. It is mostly suspected in patients who are sick and show signs of one or more organ failure with demonstrable **schistocytes** or **fragmented red cells** (Fig. 7.1).

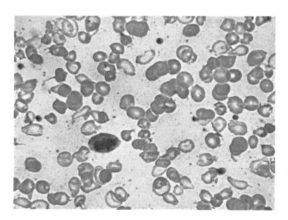

Fig. 7.1 Schistocytes on peripheral smear, 100×

A. Singh · M. Kotru (✉)
Department of Pathology, University College of Medical Sciences and GTB Hospital, New Delhi, Delhi, India

7.1 Pathogenesis

A wide variety of clinical diseases both inherited and acquired can lead to the development of microthrombi. These microthrombi formed in high-flow/high-shear vasculature (arterioles and arteries) result in partial vascular obstruction, thereby causing end organ damage along with red cell fragmentation and hemolysis. During this episode, fairly large amount of lactate dehydrogenase is detectable in blood secondary to red cell damage. Similarly, there is consumption of platelets leading to thrombocytopenia. *Hence, the formation of microthrombi is central to the development of clinical symptoms, hemolysis and thrombocytopenia.* These microthrombi are a byproduct of various mechanisms depending on the underlying disease. For example, in TTP, there are platelet aggregates in the systemic microvasculature; in HUS, platelet-fibrin thrombi are present in the renal microvasculature.

The levels of red cell fragmentation and schistocytosis show little proportionality to either the severity of endothelial damage or the degree of vascular occlusion and shear stress, few examples being disseminated intravascular coagulation (DIC), preeclampsia/eclampsia, march hemoglobinuria, and Kasabach–Merritt syndrome (Fig. 7.2).

We discuss a few important diseases under the umbrella of MAHA, before discussing the approach to the diagnosis.

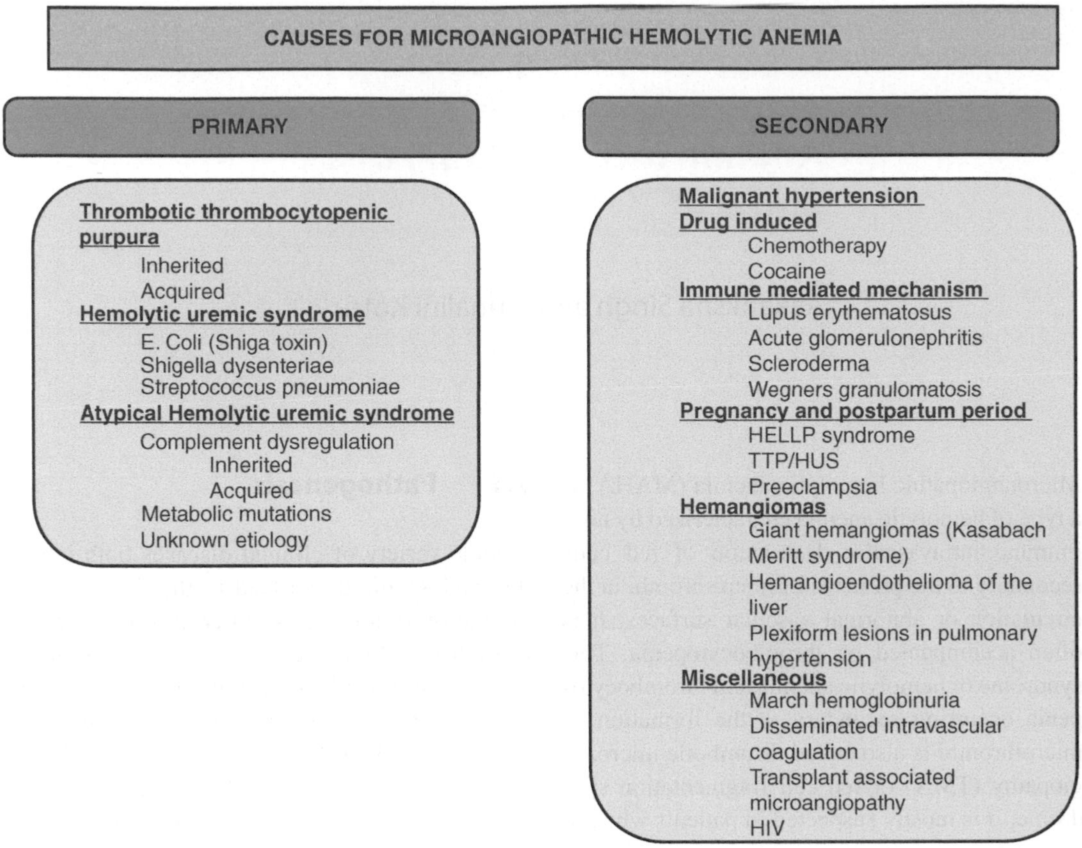

Fig. 7.2 Microangiopathic hemolytic anemia: causes

7.2 Thrombotic Thrombocytopenic Purpura (TTP)

TTP is a rare life-threatening TMA occurring due to severe deficiency in ADAMTS13 metalloproteinase.

7.2.1 Definition

Earlier, TTP remained a diagnosis of exclusion, requiring the presence of multiorgan ischemic clinical manifestations (Reynolds pentad) along with laboratory-established MAHA and thrombocytopenia. It has been long established that the above-said criterion is present only in about 10% of the patients. Also, many recent studies have demonstrated that *ADAMTS13 activity less than*

10% is specific for TTP. Hence, the diagnosis can only be confirmed on the estimation of the enzyme activity of ADAMTS13.

7.2.2 Pathophysiology

ADAMTS13 (a disintegrin and metalloproteinase with a thrombospondin type 1 motif, member 13) is central to the development of TTP. It is the 13th member of the ADAMTS family of proteins. It is a specific von Willebrand factor (VWF) cleaving protease.

The activated endothelium releases ultra-large VWF monomers, which under shear stress, partially unfold, exposing their A2 domain, the cleavage site of ADAMTS13 protease. This proteolytic cleavage leads to the formation of small multimers. The significance of this function can

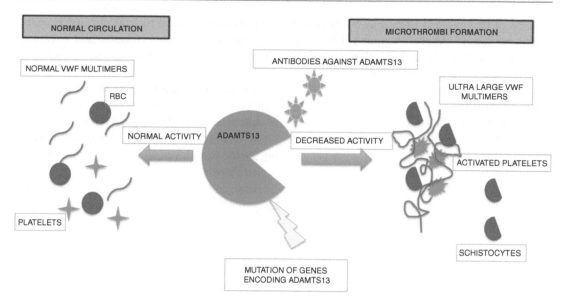

Fig. 7.3 Pathogenesis of thrombotic thrombocytopenic purpura

be observed by the unabated thrombosis in small arterioles caused by the accumulation of platelet-hyperadhesive ultra-large VWF multimers in severe ADAMTS13 deficiency (Fig. 7.3).

7.2.2.1 Causes of ADAMTS13 Deficiency

It can be both acquired and inherited.

- **Acquired** ADAMTS13 deficiency:
  Caused by the presence of **autoantibodies**, mostly. It can be either idiopathic (primary) or nonidiopathic (secondary), i.e., associated with other autoimmune conditions. They are mostly polyclonal IgGs in nature and target cysteine-rich/spacer domain of ADAMTS13.
  Anti-ADAMTS13 IgG assays may not demonstrate any IgG antibodies, in about 20–25% of acute TTP. This may be because of:
  - Immunoglobulin trapping
  - Immunoglobulin isotypes other than IgG
  - ADAMTS13 metabolism by calpains, elastases, thrombin, or plasmin
  - ADAMTS13 inhibition by free hemoglobin
- **Inherited** ADAMTS13 deficiency—
  Upshaw–Schulman syndrome (USS):
  It constitutes 2% of all cases. It is a recessively inherited (compound heterozygous more

common than homozygous) qualitative disorder of the ADAMTS13. Majority of the mutations impact the protease domain and may rarely affect ADAMTS13 secretion also. Interestingly, a mutual exclusivity is observed in mutations observed in either childhood or adult onset disease.

7.2.3 Risk Factors

Acquired TTP has a higher reported prevalence in the black ethnicity. Although, no causative link has been established, but obesity and HLA-DRB1∗11 mutation have a significant association with TTP. Whereas the presence of HLA-DRB1∗04 abates the propensity of having TTP. However, it must be borne in mind that the mere deficiency of ADAMTS13, moderate to severe, is no prelude to the TTP syndrome.

7.2.4 Epidemiology

7.2.4.1 Age

TTP has both adult and pediatric onset. Inherited TTPs generally present as early as the neonatal period or by early childhood. Surprisingly about

10–20% of the inherited TTPs may not manifest up to the second decade. Acquired TTP may rarely occur in the first decade itself, nevertheless it is a disease of the adolescent and adults.

7.2.4.2 Gender

Adult onset TTP shows a female predilection supporting its autoimmune origin with female-to-male ratio being 2 to 3:1. However, USS has no sex predilection.

7.2.5   Clinical Presentation (Fig. 7.4)

7.2.5.1 Upshaw–Schulman Syndrome

It is a rare form of inherited TTP, accounting for less than 5% of all TTP cases, and often tends to have a chronic remitting and relapsing course. A typically affected neonate may have plethora of nonspecific manifestations ranging from meco-

nium passage in utero to fetal distress, neonatal jaundice, and thrombocytopenia and occasionally may have signs and symptoms secondary to thrombosis.

For the unsuspecting pediatrician, any blood transfusion or plasma exchange may lead to complete recovery, thereby delaying the diagnosis up to a later stage in life. Another contributing factor to delayed diagnosis is the minimal schistocytosis.

However, these patients tend to have a chronic relapsing course, requiring plasma infusion every 2–4 weeks. Such should be instituted on a regular basis to prevent the development of complications.

Hereditary TTP shows increased propensity for acute and chronic renal disease as compared to acquired TTP. It is speculated that local expression of ADAMTS13 in renal endothelial cells and glomerular podocytes may provide protection

Hematological	Central Nervous System (60%)	Cardiovascular (25%)	Gastrointestinal (35%)	Renal
Severe thrombocytopenia (~30x109/L)	Headache and confusion	Isolated ECG abnormalities	Abdominal pain	Isolated proteinuria and hematuria
Microangiopathic hemolytic anemia	Seizures	Myocardial infarction (rare)	Diarrhoea	Serum creatinine level < 2mg/dl
	Stroke and coma (rare)		Mesenteric ischemia	Acute/ Advanced renal failure is unusual

Fig. 7.4 Clinical presentation of TTP

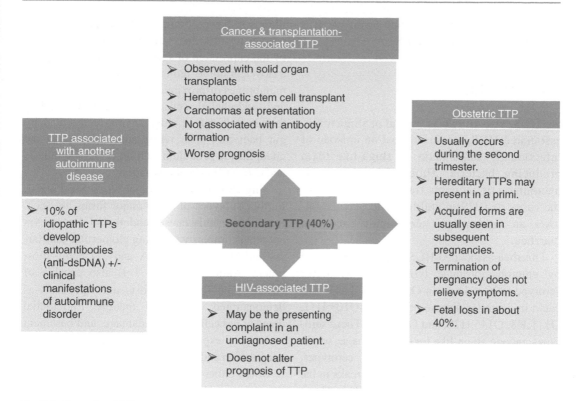

Fig. 7.5 Secondary TTPs

against VWF-platelet aggregation before the inhibitors suppress its activity. Such protection is not present in patients with genetic ADAMTS13 mutations. A list of secondary TTPs have been briefly discussed in Fig. 7.5.

Summary
Thrombotic thrombocytopenic purpura is defined by less than 10% of ADAMTS13 activity. Severe ADAMTS13 deficiency leads to the accumulation of platelet-hyperadhesive ultra-large VWF multimer complexes and subsequent thrombi formation. Caused by both acquired (autoantibodies against ADAMTS13) and inherited (Upshaw–Schulman syndrome). Clinically described by Reynolds pentad.

7.3 HUS and Atypical HUS

Hemolytic uremic syndrome (HUS) falls under the umbrella diagnosis of TMAs. Historically, HUS was regarded as one of the most common causes of acute dialysis requirement in young children. In autopsy series of children succumbing to HUS, histopathological changes in kidney ranged from TMA limited to the glomerulus to extensive involvement of arterioles.

7.3.1 Definition

HUS is a clinical syndrome of acute renal failure heralded by intravascular hemolysis (schistocytosis, raised lactate dehydrogenase levels, and consumption of haptoglobin) along with thrombocytopenia.

On the basis of etiology, two forms of HUS are observed: D+ and D− HUS.

7.4 D+ HUS

D+ HUS, also known as typical or shiga toxin-associated HUS, is caused post an episode of infection by shiga toxin or shiga-like toxin producing bacteria. Though the disease is uncommon, it accounts for majority (90%) of the cases of HUS in children and usually follows an epidemic of community acquired diarrhea.

Diarrhea-associated HUS is primarily caused by enterohemorrhagic type (70%), O157:H7 serotype (80%). The non-O157 serotypes implicated in a similar disease picture are O103:H11, O111:H8, O145:H28, and O26:H11. These serotypes encode shiga-like toxin by a phage, which infects other non-disease-causing serotypes, turning them virulent. Rarely, in outbreaks in the past, enteroaggregative *E. coli* O104:H4 has been implicated, which became virulent post acquisition of mutated prophage. Shigella dysenteriae serotype 1 has also been found to be an offending organism in non-*E. coli* cases.

The natural reservoir for these organisms happens to be the gut of cattle, and they are therefore transmitted through contaminated unpasteurized milk and dairy products, poultry, and undercooked meat. Sometimes poorly washed vegetables and fruits and nuts secondary to a contaminated water source may also be disease causing. Rarely man-to-man transmission via the feco-oral route has also been described. Since the implicating organisms propagate disease by elaborating toxin via bacteriophage, very little infecting dose almost always suffices, and it also explains the tendency to cause epidemics.

7.4.1 Pathophysiology

Central to the pathogenesis is microangiopathy, which may or may not be accompanied by thrombosis. The pathology tends to dominate around glomerular capillaries, secondarily affecting capillaries in bowel, brain, heart, and pancreas. The propensity of kidney affection can be explained by the expression of specific sphingolipid globotriaosylceramide tethered to lipid rafts of cell membranes of proximal tubular cells, podocytes, and endothelial cells. These globotriaosylceramide endocytose shiga toxins (elaborated by gut bacteria), with retrograde transport to the endoplasmic reticulum, inhibit protein synthesis and cause ribosomal disruption.

Shiga toxin is of two major types: Stx 1 and 2. Further subtypes of these major forms are seen. Stx 2 dominantly causes endothelial damage via apoptosis primarily affecting glomerular capillaries and arterioles, Stx 2A and 2D being most potent. Additionally, Stx 1 is also capable of causing endothelial necrosis and apoptosis as demonstrated on animal models. Endothelial damage via cell swelling, damage, and basement membrane exposure leads to the activation of coagulation and complement pathway. The extent to which either pathway is elaborated determines the extent of thrombus formation and/or microangiopathy with the presence of polymorphonuclear leucocytes within the vessel wall. A common feature seen in autopsy series is the increased vascular permeability, dominant cause of all clinical manifest, ischemic organ dysfunction (e.g., renal cortical necrosis) (Fig. 7.6).

7.4.2 Age

Stx-HUS principally affects young children. This age predilection can be explained by the variability in intensity and patterns of sphingolipid receptors on cell surface with age.

7.4.3 Gender

No gender predilection is seen.

7.4.4 Clinical Features

D+ HUS usually occurs 5–10 days after a preceding episode of bloody diarrhea. Shiga toxin-associated HUS is not unknown in patients

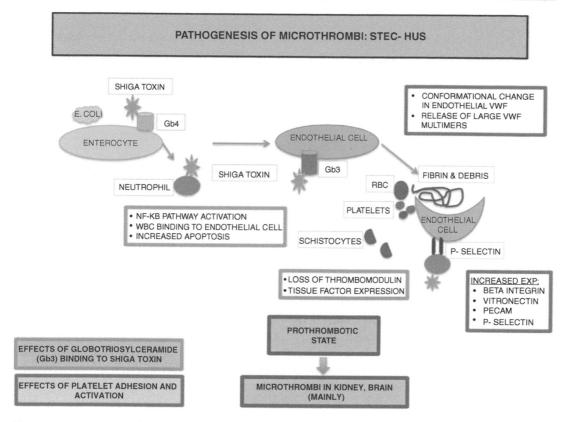

Fig. 7.6 Pathogenesis of Shiga toxin associated hemolytic uremic syndrome

without a prodrome of colitis. *E. coli* causing genitourinary tract infections have been incriminated with similar pathophysiology.

Syndrome of D+ HUS secondary to EHEC infection can be asymptomatic or have a variable clinical course. It may involve the CNS, bowels, endocrine pancreas and heart, making the clinical differentiation with other MAHAs difficult.

Hematological Features: Thrombocytopenia, though found in majority of patients, is usually not associated with purpura or bleeding. However, no direct relationship has been established with MAHA associated with reduced platelet counts to the extent of renal dysfunction. The blood picture associated with D+ HUS is usually one of the earliest features to resolve completely in about 1–2 weeks.

Renal Features: Renal manifestations can be extremely variable, ranging from asymptomatic microscopic hematuria and proteinuria to overt oliguric renal failure, which is usually accompanied by hypertension. The prognosis of this renal

infliction usually remains favorable; however, a remote possibility of renal failure years later cannot be ruled out despite complete recovery.

CNS Features: Central nervous system involvement occurs in about 20–50%. It is the most life-threatening complication. Confusion, irritability, seizures, cranial nerve palsies secondary to cerebral edema, and hemiparesis and pyramidal or extrapyramidal symptoms secondary to thrombosis are some of the CNS manifestations.

GIT Features: D+ HUS is usually preceded by bloody diarrhea which can later complicate to severe hemorrhagic colitis, bowel necrosis and perforation, peritonitis, and intussusception. Hepatomegaly and/or increased serum transaminases are frequently observed.

Endocrine Features: Transient glucose intolerance is quite commonly reported. One of the late reported complication rarely is type 1 diabetes mellitus.

CVS Features: Cardiovascular and respiratory complications are secondary to the increased vas-

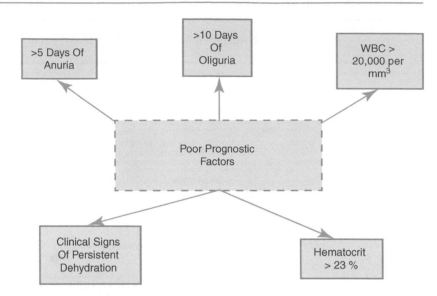

Fig. 7.7 Poor prognostic factors associated with shiga-HUS

cular permeability. Congestive heart failure, pericardial or pleural effusion, and acute respiratory distress syndrome have been well documented in literature. Though rarely reported, myocardial infarction remains a dreaded complication (Fig. 7.7).

Summary
D+ HUS is associated with a triad of MAHA, thrombocytopenia, and acute renal failure. Shiga toxin-mediated endothelial damage and complement activation is central to the pathogenesis.

7.5   D– HUS

D– HUS also known as atypical HUS (aHUS), is an encompassing term for disorders with unregulated activation of alternate pathway of complement. The reported incidence of D– HUS is about 10% in children; however, we firmly believe that it is largely underreported and misdiagnosed. Unlike D+ HUS, which has a dramatic presentation, D– HUS tends to have an unsuspecting manifest with prolonged remitting relapsing course. The child may present with nonresponsive hypertension and renal failure impending to transplantation.

D– HUS is caused by either inherited or acquired defect causing unregulated complement activation. It is largely observed that these patients give a preceding history of infection, most common being an upper respiratory tract infection. However, these are mere catalysts to an underlying complement defect.

7.5.1   Pathophysiology

Much like dense deposit disease, it affects glomeruli, arterioles, and capillaries. Doubling of basement membrane, subendothelial deposits and a spectrum of mesangioproliferative glomerulonephritis are seen without cortical necrosis. Mesangiolysis is also often observed. All these changes are secondary to endothelial damage, subendothelial edema, and rarely microangiopathy. A summary of commonly described mutations and a simplified dysregulated alternate complement pathway are illustrated in Figs. 7.8, 7.9, and 7.10.

7.5.1.1 Antifactor H Autoantibody-Associated D– HUS
Another important etiology causing atypical HUS other than mutations involving the complement pathway is the presence of autoantibodies against factor H. These antibodies are detected in

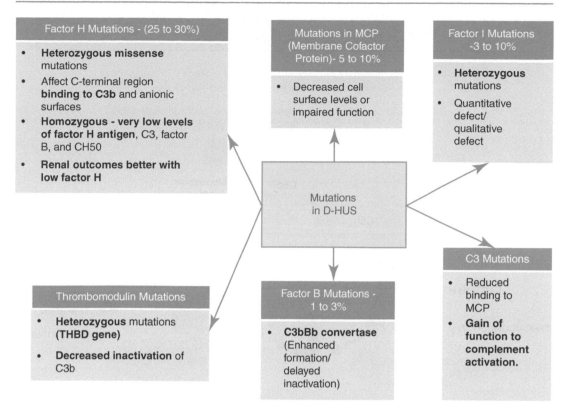

Fig. 7.8 Mutations with D– HUS

Fig. 7.9 Endothelial damage outcomes, secondary to dysregulated activation of complement pathway

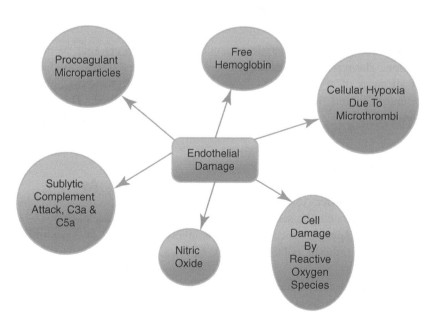

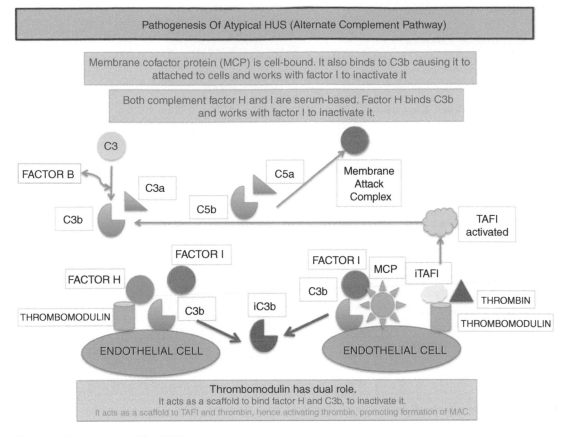

Fig. 7.10 Pathogenesis of D– HUS

the first decade and demonstrate no gender predilection. The reported incidence is about 6–10% of all cases of atypical HUS. These antibodies primarily inhibit the binding of factor H to C3 convertase.

7.5.2 Epidemiology

The ratio of carriers to manifest cases is almost about half; this can be secondary to incomplete penetrance, especially seen in mutations involving CFH, membrane cofactor protein, CFI C3, and CFB.

Thirty percent of patients of D– HUS with the above mutations may have a preceding episode of diarrhea. Additionally, the mere presence of mutations does not determine the manifestation of disease. Numerous known triggers such as coexisting autoimmune disorders, drugs, solid organ cancers, hematopoetic malignancies, and pregnancy have been described. This interaction between environmental triggers and mutations has not been completely elucidated.

7.5.3 Age

The prevalence of D– HUS is rare and has been reported at 3 per million children. Though D– HUS is commoner in children, adult cases are well documented.

7.5.4 Gender

No gender predilection has been reported.

7.5.5 Clinical Features

The onset of an acute D– HUS crisis may occur spontaneously or after stressful environmental triggers. D– HUS is not an organ-specific disease; it is multisystemic disorder, with intravascular hemolysis, low platelet count, and renal failure being common presentation.

Gastrointestinal Symptoms: D– HUS may present with an acute abdomen which may or may not be associated with bloody diarrhea. Elevated pancreatic amylase or lipase may indicate a diagnosis otherwise. Impaired glucose tolerance and abnormal liver function tests may be additional findings. Increased vascular permeability leads to mild to moderate ascites along with intestinal wall and mesenteric edema.

CNS: Glasgow coma scale rarely shows significantly impaired scores. Impaired mentum (which tends to improve and deteriorate), headache, seizures and coma have been well documented. Focal neurologic deficits may occur although these are not as frequent as in patients with TTP. Posterior reversible encephalopathy, again secondary to cerebral edema, remains one of the dreaded complications.

Hematological Features: Severe intravascular hemolysis has been documented with factor H mutations and tends to have a chronic relapsing course.

Renal: D– HUS has major affliction to kidneys. Patients tend to have a dramatic course to end stage renal disease. Associated hypertension is usually unrelenting. Young patients usually tend to undergo renal transplant, but the chances of recurrence remain exceptionally high (75–90%). Of all mutations, mutated membrane cofactor protein, tend to have the best renal prognosis, though early in onset, fewer relapses are observed and recurrence in allograft is rare.

7.5.6 Vitamin B$_{12}$ Metabolism Defects Associated with D– HUS

It is commonly associated with an inborn error of intracellular cobalamin metabolism, with functional mutations involving MMACHC gene. The clinical presentation and the age of onset depend on the type of mutation involved.

Prenatally, intrauterine growth retardation and microcephaly are observed, rarely along with fetal dilated cardiomyopathy. In infants, newborn screening remains unremarkable, but the child may show features of failure to thrive, hypotonia along with developmental delay. Hemolytic uremic syndrome starts to manifest associated with visual inattention, nystagmus, and hydrocephalous. Cor pulmonale in the absence of other causes may also bring the child to clinician's attention.

Childhood is marked by developmental regression and chronic TMA. Manifestation of the disease in adolescence is marked by progressive leukoencephalopathy, subacute combined degeneration of cord with associated thromboembolic events.

Pathogenesis: Mutations in the MMACHC gene lead to impaired function, thereby causing decreased production of methylcobalamin and adenosylcobalamin. These in turn serve as cofactors to two enzymes methionine synthase and methylmalonyl-CoA mutase, respectively. Deficient activity of these two enzymes leads to increased metabolites, homocysteine and methylmalonic acid.

Biochemical hallmarks of the disorder are raised plasma homocysteine, plasma and urine methylmalonic acid accompanied with low levels of methionine. What should alert the clinician against nutritional deficiency is the normal plasma B$_{12}$ levels in the background of megaloblastosis, hypersegmented neutrophils, schistocytosis, and thrombocytopenia. Another indicator to consider in born error of cobalamin metabolism is the poor response to intramuscular cyanocobalamin as opposed to hydroxyl cobalamin, which is curative.

7.5.7 D– HUS After Renal Transplantation

There are many implicating factors for D– HUS secondary to renal transplant, the most common being drugs. High-dose administration of calcineurin inhibitors (cyclosporine and tacrolimus) usually leads to MAHA within the first 6 months of transplant. HUS may be secondary to underlying recurrent disease or rarely may arise de novo.

Summary
D– HUS is often attributed to mutations in CFH, MCP, CFI, C3, and thrombomodulin. Primary to pathogenesis is dysregulation of the complement system (especially, the alternate pathway) leading to excessive complement activation and endothelial damage.

Drugs Causing D– HUS
Tacrolimus, cyclosporine, mitomycin C, bleomycin, cisplatin, quinine, gemcitabine, quetiapine, and cocaine.

Recent Insights
The central role of damaged endothelial cells which was assumed to be pivotal to the pathogenesis of HUS is now being disputed. Various animal models have now demonstrated that red cells or platelets may be damaged earlier.

7.6 Disseminated Intravascular Coagulation (DIC)

7.6.1 Introduction

DIC is not a disease per se; it is an outcome or a complication of any condition which leads to unregulated generalized activation of the clotting system which overwhelms the innate anticoagulant system of the body, causing the generation of vast amounts of intravascular thrombin and fibrin. The various outcomes associated with this complication are elaborated in Fig. 7.11.

7.6.2 Definition

In 2011, the International Society on Thrombosis and Hemostasis (ISTH) proposed a definition of DIC as: "DIC is an acquired syndrome characterized by the intravascular activation of coagulation without a specific localization and arising from different causes. It can originate from and cause damage to the microvasculature, which if sufficiently severe, can produce organ dysfunction."

7.6.3 Pathogenesis

Acute DIC is a consumptive state, where impaired coagulation is secondary to the generation of thrombin to such excess degrees that the natural anticoagulants are deemed ineffective. The trigger to such a response is a result of large amounts of tissue factor released intravascularly. This response results in systemic organ dysfunction secondary to fibrin thrombi predominantly in the capillaries and arterioles. It has myriad causes (Fig. 7.12).

This unregulated activation leads to drastic depletion of platelets and coagulation factors. Therefore, the laboratory parameters at this point of time indicate thrombocytopenia approximately less than 50,000/L (10–15% of cases), deranged PT and aPTT (ranging from minimal to marked prolongation), and excessive fibrin degradation products (D-dimers).

Acute DIC usually results in multiorgan dysfunction secondary to ischemia caused by the widespread fibrin thrombi observed in small vessels due to the hyper-procoagulant state. These microthrombi lead to not only ischemia but also red cell fragmentation leading to schistocytosis.

In acute DIC, the multiorgan ischemia is untenable to the amount of microvascular thrombosis. This can be explained by the enhanced vasospasm and platelet activation secondary to the consumption of endothelial relaxing factor (nitric oxide) by free hemoglobin released during intravascular hemolysis. Other indicators of red

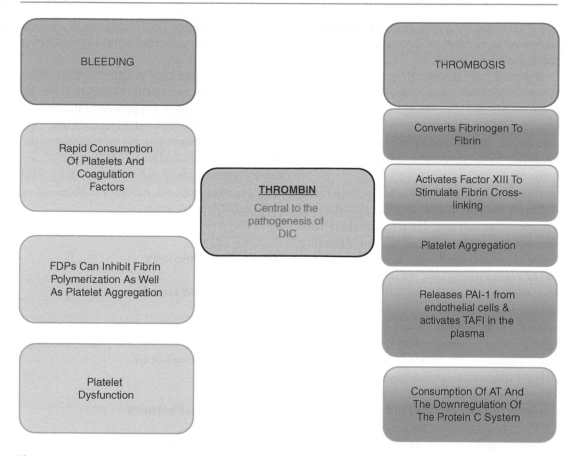

Fig. 7.11 Pathogenesis of DIC

Fig. 7.12 Causes of acute DIC

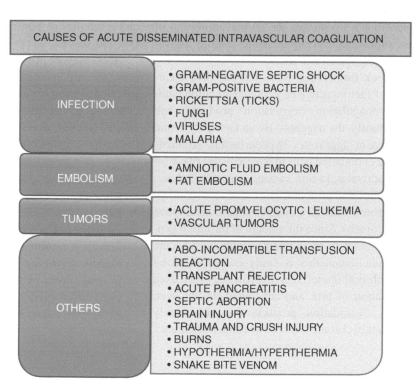

cell fragmentation accompanying schistocytosis are raised lactate dehydrogenase levels and indirect hyperbilirubinemia.

D-dimers are produced by the proteolytic action of plasmin, which cleaves polymerized fibrin monomers after the penultimate step post cross-linking by activated factor XIII. Therefore, factor XIII, thrombin and plasmin are absolutely necessary for the production of fibrin degradation products.

It must be however borne in mind that D-dimers are not specific to DIC. D-dimers are essentially an indicator that a recent clot formation has taken place. Therefore, any detectable levels of D-dimer can be seen in any cause of arterial or venous thrombosis, inflammation, healing, and subclinical thrombosis seen in states of hypertension. Impaired clearance secondary to chronic liver disease may also lead to a false-positive presumption of ongoing DIC. Therefore, the presence of D-dimers may only be suggestive, not diagnostic. However, the absence definitely rules out (high negative predictive value) the possibility of DIC.

The coagulation pathway and the contact/kininogen pathway are intimately intertwined. Unprecedented stimulation of the coagulation pathway leads to overproduction of bradykinin, such that it overcomes the normal inhibition of angiotensin-converting enzyme, leading to systemic vasospasm and shock.

Shock further aggravates the impaired clearance of factors activated in the coagulation pathway, coagulation degradation products, and importantly, the triggers—tissue factor. Systemic vasospasm aggravates hypoperfusion, stimulating the endothelial cells to release tissue plasminogen activator, in turn causing hyperfibrinolysis, with amplified protein C loop.

Chronic DIC is a compensated consumptive coagulopathy. Since the amount of thrombin generation tends to be in minute amounts, subacute and subclinical, this is easily compensated by brisk thrombopoiesis by marrow and increased production of pro- and anticoagulants by liver. Fibrin degradation products are also rarely detected in chronic DIC due to efficient clearance by the liver. Chronic DIC is commonly reported with aneurysms, vasculitis, solid organ tumors, and intrauterine death.

Therefore, laboratory parameters tend to be very subtle with chronic DIC. Bleeding is not the primary manifestation as opposed to thrombosis and shock is rarely reported. In fact, chronic DIC is incidentally detected, in the background of the above-mentioned conditions. PT and aPTT are usually normal, rarely mildly raised along with mild thrombocytopenia, making the diagnosis of chronic DIC very daunting.

7.6.4 Epidemiology

7.6.5 Age and Gender

Since DIC is a complication secondary to variable etiologies, skewed age and gender predisposition cannot be established.

7.6.6 Clinical Features

The clinical presentation of acute DIC can be extremely variable, ranging from general malaise, mucosal bleeds, petechial rashes to signs and symptoms pertaining to multiorgan dysfunction and shock.

Abnormalities of coagulation system in DIC are about the shift in balance either ways, leading to an overall dominant hematological manifestation, i.e., either hypercoagulation or hyperfibrinolysis. These clinical types are dynamic categories and may shift or change to another (Fig. 7.13).

Summary
DIC is a systemic disorder, which has a simultaneous procoagulant and fibrinolytic activation resulting in consumption coagulopathy causing organ dysfunction. Diagnosis rests on thrombocytopenia, fibrin degradation products, D-dimer, PT, aPTT, fibrinogen, and scoring systems.

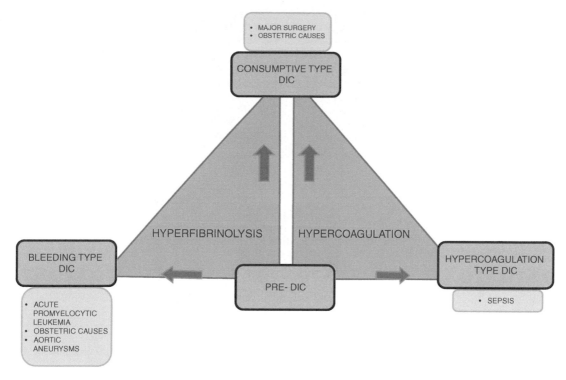

Fig. 7.13 Clinical spectrum of DIC with associated conditions

7.6.7   Laboratory Diagnosis

7.6.7.1 Baseline Investigations

Complete Blood Count: TMA is characterized by anemia that is often severe (decreased hemoglobin and hematocrit) and may be accompanied by moderate polymorphonuclear leukocytosis and severe thrombocytopenia (platelet count usually $<30 \times 10^9 \ L^{-1}$). The hematologic findings of all three disorders, namely HUS, TTP, and DIC tend to be similar, with variable degrees of thrombocytopenia. Also it should be borne in mind that the degree of thrombocytopenia does not always reflect the severity of the clinical status.

Peripheral Blood Smear: There are a few ICSH recommendations:

- Schistocytes, also known as helmet cells, are small, irregularly shaped red cells which lack a central pallor. Variable shapes are noted—triangular, crescent-shaped cells or cells with pointed projections. Nowadays, fragmented red cells are regularly being reported on auto-

mated coulters such as the DxH 800 coulter, cellular analysis system.
- These schistocytes should be reported per 1000 counted red cells, indicated in percentages.
- In the absence of an alternative diagnosis, a value as low as 1% is taken to be suggestive of thrombotic microangiopathic anemia.
- In appropriate clinical setting, 4% or more schistocytes are indicative of TMAs.
- Another factor that should be taken into account is either the absence of schistocytosis in early part of the disease or persistence post resolution of symptoms. Therefore, schistocytosis should never be used for prognostication or disease follow-up. Its presence is only of high positive predictive value (Fig. 7.14).

Reticulocyte Count: A high reticulocyte count is seen in most TMA $(120 \times 10^9 \ L^{-1})$.

Plasma Hemoglobin: Hemoglobinemia though a common feature in all TMAs, but may be more marked in HUS and aHUS.

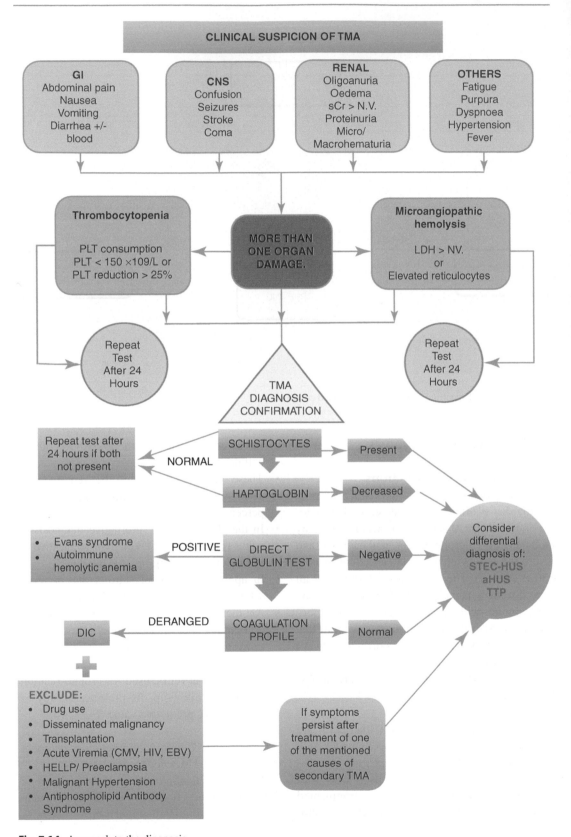

Fig. 7.14 Approach to the diagnosis

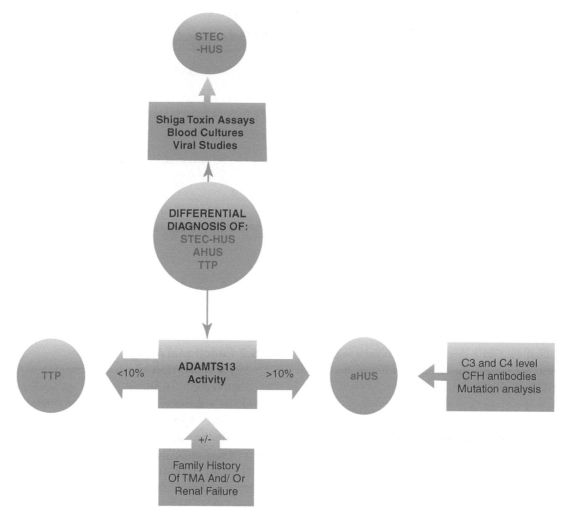

Fig. 7.14 (continued)

Serum Haptoglobin: Is usually undetectable, except in chronic DIC.

Lactate Dehydrogenase: Is elevated.

Liver Function Test: An increased indirect bilirubinemia along with elevated liver transaminases and amylase is usually observed.

Renal Function Test: At presentation, very high blood urea nitrogen and serum creatinine may be encountered, especially in HUS and aHUS.

Urine Examination: Proteinuria and hematuria are frequently observed. The urine usually contains hemoglobin and hemosiderin in addition to albumin. The same can be verified microscopically, either as individual cells or as casts.

Direct and Indirect Coombs' Test: Negative across all TMA, except in the ones associated with autoimmune diseases (SLE).

Global Coagulation Tests: Standard coagulation parameters (PT, APTT, and TT) are within normal limits in TTP and may be minimally prolonged in HUS and aHUS. It has been observed that prothrombin time is usually elevated in up to half of the patients of DIC at any point during the course of the disease. A reduction in the platelet count or clear downward trend in subsequent measurements is a sensitive sign of DIC.

The biphasic waveform of the activated partial thromboplastin time (APTT) has been associated specifically with DIC, though not being very

COAGULATION PROFILE IN VARIOUS DIFFERENTIALS				
Diagnosis	Platelet count	PT	APTT	Fibrinogen
TTP, HUS, aHUS	Decreased	N	N	N
DIC	Decreased	Increased	Increased	Decreased
ITP	Decreased	N	N	N
Cirrhosis	Decreased	Increased	Increased	N to Decreased
Heparin	N	N to Increased	Increased	N
Coumarin	N	Increased	Increased	N
HITT	Decreased	N to Increased	Increased	N

Fig. 7.15 Spectrum of coagulation profile in various differentials

sensitive. Fibrin degradation products or D-dimer tests are usually raised not only in DIC but also in HUS (Fig. 7.15).

7.6.8 Specific Investigations

7.6.8.1 TTP

ADAMTS13 Investigation
Plasma ADAMTS13 activity remains the cornerstone in the diagnosis of TTP. Screening for ADAMTS13 activity is the first test to be performed. Demonstration of less than 10% of ADAMTS13 activity is considered sine qua non to TTP. There are several assays available commercially, both functional and immunochemical, to detect ADAMTS13. The value of immunochemical assays remains limited. The activity measurement of this enzyme is based on its proteolytic activity against von Willebrand factor. For this test, ideally citrated substrate plasma is utilized, and the results are expressed as percentages against a known test citrated plasma. This test plasma is usually the pooled plasma calibrated against the World Health Organization international standard taken to be 100%.

7.6.8.2 Functional Assays for ADAMTS13

The reference methods for measuring ADAMTS13 activity are the collagen-binding activity and FRETS-VWF73-based assays. Various studies have proposed the FRETS-VWF73 assay to be superior to collagen-binding activity assay. Another advantage of performing functional assays is the detection of antibodies against ADAMTS13, which can be detected on a two-staged procedure, with additional incubation and correction with normal plasma.

7.6.8.3 Immunochemical Assays for ADAMTS13

ADAMTS13 antibody assays are essentially protein precipitation assay where IgG immunoglobulins against ADAMTS13 are used in commercial kits. A positive detection is read as a colored product, and concentration can be derived against titration with variable dilutions as against a known standard. Immunochemical assays are not diagnostic, as no absolute value carries any meaning, unless reported with functional activity.

It must be noted that the available commercial kit results are not universal and are different for different laboratories. The paucity of reliable assays should, however, not hold back the physician from instituting empirical therapy based on presumptive diagnosis.

7.6.8.4 Scoring Systems

In non-tertiary centers and in the absence of sophisticated hemostatic laboratories, a handy clinical scoring system has been proposed by Coppo et al. to rule in whether the patient has ADAMTS13 deficiency or not. The three criteria included in the scoring system are:

- Creatinine values <2.2 mg L^{-1}
- Platelet count <30 × 10^9 L^{-1}
- Detectable levels of antinuclear antibodies (ANAs)

Any two of the three given criteria when present have a specificity of 98% and a positive predictive value of 99%. This scoring system however has a very low sensitivity.

Another recently proposed scoring system is the PLASMIC score. It consists of seven criteria:

- Platelet count <30 × 10^9 L^{-1}
- Hemolysis
- Positive history of cancer
- Positive history of transplant
- MCV < 99 × 10^{-14} L
- INR < 1.5
- Creatinine <2 mg dL^{-1}

This score also has similar positive predictive value, but Coppo is considered fairly simple and a better predictor in low-risk patient profile.

7.6.9 HUS and aHUS

Shiga Toxin Assays: Should be done for all patients presenting with bloody diarrhea.

Blood Cultures or Viral Studies: To establish systemic infections.

C3 and C4 Level: There are no reliable standardized commercially available kits in market to detect abnormalities in alternative complement regulation. Decreased levels of C3 reported in about 30–50% of the patients and C4 in about 10% of the patients may be suggestive in appropriate clinical setting. Decreased levels, by no means are either sensitive or specific to aHUS. The same principle applies to patients with mutations of CFH or CFI.

CFH Antibodies: Are detected by ELISA in 5–10% of patients with aHUS.

Mutation Analysis: Detects abnormalities in about 50% of the cases. Because compound mutations are more common, all genes known to be involved in alternative complement regulation need to be analyzed. Due to its complexity and incomplete understanding of pathogenic mechanisms, genetic study is not required for the diagnosis of aHUS.

Presently the diagnosis of aHUS relies on a process of exclusion. aHUS is suspected in patients presenting with the spectrum of microangiopathic hemolysis, any degree of renal function impairment and thrombocytopenia, and the diagnosis is presumed after exclusion of TTP, HUS and secondary microangiopathies.

7.6.10 DIC

Plasma Fibrinogen: In DIC secondary to pregnancy or hematological malignancies, a reduced plasma fibrinogen level may indicate diagnosis. However, such a relation is not seen in DIC secondary to sepsis.

Fibrin-Related Markers (FRMs): Elevated fibrin degradation products (including soluble fibrin) do serve valuable indicators to DIC.

Soluble Fibrin Assays: The advantage of detecting thrombin functions over fibrinogen or FDPs appears only theoretical in clinical settings. Soluble fibrin is nonspecifically elevated secondary to many conditions such as trauma, recent surgery, or recent bleeding, and is difficult to detect owing to its short half-life.

The coagulation profile (Fig. 7.16) observed in DIC is:

- Reduced antithrombin III
- Reduced protein C
- Reduced ADAMTS13 activity

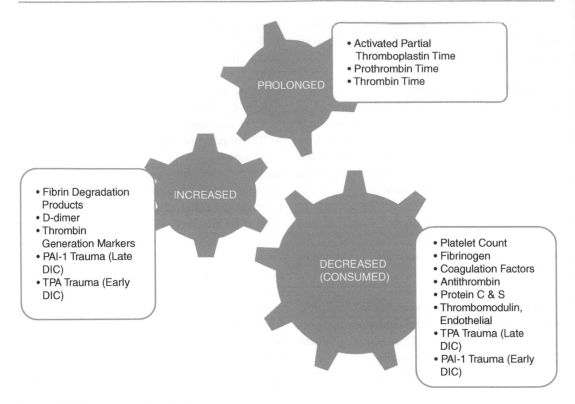

Fig. 7.16 Laboratory profile of DIC

- Elevated soluble thrombomodulin
- Elevated PAI-I
- Elevated ultra-large monomers of von Willebrand factor

It must be always kept in mind that none of these markers in isolation have any significance either diagnostically or prognostically.

A certain panel can definitely make a clinician's job easier.

- When massive bleeding is the predominant manifestation, PT, fibrinogen, and platelet count are important.
- When the presentation is mixed, then fibrinogen, FDP, and plasmin-plasmin inhibitor complex (PPIC) are important.
- When thrombosis is the predominant manifestation, then platelet count, PT, and APTT are important.
- For chronic DIC, which is incidentally detected, then soluble fibrin and the thrombin-antithrombin complex are important.

Scoring System: Various scoring systems have been proposed over the years, to help in empirical diagnosis of DIC, for example, Japanese Ministry Health, Labour and Welfare score—prognosis based, International Society of Thrombosis and Haemostasis score—useful in overt DIC, and Japanese Association of Acute Medicine score for septic DIC.

7.6.11 Treatment

7.6.11.1 Management of TTP

- *Plasma exchange*: Institution of plasma replacement causes immediate remission of signs and symptoms of TTP. Therapy should not be awaited until the diagnosis is made.
- *Steroids*: Steroids are the most appropriate treatment for acquired TTP, which is caused secondary to antibodies against ADAMTS13. Also, various treatment protocols have established superior efficacy of high-dose methylprednisolone (10 mg/kg/day for 3 days and

then 2.5 mg/kg/day) as against the standard dose (1 mg/kg/day). However, steroids are additionally added to treatment regimen, where plasma exchange remains cornerstone to treatment.

- *Rituximab*: Though the use of rituximab has not been established in primary line of treatment, clinical trials have reported significant efficacy against refractory TTP.
- *Other Immunomodulators*: Vincristine and cyclosporine A have been documented to provide theoretical advantage in refractory acquired TTP.
- *New drugs*: With our evolving understanding of the pathogenesis of TTP, certain new drugs are now being studied in clinical trials. *N-acetylcysteine*, has been proposed to decrease the size of ultra-large VWF multimers, therefore indirectly inhibits the attachment of platelets to endothelial cell. *Bortezomib*, a proteasome inhibitor, inhibits plasma cell production, indirectly inhibiting the production of antibodies. *Caplacizumab, formerly ALX-0081*, in recent trials has shown to reduce relapses.

7.6.11.2 Management of HUS

Treatment of Stx-HUS includes:
- Remains largely supportive, centered around management of clinical manifestations such as anemia, significant clinical bleeding, hypertension, renal support measures along with the prevention of systemic complications.
- Various treatment regimen including antithrombotic drugs, plasma exchange, tissue-type plasminogen activator, etc. have failed to demonstrate any efficacy.
- Eculizumab has shown effective results especially in severe refractory cases with neurological complications.

7.6.11.3 Management of aHUS
- Intensive plasma exchange (40–60 mL/kg) remains the primary management of aHUS with acute presentation. However, the response to treatment may depend on the extent to which the complement pathway is involved.

- Patients with autoantibodies against factor H should receive an immunosuppressive treatment in the form of rituximab or other immunomodulators.
- Eculizumab is a recently developed monoclonal antibody, which inhibits the production of C5a and overall inhibiting the membrane attack complex formation. It has shown promising results in aHUS post transplantation. A prolonged therapy has proved superior to single-dose treatment.
- Patients (with mutations in genes for factor H, factor I, or C3) progressing to ESRD despite multiple plasma exchanges have to be included on renal transplantation list. The chances of disease recurrence will significantly depend on the mutation involved.

7.6.11.4 Management of DIC
- Treatment of underlying cause remains the primary line of management. Only in severe cases, correction of coagulation abnormalities may be of help.
- Blood component transfusion therapy should be administered to patients with active clinical bleed or patients scheduled for any surgical intervention, despite the laboratory coagulation profile.
- Fresh frozen plasma should be administered at a bolus dose of 15 mL/kg and may be increased up to 30 mL/kg for a complete correction of coagulation profile. But this should be reserved for cases of severe DIC.
- Purified fibrinogen concentrate or cryoprecipitate may be administered for severe hypofibrinogenemia (<1 g/L), persisting post FFP transfusion, in order to maintain fibrinogen level above 1 g/L. The goal is to keep PT and aPTT to <1.5 times the normal.
- As supportive measure, packed red cells may be transfused to ensure better oxygen delivery to tissues.
- In DIC secondary to malignancies, significant vascular abnormalities or secondary to thromboembolic disease, heparin has been found useful, and also prevents complications.

- Recombinant human soluble thrombomodulin has recently found use in DIC and has shown promising results.
- In DIC secondary to severe systemic sepsis or multiorgan dysfunction, institution of activated protein C may prove beneficial.
- Tranexamic acid has shown encouraging results in hyperfibrinolysis with severe bleeding.

Recent Insights

Drug-Induced Thrombotic Microangiopathy (DI-TMA) can be either immune-mediated DI-TMA, especially seen with drugs that have the capacity to induce antibody formation against a variety of cells or can be through a direct, toxic effect (loss of VEGF expression has been implicated).

Recent Insights

TMA in the critically ill intensive care unit patients: Proinflammatory etiopathogenesis, neutrophil extracellular traps (NETs), and DNA and histones as a part with nucleosomes have shown prothrombotic tendencies, causing fibrin deposition, platelet aggregation, and adhesion.

Recent Insights

Mucin-producing adenocarcinomas (stomach and breast) have been most commonly implicated with TMA.

Suggested Reading

1. Joly BS, Coppo P, Veyradier A. Thrombotic thrombocytopenic purpura. Blood. 2017;129(21):2836–46.
2. Jokiranta TS. HUS and atypical HUS. Blood. 2017;129(21):2847–56.
3. Masias C, Vasu S, Cataland SR. None of the above: thrombotic microangiopathy beyond TTP and HUS. Blood. 2017;129(21):2857–63.
4. Kerr H, Richards A. Complement-mediated injury and protection of endothelium: lessons from atypical haemolytic uraemic syndrome. Immunobiology. 2012;217(2):195–203.

Inherited Bone Marrow Failure Syndromes

8

K. V. Karthika, Priyanka Mishra, and Hara Prasad Pati

8.1 Introduction

The inherited bone marrow failure syndromes are a heterogeneous group of disorders characterized by bone marrow failure which may or may not be associated with one or more somatic abnormality. The bone marrow failure can involve all or a single cell lineage resulting in pancytopenia or single cytopenias, respectively. Their true incidence is not clear since most of them are misdiagnosed as cases of acquired aplastic anemia. These syndromes often present in childhood but may not do so until adulthood in some cases. Inherited marrow failure syndromes need to be considered in the differential diagnosis of patients with characteristic physical abnormalities when present, along with idiopathic aplastic anemia, myelodysplastic syndrome, acute myeloid leukemia, or other characteristic solid cancers at an unusually early age. Diagnosis is confirmed by the identification of pathogenic mutations associated with each syndrome.

8.2 Classification

1. Pancytopenia
   (a) Fanconi anemia
   (b) Dyskeratosis congenita

2. Single cytopenias
   (a) Anemia
      • Diamond–Blackfan anemia
   (b) Neutropenia
      • Schwachman–Diamond syndrome*
      • Severe congenital neutropenia
   (c) Thrombocytopenia
      • Congenital amegakaryocytic thrombocytopenia*
      • Thrombocytopenia absent radii

*Although they present with neutropenia/thrombocytopenia to begin with, they eventually progress to pancytopenia (hence discussed along with pancytopenia syndromes).

8.3 Fanconi Anemia

Fanconi anemia (FA) is the most common among the inherited bone marrow failure syndromes, in which cells cannot properly repair a particularly deleterious type of DNA damage known as interstrand crosslinks (ICLs). ICLs can be caused by chemotherapeutic agents and endogenous metabolites such as acetaldehyde, malon-di-aldehyde, and nitrous acid. ICLs pose a major challenge to DNA replication and transcription. ICL lesions cause stalling of replication forks and activation of the DNA damage response and DNA repair processes, all of which are coordinated to repair ICLs and resume DNA replication. Unrepaired ICLs are par-

K. V. Karthika · P. Mishra · H. P. Pati (✉)
Department of Hematology, All India Institute of Medical Sciences, New Delhi, India

ticularly deleterious, as they prevent strand separation. This defect in DNA repair results in genomic instability and inability to repair these errors. This in turn leads to increased sensitivity to cytotoxic therapies and a predisposition to certain malignancies. This defect also causes loss of hematopoietic stem cells, resulting in bone marrow failure. The incidence of FA is approximately 1 in 100,000 to 250,000 births [1]. This condition is more common among the people of Ashkenazi Jews, with a carrier frequency of 1 in 89 [2], and black South Africans where the carrier frequency is 1 in 83 [3].

FA was first described in 1927 by the Swiss pediatrician Guido Fanconi when he described a family with three boys with birth defects and anemia [4]. The median age at diagnosis of FA in literature is around 6.6 years, with cases being reported up to the age of 49 years, the delay being due to the variable clinical presentation. Determining whether FA is the cause of bone marrow failure has important implications for management because individuals with FA require increased surveillance for hematologic and non-hematologic malignancies and other organ dysfunction. They also need to be managed with dramatically reduced doses of chemotherapy for treating malignancies and in the preparative regimen for hematopoietic cell transplantation (HCT). Additionally, the presence of FA must be confirmed or excluded when evaluating siblings as HCT donors, so that the patient does not receive hematopoietic stem cells from a sibling with FA.

8.3.1 Pathophysiology

FA is caused by mutations in one of at least 17 different FA genes (*FANCA to FANCQ*), although pathogenicity of mutations in *FANCM* has been called into question [5–9]. Mutations in these genes account for more than 95% of all known patients with Fanconi anemia. Additional genetic subtypes may be added, including those affecting RAD51 (*FANCR*), BRCA1 (*FANCS*), UBE2T (*FANCT*), and XRCC2 (*FANCU*) [10–17]. The latter group of genes are called Fanconi anemia-like genes since they do not present with the classical phenotype of FA.

In most cases, FA is inherited in an autosomal recessive manner through homozygous or compound heterozygous mutations affecting an individual FA gene. Two exceptions are the rare FA subtypes associated with mutation in *FANCB*, which is X-linked recessive, and *FANCR* (*RAD51*), which is autosomal dominant [18, 19]. Heterozygotes for mutations in FA genes other than *FANCB* and *FANCR* are considered to be unaffected carriers, although some of these individuals may have an increased susceptibility to cancer.

The methods of inactive gene function include point mutations, large deletions, and duplications. Genotype–phenotype correlations have occasionally been identified. However, it has been found that the presence of congenital malformations in one sibling does not imply that all affected siblings will have similar congenital malformations indicating the phenotypic heterogeneity of these mutations.

8.3.2 The Fanconi Anemia Pathway

The Fanconi anemia genes encode proteins involved in a common DNA repair pathway known as the Fanconi anemia pathway. These proteins are also involved in homologous recombination. This pathway functions during the S phase of the cell cycle and involves the various steps of ICL repair, namely lesion recognition, DNA incision, lesion bypass, and lesion repair [20].

The appearance of ICLs is identified by FANCM along with Fanconi anemia-associated protein 24 (FAAP24) and the histone fold proteins MHF1 (also known as FAAP16 or CENPS) and MHF2 (also known as FAAP10 or CENPX). Once bound to chromatin, FANCM forms the platform for the assembly of the Fanconi anemia core complex consisting of 14 proteins (FANCA, FANCB, FANCC, FANCE, FANCF, FANCG, FANCL, FANCM, FANCT, FAAP100, MHF1, MHF2, FAAP20, and FAAP24). The Fanconi anemia core complex serves as an ubiquitin ligase for two other Fanconi anemia proteins, FANCD2 and FANCI, which together form a heterodimer (referred to as FANCD2–I).

At the site of attachment, ubiquitylated FANCD2–Ire moves nucleotides at the replication forks to release the ICL from one of the two parental strands. This process is known as "unhooking." BRCA1 is also required for FANCD2 recruitment. FANCD2Ub through SLX4 (also known as FANCP) recruits and activates several endonucleases. After unhooking, polymerases carry out lesion bypass by inserting nucleotides opposite the ICL and extending the nascent strand (known as "extension"). This process inherently has low infidelity and hence can cause potentially introducing mutations in the genome.

Double strand breaks caused by the nucleolytic incision step of the Fanconi anemia pathway must be repaired by homologous recombination for the completion of ICL repair. The BRCA2–FANCN complex promotes RAD51mediated formation of singlestranded DNA (ssDNA) nucleofilaments. FANCJ along with BRCA1 mediates homologous recombination, thereby completing the process of ICL repair.

In patients with FA, loss of FA gene function leads to disruption of this normal repair process, genomic instability, aberrant cell cycle regulation, and cell death. These cellular effects occur both during development, leading to congenital anomalies, as well as during childhood and into adulthood leading to increased risk of bone marrow failure, organ susceptibility to toxic exposures, and cancer.

Bone marrow failure in FA is thought to occur due to premature, selective attrition of CD34$^+$ HSCs possibly due to defective DNA repair leading to increased DNA damage and cell cycle arrest; increased levels of reactive oxygen species and circulating inflammatory cytokines affecting bone marrow microenvironment; and excessive damage caused by reactive aldehydes in the absence of intact FA repair pathways.

8.3.3 Clinical Features

A wide range of congenital anomalies have been reported in patients with FA. However, a study of 370 patients by the International Fanconi Anemia Registry (IFAR) found that nearly 40% of them had no physical findings [21]. Patients with biallelic mutations in *FANCD1/BRCA2* have a very severe phenotype, including features of the vertebral, anal, cardiac, tracheal, esophageal, and limb (VACTERL) association.

1. *Skeletal*
   - Short stature is seen in almost half of all FA patients.
   - Upper limb abnormalities (40%)—most common are thumb abnormalities.
     - Thumbs can be absent or hypoplastic, supernumerary, bifid, rudimentary, short, triphalangeal or tubular.
     - Radii—Absent or hypoplastic (In FA, hypoplastic radii are associated with abnormal thumbs unlike in TAR).
     - Hands—Clinodactyly, hypoplastic thenar eminence, polydactyly, absent first metacarpal, enlarged or short fingers.
     - Ulnae can also be occasionally dysplastic.
   - Spine—Spina bifida, scoliosis, abnormal ribs, sacrococcygeal sinus, Klippel–Feil syndrome, extra vertebrae.
   - Lower limbs—Toe syndactyly, polydactyly, abnormal toes, flat feet, clubfoot, hip dislocation, Perthes disease, coxa vara, abnormal femur, thigh osteoma.
2. *Skin*
   - Hyperpigmentation or hypopigmentation on the trunk, neck, back, and intertriginous areas (café au lait spots) (>50%)
3. *Genitourinary*
   - Renal defects (20%)—such as horseshoe kidney
   - **Gonadal** abnormalities
     - Males (30%)—Undescended testes, hypospadias, abnormal or absent testis, azoospermia, phimosis, abnormal urethra, small penis, delayed development
     - Females (<5%)—Structural anomalies of the uterus; aplasia of vagina; absence of uterus, vagina, or ovary/ovaries

4. *Craniofacial*
   - Head and face—Microcephaly (25%), hydrocephalus, micrognathia, bird facies, flat head, frontal bossing, scaphocephaly, sloped forehead, choanal atresia
   - Neck—short neck, low hairline, webbed neck
   - Ophthalmic abnormalities (20%)—Microphthalmia, epicanthal folds, strabismus, hypertelorism, ptosis, slanted eyes, cataracts, epiphora, nystagmus, proptosis, small iris
   - Otic anomalies (10%)—Conductive deafness, atresia, low-set, large, small, abnormal middle ear, absent drum, canal stenosis

5. *Gastrointestinal malformations*
   - High-arched palate, atresia, imperforate anus, tracheoesophageal fistula, Meckel diverticulum, umbilical hernia, abnormal biliary radicles, megacolon, Budd–Chiari syndrome

6. *Congenital heart disease (5%)*
   - Patent ductus arteriosus, ventricular septal defect, coarctation of aorta, truncus arteriosus

7. *Low birth weight (10%)*

8. *Developmental delay (10%)*

9. *Bone marrow failure*
   Bone marrow failure in FA usually begins with single-lineage cytopenias which then progresses to pancytopenia. This progression may take several years or may occur rapidly or may not progress at all. Thrombocytopenia is usually the first cytopenia to develop. Anemia is usually the last to develop. The anemia is usually macrocytic. Sometimes there can be macrocytosis without anemia. The cumulative incidence of bone marrow failure is about 90% by the age of 40 years. However, all are not affected, for example, patients with biallelic *FANCD2/BRCA2* mutations appear less likely to develop bone marrow failure. Also, in 25% of patients, factors like additional mutations and somatic mosaicism ameliorate bone marrow failure symptoms though the risk of malignancy remains.

10. *MDS/Leukemia*
    Patients with FA are at an increased risk of developing MDS and acute myeloid leukemia, sometimes maybe the presenting finding. By the age of 50, the cumulative incidence of MDS and AML is around 40 and 15%, respectively [22]. Rarely, these patients may also develop lymphoid malignancies like ALL, Burkitt's lymphoma, etc. The risk is much higher in patients with biallelic mutations of FANCD1/BRCA2 (about 80% by the age of 10).

11. *Solid tumors*
    Patients with FA have a higher risk of developing solid malignancies and usually present at an earlier age. The median age of developing malignancy in FA patients is 16 years [23], the risk increasing with age. The most common were squamous cell cancers (SCCs) of the head, neck, esophagus, anus, and urogenital region, liver tumors as well as renal, brain, breast cancers, and other tumor types including germ cell tumors and sarcomas [21]. Yet again, patients with biallelic mutations of FANCD1/BRCA2 have an increased risk, with about 97% of patients developing at least one solid malignancy by the age of 5 years.

12. *Endocrine manifestations*
    These may be due to anatomical disruption of the hypothalamic-pituitary axis or due to conditioning regimens.
    - Short stature
    - Primary hypothyroidism
    - Adrenal dysfunction due to low ACTH secretion
    - Altered glucose metabolism, including diabetes mellitus and impaired glucose tolerance
    - Dyslipidemia
    - Infertility and delayed or abnormal progression of puberty

8.3.4 Diagnosis

Testing for FA is absolutely and urgently indicated in any child or young adult meeting any of the following criteria:

- Two or more moderate to severe cytopenias (absolute neutrophil count [ANC] <1000/μL, platelet count <50,000/μL, hemoglobin<10 g/dL with absolute reticulocyte count <40,000/μL), persistent for more than 2 weeks, and a hypocellular bone marrow (<25% of normal cellularity) in the absence of malignancy, cytotoxic therapy, or other known cause.
- Findings that satisfy criteria for the VACTERL-H association or multiple other malformations such as short stature, café au lait spots, or hypospadias, which are strongly associated with FA.
- Relative of a known patient with FA who is being evaluated as a potential donor for HCT.

Testing for FA is also recommended in the following scenarios, with the rationale that the diagnosis of FA should be established (or eliminated) prior to administration of cytotoxic chemotherapy for cancer or HCT; and if FA is present, related family members should be tested before being considered as HCT donors:

- Any patient with single-lineage or multi-lineage cytopenias without known cause with one or more congenital malformations strongly associated with FA.
- Any patient less than 40 years of age diagnosed with myelodysplastic syndrome (MDS) not attributable to other known genetic cause or to prior cytotoxic radiation or chemotherapy.
- Any patient less than 40 years of age with de novo acute myeloid leukemia (AML) not caused by another known germline predisposition and associated with the following cytogenetics: monosomy 7, deletion 7q, complex cytogenetics, gain of 1q, 3q, or 13q. The rationale is that doses of chemotherapy and/or cytotoxic agents given as part of the HCT conditioning regimen need to be dramatically reduced in a patient with FA.
- Any patient with unexplained severe toxicity to cytotoxic agents indicative of increased sensitivity without other known cause.
- Any child or young adult who develops head/neck or anorectal squamous cell carcinoma with no known attributable exposures.
- Family members of known FA patients who request genetic testing.

8.3.4.1 Stress Cytogenetics

The hallmark of FA is defective DNA repair that results in extreme sensitivity to DNA interstrand crosslinking agents. The screening laboratory test for this defect involves assessment of chromosomal breakage upon exposure of cells to diepoxybutane (DEB) or mitomycin C (MMC) [1]. This testing is performed on T lymphocytes; thus, peripheral blood is preferred as a test source over bone marrow. In settings of severe leukopenia, the testing can still be performed on cells expanded in culture. It can be performed on skin fibroblasts too.

Heparinized venous blood is taken and expanded in culture. The cells are then treated with 150 nM and 300 nM of mitomycin C. The cells are arrested at metaphase using colcemid and harvested. Increased chromosomal sensitivity results in chromatid gaps, breaks, triradial and quadriradial chromosomes. These aberrations are scored as "break events." In a typical FA patient, at 300 nM MMC, no undamaged cells should be left and most cells should have "$\geq$10 breaks/cell." This should be run along with a healthy control in whom at 300 nM, around 30% of the cells may show 1 to $\leq$5 break events/cell [24].

FA gene sequencing is recommended for all patients with a positive result from chromosomal breakage testing. The differential diagnosis of FA includes acquired aplastic anemia, paroxysmal nocturnal hemoglobinuria (PNH), other inherited bone marrow failure syndromes, other causes of pancytopenia, other chromosomal breakage syndromes, and de novo MDS. Sequencing not only helps to confirm the diagnosis but also serves to screen family members and allows for genotype–phenotype correlations.

8.3.5 Treatment

Allogeneic hematopoietic cell transplantation (HCT) is the only established curative therapy for FA-associated bone marrow failure, myelodysplastic syndromes (MDS), and leukemia. Androgen therapy is not curative, but it may be appropriate for patients with bone marrow failure awaiting HCT or those who cannot undergo HCT. Transfusion and growth factor support may be necessary in patients. These patients need to be screened routinely for MDS, leukemias, and other solid malignancies from time to time. If a patient with FA develops a malignancy that requires chemotherapy and/or radiation therapy, dose reductions or alternative regimens are likely to be necessary. These patients also require a multispeciality approach for other associated anomalies such as endocrine dysfunction and congenital abnormalities.

8.4 Dyskeratosis Congenita

Dyskeratosis congenita (DKC), also known as Zinsser-Engman-Cole syndrome, was first described in 1906. It is estimated to occur in 1 in one million people with a male to female ratio of 3:1. Approximately 2–5% of patients with bone marrow failure are identified to have DKC. It is an inherited disorder characterized by bone marrow failure, cancer predisposition, and additional somatic abnormalities. DKC and related short telomere syndromes are caused by mutations that interfere with normal maintenance of telomeres, the regions at the ends of the chromosomes that protect nucleated cells from the loss or gain of genetic material.

8.4.1 Pathophysiology

Telomeres are specialized structures at the end of chromosomes that protect the natural ends of chromosomes from loss of DNA, abnormal fusion to other chromosomes, and from activation of DNA damage pathway responses that normally would occur in response at free ends of DNA created by strand breaks. Telomeric DNA consists of tandem repeats of the TTAGGG sequence. Most of the telomeric DNA exists as duplex DNA, with a terminal single-stranded overhang of typically approximately 150–200 nucleotides of the G-rich strand. The shortening of the duplex DNA portion of telomeres is most characteristic of telomere biology disorders.

At birth, the telomere length is around 8–14 kilobase pairs. With each cell division, this length shortens. When the telomere length reaches a critical minimum, the cells can no longer divide. For this reason, the telomeres are referred to as biological clocks that keep track of the number of divisions a cell undergoes. In most somatic cells, this shortening is a normal part of ageing. However, some cells such as germ cells, epithelial cells, and malignant cells require unlimited replicative potential. This increased replicative capacity is made possible by the action of the telomerase complex, a ribonuclear protein complex (RNA and proteins) that counteracts telomere shortening by adding back DNA to the ends of chromosomes. The ability of telomerase to lengthen telomeres is regulated by several other mechanisms. The nucleoprotein factors contributing to these mechanisms, and consequently the genes encoding these factors, mutations of which lead to telomere biology disorders, have been subdivided into five categories [25]:

- *Telomerase activity*—Telomerase is a reverse transcriptase enzyme consisting of TERT, a catalytic protein; and TR, an RNA template. Its assembly requires small nucleolar ribonucleoproteins including dyskerin, NHP2, NAF1, and NOP10.
- *Telomerase trafficking and recruiting to telomeres*—Once the telomerase has been assembled, its recruitment to the telomeric site is mediated by TCAB1 and the shelterin complex which consists of the proteins TRF1, TRF2, RAP1, TIN2, TPP1, and POT1.
- *Telomere replication*—The CST complex causes extension of the telomere end in conjunction with the telomerase enzyme.
- *Telomere stability*—The RTEL1 is a DNA helicase that maintains the integrity of the

newly formed DNA duplex end of the telomere.

- *Unknown or multifactorial*—This group includes other proteins whose functional and pathologic significance have not yet been elucidated.

In telomere biology disorders (also called short telomere syndromes or telomeropathies), mutations in the genes encoding any of the above factors implicated in telomere function lead to abnormally short telomeres. This group of disorders exhibit the phenomenon of "disease anticipation" in which successive generations of affected individuals may be born with progressively shorter telomeres. Premature telomere shortening leads to premature cell death, senescence, or genomic instability, which in turn leads to impaired organ and tissue function, altered homeostasis, or inappropriate growth.

DKC is the prototypic short telomere syndrome defined by the bone marrow failure and the classic clinical triad of abnormal skin pigmentation, nail dystrophy, and oral leukoplakia. The inheritance pattern varies depending on the gene involved. It can be autosomal dominant (mutations in *ACD*, *RTEL1*, *TERC*, *TERT*, *TINF2*, and *NAF1*), autosomal recessive (mutations in *CTC1*, *NHP2*, *NOP10*, *PARN*, *RTEL1*, *STN1*, *TERT*, and *WRAP53*), or X-linked (also called Hoyeraal–Hreidarsson syndrome caused by mutations in DKC1 gene and characterized by severe phenotype with symptoms beginning in early childhood). The prevalence of DKC has been estimated to be approximately 1 in one million people in the general population [26] with a median age at diagnosis of 15 years. Approximately 2–5% of patients with bone marrow failure are identified to have DKC.

8.4.2 Clinical Features

The classical clinical findings are:
- Abnormal lacy reticular skin hyperpigmentation of the upper chest and neck (89%)
- Nail dystrophy with longitudinal ridges (88%)
- Oral leukoplakia (78%)

The other findings include:
- Bone marrow failure (86%)
- Premature graying/hair loss (16%)
- Hyperhidrosis (15%)
- Epiphora
- Developmental delay
- Pulmonary fibrosis (31%)—typically presenting in adulthood
- Endocrine manifestations such as short stature and hypogonadism
- Gastroenterological manifestations such as esophageal strictures and liver cirrhosis
- Increased predisposition to cancers including squamous cell carcinoma of the head and neck; stomach, rectal, and other gastrointestinal cancers; leukemia and myelodysplastic syndrome; and cancers of the skin, lung, and liver [27]

8.4.3 Diagnosis

The diagnosis of DKC has evolved from a purely clinical one based on classic mucocutaneous findings with or without bone marrow failure to the demonstration of telomeric dysfunction in these diseases by assays for telomere length and genetic testing for specific abnormalities that affect telomeric function. This approach enables diagnosis of probands with subtle clinical presentations.

- *Telomere length analysis*—This is done by flow-FISH (multi-color flow cytometry with fluorescence in situ hybridization) peripheral blood lymphocytes using peptide nucleic acid probes for telomeric DNA. Average telomere length below the first percentile for age is considered indicative of abnormally short telomeres and is consistent with DKC or a related telomere biology disorder.
- *Molecular sequencing*—This testing is critical for definitive establishment of a genetic diagnosis and enabling testing of first-degree relatives for potential carrier or disease status, and to determine family member eligibility to be an HCT donor. This could be done by sequential single gene testing, next generation sequencing panels or by whole exome sequencing.

8.4.4 Treatment

Historically, treatment options for patients with DKC have been limited by the rarity of the disease, few prospective studies, and predisposition to excess organ toxicities seen with conventional treatments used for other bone marrow failure conditions. However, the treatment outlook may be improving with active exploration of the roles for certain telomere-directed treatments, including androgen therapy, as well as hematopoietic cell transplantation (HCT) with reduced intensity conditioning regimens specifically designed for patients with telomere disorders.

8.5 Schwachman–Diamond Syndrome

Shwachman–Diamond syndrome (SDS, also known as Shwachman–Bodian–Diamond syndrome, Shwachman–Diamond–Oski syndrome, or Shwachman syndrome) is a rare inherited disorder associated with neutropenia which progresses to bone marrow failure along with exocrine pancreatic dysfunction and skeletal abnormalities. The disease usually presents in infancy. Among inherited bone marrow failure syndromes, SDS comes third after Fanconi anemia and DKC in frequency.

8.5.1 Genetics and Pathophysiology

SDS is an autosomal recessive disorder. About 90% of affected individuals harbor mutations in the SBDS gene situated on the long arm of chromosome 7 [28]. The protein encoded (SBDS protein) is involved in ribosomal biogenesis and mitotic spindle function. How these defects contribute to the clinical manifestations of SDS has not been established. Defects in maintaining cellular ploidy may contribute to the increased risk of leukemic transformation.

8.5.2 Clinical Features

- Bone marrow failure—usually presents as neutropenia (98%), but can also present as anemia (42%), thrombocytopenia (34%), or pancytopenia (19%).
- Steatorrhea—86%. SDS is the second most common cause of exocrine pancreatic insufficiency after cystic fibrosis. Interestingly, pancreatic function improves with age.
- Serum hepatic aminotransferase abnormalities—60%.
- Skeletal abnormalities such as osteopenia, metaphyseal dysplasia, thoracic/rib and pelvic dystrophies, short arms and legs, and duplicated distal thumb—49%.
- Short stature—56%.
- MDS/AML—The cumulative risk of developing MDS or AML in individuals with SDS was estimated to be 19% at 20 years and 36% at 30 years.
- The other less common findings include hepatic, cardiac, endocrine, neurocognitive abnormalities and increased HbF due to stress erythropoiesis.

8.5.3 Diagnosis

SDS should be suspected in an infant with growth failure, feeding difficulties, steatorrhea, neutropenia, and/or recurrent infections [29]. Diagnosis is established by demonstrating bone marrow failure with exocrine pancreatic dysfunction. Molecular diagnosis is established by identifying biallelic mutations in SBDS genes known to be deleterious, though their absence does not rule out the disease.

8.5.4 Treatment

Treatment of patients with SDS is directed at specific clinical manifestations. Management by a multidisciplinary team (e.g., gastroenterologist and hematologist, with other subspecialists as clinically indicated) provides optimal care. Allogeneic hematopoietic cell transplantation (HCT) is the only curative therapy for SDS-associated bone marrow dysfunction and/or progression to MDS or AML. However, HCT will not improve pancreatic exocrine function or a predisposition to non-hematologic abnormalities.

8.6 Congenital Amegakaryocytic Thrombocytopenia

Congenital amegakaryocytic thrombocytopenia (CAMT) is a rare bone marrow failure syndrome that initially presents with severe thrombocytopenia and can evolve into aplastic anemia and leukemia. The disorder presents in infancy and is usually not associated with physical anomalies. It is often recognized early in life on day 1 or at least within the first month. It is often initially confused with fetal and neonatal alloimmune thrombocytopenia, but the neonate fails to improve and responds only to platelet transfusion.

8.6.1 Genetics and Pathophysiology

CAMT is an autosomal recessively inherited disorder associated with mutations in the c-Mpl gene, which encodes the receptor for TPO (thrombopoietin). High levels of TPO are characteristic of CAMT. The normal function of TPO is to bind to its receptor and increase the number, size and ploidy of megakaryocytes and expression of platelet-specific markers. It is also essential to maintain the number of hematopoietic stem cells, and therefore their mutation can cause pancytopenia too, as seen in CAMT.

A recent classification was proposed in 2005 supported by several other reports based on the course on outcome of the disease as follows [30]:

(a) Type I—early onset of severe thrombocytopenia and pancytopenia. In this group, there is complete loss of functional c-Mpl due to nonsense mutations.

(b) Type II—milder form with transient increases of platelet counts up to nearly normal values during the first year of life and a late onset of bone marrow failure around the age of 3 to 6 years or later. In this group, there are partially functional receptors for the c-Mpl gene (missense mutations).

(c) Type III—there is ineffective production of megakaryocytes with no defects in the c-Mpl gene.

8.6.2 Clinical Features

Bleeding is the primary clinical manifestation: it could be cutaneous, gastrointestinal, pulmonary, and intracranial. Some patients may present with petechial purpura, cranial hematoma, or recurrent per rectal bleeding. Platelet counts among neonates are usually in the level of $150 \times 10^9/L$. Mental retardation, renal failure, high tone hearing loss, cataracts, or the development of leukemia are other associated features that may be seen in some patients though most of them lack these features.

8.6.3 Diagnosis

The primary manifestations are thrombocytopenia and megakaryocytopenia or low numbers of platelets and megakaryocytes. Mean platelet volume is typically normal. Abnormal size platelets, absence of platelet alpha granules, Dohle-like bodies or microcytosis have also been observed. There is an absence of megakaryocytes in the bone marrow. However, normal megakaryocytes in the bone marrow cannot rule out CAMT in the first year of life [31]. TPO levels are high. Genetic sequencing of c-Mpl gene is carried out for the diagnosis of probands.

8.6.4 Treatment

Currently, the only curative therapy for CAMT is a hematopoietic stem cell transplant. Platelet transfusions are reserved for patients experiencing bleeding symptoms. Prophylactic platelet transfusions may be considered for patients posing a high bleeding risk. Antifibrinolytic agents such as tranexamic acid and aminocaproic acid may be useful in mucous membrane bleeds such as oral or nasal bleeding.

8.7 Diamond–Blackfan Anemia

Diamond–Blackfan anemia (DBA) is an inherited bone marrow failure syndrome characterized by pure red cell aplasia, birth defects, and predisposition to cancer. It was first defined as a clinical syndrome by Diamond and Blackfan in 1938. However, the first case report was from Josephs in 1936.

8.7.1 Genetic Defects

RPS19, located at chromosome 19q13.2, was the first gene found to be mutated in this disorder and is essential for maturation of the 40S ribosomal subunit. It is involved in ribosomal biogenesis and is mutated in about 25% of patients with DBA leading to haplo-insufficiency of rps19 protein. Other recently identified genes include RPS24 at chromosome 10q22-q23, RPS17 at chromosome 15q25.2 and large ribosomal subunit-associated proteins such as rpl5, rpl11, and rpl35a [32, 33]. These mutations together are seen in 70% of cases. All the mutations to date have been found in one allele, resulting in severe loss of function or protein haplo-insufficiency. Mutation in GATA-1 is seen in <1% of cases and no gene disorder is identified in 30% cases [34].

8.7.2 Inheritance

Approximately 40–45% of DBA cases are familial with autosomal dominant with variable penetrance and the remainder being sporadic or familial with seemingly different patterns of inheritance. Both mild and severe forms co-exist within a pedigree (variable expressivity). It is yet to be ascertained whether the rest are recessive

forms or dominant inheritance with a reduced penetrance, or rarely gonadal mosaicism. It is important to identify family members likely to have silent forms of the disease to exclude them as stem cell transplant donors and for reproductive counseling [34].

8.7.3 Clinical Features

The incidence of DBA is estimated to be between 1/100000 and 1/200000 without ethnic predilection, with both sexes being equally affected. The birth defects associated with DBA are mainly craniofacial (50%), skeletal (39%), genitourinary (38%), and cardiac (30%) cases. The classic DBA facies described by Cathie in 1950 include hypertelorism and broad flat nasal bridge. Thumb anomalies ranging from hypoplasia of the thenar eminence to absence of the radius or forearm, duplicated, bifid or the classic triphalangeal thumb (Aase syndrome) are seen in 9–19% of the patients. A low birth weight and growth retardation are seen in about 25–30% of patients. The true prevalence of constitutional short stature is not known as it can be secondary to chronic anemia, iron overload, and corticosteroid use [35].

8.7.4 Diagnosis

The diagnostic criteria of DBA, revised at the sixth Annual Diamond Blackfan Anemia International Consensus Conference in 2005, are as below:

Diagnostic criteria
- Age less than 1 year
- Macrocytic anemia with no other significant cytopenias
- Reticulocytopenia
- Normal marrow cellularity with a paucity of erythroid precursors

Supporting criteria
Major
- Gene mutation described in "classical" DBA
- Positive family history

Minor

- Elevated erythrocyte adenosine deaminase (eADA) activity
- Congenital anomalies described in "classical" DBA
- Elevated HbF
- No evidence of another inherited bone marrow failure syndrome

Non-classical DBA—Otherwise normal individual with positive family history having a mutation shared by affected family members.

Non-classical, sporadic—Individual suspected of having DBA, but diagnostic criteria is insufficient, and reported mutation is present.

Probable DBA

1. Three diagnostic criteria are present along with a positive family history.
2. Two diagnostic criteria and three minor supporting criteria are present.
3. Positive family history and three minor supporting criteria are evident, even in the absence of diagnostic criteria.

In case anemia and reticulocytopenia are present and the bone marrow is normal, bone marrow should be repeated at a later date. The presence of additional cytopenias does not preclude the diagnosis of DBA and may be severe enough to warrant treatment [34].

8.7.4.1 Family Screening

In a family in which classical DBA is present in the parent and offspring, or in two or more siblings, the risk of recurrence in the subsequent generation is up to 50%. If the mutation of the proband is excluded in both parents, this is likely to be a new sporadic mutation with a recurrence risk related to the possibility of gonadal mosaicism. If no mutation is identified in the proband and if elevated eADA activity, Hb F and/or MCV (highly suggestive of DBA) are found in asymptomatic first-degree relatives, the recurrence risk should be considered as 50%. However the possibility of false positive results in these tests should be kept in mind. If, however, these values are normal in first-degree relatives, the recurrence risk is only 5–10% [34].

An evaluation of the family of the first identified case is necessary. All immediate family members should be evaluated with a thorough relevant history (anemia, cancer, birth defects, etc.), complete blood count including red cell indices, eADA activity, and HbF. If the proband has an identifiable mutation, then the parents and siblings need to have appropriate mutation analysis if available. The nature of any other positive findings will determine the extent of the family evaluation. Elevated eADA, increased HbF and MCV are not very strong independent criteria, but should be evaluated in the sibling donor when HSCT is planned, and if positive, mutational analysis should be carried out.

Prenatal diagnosis is possible for DBA if a mutation is identified in the family. More recently, preimplantation genetic diagnosis (PGD) is an option to greatly reduce the risk of a second affected child. This can be performed in order to select and implant embryos without the parental mutation, hence eliminating the risk for DBA. This method can also be combined with PGD for human leukocyte antigen (HLA) typing for families with an affected child in need of an HLA-matched stem cell transplant [35] after due ethical considerations.

8.7.5 Management and Follow-Up

A periodic history to assess any new complaints and physical examination with blood count monitoring is done at 4–6 month intervals in stable DBA patients. If any of these are abnormal, bone marrow aspirate, biopsy, cytogenetics, and FISH should be performed to determine early signs of evolution to MDS and AML. Radiation exposure from diagnostic tests should be minimized in these patients to minimize the risk of malignancies [34].

Corticosteroids form the cornerstone of treatment in DBA. Approximately 80% of DBA patients respond to an initial course of steroids. After starting steroids, an increase in hemoglobin is usually seen within 2–4 weeks. The dose is then tapered and maintained at the minimum dosage required for continued transfusion independence. Steroids should be discontinued in the absence of response after 4 weeks. In order to minimize their adverse effects, steroids are avoided before 1 year of age. Chelation may be required in case of iron overload secondary to frequent transfusions. In around 20% of DBA patients, steroids (or red cell transfusions) may eventually be stopped completely with continued maintenance of adequate hemoglobin levels (remission) [34, 35].

8.8 Severe Congenital Neutropenia

Severe congenital neutropenia (SCN), Kostmann syndrome, is an inherited bone marrow failure syndrome characterized by severe chronic neutropenia with maturation arrest of neutrophil precursors at the promyelocyte stage in the bone marrow. This entity was first described by Kostmann in 1956 in Swedish kindred.

8.8.1 Pathogenesis

It is proposed that Kostmann syndrome represents a defect in the regulation or production of granulocyte colony-stimulating factor (GCSF). Neutrophils from these patients have markedly increased levels of 2 cytosolic protein tyrosine phosphatases (PTPs) that contain Src-homology 2 domain (SH2 domain), Anti-Src Homology Phosphatase-1 (SHP-1) and Src Homology Phosphatase 2 (SHP2). Over-expression of these proteins alters intracellular signal transduction. A selective deficiency of anti-apoptotic BCL-2 expression in myeloid cells leads to release of mitochondrial cytochrome c, thus activating intracellular apoptotic caspase pathway [36]. Previous hypothesis that the underlying defect in Kostmann syndrome is decreased G-CSF production or its diminished binding to GCSF-R no longer holds true as studies show that there are increased GCSF-R on myeloid cells with normal binding affinity for G-CSF. The autosomal dom-

inant (60–80% cases) form of SCN is associated with inherited or spontaneous point mutation in one copy of gene encoding neutrophil elastase ELA2 [37]. A subset of SCN patients harbor acquired somatic mutations in the CSF3R gene encoding GCSF-R and have shown a strong predisposition to AML. These mutations truncate the intracellular leading to defective internalization and loss of binding sites for negative regulators leading to extended signaling of STAT5 (Signal transducer and activator of transcription 5). A subset of SCN patients are reported to have constitutive mutations in the extracellular domain of the GCSF-R that act in dominant-negative manner leading to hypo-responsiveness to G-CSF [38].

Recent studies point to recurrent homozygous germline mutation in HAX1 in SCN. The mitochondrial protein HAX1 has critical role in signal transduction and cytoskeletal control. It maintains the inner mitochondrial membrane potential and thus protects neutrophils from apoptosis. HAXI deficiency causes AR form of Kostmann disease [39].

8.8.2 Clinical Features

The classic Kostmann syndrome presents in early infancy with an equal incidence in males and females. Severe neutropenia (ANC < 200/cu mm) is brought to clinical attention after an initial infection which typically occurs shortly after birth. Common indicators to this disorder are temperature instability in neonatal period, fever, irritability and recurrent oral ulcers, gingivitis, localized infections such as pharyngitis, sinusitis, otitis media, bronchitis, pneumonia, cellulitis, cutaneous abscess, perianal abscess, lung or liver abscess, enteritis with chronic diarrhea and vomiting. Streptococcal or staphylococcal sepsis commonly occur though Pseudomonas, fungi, and Clostridium may rarely be causative. The mortality rate in the absence of appropriate medical management is around 70%. The progression to MDS and AML is seen in 7% of cases [36].

8.8.3 Diagnosis

Patients have ANCs generally below 0.2×10^9/L and neutrophils may be completely absent from peripheral blood. There may be transient rise of neutrophils during an episode of acute infection, but normal ANC is seldom reached. There may be co-existent mild anemia and thrombocytosis. A two- to four-fold increase in blood monocytes and an eosinophilia is usually common. Majority of the patients have elevated IgG levels with a normal immune response after vaccinations. Testing for anti-neutrophil antibodies is helpful to exclude autoimmune neutropenia of infancy. The bone marrow usually shows maturation arrest of myeloid precursors at stage of promyelocytes and myelocytes with few neutrophils. The promyelocytes show atypical nuclei with cytoplasmic vacuolization. Megakaryocytes are normal in number and morphology. Cytogenetics at the time of diagnosis is almost always normal. Monosomy 7 is the most frequent aberration acquired in 50% of cases with progression of disease and usually coincides with the development of MDS and AML [36].

8.8.4 Management

Management is usually supportive in the form of antibiotics and recombinant human G-CSF (rHuG-CSF) whose dosages depend on the patient's clinical course and ANC. Careful monitoring for cytogenetic abnormalities and G-CSF-R mutation is necessary to initiate rHuG-CSF. Adverse events of rHuG-CSF therapy include mild splenomegaly, osteoporosis, and malignant transformation into MDS/leukemia. HSCT remains the only currently available treatment for patients who are refractory to rHuG-CSF [36].

8.9 Thrombocytopenia with Absent Radii (TAR)

Thrombocytopenia with absent radii (TAR) syndrome is a rare autosomal recessive disease characterized by hypomegakaryocytic thrombocytopenia and bilaterally absent radii [40].

8.9.1 Genetics

Mutations in c-mpl gene coding for TPO receptor were earlier attributed to TAR, and these patients generally have elevated TPO levels. However, recent studies indicate that mutations in multifunctional transforming growth factor (TGF)-β2 gene and lack of expression of CD105 antigen on bone marrow stromal cells which is a part of the receptor complex for TGF-β1 and TGF-β3 have been implicated in this disease. The deletion on chromosome 1q21.1 described by Klopocki et al. though found to be associated is not considered sufficient to cause TAR. TAR is characterized by a defect in megakaryocyte proliferation and differentiation and the inability to form proplatelets [41].

Inheritance is autosomal recessive in the majority of cases although an autosomal dominant with variable penetrance has also been proposed. TAR syndrome phenotypically overlaps with Roberts syndrome, but while the former is compound heterozygous form of a mild and a severe mutation, Roberts syndrome is the homozygous form with severe mutation [41, 42].

8.9.2 Clinical Features

Classically, the syndrome presents in the neonatal period with severe thrombocytopenia (usually <20,000/cu mm) and bilateral aplasia of the radii, which is the most common skeletal defect, but unlike Fanconi anemia, thumbs are present. The other skeletal abnormalities include anomalies of the lower extremity and short stature. Cardiac and facial anomalies may be found in 15% to 33% and 50% of patients, respectively. Hypoplasia of the cerebellar vermis and corpus callosum and mental retardation are seen in about 7% of all cases of TAR syndrome. Thrombocytopenia and bleeding episodes may improve with age. Survival is significantly longer in patients with TAR syndrome than that of Fanconi anemia or Diamond–Blackfan anemia, with the survival curve reaching a plateau of 75% by 4 years of age. Progression to aplastic anemia is not seen though AML or MDS can occur however at a lower frequency [41].

Patients usually present with symptoms of thrombocytopenia (platelet count <10 × 10⁹/L) as early as in the first week of life. Leukocytosis (usually >35 × 10⁹/L) may be present and precedes thrombocytopenia, with a left shift and eosinophilia in about 50% of patients. Bone marrow erythropoiesis is normal or may show compensatory erythroid hyperplasia due to anemia following bleeding episodes. Bleeding is most frequent during the first 1 to 2 years of life, with increased mortality due to intracranial hemorrhage [40].

8.9.3 Management

Treatment is usually supportive in the form of platelet support. Prophylactic transfusions are restricted to patients at high risk of clinically significant hemorrhage. Leukocyte-reduced platelet concentrates or random single-donor platelets reduce risk of exposure to foreign human leukocyte antigen and alloimmunization. HSCT is an option for patients whose counts do not improve with age and life-threatening bleeds not adequately controlled with platelets [41, 42].

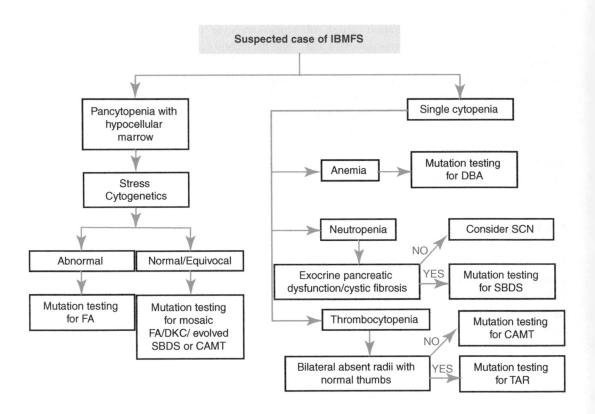

References

1. Alter BP. Inherited bone marrow failure syndromes. In: Nathan DG, Orkin SH, Ginsburg D, Look AT, editors. Nathan and Oski's hematology of infancy and childhood. Philadelphia: W.B. Saunders; 2003.
2. Verlander PC, Kaporis A, Liu Q, Zhang Q, Seligsohn U, Auerbach AD. Carrier frequency of the IVS4 + 4 AT mutation of the Fanconi anemia gene FANC in the Ashkenazi Jewish population. Blood. 1995;86:4034–8.
3. Timmers C, Taniguchi T, Hejna J, Reifsteck C, Lucas L, Bruun D, et al. Positional cloning of a novel Fanconi anemia gene, FANCD2. Mol Cell. 2001;7:241–8.
4. Lobitz S, Velleuer E. Guido Fanconi (1892-1979): a jack of all trades. Nat Rev Cancer. 2006;6(11):893–8.
5. Faivre L, Guardiola P, Lewis C, et al. Association of complementation group and mutation type with clinical outcome in fanconi anemia. European Fanconi Anemia Research Group. Blood. 2000;96:4064.
6. D'Andrea AD, Grompe M. The Fanconi anaemia/BRCA pathway. Nat Rev Cancer. 2003;3:23.

7. Litman R, Peng M, Jin Z, et al. BACH1 is critical for homologous recombination and appears to be the Fanconi anemia gene product FANCJ. Cancer Cell. 2005;8:255.
8. Reid S, Schindler D, Hanenberg H, et al. Biallelic mutations in PALB2 cause Fanconi anemia subtype FA-N and predispose to childhood cancer. Nat Genet. 2007;39:162.
9. De Rocco D, Bottega R, Cappelli E, et al. Molecular analysis of Fanconi anemia: the experience of the Bone Marrow Failure Study Group of the Italian Association of Pediatric Onco-Hematology. Haematologica. 2014;99:1022.
10. Hira A, Yoshida K, Sato K, et al. Mutations in the gene encoding the E2 conjugating enzyme UBE2T cause Fanconi anemia. Am J Hum Genet. 2015;96:1001.
11. Dong H, Nebert DW, Bruford EA, et al. Update of the human and mouse Fanconi anemia genes. Hum Genomics. 2015;9:32.
12. Rickman KA, Lach FP, Abhyankar A, et al. Deficiency of UBE2T, the E2 ubiquitin ligase necessary for FANCD2 and FANCI ubiquitination, causes FA-T subtype of Fanconi anemia. Cell Rep. 2015;12:35.
13. Virts EL, Jankowska A, Mackay C, et al. AluY-mediated germline deletion, duplication and somatic stem cell reversion in UBE2T defines a new subtype of Fanconi anemia. Hum Mol Genet. 2015;24:5093.
14. Sawyer SL, Tian L, Kähkönen M, et al. Biallelic mutations in BRCA1 cause a new Fanconi anemia subtype. Cancer Discov. 2015;5:135.
15. Wang AT, Kim T, Wagner JE, et al. A dominant mutation in human RAD51 reveals its function in DNA interstrand crosslink repair independent of homologous recombination. Mol Cell. 2015;59:478.
16. Ameziane N, May P, Haitjema A, et al. A novel Fanconi anaemia subtype associated with a dominant-negative mutation in RAD51. Nat Commun. 2015;6:8829.
17. Park JY, Virts EL, Jankowska A, et al. Complementation of hypersensitivity to DNA interstrand cross-linking agents demonstrates that XRCC2 is a Fanconi anaemia gene. J Med Genet. 2016;53:672.
18. Wang W. Emergence of a DNA-damage response network consisting of Fanconianaemia and BRCA proteins. Nat Rev Genet. 2007;8:735.
19. Meetei AR, Levitus M, Xue Y, et al. X-linked inheritance of Fanconi anemia complementation group B. Nat Genet. 2004;36:1219.
20. Kottemann MC, Smogorzewska A. Fanconi anaemia and the repair of Watson and Crick DNA crosslinks. Nature. 2013 Jan 17;493(7432):356–63.
21. Giampietro PF, Adler-Brecher B, Verlander PC, Pavlakis SG, Davis JG, Auerbach AD. The need for more accurate and timely diagnosis in Fanconi anemia. A report from the International Fanconi Anemia Registry. Paediatrics. 1993;91:1116–20.
22. Alter BP. Fanconi anemia and the development of leukemia. Best Pract Res Clin Haematol. 2014;27:214.
23. Alter BP. Cancer in Fanconi anemia, 1927-2001. Cancer. 2003;97:425.
24. Oostra AB, Nieuwint AWM, Joenje H, de Winter JP. Diagnosis of Fanconi anemia: chromosomal breakage analysis. Anemia. 2012;2012:238731.
25. Bertuch AA. The molecular genetics of the telomere biology disorders. RNA Biol. 2016;13:696.
26. https://www.dcoutreach.org/
27. Horiguchi N, Kakizaki S, Iizuka K, et al. Hepatic angiosarcoma with dyskeratosis congenita. Intern Med. 2015;54:2867.
28. Woloszynek JR, Rothbaum RJ, Rawls AS, et al. Mutations of the SBDS gene are present in most patients with Shwachman-Diamond syndrome. Blood. 2004;104:3588.
29. Dror Y, Donadieu J, Koglmeier J, et al. Draft consensus guidelines for diagnosis and treatment of syndrome. Ann N Y Acad Sci. 2011;1242:40.
30. King S, Germeshausen M, Strauss G, Welte K, Ballmaier M. Congenital amegakaryocytic thrombocytopenia (CAMT): a detailed clinical analysis of 21 cases reveal different types of CAMT. Blood/ASH Annual Meeting abstracts 2004; abstract 740; 2005. Dec, 2004. American Society of Hematology.
31. Rose MJ, Nicol KK, Skeens MA, Gross TG, Kerlin BA. Congenital amegakaryocytic thrombocytopenia: the diagnostic importance of combining pathology with molecular genetics. Pediatr Blood Cancer. 2008;50:1263–5.
32. Gazda HT, Zhong R, Long L, Niewiadomska E, Lipton JM, Ploszynska A, et al. RNA and protein evidence for haplo-insufficiency in Diamond-Blackfan anaemia patients with RPS19 mutations. Br J Haematol. 2004;127:105–13.
33. Gazda HT, Grabowska A, Merida-Long LB, Latawiec E, Schneider HE, Lipton JM, et al. Ribosomal protein S24 gene is mutated in Diamond-Blackfan anemia. Am J Hum Genet. 2006;79:1110–8.
34. Vlachos A, Ball S, Niklas D, Alter BP, Sheth S, Ugo R, et al. Diagnosing and treating Diamond Blackfan anaemia: results of an International Clinical Consensus Conference; 2008. p. 1365–2141.
35. Lipton JM, Ellis SR. Diamond Blackfan anemia: diagnosis, treatment and molecular pathogenesis. Hematol Oncol Clin North Am. 2009;23(2):261–82.
36. Welte K, Zeidler C, Dale DC. Severe congenital neutropenia. Semin Hematol. 2006;43(3):189–95.
37. Dale DC, Person RE, Bolyard AA, Aprikyan AG, Bos C, Bonilla MA, et al. Mutations in the gene encoding neutrophil elastase in congenital and cyclic neutropenia. Blood. 2000;96(7):2317–22.
38. Ward AC. The role of the granulocyte colony-stimulating factor receptor (G-CSF-R) in disease. Front Biosci. 2007;12:608–18.
39. Klein C, Grudzien M, Appaswamy G, Germeshausen M, Sandrock I, Schaffer AA, et al. HAX1 deficiency causes autosomal recessive severe congenital neutropenia (Kostmann disease). Nat Genet. 2007;39(1):86–92.
40. Alter BP, D'Andrea AD. Inherited bone marrow failure syndromes. In: Handin RI, Lux SE, Stossel TP,

editors. Blood: principles and practice of hematology. 2nd ed. Philadelphia: Lippincott Williams & Wilkins; 2003. p. 209–72.

41. Bonsi L, Marchionni C, Alviano F, Lanzoni G, Franchini M, Costa R. Thrombocytopenia with absent radii (TAR) syndrome: from hemopoietic progenitor to mesenchymal stromal cell disease? Exp Hematol. 2009;37:1–7.

42. Letestu R, Vitrat N, Massé A. Existence of a differentiation blockage at the stage of a megakaryocyte precursor in the thrombocytopenia and absent radii (TAR) syndrome. Blood. 2000;95:1633–41.

Part II

WBC Disorders

Myelodysplastic Syndrome: An Overview

Jasmita Dass and Jyoti Kotwal

9.1 Introduction

Myelodysplastic syndrome (MDS) is clonal hematopoietic stem cell disorders characterized by presence of cytopenia(s), dysplasia in ≥ 1 hematopoietic cell lineage, ineffective hematopoiesis, and an increased risk of progression to acute myeloid leukemia (AML) [1]. The diagnosis of MDS rests on the clinical features, presence of cytopenia in one or more myeloid lineages, morphological evidence of dysplasia, increased blasts in bone marrow and relevant cytogenetic abnormalities and molecular mutations. World Health organization (WHO) 2017 revised classification uses a combination of morphology, genetic features, and immunophenotype to assign a disease category to a case [2].

Anemia is the commonest feature, presents as easy fatigability, feeling of tiredness, malaise and may require blood transfusions. Severe neutropenia may present with increased infections, and moderate to severe thrombocytopenia may cause bleeding in the form of petechiae, and ecchymosis. Patients may present with a single or a combination of cytopenias [3].

9.2 Nomenclature

Since the French-American-British classification proposed in 1982 [4], cases of MDS were referred to as refractory anemia and refractory cytopenia. The same was retained through the two previous WHO classifications [5, 6]. However, this terminology of "refractory anemia" and "refractory cytopenia" has been replaced by MDS in recent classification. The entities are further defined on the basis of presence of single lineage/multilineage dysplasia, blast counts, ring sideroblasts (RS) into subdivisions of MDS. A comparative of WHO 2008 and 2017 classified cases is given in Table 9.1.

9.3 Cutoffs in MDS

The evaluation of a patient of MDS requires well-stained cellular peripheral blood (PB) and bone marrow aspirate (BMA) smears. WHO has recommended the use of May Grunwald Giemsa and Wright-Giemsa stained smears for optimal assessment of granularity [5].

9.3.1 Cutoffs for Cytopenias

The WHO 2017 classification retains the prior cutoffs for cytopenias, a hemoglobin of <10 g/dL, absolute neutrophils count (ANC) of

J. Dass · J. Kotwal (✉)
Department of Hematology, Sir Ganga Ram Hospital, New Delhi, Delhi, India

© Springer Nature Singapore Pte Ltd. 2019
R. Saxena, H. P. Pati (eds.), *Hematopathology*, https://doi.org/10.1007/978-981-13-7713-6_9

Table 9.1 A comparison of WHO 2008 [6] and WHO 2017 [2] Nomenclatures for MDS subcategories

WHO 2008 entity [6]	WHO 2017 entity [2]
Refractory cytopenia with unilineage dysplasia (RCUD; encompassing refractory anemia, refractory thrombocytopenia, and refractory neutropenia)	MDS with single lineage dysplasia (MDS-SLD)
Refractory cytopenia with multilineage dysplasia (RCMD)	MDS with multilineage dysplasia (MDS-MLD)
Refractory anemia with ring sideroblasts (RARS)	MDS with single lineage dysplasia and ring sideroblasts (MDS-RS-SLD)
Refractory cytopenia with multilineage dysplasia and ring sideroblasts* (RCMD-RS) (WHO 2001)	MDS with multilineage dysplasia and ring sideroblasts (MDS-RS-MLD)
Refractory anemia with excess blasts-1 (RAEB1)	MDS with excess blasts-1 (MDS-EB1)
Refractory anemia with excess blasts-2 (RAEB2)	MDS with excess blasts-2 (MDS-EB2)
MDS with isolated del(5q)	MDS with isolated del(5q): Expanded to include cases with one additional low-risk cytogenetic abnormality excluding monosomy 7
MDS-unclassifiable	MDS-unclassifiable: For cases of pancytopenia with 1% blasts, a documentation of 1% peripheral blood blasts is required on at least two occasions
Provisional entity: Refractory cytopenia of childhood (RCC)	Provisional entity: Refractory cytopenia of childhood (RCC)

*The entity was a part of WHO 2001 classification but was merged with RCMD in WHO 2008 classifiaction

$\leq 1.8 \times 10^9$/L, and platelet count of 100×10^9/L [7]. However, it has been recognized that some patients may have persistent cytopenias at values higher than the recommended thresholds [8, 9]. The WHO 2017 classification provides lower thresholds for such cases when characteristic morphological abnormalities or cytogenetic abnormalities are present and hemoglobin <13 g/dL in men and <12 g/dL in women or platelet count is $<150 \times 10^9$/L [2]. In addition, all cases of MDS should have an absolute monocyte count of $<1 \times 10^9$/L [2, 5, 6]. A platelet count of $>450 \times 10^9$/L may be present in patients of MDS with del(5q) abnormality or cases associated with t(3,3)(q21.3;q26.2) or inv(3) (q21.3;q26.2) and does not warrant a classification to myelodysplastic syndrome/myeloproliferative neoplasm (MDS/MPN) [2].

9.3.2 Cutoffs for Dysplasia and Blasts

The second hallmark of MDS is the morphological evidence of dysplasia in ≥ 1 myeloid cell line. The WHO 2017 classification has retained a cutoff of $\geq 10\%$ dysplasia in either erythroid, myeloid, or megakaryocytic lineage. It, however, recognizes the fact that some normal individuals may harbor dysplasia in >10% cells [2]. Parmentier et al. [10] showed that >10% dysmyelopoiesis could be seen in 45% marrows of normal stem cell donors, 26% have bi-lineage, and 7% have tri-lineage dysplasia. In contrast to the age-related increase in MDS, it was seen that young donors were more likely to have dysplasia in myeloid and megakaryocytic lineage [10]. Certain abnormalities like pseudo Pelger–Huet abnormality and megakaryocytic abnormalities (karyorrhexis, multinuclearity, nuclear fragmentation, and micromegakaryocytes) are more specific for MDS [11, 12]. Reproducibility of dysplasia, however, tends to be poor even when experienced hematopathologists examine the slides [13]. Moreover, cases with subtle dysplasia limited to one lineage require a stringent exclusion of reactive mimics of MDS [10].

Myeloblasts constitute <20% of all nucleated cells. Peripheral blood and bone marrow blast percentages decide the categorization of MDS into individual subdivisions [2]. Morphological features of dysplasia are described in Table 9.2.

Table 9.2 Morphological features of dysplasia in MDS [2]

Dysmyelopoiesis	Dyserythropoiesis	Dysmegakaryopoiesis
Pseudo Pelger–Huet abnormality and hyposegmented neutrophils Hypogranularity Small or unusually large size Nuclear hypersegmentation Dohle bodies Auer rods Pseudo Chediak Higashi granules	Nuclear budding Irregular nuclear membrane Inter-nuclear bridging Karyorrhexis Multinuclearity Megaloblastosis Ring sideroblasts Cytoplasmic vacuolization Per-iodic acid Schiff positivity	Micromegakaryocytes Nuclear hypolobation and monolobation Multinuclear megakaryocytes with presence of widely separated nuclei

9.3.3 Cutoffs for Ring Sideroblasts

Cases of MDS may show the presence of ring sideroblasts (RS) defined as >5 granules encircling >1/3rd of the nuclear membrane [14]. The earlier WHO 2008 classification warranted ≥15% RS to be considered as significant [6] but the WHO 2017 classification incorporates the genetic data for SF3B1 mutations [2]. In cases where RS are present but are 5–15%, the presence of SF3B1 mutations should be ideally assessed and if present, they are adequate to classify a case as MDS-single lineage dysplasia with RS or MDS-multilineage dysplasia with RS [2, 15, 16]. This is the only mutation that impacts the classification of MDS as it has been strongly found to be associated with this subcategory of MDS [17–19]. The RS threshold has been lowered as cases with SF3B1 mutations may present with as low as 1% RS [19]. However, if the SF3B1 mutation testing cannot be performed, a threshold of ≥15% should be adhered to [2].

Clonal cytogenetic abnormalities are present in ~50% of all patients of MDS [2, 6, 20, 21]. The incidence is higher in patients with therapy-related MDS at ~80% [21]. Del(5q) is the commonest abnormality seen in MDS with an incidence of ~10–15%. On one extreme, it is associated with good prognosis and a good response to lenalidomide therapy [22, 23] and at the other extreme, it is enriched in therapy-related MDS and is associated with a short overall survival and high risk of progression to acute

myeloid leukemia [24–26]. Hence, for the diagnosis of MDS with isolated del(5q), it is important that all therapy-related MDS be classified first and the strict diagnostic criteria of the entity are then adhered to. Del(5q) is associated with a distinct clinical syndrome with presence of macrocytosis, normal or high platelet count, and presence of hypolobated or monolobated megakaryocytes on the BM examination [2, 6]. Trisomy 8, del(20q), and loss of chromosome Y are seen in 10%, 5–8%, and ~5% cases of MDS but are not sufficient to warrant a diagnosis of MDS as they are not specific to MDS [2]. The list of cytogenetic abnormalities which can lead to a classification of MDS in MDS-U is presented in Table 9.3 [2]. These abnormalities should be demonstrated only by conventional karyotype and not by FISH or sequencing [2]. Loss of 17p is associated strongly with TP53 mutations and manifests morphologically as pseudo Pelger–Huet anomaly and vacuolation in neutrophils [2].

9.3.4 Exclusion Criteria

A diagnosis of MDS should not be made if the assessment is made during an acute infection. Vitamin B12/folate, copper deficiencies should be excluded. Patients exposed to heavy metals such as arsenic, lead, and zinc may also show marked dysplasia [2, 5, 6]. Copper deficiency causes cytopenias with cytoplasmic vacuolization in the erythroid precursors and presence of

Table 9.3 List of unbalanced mutations and balanced translocations considered as presumptive evidence of MDS [2]

Unbalanced chromosomal abnormality	MDS	Therapy-related MDS	Balanced chromosomal abnormality	MDS	Therapy-related MDS
−7/del (7q)	10%	50%	t(11;16)(q23.3;p13.3)		3%
del(5q)	10%	40%	t(3;21)(q26.2;q22.1)		2%
i(17q)/t(17p)	3–5%	25–30%	1(1;3)(p36.3;q21.2)	1%	
−13/del(13q)	3%		t(2;11)(p21;q23.3)	1%	3%
del(11q)	3%		inv(3)(q21.3q26.2)/ t(3;3)(q21.3;q26.2)	1%	
del(12p)/t(12p)	3%		t(6;9)(p23;q34.1)	1%	
del(9q)	1–2%				
idic(X) (q13)	1–2%				

Table 9.4 Diagnostic criteria for various subcategories of MDS according to WHO 2017 classification [2]

Category	Number of cytopenias	Lineages with dysplasia	Ring sideroblasts	PB blasts	BM blast
MDS-SLD	1–2	1	<15%; <5%[a]	<1%	<5%
MDS-MLD	1–3	2–3	<15%; <5%[a]	<1%	<5%
MDS-RS-SLD	1–2	1	≥15%; ≥5%[a]	<1%	<5%
MDS-RS-MLD	1–3	2–3	≥15%; ≥5%[a]	<1%	<5%
MDS with isolated del(5q)	1–2	1–3	<15%/≥15%	<1%	<5%
	Del(5q) may be present alone or in concert with one additional chromosomal anomaly as long as it is not −7 or del(7q)				
MDS-EB1	1–3	1–3	<15%/≥15%	2–4%	5–9%
MDS-EB2	1–3	1–3	<15%/≥15%	5–19%	10–19%
				Auer rods	
MDS-U (a) with 1% blasts	1–3	1–3	<15%/≥15%	1%[b]	<5%
(b) SLD and pancytopenia	3	1	<15%/≥15%	<1%	<5%
(c) MDS defining cytogenetic abnormality	1–3	0	<15% as cases with ≥15% RS are MDS-SLD	<1%	>5%
RCC	1–3	1–3	None	<2%	<5%

[a]5–<15% RS are acceptable for classification as MDS-RS-SLD and MDS-RS-MLD if SF3B1 mutation is present
[b]1% PB blasts should be documented on at least two occasions

RS [27–29]. Copper deficiency may be precipitated by zinc excess and should be considered in patients receiving supplemental zinc [30]. In addition, tuberculosis [31] and autoimmune diseases [32] may also be associated with myelodysplasia on morphology and they should be excluded if other suggestive features are present. Mycophenolate mofetil, tacrolimus, and ganciclovir may cause pseudo Pelger–Huet abnormality [33, 34], and isoniazid in absence of pyridoxine may cause ring sideroblasts [35]. Patients should not be evaluated within a short period of chemotherapeutic agents or granulocyte colony stimulating factor (G-CSF) therapy [2, 5, 6]. Other clinical mimics of MDS are paroxysmal nocturnal hemoglobinuria (PNH), large granular lymphocytic leukemia, and hairy cell leukemia [2].

9.4 Diagnostic Criteria for WHO 2017 Classification of MDS [2]

The diagnostic criteria as per WHO 2017 to divide MDS into various subcategories are given in Table 9.4.

An algorithmic approach to the subclassification of MDS is presented in Fig. 9.1.

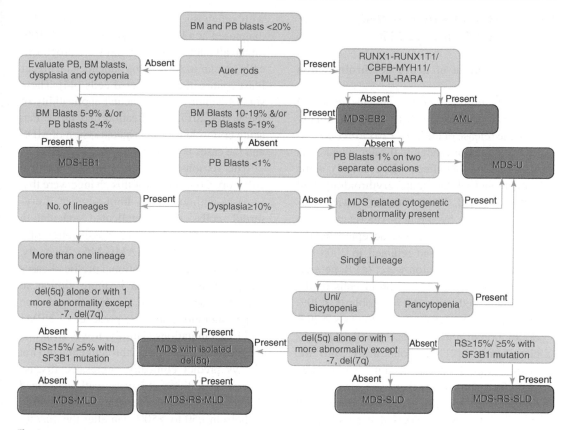

Fig. 9.1 An algorithmic approach to sub-classification of de novo MDS

9.5 Evaluation of a Case of MDS

Evaluation of a patient suspected as MDS requires a peripheral blood sample for a complete blood count, reticulocyte count, and smear evaluation. A 200 cell differential on well-stained PB smears and 500 cell myelogram on BM smears is mandatory [2]. Blood smears should be prepared within 2 h of sample collection and in cases of very low counts, buffy coat smears may be used for differential counts on the peripheral smear [2].

A bone marrow examination procedure should always include an aspiration and bone marrow biopsy (BMBx), and additional samples should be collected in heparin and EDTA to send for karyotyping, fluorescence-in-situ hybridization (FISH), and for molecular workup [2]. Additional stains may be required on BMA smears to identify erythroid dysplasia. These include Perl's stain to look for RS and Per-iodic acid Schiff stain (PAS) to identify dysplastic erythroid cells [2]. Normally erythroid cells are negative for PAS but dysplastic erythroid cells may show diffuse cytoplasmic positivity or diffuse granular positivity or block positivity [12]. BMBx is extremely important in MDS presenting with marrow fibrosis for evaluation of megakaryocytic dysplasia and blast counts in borderline cases using immunohistochemistry (IHC) for CD34 and CD117. IHC for CD61 or CD42b may be applied to identify micromegakaryocytes and megakaryocytic dysplasia [36]. Though WHO has not made immunophenotyping mandatory, it should also be considered in the evaluation of MDS as it can give objective clues in difficult cases, especially the low-grade MDS cases with blasts <5% and RS <15% [37–40]. The evaluation for PNH clone should be done in low-grade MDS cases [41].

9.6 Other Changes in WHO Classification, 2017

1. **Reclassification of acute erythroleukemia to MDS**

   With the proposal of the updates in WHO 2008 classification in 2016 [16] and finally with the release of the WHO 2017 revised edition [2], a major change in the acute leukemia classification that affects MDS directly is the abolishment of the acute erythroid/myeloid leukemia (AML-M6a). This entity was originally defined by French-American-British classification [42] but was accepted by the WHO in 2001 [5] and retained in 2008 [6]. The criteria of definition were: (a) Bone marrow containing ≥50% erythroid cells of the total nucleated cells; (b) Myeloblasts ≤20% of all nucleated cells; (c) Myeloblasts ≥20% of all non-erythroid cells. The WHO 2017 classification [2] has done away with the "non-erythroid blast count" altogether. Therefore, most cases that were classified in pre-2016 era as AML-M6a would now fall into the category of MDS with excess blasts.

   The prognostic similarity of AML-M6a and MDS has been shown by two series from MD Anderson Cancer center [43] and Grupo Español de Síndromes Mielodisplásicos (GESMD) [44] published in the same issue of Modern Pathology in 2016. In the former series, 77 AML-M6a cases were compared to 279 de novo MDS-refractory anemia with excess blasts cases. Patients of AML-M6a treated with intensive AML chemotherapy did not perform better than patients treated with lower intensity therapy or only supportive care. In addition, on multivariate analysis, very high R-IPSS and high R-IPSS were independent risk factors for short overall survival while a diagnosis of AML-M6a was not a risk factor [43]. In the second series, AML-M6a patients were compared to erythroid predominant refractory anemia with excess blasts 1 and 2 (RAEB1 and RAEB2) patients separately and there was no prognostic difference between them. Only high-risk karyotype as defined by R-IPSS and IPSS was associated with prognosis. Even patients of AML-M6a diagnosed at a low blast percentage of 5–10% on the all nucleated cell count were prognostically similar to AML-M6a patients with higher blast counts in all nucleated cells [44]. These studies demonstrate the actual applicability of the WHO 2017 classification and prove that acute erythroleukemia is an extension of MDS and the cases are better classified in MDS.

   The reasons considered by the Clinical Advisory Committee for this change were that in cases with extremely high number of erythroid cells, the complicated calculation would sometimes lead to a classification of a case with ≤5% blasts as AML-M6a. Secondly, the cytogenetic and mutational profile of cases classified as AML-M6a is more similar to MDS than de novo AML, such as the presence of p53 mutations and rare presence of NPM1 and FLT3 mutations. Thirdly, it was seen that diagnosis of a case as erythroleukemia did not always predict clinically aggressive disease course. In addition, it is very well recognized that a slight change in percentage of erythroid cells from <50 to ≥50% can alter the diagnosis and may result from many variables including nutritional deficiency, erythropoietin supplementation, or inter-/intra-observer variation. There are problems pertaining to poor reproducibility and lack of consistency [15, 45–48]. Therefore, the entity of erythroleukemia/AML-M6a has been abolished by WHO 2017 classification [2]. This change in classification means that cases with 70% erythroid cells, 12% myeloblasts and >20% non-erythroid blasts will now be classified as MDS-EB2 and not as AML-M6a. The entity of pure erythroid leukemia (PEL) will however continue to be a part of the AML classification. To classify a case as PEL, there should be ≥80% erythroblasts and ≥30% pro-erythroblasts [2]. An approach to the cases with ≥50% erythroblasts in the bone marrow is being presented in Fig. 9.2.

2. **Identification of myeloid neoplasms with germline mutations**

   This category has been incorporated by WHO 2017 to address the familial cases of MDS

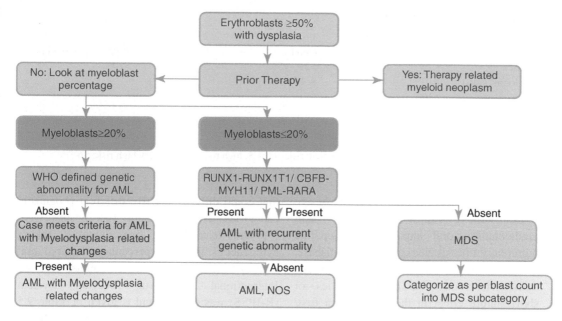

Fig. 9.2 Approach to a case with ≥50% erythroid cells and dysplasia on the bone marrow

and AML [2]. MDS/AML associated with inherited marrow failure syndromes like Fanconi anemia, dyskeratosis congenita, etc. had been recognized since long but now other disorders with an inherited predisposition to MDS and AML have been identified [2]. Of these, common ones are MDS/AML with RUNX1 mutations, ETV6 mutations, ANKRD26 and DDX41 mutations [2]. The reported neoplasms associated with DDX41 mutations include MDS-MLD, MDS-EB, and MDS with isolated del(5q), and they appear to have a long latency [49]. Cases with RUNX1 mutations have monoallelic germline RUNX1 mutations and have a bleeding tendency out of proportion to the platelet counts [50]. The median patient age is lower at 33 years and they exhibit the phenomenon of anticipation with the disease manifesting at an earlier age in the subsequent generations [51, 52]. The other myeloid neoplasms with germline predisposition may have ANKRD26 or ETV6 mutations [2]. Of the cases associated with organ dysfunction, germline GATA2 mutations are very interesting as they can present with 4 syndromes—MonoMAC syndrome, Emberger syndrome with a predisposition to MDS, familial MDS/AML, and dendritic cell, monocyte, B- and NK-lymphoid (DCML) deficiency with vulnerability to viral infections [53, 54]. The patients may present with MDS at a median age of 29 years, and MDS may be the first manifestation of the disease [55]. GATA2 mutations have been found in 5% cases of RCC and were associated with monosomy 7 or trisomy 8. If all childhood MDS cases are considered, GATA2 mutations are seen in ~15% of advanced and ~7% of all MDS cases. Bone marrow features in such cases include marrow hypocellularity, multilineage dysplasia with dysmegakaryopoiesis and reticulin fibrosis [56]. A clue to detection is an almost complete absence of monocytes, B cells, and NK cells on flow cytometry [53, 54, 57].

These disorders should be considered in individuals presenting with MDS/acute leukemia if they have either (a) a personal history of multiple cancers or (b) pre-existent thrombocytopenia, bleeding tendency or macrocytosis or (c) a first/second-degree relative with a hematological malignancy or (d) first/second-degree relative with a solid tumor consistent with germ line predisposition such as sarcoma,

Table 9.5 R-IPSS risk scoring in MDS [8]

Variable	0	0.5	1	1.5	2	3	4
Cytogenetics	Very good	–	Good	–	Intermediate	High	Very high
BM blast%	≤2%	–	>2%–<5%	–	5–10%	>10%	–
Hemoglobin (g/dL)	≥10	–	8–10	<8	–	–	–
Platelets (×10⁹/L)	≥100	50–100	–	–	--	–	–
ANC (×10⁹/L)	≥0.8	<0.8	–	–	–	–	–

Very low R-IPSS: ≤1.5; low risk: >1.5–3; intermediate risk: >3–4.5; high risk: >4.5–6; very high risk: >6

early-onset breast cancer at <50 years of age or brain tumors or (e) abnormal nails or skin pigmentation, oral leukoplakia, idiopathic pulmonary fibrosis, unexplained liver disease, lymphoedema, atypical infections, immune deficiencies, congenital limb anomalies, or short stature either in the patient or a first/second-degree relative or (f) failure of mobilization of a related donor using standard protocol or if such a donor is being considered and the patient meets any of the criteria from a to e [2, 58].

Recognition of these disorders is important for the treatment, family counseling, and anticipating other issues that might arise later in the course of the disease.

9.7 Determining Prognosis in MDS

Prognosis in MDS was determined using various prognostic scoring systems. The most used was International Prognostic Scoring System (IPSS) that was derived from cases classified according to FAB classification and included patients of CMML. It could be applied only to patients at first presentation and included categories of number of cytopenias, blast percentage, and karyotype [7]. After the WHO 2001 classification, a new prognostic scoring system called WHO classification-based prognostic scoring system (WPSS) that incorporated WHO classification subtype, karyotype and transfusion requirement was validated in 2005 [59].

In 2012, Greenberg et al. analyzed over 7000 cases of MDS to derive a better prognostic system

that could differentiate five different prognostic categories. The cytogenetic risk groups were expanded from three to five categories. Taking cytogenetics, BM blast percentage, hemoglobin, neutrophil count and platelet counts, Revised International Prognostic Scoring System (R-IPSS) was devised and is given in Table 9.5 [8]. These risk categories correlate both with better survival and also predict evolution to AML. R-IPSS has shown a very good correlation with WPSS in a large study [60]. The WHO 2017 revised classification has not lowered the blast threshold to ≤2% for low-risk MDS as the reproducibility would be low [2, 15, 16].

Additional scoring system for low-grade MDS was proposed by M.D. Anderson cancer center as M.D. Anderson Lower-Risk MDS Prognostic Scoring System (MDA-LR). This system incorporates BM blast percentage, cytogenetics, hemoglobin, platelet count, and patient age [61].

9.8 Flow Cytometry in MDS

Flow cytometry in MDS has been studied extensively. The aberrant maturational patterns on granulocytes are abnormal CD11b-CD16, abnormal CD13-CD16, abnormal CD11b-CD13 patterns while on monocytes, CD11b-HLADR pattern is most frequently abnormal. A reduction in normally expressed antigen like CD10 on granulocytes and CD33 on monocytes is also considered as an abnormality [62, 63]. The second set of abnormalities pertains to aberrant antigen expression like CD7, CD2, CD56, and CD5 on either granulocyte, monocytes, or myeloblasts [39, 63]. A different approach was utilized by

Ogata et al. who limited the study to myeloblasts and B-cell progenitors in low-grade MDS patients. Their study explored percentage of CD34 positive myeloblasts, percentage of CD34 positive B-cell progenitors in all CD34 positive cells, lymphocyte/myeloblast CD45 mean fluorescent intensity, and granulocyte/lymphocyte SSC peak channel ratio to come to the Ogata score. A score of ≥2 is associated with MDS [37]. This Ogata mini-panel has a high positive predictive value and specificity for MDS at ~90% but the sensitivity and negative predictive value is relatively lower at ~70% to identify low-grade MDS and differentiate them from non-clonal cytopenias [38].

Flow cytometry has been applied extensively to MDS but is still not considered mandatory in a patient's evaluation as there is a lack of standardization in the panels used. An attempt to bring about this standardization was taken up by European leukemia Net with the first guideline in 2012 [64] and the most recent in 2014 [65]. These guidelines require ≥3 abnormalities in the set of markers affecting granulocytic or monocytic maturation and also the Ogata parameters. Flow cytometry findings if studied should always be reported as a part of an integrated report incorporating morphology and cytogenetic data [65].

9.9 Genetic Landscape of MDS

Over the last 5 years, there has been a massive surge in publications pertaining to mutations in MDS using next generation sequencing (NGS) [17–19, 34, 66–71]. The mutations described affect the epigenetic regulation and spliceosome machinery, and others affect the cohesin complex while some are the mutations of the transcription factors [66, 67]. Using NGS, mutations have been discovered in ~90% of all MDS cases. The epigenetic pathway comprises of two main subdivisions—the CpG islands and hypermethylation and the histone modification. The methylation pathway is controlled by the methyltransferase DNMT3A and DNA hydroxymethylation genes TET2, IDH1, and IDH2. Histone pathway comprises genes EZH2, ASXL1, and UTX. The tran-

scription factor mutations affect RUNX1, ETV6, GATA2, and PHF6. Kinase signaling mutations affect KRAS, NRAS, JAK2, and CBL. Cohesin complex mutations occur in STAG2, SMC3, and RAD1 genes [66–68]. Mutations in the epigenetic regulators occur in ~45% of all cases of MDS while spliceosome pathway is affected in ~50% of all cases of MDS. About 25% patients exhibit mutations both in the spliceosome machinery and in the epigenetic pathway [69]. TP53 is affected in ~5% cases and is consistently associated with a poor prognosis [69]. TP53 mutations are also associated with complex karyotype, monosomies, and abnormalities of chromosome 7 [70]. Patients of MDS with isolated del(5q) may also harbor p53 mutations at diagnosis and such patients show a higher rate of progression in lenalidomide therapy. Even subclonal TP53 mutations impact prognosis and in the setting of del(5q), even IHC has been used to pick up TP53 mutations using a cutoff of ≥2% positive cells. This cutoff correlated with TP53 mutations detected by NGS could predict evolution to AML and was associated with lower overall survival [34]. Therefore, testing for TP53 in patients with del(5q), a low or intermediate-1 IPSS score has been recommended by European Leukemia Net guidelines in 2013 as these patients may not perform well on lenalidomide therapy [72].

Patients with 3 or more than 3 driver mutations have a lower leukemia-free survival than patients with 0–2 mutations. This impact on leukemia-free survival is regardless of whether the mutation is subclonal or clonal [66]. Mutations affecting TP53, ASXL1, RUNX1, ETV6, and EZH2 have a negative impact on overall survival even in very low risk, low-risk, and intermediate R-IPSS risk categories [70]. A few papers have explored the impact of these mutations with response to hypomethylating agents. The most data exists for TET2 mutations as a predictor of better response to hypomethylating agent therapy [71, 73, 74]. In one series, patients who were TET2+/ASXL1 negative were shown to have the best chance of responding to hypomethylating agents [71]. These mutations also affect overall survival in patients who undergo stem cell transplantation. In a series of

Table 9.6 A comparison of the characteristics of ICUS, CCUS and MDS

	ICUS	CCUS	Low-grade MDS	High-grade MDS
Clonality	Absent	Present	Present	Present
Cytopenias	Present	Present	Present	Present
Dysplasia	Absent	Absent	Present	Present
BM blast %	<5	<5	<5	5–19%

~87 patients who underwent stem cell transplantation, ~46% patients had mutations in TP53, TET2 and DNMT3A mutations, and the overall survival in these patients was ~19% compared to ~59% in patients who lacked these mutations. Among these mutations, TP53 had the worst impact on overall survival [68]. In contrast, SF3B1 mutations are associated with good overall survival and fewer cytopenias [17–19]. These mutations are strongly associated with RS, and SF3B1 mutations are the only ones that have been incorporated in WHO 2017 classification to classify a patient as MDS-RS-SLD and MDS-RS-MLD in presence of 5–<15% RS [2]. In addition, these are also a target for small molecule inhibitors like luspatercept that are in trial and have shown an excellent response if a patient shows the SF3B1 mutation [75].

Since these mutations have also been described in normal individuals without MDS [**Clonal hematopoiesis of indeterminate potential (CHIP)**] [76–79], the presence of these alone is not sufficient to classify a patient as MDS. This is also applicable to patients who have unexplained cytopenias and do not meet the diagnostic criteria for MDS [2, 80]. With the advent of NGS, three large series of patients were found to have age-related clonal hematopoiesis designated as CHIP [76–78]. This was found to be associated with all-cause mortality but all patients do not progress to MDS or AML.

Idiopathic cytopenia of undetermined significance (ICUS): The term ICUS was proposed for those patients in whom a diagnosis of MDS could not be established but is possible. An individual case can be classified as ICUS if there are cytopenias including hemoglobin of <11 g/dL, ANC of <1.5 × 10⁹/L, and platelet count of <150 × 10⁹/L that persist for a minimum of 6 months, do not meet diagnostic criteria for MDS and cannot be explained by any other pos-

sible causes. The patient requires extensive evaluation to establish this diagnosis. There is a subset of ICUS patients who can be shown to have clonal hematopoiesis if genetic mutations can be demonstrated [80]. These cases can be called as clonal cytopenia of undetermined significance (CCUS) [81]. It is understandable that with the wide application of newer tools like flow cytometry and application of NGS, many cases of ICUS would move to categories of MDS and CCUS. Based on the presence of cytopenias, clonality, BM blast percentage, and dysplasia, the spectrum of these disorders and MDS is given in Table 9.6.

9.10 Conclusions

The WHO 2017 classification has revamped MDS and each entity is being described as MDS with rather than "refractory anemia" or "refractory cytopenia". There have been important changes specially pertaining to MDS-RS-SLD, and there has been a re-recognition of the entity of MDS-RS-MLD which derives from the earlier RCMD-RS in WHO 2001 classification. This has been possible due to incorporation of SF3B1 mutations for identification of these categories if there are 5–<15% RS. Another important change has been inclusion of one additional chromosomal anomaly in del(5q) as long as it is not −7 or del(7q). Minor changes are that PB blasts ~1% have to be documented on two separate occasions if considering a diagnosis of MDS-U. In addition, the entity of acute erythroleukemia has been abolished and most of these cases would now be classified as MDS. There is now a recognition that many myeloid neoplasms with germline mutations exist and that these have an important impact on patient outcome. Flow cytometry although not mandatory to the patient evaluation in MDS should be considered especially in patients with low-grade MDS lacking RS. There has been a massive surge in the genetic knowledge of MDS with the advent of NGS. This information has an impact on prognosis and possibly on response to hypomethylating agent therapy and may form a part of every patient's evaluation if the cost of the testing reduces in the future. The advent of NGS has also led to the discovery of CHIP adding to the complexity associated around MDS.

References

1. Cazzola M, Malcovati L. Myelodysplastic syndromes—coping with ineffective hematopoiesis. N Engl J Med. 2005;352:536–8.
2. Swerdlow SH, Campo E, Harris NL, et al., editors. WHO classification of tumours of haematopoietic and lymphoid tissues. Revised 4th ed. Lyon: IARC; 2017.
3. Hamblin T. Clinical features of MDS. Leuk Res. 1992;16:89–93.
4. Bennett JM, Catovsky D, Daniel MT, et al. Proposals for the classification of the myelodysplastic syndromes. Br J Haematol. 1982;51:189–99.
5. Jaffe ES, Harris NL, Stein H, Vardiman JW, editors. World Health Organization classification of Tumours: pathology and genetics of tumours of haematopoietic and lymphoid tissues. Lyon: IARC; 2001.
6. Swerdlow SH, Campo E, Harris NL, et al., editors. WHO classification of tumours of haematopoietic and lymphoid tissues. Lyon: IARC; 2008.
7. Greenberg P, Cox C, Le Beau MM, et al. International scoring system for evaluating prognosis in myelodysplastic syndromes. Blood. 1997;89:2079–88.
8. Greenberg PL, Tuechler H, Schanz J, et al. Revised international prognostic scoring system for myelodysplastic syndromes. Blood. 2012;120:2454–65.
9. Verburgh E, Achten R, Louw VJ, et al. A new disease categorization of low-grade myelodysplastic syndromes based on the expression of cytopenia and dysplasia in one versus more than one lineage improves on the WHO classification. Leukemia. 2007;21:668–77.
10. Parmentier S, Schetelig J, Lorenz K, Kramer M, Ireland R, Schuler U, et al. Assessment of dysplastic hematopoiesis: lessons from healthy bone marrow donors. Haematologica. 2012;97(5):723–30.
11. Bain BJ, Clark DM, Wilkins B. Bone marrow pathology. 4th ed. Hoboken, NJ: Wiley-Blackwell; 2010.
12. Bain BJ. Leukaemia diagnosis. 4th ed. Hoboken, NJ: Wiley-Blackwell; 2010.
13. Ramos F, Fernandez-Ferrero S, Suarez D, Barbon M, Rodriguez JA, Gil S, et al. Myelodysplastic syndrome: a search for minima diagnostic criteria. Leuk Res. 1999;23(3):283–90.
14. Mufti GJ, Bennett JM, Goasguen J, Bain BJ, Baumann I, Brunning R, et al. Diagnosis and classification of myelodysplastic syndrome International Working Group on Morphology of myelodysplastic syndrome (IWGM-MDS) consensus proposals for the definition and enumeration of myeloblast and ring sideroblasts. Haematologica. 2008;93:1712–7.
15. Arber DA, Hasserjian RP. Reclassifying myelodysplastic syndromes: what's where in the new who and why. Hematol Am Soc Hematol Educ Prog. 2015;2015:294–8.
16. Arber DA, Orazi A, Hasserjian R, et al. The 2016 revision to the World Health Organization classification of myeloid neoplasms and acute leukemia. Blood. 2016;127:2391–405.
17. Papaemmanuil E, Cazzola M, Boultwood J, et al. Somatic SF3B1 mutation in myelodysplasia with ring sideroblasts. N Engl J Med. 2011;365(15):1384–95.
18. Visconte V, Makishima H, Jankowska A, et al. SF3B1, a splicing factor is frequently mutated in refractory anemia with ring sideroblasts. Leukemia. 2012 Mar;26:542–5.
19. Malcovati L, Karimi M, Papaemmanuil E, et al. SF3B1 mutation identifies a distinct subset of myelodysplastic syndrome with ring sideroblasts. Blood. 2015;126(2):233–41.
20. Pozdnyakova O, Miron PM, Tang G, et al. Cytogenetic abnormalities in a series of 1,029 patients with primary myelodysplastic syndromes: a report from the US with a focus on some undefined single chromosomal abnormalities. Cancer. 2008;113:3331–40.
21. Haase D, Germing U, Schanz J, Pfeilstocker M, Nosslinger T, Hildebrandt B, et al. New insights into the prognostic impact of the karyotype in MDS and correlation with subtypes: evidence from a core dataset of 2124 patients. Blood. 2007;110:4385–95.
22. Fenaux P, Giagounidis A, Selleslag D, et al. A randomized phase 3 study of lenalidomide versus placebo in RBC transfusion-dependent patients with low-/intermediate-1-risk myelodysplastic syndromes with del5q. Blood. 2011;118:3765–76.
23. List A, Dewald G, Bennett J, et al. Lenalidomide in the myelodysplastic syndrome with chromosome 5q deletion. N Engl J Med. 2006;355:1456–65.
24. Christiansen DH, Andersen MK, Pedersen-Bjergaard J. Mutations with loss of heterozygosity of p53 are common in therapy-related myelodysplasia and acute myeloid leukemia after exposure to alkylating agents and significantly associated with deletion or loss of 5q, a complex karyotype, and a poor prognosis. J Clin Oncol. 2001;19:1405–13.
25. Jädersten M, Saft L, Pellagatti A, et al. Clonal heterogeneity in the 5q-syndrome: p53 expressing progenitors prevail during lenalidomide treatment and expand at disease progression. Haematologica. 2009;94:1762–6.
26. Möllgård L, Saft L, Treppendahl MB, et al. Clinical effect of increasing doses of lenalidomide in high-risk myelodysplastic syndrome and acute myeloid leukemia with chromosome 5 abnormalities. Haematologica. 2011;96:963–71.

27. Gregg XT, Reddy V, Prchal JT. Copper deficiency masquerading as myelodysplastic syndrome. Blood. 2002;100:1493–5.

28. Fong T, Vij R, Vijayan A, et al. Copper deficiency: an important consideration in the differential diagnosis of myelodysplastic syndrome. Haematologica. 2007;92:1429–30.

29. Halfdanarson TR, Kumar N, Li CY, et al. Hematological manifestations of copper deficiency: a retrospective review. Eur J Haematol. 2008;80:523–31.

30. Monte SW, Sara AM, Michael LM, et al. Zinc-induced copper deficiency: a report of three cases initially recognized on bone marrow examination. Am J Clin Pathol. 2005;123:125–31.

31. Kar R, Rao S, Saxena R. Myelodysplastic syndromes: classification and prognostic scoring systems and their applicability in Indian scenario-experience from a tertiary care center. Hematology. 2009;14:145–9.

32. Braun T, Fenaux P. Myelodysplastic syndromes (MDS) and autoimmune disorders (AD): cause or consequence? Best Pract Res Clin Haematol. 2013;26:327–36.

33. Endi W, Elizabeth B, Imran S, et al. Pseudo–Pelger-Huët anomaly induced by medications: a clinico-pathologic study in comparison with myelodysplastic syndrome–related Pseudo–Pelger-Huët anomaly. Am J Clin Pathol. 2011;135:291–303.

34. Taegtmeyer AB, Halil O, Bell AD, et al. Neutrophil dysplasia (acquired pseudo-pelger anomaly) caused by ganciclovir. Transplantation. 2005;80:127–30.

35. Sharp RA, Lowe JG, Johnston RN. Anti-tuberculous drugs and sideroblastic anaemia. Br J Clin Pract. 1990;44:706–7.

36. Valent P, Orazzi A, Büschner G, et al. Standards and impact of hematopathology in myelodysplastic syndromes (MDS). Oncotarget. 2010;1:483–96.

37. Ogata K, Della Porta MG, Malcovati L, Picone C, Yokose N, Matsuda A, et al. Diagnostic utility of flow cytometry in low-grade myelodysplastic syndromes: a prospective validation study. Haematologica. 2009;94:1066–74.

38. Della Porta MG, Picone C, Pascutto C, Malcovati L, Tamura H, Handa H, et al. Multicenter validation of a reproducible flow cytometric score for the diagnosis of low-grade myelodysplastic syndromes: results of a European LeukemiaNET study. Haematologica. 2012;97:1209–17.

39. Kern W, Haferlach C, Schnittger S, Haferlach T. Clinical utility of multiparameter flow cytometry in the diagnosis of 1013 patients with suspected myelodysplastic syndrome: correlation to cytomorphology, cytogenetics, and clinical data. Cancer. 2010;116:4549–63.

40. Kern W, Bacher U, Haferlach C, et al. Multiparameter flow cytometry provides independent prognostic information in patients with suspected myelodysplasti syndromes: a study on 804 patients. Cytometry B Clin Cytom. 2015;88:154–64.

41. Wang SA, Pozdnyakova O, Jorgensen JL, et al. Detection of paroxysmal nocturnal hemoglobinuria clones in patients with myelodysplastic syndromes and related bone marrow diseases, with emphasis on diagnostic pitfalls and caveats. Haematologica. 2009;94:29–37.

42. Bennett JM, Catovsky D, Daniel MT, et al. Proposals for the classification of the acute leukemias. French-American-british (FAB) co-operative group. Br J Haematol. 1976;33:451–8.

43. Wang SA, Patel KP, Pozdnyakova O, et al. Acute erythroid leukemia with <20% bone marrow blasts is clinically and biologically similar to myelodysplastic syndrome with excess blasts. Mod Pathol. 2016;29:1221–31.

44. Calvo X, Arenillas L, Luno E, et al. Erythroleukemia shares biological features and outcome with myelodysplastic syndromes with excess blasts: a rationale for its inclusion into future classifications of myelodysplastic syndromes. Mod Pathol. 2016;29: 1541–51.

45. Santos FP, Faderl S, Garcia-Manero G, et al. Adult acute erythroleukemia: an analysis of 91 patients treated at a single institution. Leukemia. 2009;23(12):2275–80.

46. Bacher U, Haferlach C, Alpermann T, Kern W, Schnittger S, Haferlach T. Comparison of genetic and clinical aspects in patients with acute myeloid leukemia and myelodysplastic syndromes all with more than 50% of bone marrow erythropoietic cells. Haematologica. 2011;96(9):1284–92.

47. Hasserjian RP, Zuo Z, Garcia C, et al. Acute erythroid leukemia: a reassessment using criteria refined in the 2008 WHO classification. Blood. 2010;115(10):1985–92.

48. Bacher U, Haferlach C, Alpermann T, et al. Comparison of genetic and clinical aspects in patients with acute myeloid leukemia and myelodysplastic syndromes all with more than 50% of bone marrow erythropoietic cells. Haematologica. 2011;96:1284–92.

49. Polprasert C, Schulze I, Sekeres MA, et al. Inherited and somatic defects in DDX41 in myeloid neoplasms. Cancer Cell. 2015;27:658–70.

50. Owen C, Barnett M, Fitzgibbon J. Familial myelodysplasia and acute myeloid leukaemia—a review. Br J Haematol. 2015;140:123–32.

51. Nickels EM, Soodalter J, Churpek JE, et al. Recognizing familial myeloid leukemia in adults. Ther Adv Hematol. 2013;4:254–69.

52. West AH, Godley LA, Churpek JE. Familial myelodysplastic syndrome/acute leukemia syndromes: a review and utility for translational investigations. Ann N Y Acad Sci. 2014;1310:111–8.

53. Collin M, Dickinson R, Bigley V. Haematopoietic and immune defects associated with GATA2 mutation. Br J Haematol. 2015;169:173–87.

54. Hsu AP, McReynolds L, Holland SM. GATA2 deficiency. Curr Opin Allergy Clin Immunol. 2015;15:104–9.

55. Micol JB, Abdel-Wahab O. Collaborating constitutive and somatic genetic events in myeloid malignancies: ASXL 1 mutations in patients with germline GATA2 mutations. Haematologica. 2014;99:201–3.

56. Wlodarski MW, Hirabayashi S, Pastor V, et al. Prevalence, clinical characteristics, and prognosis of GATA2-related myelodysplastic syndromes in children and adolescents. Blood. 2016;127:1387–97.

57. Calvo KR, Vinh DC, Marie I, et al. Myelodysplasia in autosomal dominant and sporadic monocytopenia immunodeficiency syndrome: diagnostic features and clinical implications. Haematologica. 2011;96:221–5.

58. Churpek JE, Lorenz R, Nedumgottil S, et al. Proposal for the clinical detection and management of patients and their family members with familial myelodysplastic syndrome/acute leukemia predisposition syndromes. Leuk Lymphoma. 2013;54:28–35.

59. Malcovati L, Germing U, Kuendgen A, et al. Time-dependent prognostic scoring system for predicting survival and leukemic evolution in myelodysplastic syndromes. J Clin Oncol. 2007;25:3503–10.

60. Della Porta MG, Tuechler H, Malcovati L, et al. Validation of WHO classification-based Prognostic Scoring System (WPSS) for myelodysplastic syndromes and comparison with the revised International Prognostic Scoring System (IPSS-R). A study of the International Working Group for Prognosis in Myelodysplasia (IWG-PM). Leukemia. 2015;29:1502–13.

61. Garcia-Manero G, Shan J, Faderl S, et al. A prognostic score for patients with lower risk myelodysplastic syndrome. Leukemia. 2008;22:538–43.

62. Bowen KL, Davis BH. Abnormal patterns of expression of CD16 (FcR-III) and CD11b (CRIII) antigens by developing neutrophils in the bone marrow of patients with myelodysplastic syndrome. Lab Hematol. 1997;3:292–8.

63. Stetler-Stevenson M, Arthur DC, Jabbour N, Xie XY, Molldrem J, Barrett AJ, et al. Diagnostic utility of flow cytometric immunophenotyping in myelodysplastic syndrome. Blood. 2001;98:979–87.

64. Westers TM, Ireland R, Kern W, Alhan C, Balleisen JS, Bettelheim P, et al. Standardization of flow cytometry in myelodysplastic syndromes: a report from an international consortium and the European LeukemiaNet Working Group. Leukemia. 2012;26(7):1730–41.

65. Porwit A, van de Loosdrecht AA, Bettelheim P, Brodersen LE, Burbury K, Cremers E, et al. Revisiting guidelines for integration of flow cytometry results in the WHO classification of myelodysplastic syndromes-proposal from the International/European LeukemiaNet Working Group for Flow Cytometry in MDS. Leukemia. 2014;28(9):1793–8.

66. Papaemmanuil E, Gerstung M, Malcovati L, et al. Clinical and biological implications of driver mutations in myelodysplastic syndromes. Blood. 2013;122:3616–27.

67. Haferlach T, Nagata Y, Grossmann V, et al. Landscape of genetic lesions in 944 patients with myelodysplastic syndromes. Leukemia. 2014;28:241–7.

68. Bejar R, Stevenson KE, Caughey B, et al. Somatic mutations predict poor outcome in patients with myelodysplastic syndrome after hematopoietic stem-cell transplantation. J Clin Oncol. 2014;32:2691–8.

69. Bejar R, Steensma DP. Recent developments in myelodysplastic syndromes. Blood. 2014;124:2793–803.

70. Bejar R, Stevenson K, Abdel-Wahab O, Galili N, Nilsson B, Garcia-Manero G, et al. Clinical effect of point mutations in myelodysplastic syndromes. N Engl J Med. 2011;364:2496–506.

71. Bejar R, et al. TET2 mutations predict response to hypomethylating agents in myelodysplastic syndrome patients. Blood. 2014;124:2705–12.

72. Malcovati L, Hellström-Lindberg E, Bowen D, et al. Diagnosis and treatment of primary myelodysplastic syndromes in adults: recommendations from the European LeukemiaNet. Blood. 2013;122:2943–64.

73. Itzykson R, Thepot S, Quesnel B, et al. Prognostic factors for response and overall survival in 282 patients with higher-risk myelodysplastic syndromes treated with azacitidine. Blood. 2011;117:403–11.

74. Traina F, Visconte V, Elson P, et al. Impact of molecular mutations on treatment response to DNMT inhibitors in myelodysplasia and related neoplasms. Leukemia. 2014;28:78–87.

75. Platzbecker U, Germing U, Götze KS, et al. Luspatercept for the treatment of anaemia in patients with lower-risk myelodysplastic syndromes (PACE-MDS): a multicentre, open-label phase 2 dose-finding study with long-term extension study. Lancet Oncol. 2017;18:1338–47.

76. Xie M, Lu C, Wang J, et al. Age-related mutations associated with clonal hematopoietic expansion and malignancies. Nat Med. 2014;20:1472–8.

77. Genovese G, Kahler AK, Handsaker RE, et al. Clonal hematopoiesis and blood-cancer risk inferred from blood DNA sequence. N Engl J Med. 2014;371(26):2477–87.

78. Jaiswal S, Fontanillas P, Flannick J, et al. Age-related clonal hematopoiesis associated with adverse outcomes. N Engl J Med. 2014;371(26):2488–98.

79. Kwok B, Hall JM, Witte JS, et al. MDS associated somatic mutations and clonal hematopoiesis are common in idiopathic cytopenias of undetermined significance. Blood. 2015;126(21):2355–61.

80. Valent P, Hprny H-P, Bennett JM, et al. Definitions and standards in the diagnosis and treatment of the myelodysplastic syndromes: consensus statements and report from a working conference. Leuk Res. 2007;31:727–36.

81. Steensma DP, Bejar R, Jaiswal S, et al. Clonal hematopoiesis of indeterminate potential and its distinction from myelodysplastic syndromes. Blood. 2015;126(1):9–16.

Acute Myeloid Leukemia: An Update

10

Deepshi Thakral and Ritu Gupta

10.1 Introduction

Acute myeloid leukemia (AML) is a rapidly progressing aggressive malignancy of the hematopoietic myeloid progenitor cells most commonly found in older adults. It is characterized by an impaired differentiation and aberrant clonal proliferation of immature myeloid precursors in the bone marrow that result in the accumulation of nonfunctional myeloblasts, impaired hematopoiesis, bone marrow failure, and peripheral blood cytopenias, thus increasing the risk of severe infections, anemia, bleeding, and other complications in patients [1, 2]. Classically, morphology, immunophenotyping, and cytogenetic approaches have been used for the diagnosis and classification of AML (French-American-British (FAB) classification) [3, 4]. With the advent of whole genome sequencing, the complexity of AML emerged wherein heterogeneous and competent clones evolve and coexist at any time during the disease course [5–8]. Recurrent somatic mutations have been identified in AML, and the number of leukemia-associated genes is increasingly comprehensive [9, 10]. Henceforth, the WHO incorporated molecular alterations, in addition to the conventional methods for AML

classification to establish clonality, identify molecular translocations and risk stratification of patients (2008–2009) and further revised in 2016 [11–14]. Thereafter, a paradigm shift from a morphologic classification of AML to one guided by causative genomic changes has been witnessed [15]. For the past four decades, the standard of care for AML has been 3 + 7 combination chemotherapy, with 3 days of anthracycline and 7 days of cytarabine [16, 17]. Although many patients with AML respond to induction chemotherapy, refractory disease is common, and relapse represents the major cause of treatment failure despite intensive therapy. Targeted therapies are emerging as treatment modalities and several clinical trials are ongoing [18, 19].

10.2 Epidemiology

The annual incidence of acute myeloid leukemia worldwide is ~2.5–3 cases per 100,000 population per year with the highest incidence in the USA, Australia, and Europe [11]. The National Cancer Institute's (NCI's) Surveillance, Epidemiology, and End Results (SEER) Program estimated an incidence of 21,380 cases of AML, representing 1.3% of all new cancer cases in the United States in 2017 [20]. The incidence of AML was documented as 4.2 new cases and 2.8 deaths per 100,000 in 2014 with 68 years as the median age at diagnosis. Death rate from AML was estimated at 1.8% of the total deaths from cancer in

D. Thakral · R. Gupta (✉)
Laboratory Oncology Unit, Dr. B.R.A. IRCH,
All India Institute of Medical Sciences,
New Delhi, India
e-mail: drritu.laboncology@aiims.edu

© Springer Nature Singapore Pte Ltd. 2019
R. Saxena, H. P. Pati (eds.), *Hematopathology*, https://doi.org/10.1007/978-981-13-7713-6_10

the United States with higher incidence among older adults (65 years and above) and 72 years as the median age at death. The age-adjusted incidence of AML was found to be higher in men than in women (3:2). AML accounts for 15–20% of all cases of childhood acute leukemia, generally peak incidence observed in early 3–4 years of life [11].

The risk factors for AML include cigarette smoke as a major source of benzene [21, 22], exposure to high-dose or chronic low-dose ionizing radiations and treatment with cytotoxic chemotherapy [2]. In fact, the WHO categorized therapy-related AML (t-AML) as a subtype, which occurs as a complication after long-term exposure to cytotoxic chemotherapy with either alkylating agents or DNA topoisomerase II inhibitors [23, 24]. Other etiological factors include past history of blood disorders (e.g., myelodysplastic syndrome, polycythemia vera), certain genetic disorders (e.g., Down syndrome, Fanconi anemia) [25], and in rare cases immunosuppression subsequent to stem cell transplantation [26, 27]. About 60–80% of newly diag-

nosed adult AML patients achieve complete remission (CR) with intensive induction chemotherapy and a 5-year relative survival rate of 26.9% [20]. Reduced survival rate among older adults with AML is attributed to chemotherapy-related complications [28, 29]. The morbidity and mortality in post-induction chemotherapy phase of AML is influenced by various adverse prognostic factors such as infections, involvement of central nervous system, and smoking [30–33].

10.3 Clinical Characteristics

The clonal neoplastic expansion of hematopoietic cells that normally differentiate into various cell types including granulocyte, monocyte, erythrocyte, and megakaryocyte progenitors results in accumulation of myeloblasts and other immature myeloid cells and deficit of mature functional white blood cells, red blood cells, and platelets in the bone marrow of AML patients (Fig. 10.1).

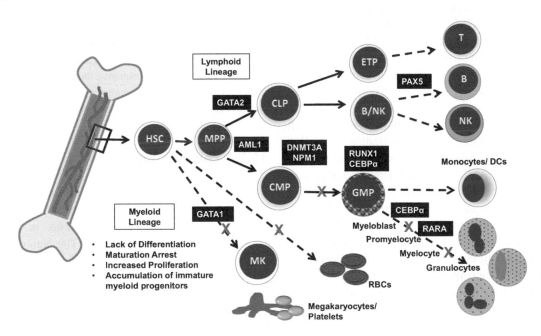

Fig. 10.1 Pathogenesis of AML. Diagrammatic representation shows various stages of myeloid and lymphoid lineage commitment from a common progenitor. Few key transcription factors involved in hematopoiesis are highlighted in black. Recurrent genetic abnormalities and mutations in these and several other target genes drive AML disease progression. (Myeloid cell differentiation arrest at different steps is marked by cross). Adapted from [11, 38, 39]. *HSC* hematopoietic stem cell; *MPP* multipotent progenitor; *CMP* common myeloid progenitor; *CLP* common lymphoid progenitor; *GMP* granulocyte/macrophage progenitor; *MK* megakaryocyte progenitor; *ETP* early T-cell precursor; *T* T lymphocyte; *B* B lymphocyte; *NK* natural killer cell

The early signs and symptoms of AML may include fever, loss of appetite, or weight loss. The increased susceptibility of AML patients to infections is attributed to the absence of normal WBCs and incapacitated leukemia cells [2]. Furthermore, anemia in these patients can cause fatigue, shortness of breath, and weakness. A lack of platelets can lead to easy bruising, bleeding, petechiae, or even a severe trauma. Sternal tenderness and splenomegaly are common in AML, but it is typically mild and asymptomatic. The leukemia cells may also present extramedullary tumor proliferation, including the central nervous system (brain and spinal cord), skin, and gum tissue. In rare cases, the first sign of leukemia may be observed as a development of a solid leukemic mass or tumor outside of the bone marrow, called a chloroma [34, 35]. As an acute leukemia, AML progresses rapidly and, if left untreated, can be fatal within weeks or months.

AMLs and to distinguish poorly differentiated monoblastic leukemia) is sufficient for diagnosis in majority of the cases. Chromosomal abnormalities such as translocations, deletion, or trisomy in a specific type of AML are also criteria irrespective of blast percentage [36]. Other cytogenetic approach such as fluorescence-in-situ-hybridization (FISH) enables detection and diagnosis of subtype of leukemia. The molecular testing for genetic mutations can facilitate prognostication for chemotherapy and/or bone marrow/stem cell transplantation [37]. Overall, for AML diagnosis, first screening is for the distinction of an acute leukemia from other hematological neoplastic diseases and reactive disorders. Next step is to differentiate acute myeloid leukemia (AML) from acute lymphoblastic leukemia (ALL). Finally, AML and ALL are classified into categories that define treatment, prognostication, and risk stratification.

10.4 Diagnosis of AML

Various factors including clinical history, presentation, age, and medical condition of the patient are taken into consideration for the choice of laboratory investigations, which may be used for the diagnosis of AML. Investigation of the bone marrow biopsy/aspirate collected from either of the pelvic bone remains the gold standard for AML diagnosis. While light microscopy allows examination of marrow or blood smears for abnormal WBCs, flow cytometry or immunophenotyping and immune/cytochemistry are used to differentiate AML from other types of leukemia and classify the subtype of AML based on unique combinations of cell surface markers expressed on leukemia cells. According to the WHO criteria, 20% blasts of the total cells in the bone marrow or blood is a prerequisite for the diagnosis of AML [13]. A unique morphological characteristic feature seen in myeloid leukemia blasts is Auer rods that can distinguish it from other leukemia [11]. A positive enzyme cytochemistry with myeloperoxidase (MPO) along with a nonspecific esterase stain (used to identify a monocytic component in

10.5 Classification of AML

Ever since Otto Naegeli first characterized the myeloblasts in 1990 [40], the classification system for AML diagnosis has evolved toward a stepwise approach. The French-American-British (FAB) classification of AML proposed in 1976 by Bennett et al. [3] was introduced by a group of French, American, and British leukemia experts. The various categories of AML subtypes from M0 to M7 in FAB classification were based on morphology showing the origin of leukemia cell, its stage of differentiation, and maturity. AML subtypes M0–M1 include the minimally differentiated or undifferentiated AML; M2 subtype is mostly associated with cytogenetic abnormalities t(8;21)(q22;q22) or t(6;9); M3 is identified with PML-RARA t(15;17)(q22;q21); and M4 is associated with combination myeloblastic-monoblastic leukemia with or without eosinophilia and inv(16), t(16;16). The del(11q), t(9;11), t(11;19) karyotypes are seen in M5 subtype, whereas AML-M6 initiates from early red blood cell precursors and AML-M7 from megakaryocytes. Eventually, the cytogenetic abnormalities that are associated with each subtype were deciphered [36, 41, 42].

Table 10.1 AML subcategorization according to the revised 2016 WHO classification

1. AML with recurrent genetic abnormalities	
(i)	AML with t(8;21)(q22;q22.1); *RUNX1-RUNX1T1*
(ii)	AML with inv(16)(p13.1q22) or t(16;16)(p13.1;q22); *CBFB-MYH11*
(iii)	APL with *PML-RARA*
(iv)	AML with t(9;11)(p21.3;q23.3); *MLLT3-KMT2A*
(v)	AML with t(6;9)(p23;q34.1); *DEK-NUP214*
(vi)	AML with inv(3)(q21.3q26.2) or t(3;3)(q21.3;q26.2); *GATA2, MECOM*
(vii)	AML (megakaryoblastic) with t(1;22)(p13.3;q13.3); *RBM15-MKL1*
(viii)	Provisional entity: AML with *BCR-ABL1*
(ix)	AML with mutated *NPM1*
(x)	AML with biallelic mutations of *CEBPA*
(xi)	Provisional entity: AML with mutated *RUNX1*

2. AML with myelodysplasia-related changes	
• Cytogenetic abnormalities sufficient to diagnose AML with myelodysplasia-related changes when >20% PB or BM blasts are present and prior therapy has been excluded	
• Complex karyotype (3 or more abnormalities)	

Balanced abnormalities	**Unbalanced abnormalities**
(i) 27/del(7q)	(ii) t(11;16)(q23.3;p13.3)
(ii) del(5q)/t(5q)	(iii) t(3;21)(q26.2;q22.1)
(iii) i(17q)/t(17p)	(iv) t(1;3)(p36.3;q21.2)
(iv) 213/del(13q)	(v) t(2;11)(p21;q23.3)
(v) del(11q)	(vi) t(5;12)(q32;p13.2)
(vi) del(12p)/t(12p)	(vii) t(5;7)(q32;q11.2)
(vii) idic(X)(q13)	(viii) t(5;17)(q32;p13.2)
	(ix) t(5;10)(q32;q21.2)
	(x) t(3;5)(q25.3;q35.1)

3. Therapy-related myeloid neoplasms	

4. AML, NOS	
(i)	AML with minimal differentiation
(ii)	AML without maturation
(iii)	AML with maturation
(iv)	Acute myelomonocytic leukemia
(v)	Acute monoblastic/monocytic leukemia
(vi)	Pure erythroid leukemia
(vii)	Acute megakaryoblastic leukemia
(viii)	Acute basophilic leukemia
(ix)	Acute panmyelosis with myelofibrosis

5. Myeloid sarcoma	

6. Myeloid proliferations related to Down syndrome	
Transient abnormal myelopoiesis (TAM)	
Myeloid leukemia associated with Down syndrome	

Subsequently, the World Health Organization (WHO) classification of AML came into existence in 1999 by Harris et al. [14]. The WHO classification included chromosomal translocations, evidence of dysplasia, and eventually recurrent gene mutations [11–13]. Even though the WHO classification is highly recommended, FAB staging system is still used widely despite its limitation of not predicting prognostically significant AML subtypes. The recently revised 2016 WHO classification of acute myeloid leukemia and related precursor neoplasms [11] defined six broad categories, each comprising subcategories (shown in Table 10.1), described briefly as follows:

1. *AML with recurrent genetic abnormalities*

According to the 2016 WHO classification of AML, the first broad category encompasses recurrent genetic abnormalities that include eight entities of balanced cytogenetic abnormalities or gene fusions and three gene-specific mutations [11]. Most of these subcategories are characterized by unique morphological, immunophenotypic, cytogenetic, and molecular features as described. Besides these 11 entities, several additional balanced abnormalities have been documented in rare cases of AML, which are still not separate entities [43].

(i)   *AML   with   t(8;21)(q22;q22.1); RUNX1-RUNX1T1*

AML with t(8;21) chromosomal translocation is the most frequent anomaly in younger patients, rare in elderly, and account for 1–5% cases of AML [44]. The bone marrow and peripheral blood show the presence of large myeloblasts with abundant basophilic cytoplasm, often filled with azurophilic granulations. The bone marrow biopsy shows sheets of immature cells with increased normal eosinophil precursors and basophils. Promyelocytes, myelocytes, and mature granulocytes with abnormal nuclear segmentation and variable dysplasia are also seen. These cells may show cytoplasmic staining defects including homogeneous salmon-colored granules. Auer rods are frequently noted. Monocytic component is usually absent with erythroblasts and megakaryocytes showing normal morphology. Immunophenotypic profile shows expression of CD34, CD13, MPO, and HLA-DR with variable CD33. Aberrant expression of CD19 (B-cell surface marker) and PAX5 is seen in most cases, and occasionally CD79a may be expressed. CD56 expression in a subset of cases may be associated with adverse prognosis.

The chromosomal translocation results in fusion of runt-related transcription factor 1 (*RUNX1*) [aka acute myeloid leukemia 1 protein (*AML1*) or core-binding factor subunit alpha-2 (*CBFA2*)] and RUNX1 translocation partner 1 (*RUNX1T1* aka *ETO*) on chromosome 21 and 8, respectively [45]. This *RUNX1-RUNX1T1* fusion transcript, which is consistently detected in these cases result in transcriptional repression of target genes that are regulated by CBF transcription factor RUNX1 and subsequent maturation arrest of hematopoietic progenitor cells, which would otherwise normally differentiate into granulocytic and monocytic lineages. Although cases of AML with t(8;21) are associated with relatively favorable prognosis and, in particular, with a good response to high-dose cytarabine (ara-C), high WBC count >20 billion/L at the presentation or presence of *KIT* mutations in exons 8 and 17 seem to be associated with intermediate to worse prognosis seen in 20–30% cases [46]. These patients benefit from allogeneic stem cell transplantation during the first remission. Other cytogenetic abnormalities seen in >70% of cases include del(9q) with loss of 9q22 and loss of a sex chromosome. Additionally, mutations reported in a subset of AML cases include *ASXL1* (~10% cases), *ASXL2* (20–25% cases in all age groups), *KRAS*, *NRAS* (30%), and rarely *FLT3*. Monitoring of MRD post-therapy in these cases is beneficial, and detection of *RUNX1-RUNX1T1* fusion transcript during remission by quantitative RT-PCR is suggested.

(ii) *AML with inv(16)(p13.1q22) or t(16;16) (p13.1;q22);CBFB-MYH11*

AML with inv(16) or t(16;16) genetic abnormality usually shows distinct morphology of acute myelomonocytic leukemia with abnormal eosinophilia irrespective of the blast count. The occurrence is 5–8% in younger AML patients, and much lower frequency is seen in older adults [11]. The incidence of extra medullary disease in these cases is relatively higher than most AML. Myeloid sarcoma and involvement of CNS are associated with relapse. Most striking morphological characteristics include abnormal eosinophils with enlarged, irregularly shaped basophilic colored granules in the bone marrow that are absent in peripheral blood. Nuclear hyposegmentation is seen in mature eosinophils. Marked reduction in neutrophils is notable. Normal myeloblasts, monoblasts, and mature monocytes are present in bone marrow and peripheral blood. Auer rods are occasionally present in myeloblasts. Exclusive lineage of only granulocytic maturation or only monocytic differentiation is reported in rare cases. Complex immunophenotypic profile showing several subsets including immature blasts (CD34, CD117), granulocytic (CD13, CD33, MPO, CD15), and monocytic (CD14, CD64, CD11b, CD11c, CD4, CD36, and lysozyme) populations is seen. The chromosomal breakpoint in t(16;16) is mapped to the core binding factor beta subunit (*CBFB*) at 16q22 and gene encoding smooth muscle myosin heavy chain (*MYH11*). The inv(16) is a pericentric inversion of chromosome 16. Together with AML t(8;21), these two AML categories are referred to as the core binding factor leukemia and are associated with favorable prognosis [47]. Likewise, presence of trisomy 8, *KIT*, and *FLT3* mutations in these cases is associated with poor prognosis. The fusion transcript CBFB-MYH11 is detected by FISH and RT-PCR at diagnosis and shows a decreasing trend during the course of therapy.

(iii) *APL with PML-RARA*

APL with PML-RARA is a well-characterized AML entity with predominance of abnormal promyelocytes. Accounting for 5–8% of AML cases in young adults, almost 70% cases present as typical or hypergranular APL and the remaining cases usually belong to microgranular variant, which generally present with leukocytosis [11]. The clinical presentation of APL is commonly associated with disseminated intravascular coagulation and increased fibrinolysis leading to early mortality. Common morphological features of both APL variants include abnormal promyelocytes with bilobed nuclei. Densely packed large granules are seen in the cytoplasm in most hypergranular APL cases with few cells showing dust-like granules that are detected on Romanowsky stain. Randomly distributed bundles of Auer rods, which are relatively larger than seen in other AML may be present. In contrast, microgranular APL is marked by hypogranular appearance of the cytoplasm because of the submicroscopic granules. The leukemic promyelocytes in both variants show strong MPO positivity. Immunophenotypically, APL with PML-RARA shows bright CD33, variable CD13, and reduced or absent CD34, HLA-DR, CD18, CD11b, CD11c, CD117, CD15, and CD65 expression. Expression of CD2 in microgranular variant or minor transcript of PML-RARA is associated with FLT3-ITD mutation, and CD56 expression in few APL cases is associated with adverse prognosis.

Promyelocytic leukemia gene (*PML*) is located on chromosome 15 and retinoic acid receptor alpha (*RARA*) on chromosome 17, and the *PML-RARA* fusion results from a recurrent, balanced translocation between chromosomes 15 and 17, denoted as t(15;17)(q22;q12) [48]. The breakpoints within the PML gene in intron 6, exon 6, and intron 3 give rise to PML-RARα isoforms referred to as long (L or bcr1), variant (V or bcr2), and short (S or bcr3). RT-PCR for *PML-RARA* fusion transcript is used in conjunction with the investigation of therapy response to all-trans-retinoic acid (ATRA) and arsenic trioxide as diagnostic measure for MRD monitoring in acute APL. Submicroscopic insertion of RARA, considered to be cryptic t(15;17) are included in this category of AML. In a subset of cases with morphological features similar to APL, variant translocations of RARA with other fusion partners (*ZBTB16*, *NPM1*, *NUMA1*, and *STAT5B*) have been documented [49]. Most cases of APL respond to treatment with the combination of tretinoin (all-trans retinoic acid) and arsenic oxide with the exception of cases with variant RARA translocations. In addition to the standard therapy of ATRA and arsenic oxide, anthracycline is administered to high-risk patients.

(iv) *AML with t(9;11)(p21.3;q23.3); KMT2A-MLLT3*

AML with t(9;11) accounts for about 2% of adult AML and almost 12% of pediatric AML with intermediate prognosis. Clinical presentation may show involvement of extramedullary sites such as skin, gingiva, and tissue infiltration; myeloid sarcoma and disseminated intravascular coagulation may be present. Bone marrow smear shows abundant monoblasts and promonocytes with pale cytoplasm containing azurophilic granules. Strongly positive nonspecific esterase reaction with absent MPO reactivity is a hallmark of AML with t(9;11). Immunophenotyping reveals bright expression of CD33, HLA-DR, CD4, and CD65. Weak expression of CD13, CD14, and CD34 is seen in pediatric population. In most adult AML with t(9;11) cases, CD14, CD4, CD11b, CD11c, CD36, CD64, and lysozyme expression is reported with variable expression of CD34, CD117, and CD56. The *KMT2A* gene (aka *MLL*) encodes a histone methyltransferase, which regulates gene transcription by chromatin remodeling. *KMT2A* on chromosome 11 is known to be associated with several partner genes [49]. Most AML with balanced translocations involving *KMT2A* other than t(9;11) are primarily grouped

as AML, NOS. *MECOM* overexpression is reported in ~40% cases of this AML subtype and is associated with adverse prognosis.

(v) *AML with t(6;9)(p23;q34.1); DEK-NUP214*

AML with t(6;9) is a rare subtype detected in about 0.7–1.8% of both pediatric and adult AML cases and is associated with poor prognosis [11]. Low WBC count is generally seen in adults, whereas severe anemia and thrombocytopenia may be present in pediatric population. Residual myeloid maturation with dysplastic features are present in the bone marrow, and blast cells display similar features of acute myelomonocytic leukemia and occasionally show Auer rods. Nucleated RBCs with variable size and shape, hypogranular neutrophils, and platelets may be present in circulation. Basophilia, erythroid hyperplasia, and dyserythropoiesis with occasional ring sideroblasts are common characteristics of AML with t(6;9). Immunophenotypic profile of blasts include nonspecific myeloid markers CD33, CD13, HLA-DR, MPO, CD9, CD38, and CD123 and variable expression of CD117, CD15, CD64, and CD34. Terminal deoxynucleotidyl transferase (TdT) may show positivity in few cases. This balanced translocation occurs between DEK oncogene (DEK) at chromosome 6 that encodes a protein involved in chromatin remodeling and DNA repair and nucleoporin 214 kDa (NUP214) gene at chromosome 9 that encodes a component of the nuclear core complex. DEK-NUP214 fusion protein acquires aberrant function by alteration of nuclear transport [42]. Monitoring of DEK-NUP214 fusion transcript is suggested in these patients although response to conventional chemotherapy is not very promising and allogeneic stem cell transplantation is beneficial. Frequency of FLT3-ITD mutations is reported to be 70–80% but poor prognosis of AML with t(6;9) is independent of FLT3 status.

(vi) *AML with inv(3)(q21.3q26.2) or t(3;3)*
      (q21.3;q26.2); GATA2, MECOM
      AML with inv(3) or t(3;3) represents
      1–2% of AML cases in adults with rare
      occurrence in children. Common clinical
      features include anemia, normal to ele-
      vated platelets, and occasional hepato-
      splenomegaly [11]. Multilineage
      dysplasia including hypogranular neutro-
      phils with hyposegmented nucleus and
      large hypogranular platelets are com-
      monly seen in peripheral blood smears.
      Heterogenous morphology including
      undifferentiated myeloid blasts, mature
      myeloid and monoblasts, and mono- or
      bilobated megakaryocytes or other dys-
      plastic features as dyserythropoiesis are
      seen in the bone marrow. Few studies
      have documented flow cytometry-based
      evaluation, and generic markers for blasts
      including CD34, CD13, CD33, HLA-DR,
      CD117, and CD38 are described. A sub-
      set of cases show megakaryocytic differ-
      entiation markers, CD41 and CD61, and
      aberrant expression of CD7 in few cases
      is reported. Most common genetic abnor-
      malities of long arm of chromosome 3
      include inv(3)(q21.3q26.2) or t(3;3)
      (q21.3;q26.2). Gene translocation inv(3)
      or t(3;3) results in repositioning of
      GATA2 enhancer that activates MECOM
      expression resulting in overexpression of
      this gene and leukemia onset, also confer-
      ring GATA2 haploinsufficiency (*MECOM*
      or MDS1 and EVI1 complex locus pro-
      tein is a transcriptional regulator that may
      be involved in hematopoiesis, apoptosis,
      and cell differentiation and proliferation).
      Secondary myelodysplasia-associated
      karyotypic abnormalities [(27/del(7q),
      del(5q)/t(5q)] and complex karyotypes
      are reported in 75% of cases. High occur-
      rence of gene mutations (>98% cases) in
      NRAS, KRAS, CBL, KIT, NF1, PTPN11,
      GATA2, RUNX1, SF3B1, and *FLT3* is
      common. Poor response to standard AML
      therapy and worse prognosis in this AML
      subtype is further complicated by the

presence of complex karyotype monosomy 7. BCR-ABL-positive cases may
acquire these abnormalities of chromosome 3 and are considered aggressive
chronic myeloid leukemia.

(vii) *AML (Megakaryoblastic) with t(1;22)*
      (p13.3;q13.3); RBM15-MKL1
      A rare form of AML that is predomi-
      nantly seen in infants without trisomy 21
      (Down syndrome), AML with t(1;22), the
      principal translocation of acute mega-
      karyoblastic leukemia, accounts for <1%
      of all AML cases [11]. Clinically, pres-
      ence of a soft tissue mass along with hep-
      atosplenomegaly, osteolytic lesions,
      anemia, and thrombocytopenia are com-
      mon features with occasional cases pre-
      senting with myeloid sarcoma without
      bone marrow involvement. Common
      morphological features include mega-
      karyoblasts with agranular basophilic
      cytoplasm, micromegakaryocytes, mar-
      row fibrosis with clumps of megakaryo-
      blasts, and more condensed nuclear
      chromatin with rare nucleolation. Similar
      to other AML with megakaryoblastic
      morphology, CD45, CD34, and HLA-DR
      may be negative with variable CD13 and
      CD33. Blasts are negative with MPO
      antibodies, and lymphoid markers (TdT)
      are absent. One or more of the platelet
      glycoproteins markers such as CD41,
      CD61, and CD42b may be positive.
      Chromosomal rearrangement t(1;22)
      results in the fusion of RNA-binding
      motif protein-15 (*RBM15*) gene with
      megakaryoblastic leukemia-1 (*MKL1*)
      gene, which encodes a DNA binding
      motif involved in chromatin remodeling
      and extracellular signaling pathways. The
      fusion transcript *RBM15-MKL1* can be
      detected by molecular methods. The
      response to treatment and risk category of
      this type of AML remains controversial.

(viii) *Provisional entity: AML with*
       BCR-ABL1
       Rare cases of *de novo* AML with BCR-
       ABL1 fusion t(9;22)(q34.1;q11.2)

accounting for <1% of AML cases is included in the revised 2016 WHO classification as a provisional entity [11]. Major features that distinguish AML with BCR-ABL1 from CML, ALL, or MPAL include less frequent basophilia and splenomegaly and 80% marrow cellularity as opposed to 95–100% seen in other leukemia. Blast cells in AML with BCR-ABL1 show positivity for CD34, CD13, and CD33 with aberrant expression of CD19, CD7, and TdT. Most cases demonstrate BCR-ABL1 fusion transcript p210 (b2a2 and b3a2 fusions), and in rare cases, p190 is reported. In addition, t(9;22) translocation may be cryptic along with other cytogenetic abnormalities (monosomy 7 or trisomy 8). Another distinguishing feature is the occasional detection of AML-associated mutations such as *NPM1* and *FLT3-ITD* in AML with *BCR-ABL1* than in CML. Recent findings of loss of genes (*IKZF1*, *CDKN2A*) and cryptic deletions (*IGH*, *TRG*) exclusively in *de novo* AML may have diagnostic utility. Poor response to conventional AML therapy in these patients can be improved by the administration of tyrosine kinase inhibitors followed by allogeneic hematopoietic stem cell transplantation.

Although chromosomal abnormalities in AML provide significant information for prognostication and risk stratification of patients, almost 50% of adults with AML show a cytogenetically normal karyotype (CN-AML) [50]. Therefore, gene mutational analysis in AML has become a primary focus of investigation. Screening of AML-associated gene mutations is not mandatory for the initial diagnosis of AML but is significant for defining prognostic implications, risk stratification, identification of novel drug targets, and germline mutations for screening of family members and is no more restricted to cytogenetically normal AML cases.

(ix) **AML with mutated NPM1**

Nucleophosmin 1 (*NPM1*) is the most commonly detected mutation accounting for 27–35% adult and 2–8% childhood AML with 45–64% occurrence in cytogenetically normal karyotype and predominance in females [11, 51, 52]. Majority of AML cases with mutated *NPM1* present with anemia, thrombocytopenia, and high WBC count. Extramedullary involvement of gingiva, skin, and lymph nodes is commonly seen. *NPM1* mutation is recurrently seen in 80–90% of acute monocytic leukemia and also in pure erythroid leukemia. Monocytic differentiation is a common characteristic in adults, whereas myelomonocytic differentiation with rare erythroleukemia is seen in children. Characterized by high expression of CD33, CD117, CD123, and CD110 and low or absent CD13 and HLA-DR, immature myeloid or monocytic features (CD14, CD36, CD64) are commonly seen in AML with mutated NPM1. Cases with non-monocytic morphology are predominantly CD34 and HLA-DR negative and demonstrate cup-like nuclear invaginations. CD34-positive cases are less common and associated with adverse prognosis.

The *NPM1* gene is located on chromosome 5q35.1 that encodes a protein with several properties including chaperone between nucleus and cytoplasm, ribosome biogenesis, centrosomal duplication, and regulation of TP53 tumor suppressor pathway. Normally localized in the nucleoli, mutations in exon 12 in patients result in aberrant localization of NPM1 in the cytoplasm that can be detected by immunohistochemistry. Approximately 55 molecular variants of *NPM1* exon 12 mutations have been identified of which more than 95% occur as a 4-base pair insertion at position 960. Eighty percent of these cases show mutation A (TCTG duplication), while mutation B and D (CATG or CCTG duplication, respectively) account for ~10% and 5% of cases, respectively. Rare *NPM1* mutations outside exon 12 have also been reported in exon 11 and exon 9 [53–55]. Given the multifaceted functions of NPM1, several pathways may be affected; however, the contribution of these mutations in leukemogenesis remains unclear. AML with mutated *NPM1* is primarily seen in CN-AML cases; however, chromosomal abnormalities have been reported in 5–15% of AML cases [gain of chr8 and del(9q)]. In the absence of *FLT3-ITD* and/ or *DNMT3A* mutations, AML with mutated NPM1 has a favorable prognosis. Multiplex PCR-based detection is performed to evaluate *NPM1* and *FLT3-ITD* mutation status in new cases of AML. Cooccurrence of other secondary mutations including *IDH1, IDH2, KRAS, NRAS, TET2*, and cohesion complex genes is common.

(x) **AML with biallelic mutation of CEBPA**
A tumor suppressor gene located on chromosome 19q13.1, CCAAT/ enhancer-binding protein alpha (*CEBPA*), encodes a transcription factor involved in the differentiation of mainly granulocytes and various other developmental processes. Biallelic mutation of *CEBPA* in AML cases occur more commonly in children than adults with 4–9% of overall incidence [11]. These cases present with increased hemoglobin levels, decreased platelets, and lower LDH levels. Morphologically, myeloblasts with and without differentiation are more common than myelomonocytic or monocytic differentiation. Myeloblasts show aberrant expression of CD7 with no other definitive markers known in AML with biallelic *CEBPA* mutations. A quarter of these patients have multilineage dysplasia but without any prognostic significance. Immunophenotypically, blasts show expression of CD13, CD33, CD65, CD11b, and CD34. High frequency of HLA-DR, CD7, and CD15 with lower frequency of blasts expressing CD56 is seen in cases with biallelic than monoallelic *CEBPA*. Approximately, 100 mutations are documented along the entire coding region of *CEBPA* gene, and identification of these mutants is challenging because of the spectrum of mutations as well as intrinsic characteristics of the gene. CEBPA double-mutated cases usually contain biallelic mutations at N- and C-terminal and are associated with a favorable clinical outcome. Also, better prognostic significance of AML with *CEBPA* mutation is indicated in the absence of *FLT3-ITD* mutations and lack of any cytogenetic abnormalities. About 10% cases show single karyotypic abnormality, 39% cases show *GATA2* mutations, and 5–9% have *FLT3-ITD* mutations. Familial syndrome is not uncommon as germline mutations may occur in *CEBPA*.

(xi) **Provisional entity: AML with mutated RUNX1**
AML with mutated *RUNX1* is included as a provisional entity in the 2016 WHO classification. With an incidence of 4–16%, this category includes cases of *de novo* AML that fail to meet criteria for other WHO AML types (especially AML-MRC and t-AML) [11]. Clinical presentation includes low hemoglobin and LDH levels with lower WBC count. *RUNX1* mutations are common among older patients with up to 65% AML cases with minimal differentiation. These missense or frameshift mutations are mapped to exons 3 to 5 or the transactivation domain from exons 6 to 8. Common cytogenetic abnormalities include monosomy 7 and trisomy 8 and 13. Cooperative mutations with *RUNX1* include *ASXL1, KMT2A-PTD, FLT3-ITD, IDH1*, and *IDH2*. Associated with a worse prognosis, AML patients with mutated *RUNX1*

may benefit from allogeneic stem cell transplantation.

2. *AML with myelodysplasia-related changes (AML-MRC)*

AML-MRC is a revised category in the 2016 WHO classification, which is assigned based on the following criteria: (i) ≥20% blasts in peripheral blood or bone marrow; (ii) either prior history of MDS or MDS/MPN neoplasms or MDS-related cytogenetic abnormalities or multilineage dysplasia in the absence of mutations including *NPM1* or *bCEBPA*; and (iii) exclusion of prior history of cytotoxic or radiation therapy for an unrelated disease or subcategories of recurring genetic abnormalities [11]. Primarily seen in older patients, AML-MRC accounts for 24–35% of all AML cases. Patients presenting with severe pancytopenia, 20–29% marrow blasts and a clinical course for ≥2 months are eligible for treatment although with poor risk and overall survival. Morphology from peripheral blood or bone marrow smears should show the presence of multilineage dysplasia in ≥50% of the cells in at least two hematopoietic cell lineages. More common morphological features in AML-MRC are similar to AML with maturation or acute myelomonocytic leukemia. Multilineage dysplasia is also reported in hypocellular AML and AML without maturation.

Exclusive immunophenotypic profile is not established for AML-MRC so far. Therefore, generic markers are used for identification, which include CD34+, CD117+, CD13+, and CD33+ for blasts and myeloid lineage. Alterations in the expression of several other markers such as reduced expression of CD117, CD38, HLA-DR, and CD135 have been associated with multilineage dysplasia, and abnormal expression of CD7, CD10, and CD56 may be present. Often expression of monocytic differentiation markers including CD4 and CD14 is seen and CD14 or CD11b may be associated with a poor prognosis or high-risk complex cytogenetic abnormalities. Complex karyotype of three or more MDS-associated cytogenetic abnormalities include unbalanced

abnormalities [(27/del(7q), del(5q)/t(5q), i(17q)/t(17p), 213/del(13q), del(11q), del(12p)/t(12p), idic(X)(q13)] and balanced abnormalities [t(11;16)(q23.3;p13.3), t(3;21) (q26.2;q22.1), t(1;3)(p36.3;q21.2), t(2;11) (p21;q23.3), t(5;12)(q32;p13.2), t(5;7) (q32;q11.2), t(5;17)(q32;p13.2), t(5;10) (q32;q21.2), t(3;5)(q25.3;q35.1)]. Unbalanced cytogenetic abnormalities are most prevalent and result in loss of genetic material, whereas most of the balanced abnormalities in AML-MRC overlap with therapy-related AML. Therefore, exclusion of any history of cytotoxic chemotherapy or radiotherapy is mandatory before assigning AML-MRC subcategory. Additionally, gene mutations including *ASXL1*, *TP53*, and *U2AF1* are common, and *TP53* is associated with a complex karyotype and poor risk. Overall, patients with complex karyotype and multilineage dysplasia have poor prognosis than those with AML, not otherwise specified.

3. *Therapy-related myeloid neoplasms*

Therapy-related AML (t-AML) is a well-known entity that includes cases exposed to chemotherapy, radiation, immunosuppressive therapy, or their combination for a previous neoplastic or non-neoplastic condition [11, 23]. These neoplasms are believed to originate as a result of direct effect of mutational events induced by cytotoxic therapy in hematopoietic stem cells or the bone marrow microenvironment and selection of myeloid clone that is prone to high-risk genetic abnormalities. Therapy-related myeloid neoplasms account for almost 20% of all cases of AML, MDS, and MDS/MPN. Seventy percent of these cases have treatment history for solid tumor and 30% for hematological neoplasm (breast cancer and non-Hodgkin lymphoma account for majority of the cases). Although t-MNs are not age-dependent, an increasing trend of risk associated with alkylating agents and age is documented. Although several cytotoxic drugs including mycophenolate mofetil, hydroxycarbamide, purine analogs, L-asparaginase, radioisotopes, growth factors possess leukemogenic properties, direct

Table 10.2 Subcategories of therapy-related AML

	Type I	Type II
Exposure to cytotoxic drug type	Alkylating agent (cisplatin, carboplatin, nitrogen mustard, cyclophosphamide, mitomycin C, procarbazine, dacarbazine, chlorambucil, busulfan) Ionizing radiations	DNA topoisomerase II inhibitors (etoposide, doxorubicin, daunorubicin, mitoxantrone, actinomycin)
Drug exposure	5–10 years	1–5 years
Incidence	70% cases	20–30% cases
Cytopenia	One or more	–
Morphology	Macrocytic anemia, poikilocytosis Dysplastic changes in neutrophils Basophilia frequently seen	Monoblastic or myelomonocytic similar to *de novo* acute leukemia, myelodysplasia (rare)
Cytogenetic abnormalities and mutations	Unbalanced, loss or deletion of Chr5q and/or 7, complex karyotypes, mutation or loss of TP53	Balanced chromosomal translocation in Chr11q23 (*KMT2A*) and 21q22.1 (*RUNX1*)
Prognosis	Adverse	Favorable

evidence in t-MNs is still awaited. Two clinical subcategories of t-MNs exist without well-defined boundaries between these subsets (Table 10.2).

With an overall 5-year survival rates of <10%, the prognosis of t-MNs is generally poor and influenced by the preexisting comorbidity and associated cytogenetic abnormalities. Similar to AML-MRC, cases with balanced chromosomal translocations have a better prognosis relative to unbalanced abnormalities.

4. *AML, NOS*

AML, Not Otherwise Specified (NOS) is a WHO category representing 25–30% of all AML cases that include cases (i) lacking any cytogenetic or clinical features of specific disease categories (AML with recurrent genetic abnormalities, AML-MRC, t-AML, myeloid dysplasia associated with Down syndrome); (ii) show morphological characteristics of leukemia indicating the major lineages involved with the maturation status; and (iii) >20% myeloblasts in the peripheral blood and bone marrow [11]. The subgroups of AML, NOS as listed below are prognostically insignificant when AML with mutated *NPM1* and *CEBPA* are excluded. For inclusion of any case into

AML, NOS, cytogenetic studies and mutational analysis are recommended for prognostication.

   (i) AML with minimal differentiation (<5% of AML cases)

  (ii) AML without maturation (5–10% cases)

 (iii) AML with maturation (~10% cases)

 (iv) Acute myelomonocytic leukemia (5–10% cases)

  (v) Acute monoblastic/monocytic leukemia (<5% of AML cases)

 (vi) Pure erythroid leukemia (rare)

 (vii) Acute megakaryoblastic leukemia (<5% of AML cases)

(viii) Acute basophilic leukemia (rare)

 (ix) Acute panmyelosis with myelofibrosis (rare)

5. *Myeloid sarcoma*

Myeloid sarcoma (also known as chloroma or granulocytic sarcoma), an extramedullary growth of myeloid blasts with or without maturation, located at any site other than the bone marrow, is diagnostic of AML. These extramedullary tumors can occur in the skin, mucous membranes, CNS, bones, lymph nodes, gastrointestinal tract, and gonads. With few reports on its epidemiology, myeloid sarcoma may either present as a first sign of acute leukemia or constitute acute transformation of MDS, MDS/MPN, or MPN and occasionally occur in cases with history of prior treatment for myeloid disease [11]. The tissue architecture of tumor masses is effaced and similar to an interfollicular pattern in lymph nodes formed by sheets of myeloblasts with or without the characteristics of promyelocytic or neutrophilic maturation or myelomonocytes/monocytes.

Immunophenotypically, CD33, CD34, CD117, and CD68 markers are commonly expressed on tumors with immature myeloid profile. CD45, MPO, and TdT staining is inconsistent. Promyelocytic cases express MPO and CD15 but lack CD34 and TdT; myelomonocytic tumors express CD68 with subsets positive for MPO. Erythroid (strongly positive for glycophorin A and C) or megakaryoblastic (CD61, LAT, von Willebrand factor) myeloid sarcomas are rare. Positivity for cytoplasmic NPM1 is observed in ~16% cases, and aberrant B- or T-cell markers are observed in rare cases. Variable degree of CD56 expression is seen in ~20% of myeloid sarcoma cases. Cytogenetic abnormalities associated with myeloid sarcoma occur in ~55% of the cases. Common chromosomal aberrations include trisomy 4, 8, and 11, monosomy 7 and 16, KMT2A-MLLT3, inv(16), and loss of 16q, 5q, and 20q. Majority of the cases with skin involvement are associated with monocytic features and NPM1 mutations. FLT3-ITD mutations have also been reported. Low-dose radiation therapy may show promising results in cases of life-threatening myeloid sarcomas but not for routine management of the patients.

6. *Myeloid proliferations related to Down syndrome*

Infants and children with Down syndrome (trisomy 21) are at increased risk for acute leukemia. Generally, the incidence ratio of ALL:AML in children <4 years is 4:1 but with Down syndrome is 1.0:1.2. High occurrence of acute megakaryoblastic leukemia is reported in ~70% cases. The myeloid proliferations in these cases are distinct from other types of acute megakaryoblastic leukemia including GATA1 mutations and therefore grouped as a separate category [11].

10.5.1 Transient Abnormal Myelopoiesis (TAM)

Spontaneously resolving (within 3 months) myeloproliferative disorder termed as transient abnormal myelopoiesis (TAM) is documented in about 10% of neonates with Down syndrome. Presentation is early on within 1 week of birth in majority of the cases with trisomy 21. Leukocytosis and thrombocytopenia are common with occasional hepatosplenomegaly in newborns presenting with TAM. Dysplasia is seen in components of marrow with blasts usually showing characteristics of megakaryoblasts detected from basophilic cytoplasm with coarse basophilic granules. Common immunophenotypic markers include CD33, CD13, HLA-DR, CD117, CD34, and CD4(dim). Megakaryocytic differentiation markers CD41, CD42, CD61, CD71, and CD110 are expressed often with aberrant CD7 and CD56. Megakaryocyte transcription factor GATA1 and JAK3 acquired mutations are strongly associated with both TAM and myeloid leukemia of Down syndrome. About 20–30% of TAM cases eventually develop non-transient AML.

10.5.2 Myeloid Leukemia Associated with Down Syndrome

Greater than 50% of AML in children below the age of 5 years with Down syndrome are megakaryoblastic leukemia [11]. Blasts with features of megakaryoblasts in this AML type accumulate in the blood, bone marrow, spleen, and liver. Individuals with Down syndrome present with a prolonged MDS-like phase, and therefore, this category includes both MDS and AML cases. The bone marrow leukemic blasts show irregular nuclei and basophilic cytoplasm with MPO-negative granules. Dyserythropoiesis and dysgranulopoiesis may be noted in the blood and marrow. Immunophenotypic profile is similar to TAM with possibly less CD34 and HLA-DR expression. Karyotypic abnormalities in addition to trisomy 21 include complete or partial trisomies of chromosomes 1 and 8 and monosomy 7. Several gene mutations including *GATA1*, *CTCF*, *EZH2*, *JAK2*, *JAK3*, *MPL*, *SH2B3*, and *RAS* are implicated. Prognosis in these cases of AML is age-related.

10.6 Genomic Classification and Prognosis in AML

The prognostic significance in AML became evident from karyotyping in leukemic blasts by chromosome banding methods. Favorable cytogenetic abnormalities included t(8:21), inv(16), and t(15:17), whereas complex karyotype was associated with unfavorable or adverse prognosis, and individuals with diploid karyotype were included in intermediate-risk category [36]. A majority (~55%) of the newly diagnosed AML cases are challenging with cytogenetically normal karyotype (CN-AML). Somatic mutations emerged as an independent prognostic factor for assigning risk categories in CN-AML [50, 56] that led to the inclusion of AML with mutated *NPM1* and *CEBPA* as full entities and mutated *RUNX1* as provisional entity in the revised 2016 WHO classification [11].

The transition from conventional Sanger sequencing method to next-generation sequencing of AML genome has revealed the molecular intricacies and complexity of AML with normal karyotype [5, 8]. As our understanding of gene mutations

in AML has evolved, it is evident that in addition to aberrant myeloid differentiation (resulting from rearrangements and mutations in genes such as *RUNX1*, *CBFB*, and *RARA*), a second-hit is necessary for the survival of neoplastic clone (mutation in *FLT-3*, *KIT*, *NRAS*, or *KRAS* promote proliferation) [57]. Moreover, mutations in epigenetic regulators (*ASXL1*, *DNMT3A*, *IDH1*, *IDH2*, and *TET2*) are commonly detected in almost half of the AML cases and are being evaluated as potential therapeutic drug targets [58, 59]. Subsequently, few systematic studies based on massively parallel sequencing have deciphered the gene mutation map of driver events in AML and proposed a genomic classification of AML with correlation to clinical outcome [15].

Therefore, comprehensive genomic profiling in AML has become a critical approach for improved diagnosis, prognostic risk stratification, eligibility for targeted therapy, minimal residual disease (MRD) detection, and monitoring for improved patient management and care (Table 10.3). Nonetheless, search for additional prognostic markers, especially in pediatric AML, is ongoing.

10.7 Targeted Therapies in AML and Clinical Implications

For the past four decades, standard treatment of AML has been intensive induction therapy, which is occasionally followed by hematopoietic stem cell transplantation (HSCT). Since AML patients do benefit from HSCT, this suggests a role of the immune system in the eradication of leukemic cells [37, 60]. The information generated from next-generation sequencing has revealed genetic abnormalities and mutations in hematopoietic stem cells as the key drivers of AML progression [61]. These mutated genes give rise to AML-specific neo-antigens (ASNAs), and aberrant expression of self-antigens generate AML-associated antigens (AAAs), both are presented as peptides by major histocompatibility complex (MHC class I and class II) on the surface of tumor

Table 10.3 Functional categorization of genetic alterations in AML

Category	Function	Genetic alteration	Clinical significance
Class I	Transcription factor (TF) Fusions	t(8;21)	Favorable risk
		inv(16) or t(16;16)	Favorable risk
		t(15;17)	Favorable risk (in the absence of FLT3∗)
		t(9;11)	Intermediate to adverse risk
Class II	Nucleophosmin 1	Mutated NPM1	Favorable risk (in the absence of FLT3∗)
Class III	Tumor suppressor genes	TP53	Associated with adverse prognosis
		PHF6	Associated with adverse prognosis
Class IV	DNA methylation-related genes	DNMT3A	Adverse prognosis in CN-AML
		IDH1/IDH2	IDH1/2 anti-metabolite enzyme inhibitors in phase I (AG-120 and 221)
		TET1/TET2	Associated with adverse prognosis
Class V	Activated signaling genes	FLT3	Midostaurin, a multi-kinase inhibitor approved by FDA for oral use
		KIT	Adverse prognosis in CBF AML
		KRAS/NRAS	Diagnostic markers
Class VI	Myeloid TF genes	CEBPA	Favorable risk (in the absence of FLT3∗)
		RUNX1	Associated with adverse prognosis
Class VII	Chromatin-modifying genes	ASXL1 EZH2 KMT2A fusions KMT2A-PTD	Associated with adverse prognosis
Class VIII	Cohesin complex genes	RAD21 SMC1/ SMC2 STAG2	Under investigation
Class IX	Spliceosome complex genes	SRSF2 U2AF1 ZRSR2	Associated with adverse prognosis

Adapted from The Cancer Genome Atlas (TCGA) project [1, 11]
FLT3∗ FLT3 mutation; CBF core binding factor

cells and recognized and eliminated by cytotoxic CD8 T cells with help from CD4 T lymphocytes [62, 63].

A massive parallel sequencing study revealed the lowest neoantigen burden in AML and CLL [64, 65], indicating potentially poor immunogenicity and weak recognition by T cells to generate a robust antigen-specific cytotoxic immune response, a potential factor for refractory disease or AML relapse. As elimination of leukemic stem cells is critical for minimizing relapse in AML patients, harnessing the immune system by modulation of immune response and designing immunotherapies for eradication of AML neoplastic clones hold great potential but with major challenges [60, 66].

Several immune-evasion mechanisms of AML have been described [67, 68]. Loss of

tumor antigen expression, modulation of immune regulatory checkpoint molecules, and activation of antiapoptotic pathways are few intrinsic mechanisms that directly impact the extrinsic effects such as increased frequency of functional regulatory T cells, immunosuppressive microenvironment, and defective cytotoxic activity. Dysfunctional cytotoxic T cells in AML show an exhausted phenotype with increased expression of PD-1 and TIM-3 [69]. In AML patients, increased TIM-3 and PD-L1 expression on AML blasts facilitates their escape from immune clearance during treatment and relapse and induces resistance to treatment. Therefore, several clinical trials are evaluating the efficacy of checkpoint blockade with monoclonal antibodies combined with CTLA-4, PD-1, or PD-L1 in AML [70, 71].

In addition to immune checkpoint inhibitors, several new molecularly targeted therapies including bispecific T-cell engager antibodies, tyrosine kinase inhibitors, metabolic and pro-apoptotic agents, hypomethylating agents, and chimeric antigen receptor (CAR) T-cell therapy are currently being investigated within clinical trials in combination with standard chemotherapy [66, 72]. Bispecific antibodies are fusion molecules consisting of the binding specificities and functions of two antibodies, one targeting a tumor-associated surface antigen and second a surface antigen on the effector cells (T cells or NK cells) [70]. The tumor cells are brought in close proximity to the effectors in the presence of these bispecific antibodies facilitating the activation of cytotoxic effector function. Several AML targets for which bispecific antibodies have been developed include CD33, CD123, WT1, CD13, CD15, CD30, CD45, CD47, C-type lectin-like molecule 1 (CLL1), FLT-3, and angiogenic growth factors.

Another targeted therapy for AML includes small molecule synthetic tyrosine kinase inhibitors (TKIs) including (1) EGFR tyrosine kinase family, (2) split kinase domain receptor kinase subgroup, and (3) inhibitors of tyrosine kinases from multiple subgroups (e.g., Gleevec). After the success of Gleevec in CML and Ph + ALL, FDA has recently approved midostaurin (a multikinase FLT3 inhibitor) for oral use in the treatment of AML [73]. Another promising target, the hypomethylating agents, azacitidine and decitabine (cytidine nucleoside analogs), both approved by the FDA for the treatment of myelodysplastic syndromes (MDS), had shortcomings including treatment failure, nonresponders, and eventually relapse because of inability to eradicate the malignant clone [74, 75]. Therefore, current combination therapies with hypomethylating agents in patients with intermediate- and high-risk MDS include investigational treatments targeting epigenetic regulation, immunomodulation, deregulated hematopoiesis, the tumor microenvironment, apoptosis, immune evasion, or other markers of leukemogenesis [76].

After the success of chimeric antigen receptor (CAR) T-cell therapy in the treatment of some of the most refractory leukemia, the efficacy of this targeted immunotherapy is being harnessed for the treatment of AML. CARs are genetically engineered cell surface receptors that are a combination of extracellular antibody binding domain for MHC-independent antigen binding and intracellular effector cell signaling for optimal and highly potent cytotoxic effector cell function. Since its inception in 1989 [77], the most prominent target antigen for CAR T-cell therapy is CD19 in B-cell malignancies [78]. In AML patients, target specificity remains a major concern although CD33 expression is seen persistently in majority of cases. Preclinical investigation of dual-targeting strategies of CD33 and CD123 was superior to monospecific approaches in terms of specific cytotoxicity and could contribute to efficacy and safety in CAR T-cell therapy in AML [78–80]. The impact of CAR T-cell therapy lies in its potential for the induction of remission and long-term disease control.

At present, combinatorial approaches to prevent AML relapse are primarily confined to clinical trials and include the testing of risk-targeted sequential strategies of induction, consolidation, HSCT, and maintenance therapies (e.g., with hypomethylating agents and/or targeted inhibitors). Moreover, evaluation of ASNAs and AAAs as source of neoantigens, transcriptomic and proteomic analysis to fully characterize the AML surfaceome, and dual-targeting approaches to improve the specificity of treatment with minimal toxicities are underway [18].

10.8 AML Monitoring During and Post-treatment: Futuristic Approach

A systematic stepwise approach that integrates morphology, immunophenotyping, cytogenetic, and molecular genetics is needed for diagnosis and classification of AML cases (Fig. 10.2). Specifically, in cases with <20% bone marrow blasts, cytogenetic studies are essential for the identification of recurrent cytogenetic abnormalities to minimize misdiagnosis. An ideal report should be comprehensive with all diagnostic data

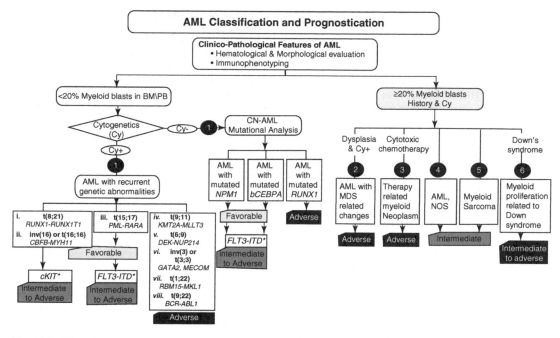

Fig. 10.2 Flow chart depicting an algorithmic approach for AML Classification and Prognostication

indicating the potential risk factors (Fig. 10.2). Moreover, the simultaneous detection of NGS-based somatic mutations associated with candidate target genes of the neoplastic clone may serve as potential genetic biomarkers and targets for therapeutic intervention in AML. In addition, these leukemia-associated genes may facilitate the prediction of response to treatment by real-time functional testing and personalized medicine in specific AML subtypes [81].

References

1. Hartmut Döhner MD, Daniel J, Weisdorf MD, Clara D, Bloomfield MD. Acute myeloid leukemia. N Engl J Med. 2015;373(12):1036–52.
2. Estey E, Döhner H. Acute myeloid leukaemia. Lancet. 2006;368(9550):1894–907.
3. Bennett JM, Catovsky D, Daniel M-T, Flandrin G, Galton DAG, Gralnick HR, et al. Proposals for the classification of the Acute Leukaemias French-American-British (FAB) Co-operative Group. Br J Haematol. 1976;33(4):451–8.
4. Bennett JM, Catovsky D, Daniel MT, Flandrin G, Galton DA, Gralnick HR, et al. Proposed revised criteria for the classification of acute myeloid leukemia. A report of the French-American-British cooperative group. Ann Intern Med. 1985;103(4):620–5.

5. Mardis ER, Ding L, Dooling DJ, Larson DE, McLellan MD, Chen K, et al. Recurring mutations found by sequencing an acute myeloid leukemia genome. N Engl J Med. 2009;361(11):1058–66.
6. Ding L, Ley TJ, Larson DE, Miller CA, Koboldt DC, Welch JS, et al. Clonal evolution in relapsed acute myeloid leukaemia revealed by whole-genome sequencing. Nature. 2012;481(7382):506–10.
7. Klco JM, Spencer DH, Miller CA, Griffith M, Lamprecht TL, O'Laughlin M, et al. Functional heterogeneity of genetically defined subclones in acute myeloid leukemia. Cancer Cell. 2014;25(3):379–92.
8. Ley TJ, Mardis ER, Ding L, Fulton B, McLellan MD, Chen K, et al. DNA sequencing of a cytogenetically normal acute myeloid leukaemia genome. Nature. 2008;456(7218):66–72.
9. Martelli MP, Sportoletti P, Tiacci E, Martelli MF, Falini B. Mutational landscape of AML with normal cytogenetics: biological and clinical implications. Blood Rev. 2013;27(1):13–22.
10. Welch JS, Ley TJ, Link DC, Miller CA, Larson DE, Koboldt DC, et al. The origin and evolution of mutations in acute myeloid leukemia. Cell. 2012;150(2):264–78.
11. Swerdlow SH, Campo E, Pileri SA, Harris NL, Stein H, Siebert R, et al. The 2016 revision of the World Health Organization classification of lymphoid neoplasms. Blood. 2016;127(20):2375–90.
12. Swerdlow SH, Campo E, Harris NL, Jaffe ES, Pileri SA, Stein H, Thiele J, Vardiman J. WHO classification of tumours of haematopoietic and lymphoid

tissues. In: WHO classification of tumours, vol. 2. 4th ed; 2008. p. 439.

13. Vardiman JW, Harris NL, Brunning RD. The World Health Organization (WHO) classification of the myeloid neoplasms. Blood. 2002;100:2292–302.

14. Harris NL, Jaffe ES, Diebold J, Flandrin G, Muller-Hermelink HK, Vardiman J, et al. World Health Organization classification of neoplastic diseases of the hematopoietic and lymphoid tissues: report of the Clinical Advisory Committee meeting—Airlie House, Virginia, November 1997. J Clin Oncol. 1999;17(12):3835–49.

15. Papaemmanuil E, Gerstung M, Bullinger L, Gaidzik VI, Paschka P, Roberts ND, Potter NE, Heuser M, Thol F, Bolli N, Gundem G, Van P, et al. Genomic classification and prognosis in acute myeloid leukemia. N Engl J Med. 2016;374:2209–21.

16. Komanduri KV, Levine RL. Diagnosis and therapy of acute myeloid leukemia in the era of molecular risk stratification. Annu Rev Med. 2016;67(1):59–72.

17. Roboz GJ. Current treatment of acute myeloid leukemia. Curr Opin Oncol. 2012;24:711–9.

18. Lichtenegger FS, Krupka C, Haubner S, Köhnke T, Subklewe M. Recent developments in immunotherapy of acute myeloid leukemia. J Hematol Oncol. 2017;10(1):142.

19. Nagler E, Xavier MF, Frey N. Updates in immunotherapy for acute myeloid leukemia. Transl Cancer Res. 2017;6(1):86–92. http://tcr.amegroups.com/article/view/12205/10186.

20. seer.cancer.gov; Accessed 10 Dec 2017.

21. Fircanis S, Merriam P, Khan N, Castillo JJ. The relation between cigarette smoking and risk of acute myeloid leukemia: an updated meta-analysis of epidemiological studies. Am J Hematol. 2014;89(8):E125.

22. Wang P, Liu H, Jiang T, Yang J. Cigarette smoking and the risk of adult myeloid disease: a meta-analysis. PLoS One. 2015;10(9).

23. Godley LA, Larson RA. Therapy-related myeloid leukemia. Semin Oncol. 2008;35(4):418–29.

24. Yin CC, Medeiros LJ, Bueso-Ramos CE. Recent advances in the diagnosis and classification of myeloid neoplasms—comments on the 2008 WHO classification. Int J Lab Hematol. 2010;32:461–76.

25. Mezei G, Sudan M, Izraeli S, Kheifets L. Epidemiology of childhood leukemia in the presence and absence of Down syndrome. Cancer Epidemiol. 2014;38:479–89.

26. Thalhammer-Scherrer R, Wieselthaler G, Knoebl P, Schwarzinger I, Simonitsch I, Mitterbauer G, et al. Post-transplant acute myeloid leukemia (PT-AML). Leukemia. 1999;13(3):321–6.

27. Morton LM, Gibson TM, Clarke CA, Lynch CF, Anderson LA, Pfeiffer R, et al. Risk of myeloid neoplasms after solid organ transplantation. Leukemia. 2014;28(12):2317–23.

28. Nazha A, Ravandi F. Acute myeloid leukemia in the elderly: do we know who should be treated and how? Leuk Lymphoma. 2014;55:979–87.

29. Kantarjian H, Ravandi F, O'Brien S, Cortes J, Faderl S, Garcia-Manero G, et al. Intensive chemotherapy does not benefit most older patients (age 70 years or older) with acute myeloid leukemia. Blood. 2010;116(22):4422–9.

30. Zeichner SB, Arellano ML. Secondary adult acute myeloid leukemia: a review of our evolving understanding of a complex disease process. Curr Treat Options Oncol. 2015;16:37.

31. Rozovski U, Ohanian M, Ravandi F, Garcia-Manero G, Faderl S, Pierce S, et al. Incidence of and risk factors for involvement of the central nervous system in acute myeloid leukemia. Leuk Lymphoma. 2015;56(5):1392–7.

32. Pui CH, Howard SC. Current management and challenges of malignant disease in the CNS in paediatric leukaemia. Lancet Oncol. 2008;9:257–68.

33. Tacke D, Buchheidt D, Karthaus M, Krause SW, Maschmeyer G, Neumann S, et al. Primary prophylaxis of invasive fungal infections in patients with haematologic malignancies. 2014 update of the recommendations of the infectious diseases working Party of the German Society for Haematology and Oncology. Ann Hematol. 2014;93:1449–56.

34. Falini B, Lenze D, Hasserjian R, Coupland S, Jaehne D, Soupir C, et al. Cytoplasmic mutated nucleophosmin (NPM) defines the molecular status of a significant fraction of myeloid sarcomas. Leukemia. 2007;21:1566–70.

35. Pileri SA, Ascani S, Cox MC, Campidelli C, Bacci F, Piccioli M, et al. Myeloid sarcoma: clinicopathologic, phenotypic and cytogenetic analysis of 92 adult patients. Leukemia. 2007;21(2):340–50.

36. Rowley JD. Chromosomal translocations: revisited yet again. Blood. 2008;112(6):2183–9.

37. Koreth J, Schlenk R, Kopecky KJ, Honda S, Sierra J, Djulbegovic BJ, et al. Allogeneic stem cell transplantation for acute myeloid leukemia in first complete remission: systematic review and meta-analysis of prospective clinical trials. JAMA. 2009;301(22):2349–61.

38. Cammenga J. Gatekeeper pathways and cellular background in the pathogenesis and therapy of AML. Leukemia. 2005;19:1719–28.

39. Koeffler HP, Leong G. Preleukemia: one name, many meanings. Leukemia. 2017;31:534–42.

40. Naegeli O. Ueber rothes Knochenmark und Myeloblasten. Dtsch Med Wochenschr. 1900;26(18):287–90.

41. Grimwade D, Walker H, Oliver F, Wheatley K, Harrison C, Harrison G, et al. The importance of diagnostic cytogenetics on outcome in AML: analysis of 1,612 patients entered into the MRC AML 10 trial. Blood. 1998;92(7):2322–33.

42. Scandura JM, Boccuni P, Cammenga J, Nimer SD. Transcription factor fusions in acute leukemia: variations on a theme. Oncogene. 2002;21(21 REV. ISS. 2):3422–44.

43. Huret JL, Ahmad M, Arsaban M, Bernheim A, Cigna J, Desangles F, et al. Atlas of genetics and cytogenetics in oncology and haematology peer reviewed internet encyclopedia/journal/database. Chromosome Res. 2009;17:S14–5. http://AtlasGeneticsOncology.org.

44. Downing JR. The AML1-ETO chimaeric transcription factor in acute myeloid leukaemia: biology and clinical significance. Br J Haematol. 1999;106:296–308.
45. Licht JD. AML1 and the AML1-ETO fusion protein in the pathogenesis of t(8;21) AML. Oncogene. 2001;20:5660–79.
46. Paschka P, Marcucci G, Ruppert AS, Mrózek K, Chen H, Kittles RA, et al. Adverse prognostic significance of KIT mutations in adult acute myeloid leukemia with inv(16) and t(8,21): a Cancer and Leukemia Group B Study. J Clin Oncol. 2006;24(24):3904–11.
47. Speck NA, Gilliland DG. Core-binding factors in haematopoiesis and leukaemia. Nat Rev Cancer. 2002;2(7):502–13.
48. de Thé H, Chomienne C, Lanotte M, Degos L, Dejean A. The t(15,17) translocation of acute promyelocytic leukaemia fuses the retinoic acid receptor α gene to a novel transcribed locus. Nature. 1990;347(6293):558–61.
49. Melnick A, Licht JD. Deconstructing a disease: RARα, its fusion partners and their roles in pathogenesis of acute promyelocytic leukemia. Blood. 1999;93(10):3167–215.
50. Schlenk RF, Döhner K, Krauter J, Fröhling S, Corbacioglu A, Bullinger L, et al. Mutations and treatment outcome in cytogenetically Normal acute myeloid leukemia. N Engl J Med. 2008;358(18):1909–18.
51. Falini B, Mecucci C, Tiacci E, Alcalay M, Rosati R, Pasqualucci L, et al. Cytoplasmic nucleophosmin in acute myelogenous leukemia with a normal karyotype. N Engl J Med. 2005;352(3):254–66.
52. Döhner K, Schlenk RF, Habdank M, Scholl C, Rücker FG, Corbacioglu A, et al. Mutant nucleophosmin (NPM1) predicts favorable prognosis in younger adults with acute myeloid leukemia and normal cytogenetics: interaction with other gene mutations. Blood. 2005;106(12):3740–6.
53. Rau R, Brown P. Nucleophosmin (NPM1) mutations in adult and childhood acute myeloid leukaemia: towards definition of a new leukaemia entity. Hematol Oncol. 2009;27:171–81.
54. Verhaak RGW, Goudswaard CS, Van Putten W, Bijl MA, Sanders MA, Hugens W, et al. Mutations in nucleophosmin (NPM1) in acute myeloid leukemia (AML): association with other gene abnormalities and previously established gene expression signatures and their favorable prognostic significance. Blood. 2005;106(12):3747–54.
55. Heath EM, Chan SM, Minden MD, Murphy T, Shlush LI, Schimmer AD. Biological and clinical consequences of NPM1 mutations in AML. Leukemia. 2017;31:798–807.
56. Ghanem H, Tank N, Tabbara IA. Prognostic implications of genetic aberrations in acute myelogenous leukemia with normal cytogenetics. Am J Hematol. 2012;87:69–77.
57. Jan M, Snyder TM, Corces-Zimmerman MR, Vyas P, Weissman IL, Quake SR, et al. Clonal evolution of preleukemic hematopoietic stem cells precedes

58. Figueroa ME, Lugthart S, Li Y, Erpelinck-Verschueren C, Deng X, Christos PJ, et al. DNA methylation signatures identify biologically distinct subtypes in acute myeloid leukemia. Cancer Cell. 2010;17(1): 13–27.
59. Abdel-Wahab O, Levine RL. Mutations in epigenetic modifiers in the pathogenesis and therapy of acute myeloid leukemia. Blood. 2013;121:3563–72.
60. Austin R, Smyth MJ, Lane SW. Harnessing the immune system in acute myeloid leukaemia. Crit Rev Oncol Hematol. 2016;103:62–77.
61. Bonnet D, Dick JE. Human acute myeloid leukemia is organized as a hierarchy that originates from a primitive hematopoietic cell. Nat Med. 1997;3(7):730–7.
62. Gillis S, Smith KA. Long term culture of tumour-specific cytotoxic T cells. Nature. 1977;268(5616):154–6.
63. Rooney MS, Shukla SA, Wu CJ, Getz G, Hacohen N. Molecular and genetic properties of tumors associated with local immune cytolytic activity. Cell. 2015;160(1–2):48–61.
64. Rajasagi M, Shukla SA, Fritsch EF, Keskin DB, DeLuca D, Carmona E, et al. Systematic identification of personal tumor-specific neoantigens in chronic lymphocytic leukemia. Blood. 2014;124(3): 453–62.
65. Chalmers ZR, Connelly CF, Fabrizio D, Gay L, Ali SM, Ennis R, et al. Analysis of 100,000 human cancer genomes reveals the landscape of tumor mutational burden. Genome Med. 2017;9(1):34.
66. Ferrara F. New agents for acute myeloid leukemia: is it time for targeted therapies? Expert Opin Investig Drugs. 2012;21(2):179–89.
67. Teague RM, Kline J. Immune evasion in acute myeloid leukemia: current concepts and future directions. J Immunother Cancer. 2013;1.
68. Elias S, Yamin R, Golomb L, Tsukerman P, Stanietsky-Kaynan N, Ben-Yehuda D, et al. Immune evasion by oncogenic proteins of acute myeloid leukemia. Blood. 2014;123(10):1535–43.
69. Zhou Q, Munger ME, Veenstra RG, Weigel BJ, Hirashima M, Munn DH, et al. Coexpression of Tim-3 and PD-1 identifies a CD8+ T-cell exhaustion phenotype in mice with disseminated acute myelogenous leukemia. Blood. 2011;117(17):4501–10.
70. Hoseini SS, Cheung NK. Acute myeloid leukemia targets for bispecific antibodies. Blood Cancer J. 2017;7:e552.
71. Krupka C, Kufer P, Kischel R, Zugmaier G, Lichtenegger FS, Köhnke T, et al. Blockade of the PD-1/PD-L1 axis augments lysis of AML cells by the CD33/CD3 BiTE antibody construct AMG 330: reversing a T-cell-induced immune escape mechanism. Leukemia. 2016;30(2):484–91.
72. Kavanagh S, Murphy T, Law A, Yehudai D, Ho JM, Chan S, et al. Emerging therapies for acute myeloid leukemia: translating biology into the clinic. JCI Insight. 2017;2(18):e95679.

human acute myeloid leukemia. Sci Transl Med. 2012;4(149):149ra118.

73. Levis M. Midostaurin approved for FLT3-mutated AML. Blood. 2017;129(26):3403–6.
74. Estey EH. Epigenetics in clinical practice: the examples of azacitidine and decitabine in myelodysplasia and acute myeloid leukemia. Leukemia. 2013;27:1803–12.
75. Cruijsen M, Lübbert M, Wijermans P, Huls G. Clinical results of Hypomethylating agents in AML treatment. J Clin Med. 2014;4(1):1–17.
76. Dombret H, Gardin C. An update of current treatments for adult acute myeloid leukemia. Blood. 2016;127(1):53–61.
77. Gross G, Waks T, Eshhar Z. Expression of immunoglobulin-T-cell receptor chimeric molecules as functional receptors with antibody-type specificity. Proc Natl Acad Sci. 1989;86(24):10024–8.
78. Jackson HJ, Rafiq S, Brentjens RJ. Driving CAR T-cells forward. Nat Rev Clin Oncol. 2016;13:370–83.
79. Pizzitola I, Anjos-Afonso F, Rouault-Pierre K, Lassailly F, Tettamanti S, Spinelli O, et al. Chimeric antigen receptors against CD33/CD123 antigens efficiently target primary acute myeloid leukemia cells in vivo. Leukemia. 2014;28(8):1596–605.
80. Ehninger A, Kramer M, Röllig C, Thiede C, Bornhäuser M, Von Bonin M, et al. Distribution and levels of cell surface expression of CD33 and CD123 in acute myeloid leukemia. Blood Cancer J. 2014;4(6):e218.
81. Lam SS-Y, He AB-L, Leung AY-H. Treatment of acute myeloid leukemia in the next decade—towards real-time functional testing and personalized medicine. Blood Rev. 2017;31:418. http://linkinghub.elsevier.com/retrieve/pii/S0268960X17300541.

Molecular Biology of B- and T-ALL

11

Jay Singh, Rajive Kumar, and Anita Chopra

11.1 Introduction

Acute lymphoblastic leukemia (ALL) is traditionally classified into precursor B-, precursor T-, and B-cell (Burkitt) and then subclassified on the basis of recurrent cytogenetic changes that include aneuploidy and translocations (75% of precursor B and 15% of T-ALL patients) [1].

ALL is biologically heterogeneous. Improving outcome of treatment for such a heterogeneous group is what has driven much of the research into the biology of the disease. Elucidation of biologically and prognostically important molecular cytogenetic groups enabled stratification of patients in clinical trials that used chemotherapeutic agents developed in the 1950s through the 1980s. The steady improvement in the 5-year survival that this approach led to enabled predictions to be made that the survival rate in children with ALL would climb to over 90% [2]. High-resolution genomic methods like microarray analysis of gene expression, DNA copy number assays, and next-generation sequencing now contributing majorly toward this goal are also revealing new diseases and new targets of therapy and

have thus brought ALL into the realm of targeted therapy and precision medicine [3].

Together, molecular cytogenetic and genomic methods of study have shown ALL to be a heterogeneous group of genetic diseases driven by sentinel genetic alterations (generally chromosome rearrangements and aneuploidy) and cooperating copy number and sequence mutations in genes that encode transcription factors regulating lymphoid development, tumor suppressors, protein regulators of the cell cycle and perturb cytokine receptor, kinase, and Ras signaling; and epigenetic/chromatin modifications. Several of these pathways, particularly kinase-activating lesions and epigenetic alterations, are candidates for novel precision medicine therapies [3, 4].

Based on the background, this chapter summarizes the key features of the major molecular subgroups of B-cell precursor ALL (BCP-ALL) and T-ALL. Table 11.1 represents WHO classification of acute lymphoblastic leukemia, 2016.

11.2 Precursor B-ALL (B-Cell Precursor ALL; BCP-ALL)

Approximately 75% of BCP-ALL patients can be risk-stratified in treatment protocols, based on NCI recommendations combined with chromosomal changes—BCR-ABL1, ETV6-RUNX1, E2A-PBX1, MLL rearrangements, hyperdiploid and hypodiploid karyotypes—into

J. Singh · A. Chopra (✉)
Laboratory Oncology Unit, Dr. BRAIRCH, AIIMS, New Delhi, Delhi, India
e-mail: dranitachopra@aiims.edu

R. Kumar
Mahavir Cancer Sansthan, Patna, Bihar, India

© Springer Nature Singapore Pte Ltd. 2019
R. Saxena, H. P. Pati (eds.), *Hematopathology*, https://doi.org/10.1007/978-981-13-7713-6_11

Table 11.1 WHO classification of acute lymphoblastic leukemia, 2016 [5]

B-cell lymphoblastic leukemia/lymphoma, not otherwise specified

B-cell lymphoblastic leukemia/lymphoma, with recurrent genetic abnormalities

    B-cell lymphoblastic leukemia/lymphoma with hypodiploidy

    B-cell lymphoblastic leukemia/lymphoma with hyperdiploidy

    B-cell lymphoblastic leukemia/lymphoma with t(9;22)(q34;q11.2)[*BCR-ABL1*]

    B-cell lymphoblastic leukemia/lymphoma with t(v;11q23)[*MLL* rearranged]

    B-cell lymphoblastic leukemia/lymphoma with t(12;21)(p13;q22)[*ETV6-RUNX1*]

    B-cell lymphoblastic leukemia/lymphoma with t(1;19)(q23;p13.3)[*TCF3-PBX1*]

    B-cell lymphoblastic leukemia/lymphoma with t(5;14)(q31;q32)[*IL3-IGH*]

    B-cell lymphoblastic leukemia/lymphoma with intrachromosomal amplification of chromosome 21 (iAMP21)[a]

    B-cell lymphoblastic leukemia/lymphoma with translocations involving tyrosine kinases or cytokine receptors ("BCR-ABL1–like ALL")[a]

T-cell lymphoblastic leukemia/lymphomas

    Early T-cell precursor lymphoblastic leukemia[a]

[a]Provisional entity

Table 11.2 Common sentinel cytogenetic abnormalities in acute lymphoblastic leukemia

Cytogenetic abnormalities	Frequency	Clinical significance
t(9;22); *BCR-ABL1*	1–3% in children; 25–30% in adults	Poor prognosis
t(v;11q23); *MLL* rearrangements	75% of infants; 1–2% in older children; 4–9% in adults	Poor prognosis
t(12;21); *TEL-AML1*	25% in children; 0–4% in adults	Good prognosis
t(1;19); *E2A-PBX1*	1–6% in children; 1–3% in adults	Intermediate to favorable prognosis
Hyperdiploidy (>50 chromosomes)	25–30% in children; 7–8% in adults	Favorable prognosis
Hypodiploidy (<44 chromosomes)	6% in children; 7–8% in adults	Poor prognosis

1. Ph-positive ALL
2. ERG-deleted ALL
3. B-ALL with intrachromosomal amplification of chromosome 21 (iAMP21)
4. Ph-like ALL

Brief accounts of the other entities can be checked from one of the reviews cited in the text [5].

11.2.1 Ph-Positive ALL

"low" (high hyperdiploidy with favorable chromosome trisomies or (ETV6-RUNX1)), "standard/intermediate," "high," or "very high" (hypodiploidy, BCR-ABL1, and induction failure) risk groups (Table 11.2) [6–10]. More recently, IKZF1 mutation/deletion, predictive of poor outcome, has been recommended for risk stratification in treatment protocols [11].

About 25% of genetically unclassified children and a greater proportion of adults having no known cytogenetic abnormality constitute the *B-other* group [6, 12–14], referred to in the WHO 2016 book as *B-cell lymphoblastic leukemia/lymphoma, not otherwise specified*. With recent work showing a large proportion of this to be comprised of BCR-ABL-like, CRLF2-rearranged (non-BCR-ABL-like), ERG-dysregulated, iAMP21, and others, the size of the true B-other group has got reduced [15].

The following entities are considered in some detail below:

The t(9,22)(q34;q11) translocation or "Philadelphia" chromosome is the most common and a highly unfavorable sentinel abnormality in ALL and is present in 20–30% adults and 2–3% children with BCP-ALL. The translocation results in a fusion gene BCR-ABL that encodes an oncogenic protein that has constitutively active tyrosine kinase activity, which by altering signaling pathways regulates cell survival and proliferation and self-renewal of stem cells [16]. The p190 BCR-ABL transcript is more commonly seen (50–80% patients) in BCP-ALL, though the p210 transcript, that is characteristic of chronic myeloid leukemia (CML), may also be present; both p190 and p210 L transcripts may coexist (Fig. 11.1).

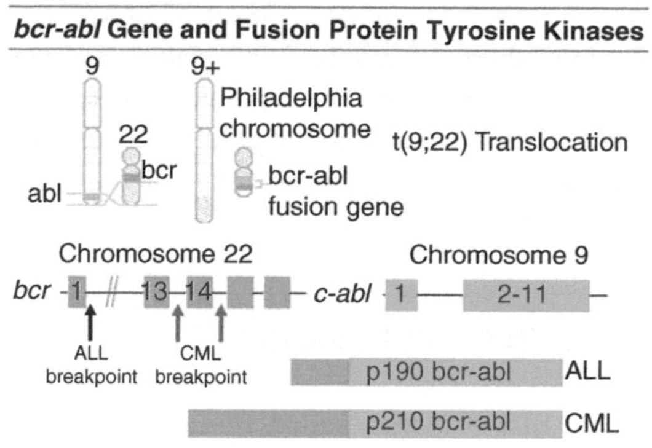

bcr-abl Gene and Fusion Protein Tyrosine Kinases

Fig. 11.1 P210 and 0190 transcripts in Ph+ ALL

Though Ph+ ALL has been frequently treated with intensive chemotherapy followed by hematopoietic stem cell transplantation, the prognosis of Ph+ BCP-ALL has been unsatisfactory with a 5-year event-free survival of approximately 50% in both children and adults. Tyrosine kinase inhibitors (TKIs), such as imatinib and dasatinib that target BCR-ABL1 fusion protein, have significantly improved treatment outcome; this is not true of all patients, which indicates the need to identify more biological features of the disease that could explain the heterogeneity.

To determine oncogenic lesions that work with BCR-ABL1 to induce ALL, Mulligan et al., 2008 [17] performed a genome-wide analysis of a large cohort of ALL patients, including BCR-ABL1 BCP-ALL. IKZF1 gene was found to be deleted in over 80% of BCR-ABL1 ALL patients. IKZF1 gene encodes IKAROS, a zinc-finger transcription factor associated with chromatin remodeling, which is expressed in fetal and adult hematopoietic system and functions as a regulator of lymphocyte proliferation and differentiation.

IKZF1 gene deletion could be of the whole gene or involve only the starting codon located in exon 2, resulting in haploinsufficiency. Additionally, there could be loss of the DNA-binding domain in exons 4–7 (what is called isoform 6) exerting a dominant negative effect over the unaffected allele, causing a loss of the tumor suppressor function of the wild-type IKZF1.

Studies have shown that in both Ph-negative BCP-ALL, in which it is fourfold less frequent,

and Ph+ ALL patients, presence of IKZF1 deletion of any kind affects the outcome adversely, partially offsetting the positive effect even of imatinib [18–20].

IKZF1 deletion thus marks patients who will do particularly poor and have a high chance of relapse even in the poor prognosis Ph+ ALL [20]. IKZF1-deleted patients thus are candidates for more intensive and/or alternative therapy.

Additional interest in *IKZF1* alteration stems from the demonstration in animal models that this molecular lesion has a stem cell-like phenotype, aberrant expression and signaling of adhesion molecules, adhesion of the leukemic cell to stem cell niche in the bone marrow, and poor treatment response. Churchman et al., 2015 [21] showed that FAK1, a cytoplasmic, non-receptor protein tyrosine kinase involved in integrin-mediated signaling arising from binding of integrin to extracellular matrix proteins, upregulated in Ph+ B-ALL, is further overexpressed in IKZF1-altered cells; it is also a potential therapeutic target. They demonstrated that a FAK inhibitor VS-4718 potently inhibits aberrant FAK signaling and leukemic cell adhesion, thereby potentiating responsiveness to tyrosine kinase inhibitors, inducing cure in vivo. Thus, targeting FAK with VS-4718 has emerged as a promising way of overcoming the deleterious effects of FAK overexpression in Ph+ B-ALL, especially in abrogating the Ikaros alteration-induced adhesive phenotype; this warrants evaluation in clinical trials of combined ABL and FAK inhibition in Ph+ B-ALL, regardless of *IKZF1* status.

11.2.2 ERG-Deleted ALL

In a comparative genomic hybridization analysis of a group of NCI high-risk ALL patients who had a distinct gene signature but lacked a sentinel chromosomal cytogenetic change [22], Mulligan et al. [23] showed ERG deletion as defining genetic lesion in them. The ERG gene is located on chromosome 21 and is a member of the erythroblast transformation-specific (ETS) (v-ets erythroblastosis virus E26 oncogene homolog) family of transcriptions factors involved in the regulation of embryonic development, cell proliferation, differentiation, angiogenesis, inflammation, and apoptosis. ERG has been shown to regulate hematopoiesis, and the differentiation and maturation of megakaryocytic cells are involved in chromosomal translocations TMPSSR2-ERG and NDRG1-ERG in prostate cancer, EWS-ERG in Ewing's sarcoma, and FUS-ERG in acute myeloid leukemia.

The frequency of ERG-deleted ALL has been reported to be approximately 3–7% of all BCP-ALL [24]. It is frequently associated with IKZF deletion, but whereas IKZF deletion is an adverse factor in Ph+ ALL and Ph-like ALL, it does not impact the favorable outcome of ERG-deleted ALL. ERG-deleted BCP-ALL has CD2 positivity and shows dysmorphic monocytes [24].

11.3 Newly Recognized B-ALL Subtypes (WHO)

In 2016 WHO classification of tumors of hematopoietic and lymphoid tissues, two new provisional B-ALL subtypes have been recognized: B-lymphoblastic leukemia/lymphoma with iAMP21 and B-lymphoblastic leukemia/lymphoma, BCR-ABL1-like. These two new entities identify B-ALL patients with inferior clinical outcome and who may benefit from more aggressive or targeted therapy [5].

11.3.1 B-ALL with Intrachromosomal Amplification of Chromosome 21 (iAMP21)

Intrachromosomal amplification of chromosome 21 (iAMP21) accounts for 2% of pediatric B-ALL. It is more common in older children and adolescents, but rare in adults. This leukemia is recognized by FISH with a RUNX1 probe that reveals extra signals (≥5 copies per interphase nucleus, or ≥3 copies on a single abnormal chromosome 21 in metaphase FISH) [25]. This makes chromosome 21 unstable and has been shown to be a primary genetic event [26]. Patients with this abnormality present with leukopenia and display common B-lymphoblast immunophenotype with a subset of blasts displaying aberrant myeloid-associated antigen expression. These patients have poor event-free and overall survival when treated with standard risk therapy that improves with more aggressive chemotherapy [27].

11.3.2 BCR-ABL1-Like ALL

BCR-ABL1-like also called Ph-like ALL is a newly described subtype of BCP-ALL defined by a GEP similar to that of Ph+ ALL, produced in the absence of BCR-ABL1 translocation, by kinase-activating alterations, amenable to treatment with currently available TKIs. It is characterized by alterations of B-lymphoid transcription factors, a high frequency of IKZF1 alterations and a high risk of relapse when treated with conventional chemotherapy [13, 28–30].

The disease constitutes 10–20% of BCP-ALL in children [13] and over 25% of young adults [31]. Ph-like subgroup is thus more common than Ph+ ALL and has emerged the most common childhood ALL with poor prognosis [13]. Ph-like ALL was discovered independently by two groups. Mullighan et al. (2009) discovered that BCP patients whose poor prognosis could be predicted by copy number alterations of IKZF1, but not other genes encoding transcriptional regulators of B-lymphocyte development and differentiation, had GEP similar to that of BCR-ABL+ ALL [17, 19, 23].

Some B-other patients share a GEP with Ph + B-ALL which was shown independently by den Boer et al. (2009) [13], who studied the subjects from an alternative perspective of using a classifier based on GEP and then characterizing the genetic abnormalities thus revealed by comparative genomic hybridization and molecular cytogenetics. GEP analysis of high-risk ALL employing ROSE outlier-identifying program has also shown Ph-like ALL as unique group. Using a candidate gene approach, identified in 10.7% BCR-ABL1-negative ALL, mutations in JAK1, JAK2, and JAK3, especially JAK2, as oncogenic drivers producing BCR-ABL gene signature in the absence of BCR-ABL translocation. JAK mutation nearly always coexisted with CRLF2 gene lesions. Conversely, only about half the CRLF2-mutated patients had JAK mutation. CRLF2 abnormality has been reported also in half the BCR-ABL-ALL patients. Using transcriptome and whole genome approaches [32], the same group of investigators showed, employing functional assays, that in patients without JAK mutations, the disease was driven in all but 9% of 154 BCR-ABL patients, by activated kinases, resulting from 30 chromosomal rearrangements or sequence mutations that dysregulated 13 cytokine receptor and kinase signaling [29]. Gene expression data from transcriptome sequencing showed that patients with ABL-class, EPOR, or JAK2 rearrangements clustered separately from those with other JAK-STAT or Ras pathway alterations. Based on this, BCR-ABL-like ALL patients could be put into several key subgroups with therapeutic implications: (1) ABL class rearrangements (~13%) targeting ABL1, ABL2, CSF1R, and PDGFRB which are sensitive to ABL1 inhibitors; (2) EPOR

(involving IGH, IGL) and JAK2 (several 5′ fusion partner genes) rearrangements (~11%), sensitive to JAK inhibitors; (3) CRLF2 rearrangements (~50%), frequently with concomitant activating JAK point mutations, that may also be sensitive to JAK inhibition; (4) other JAK-STAT activating mutations (11%) and deletions, including those involving IL7R, FLT3, etc. (e.g., JAK inhibitors for patients with IL7-R mutation); and (5) infrequent targets of rearrangement (less common kinase alterations) including NTRK3 (ETV6-NTRK3; sensitive to crizotinib). In addition, approximately 4% patients had RAS pathway mutations, but no other kinase lesions and several were associated with hypodiploidy. Genomic studies also revealed non-kinase lesions, including rearrangement of transcriptional regulators and chromatin modifiers, consistent with the notion that deregulation of multiple pathways, including kinase signaling, lymphoid maturation, and epigenetic modification contribute to leukemogenesis (Fig. 11.2) [31].

Fig. 11.2 Flowchart for the diagnosis of BCR-ABl1-like ALL

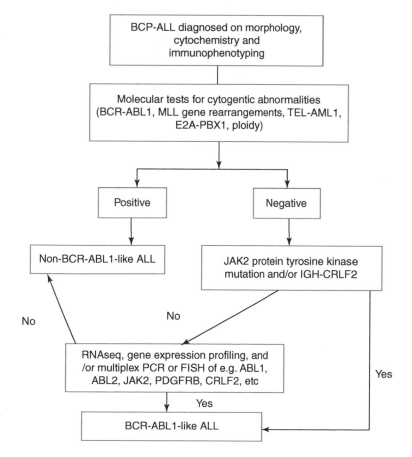

11.4 T-Acute Lymphoblastic Leukemia

11.4.1 Introduction

T-cell transformation, that has been shown to arise from transformation of T-cell progenitors blocked early or late in differentiation, is a multi-step process in which different genetic alterations in key cellular pathways cooperate to produce the T-ALL phenotype. It has been estimated that every T-ALL patient probably has over 10 genetic lesions that cooperate to alter normal mechanisms that control cell growth, proliferation, survival, differentiation, metabolism, epigenetic control, and homing properties in normal developing T-cells [33, 34].

Current understanding of the molecular basis of T-ALL has come largely from analysis of recurrent chromosomal translocations and intrachromosomal rearrangements that are present in about half the T-ALL cases. In addition, translocations have been uncovered in genomic studies. These abnormalities typically juxtapose strong promoter and enhancer elements located in the *TCRB* (7q34) or *TCRA-TCRD* (14q11) loci, responsible for high levels of expression of T-cell receptor genes, next to a small number of developmentally important transcription factor genes, including basic helix-loop-helix (bHLH) family members such as *TAL1*, *TAL2*, *LYL1*, and *BHLHB1*; LIM-only domain (LMO) genes such as *LMO1* and *LMO2*; the *TLX1/HOX11*, *TLX3/HOX11L2*, *NKX2.1*, *NKX2.2*, *NKX2.5*, and *HOXA* homeobox (HOX) genes; *MYC*; *MYB*; and *TAN1*, a truncated and constitutively activated form of the NOTCH1 receptor [33, 35]. It has been shown that aberrant activation of these key transcription factor genes often in the absence of chromosomal rearrangements is the principal transforming event in the disease. Apart from promoter swap due to translocations in the TCR loci as mentioned above, oncogene activation occurs also due to gene fusion encoding chimeric proteins (Graux et al. 2006) [36].

Gene expression profiling studies have revealed a limited number of well-defined molecular groups of T-ALL [35–39], which share unique gene expression signatures that indicate distinct stages of arrest during T-cell development. Early immature T-ALLs, an amalgam of pro- and pre-T-ALL immunological groups proposed by EGIL [40], show an early block at the double-negative stage of thymocyte development [35, 38, 41]. In contrast, early cortical T-ALLs are characteristically CD1a, CD4, and CD8 positive and are typically associated with the activation of the *TLX1*, *TLX3*, *NKX2.1*, and *NKX2.2* homeobox genes [35, 41]. Finally, late-cortical thymocyte T-ALLs express CD4, CD8, and CD3 and show activation of the *TAL1* transcription factor oncogene [33, 35]. Immature T-ALL often is CD34+ and CD7+ while lacking CD3, CD4, and CD8; the reverse is not always true as cortical and mature T-ALL patients may be CD34+ [42].

Type A and Type B Genetic Alterations: The driving lesions in the leukemogenic process, the so-called type A genetic alterations, are mutually exclusive genomic rearrangements, mainly translocations. They define specific T-ALL subgroups: (1) TAL/LMO; (2) TLX1, TLX3, and HOXA (MLL, CALM-AF4, and SET-NUP214), NKX2.1/NKX2.2; (3) MEF2C; and (4) MYB.

The much more numerous type B abnormalities such as chromosome translocations, mutations, and genomic imbalances cooperate with the driving type A lesions and are present in diverse genetic subgroups. These include CDKN2A/2B, Notch1, FBXW7, PHF6, PTEN, FBXW7, RUNX1, EZH2, SUZ12, NRAS, JAK1, IL7R, ETV6, BCL11b, LEF1, and WT1.

Table 11.3 lists cytogenetic and molecular changes in T-ALL.

The above can be considered from another perspective, that of the systems and processes affected by the molecular cytogenetic changes.

1. Transcription factor oncogenes
2. Notch1 pathway
3. Cell cycle
4. Transcription factor tumor suppressors
5. Signal transduction
6. Chromatin remodeling
7. Ribosomal proteins and translation

Table 11.3 Cytogenetic and molecular changes in T-ALL (based on [29, 33, 41])

	Involved gene(s) oncogene	Protein(s)	Function of fusion gene or expressed oncogene	Consequence of rearrangement/mutation
t(**7**;10)(q34;q24) and t(10;**14**)(q24;q11) *(T-cell receptor α, β, and δ are involved)*	*TLX1 (HOX11)*	Class II homeodomain-containing	Transcription factor	Ectopic TLX1 expression driven by TCR enhancer
t(5;**14**)(q35;q11) *(T-cell receptor δ at 14q11)* t(5;**14**)(q35;q32) (cryptic)[a] *(BCL11B at 14q32)*	*TLX3 (HOX11L2)*	Class II homeodomain-containing	Transcription factor	Ectopic TLX3 expression driven by TCR enhancer Ectopic TLX3 expression driven by BCL11B
inv(**7**)(p15q34), t(**7**;**7**)	*HOXA cluster*	Class II homeodomain-containing	Transcription factor	
t(1;**14**)(p32;q11) and t(1;**7**)(p32;q34)	TAL1	bHLH type II (basic helix-loop-helix)	Transcription factor	Ectopic TAL1 expression driven by TCR enhancer
t(**7**;19)(q34;p13)	*LYL1*	bHLH type II	Transcription factor	
t(11;**14**)(p13;q11) and t(**7**;11)(q35;p13)	LMO2	LIM-only domain	Protein–protein interaction	
t(1;**7**)(p34;q34)	LCK	SRC family of tyrosine kinase		
(**7**;9)(q34;q34.3)	*Notch1*	Notch receptor family	Cell fate determination, differentiation	
t(**7**;12)(q34;p13) and t(12;**14**)(p13;q11)	*CCND2*	D-type cyclin	Cell cycle activator	
1p32 deletion (cryptic)	*SIL/TAL1*	bHLH type II		Ectopic TAL1 expression driven by STIL promoter
t(10;11)(p13;q14) (often cryptic) CALM/AF10[b] (HOXA group)	*CALM/*	ENTH motif containing		
	AF10	Zinc fingers/leucine zipper containing		
t(11;19)(q23;p13)MLL/ENL[b] (HOXA group)	*MLL/*	Mammalian homolog of *Drosophila trithorax*		
	ENL	Nuclear targeting sequence containing		
t(6;11)(q27;q23)	*MLL/AF6*	GLGF motif containing		
t(10;11)(p13;q23)	*MLL/AF10*	See earlier		
t(X;11)(q13;q23)	*MLL/AFX1*	Forkhead family		
t(4;11)(q21;q23)	*MLL/AF4*	Nuclear targeting sequence containing		
t(9;9)(q34;q34) (episomal)[c] Amplification	*(NUP214-ABL1) NUP214/*	Nuclear pore complex component		
	ABL1	Intracellular tyrosine kinase	ABL1—signal transduction	
t(9;14)(q34;q32) (cryptic)	*EML1/ABL1*	Echinoderm microtubule-associated/…		

(continued)

Table 11.3 (continued)

	Involved gene(s) oncogene	Protein(s)	Function of fusion gene or expressed oncogene	Consequence of rearrangement/ mutation
t(9;12)(q34;p13)	*ETV6(TEL)/ ABL1*	ETS DNA binding containing		
(9;12)(p24;p13)	*ETV6(TEL)/ JAK2*	…/Intracellular tyrosine kinase	JAK2—Signal transduction	
inv14(q13;q32.33) t(7;14)(q34;q13)	*NKX2.1*			
t14;20 (q11;p11)	*NKX2.2*			
t(4;11)(q21;p15)	*NUP98/*	Nuclear pore complex component		
	RAP1GDS1	Cytoplasmic		
del9p21 (homozygous/ hemizygous)	*CDKN2A/p15* and *CDKN2B/ p16* loci *P16*	INK4/ARF		
del(9)(q34.11q34.13)[d]	*SET-NUP214*	SET	Chromatin remodeling and transcriptional activation	
NOTCH1	*NOTCH1*	Notch receptor family	Cell fate determination, differentiation	
FLT3 ITD	*FLT3*	Receptor tyrosine kinase	Development of hematopoietic stem cells	
N-RAS	*N-RAS*	Signaling protein	Signal transduction	

Notes: (1) Normal thymic expression: TLX1 and TLX3 are not expressed; TAL1, LYL1, and LMO2 are expressed in early stages. (2) Homeobox family members: TLX1, TLX3, HOXA, HOXA (CALM-AF10), HOXA (MLL-ENL), HOXA (SET-NUP214, NKX2.1, and NKX2.2. (3) Duplications (*MYB*) and amplifications also occur

[a]TLX3 is juxtaposed to the distal region of BCL11B, a gene universally expressed during T-cell differentiation. Other variants have been described

[b]HOXA group because of elevated expression of HOXA genes

[c]Fusion of NUP214 to ABL1 on amplified episomes, hence described as episomal *NUP214-ABL1* amplification, is an example of a genetic change that is acquired during leukemic growth

[d]SET-NUP214 is very similar to the DEK-NUP214 fusion as previously identified in t(6;9)(p23;q34)[+] patients with AML [43]

11.4.2 Biological Subgroups of T-ALL

There are three clinically relevant biological groups of T-ALL defined by distinct gene expression and having immunophenotypes that reflect thymocyte arrest at different stages of development. These include early immature T-ALL including ETP-ALL and early cortical/thymic and mature T-ALL [44].

Early immature T-ALL, including early thymic precursor T-ALL (ETP-ALL) is discussed below.

11.4.3 Early Immature T-ALL, Including Early Thymic Precursor T-ALL (ETP-ALL)

Immunological underpinnings: Assessment of T-ALL by immunophenotypic analysis has allowed prognostically relevant classification of the disease into developmental groups, based on maturity. The EGIL classification system (1995) distinguishes pro-T (CD7[+], CD2[−], CD5[−]), pre-T (CD7[+], CD2[+] and/or CD5[+] and/or CD8[+], CD1a being negative), cortical-T (CD1a[+]), and mature

T-cell stages (mCD3$^+$). More recent studies have not made a distinction between pro-T (CD1a$^-$, CD5$^-$) and pre-T (CD1a$^-$, CD5$^+$) ALL (EGIL), and instead, combine pro- and pre-T-ALLs, to make an early or immature T-cell ALL group (CD1a$^-$, CD5$^{-/+}$), while retaining the remaining two groups, thymic (cortical) and mature T-ALL. In contrast to the CD1a$^+$ thymic (cortical) T-ALL that has been shown in most studies to carry a relatively better prognosis, immature T-ALL cases (pro-/pre-T-cell immunophenotype; CD5$^{+/-}$, CD1a$^-$, CD8) have a lower remission induction, early relapse, and shortened overall survival [40, 41].

Immature T-ALL as a transcriptionally defined entity: Ferrando et al., 2002 [35], in the first gene expression profiling study in T-ALL showed the existence of a transcriptionally defined immature group of T-ALLs whose gene expression indicated arrest at an early stage of T-cell differentiation. This group had high expression of LYL1 and coexpression of LMO2 genes and was positive for early hematopoietic marker CD34 and myeloid antigens CD13 and CD33 and generally CD4 and CD8 negative. This immature T-ALL group was shown to be lacking deletion of short arm of chromosome 9 that deletes CDKN2A/B gene in over 70% T-ALL. These findings have been confirmed in other studies [37, 39].

Transcriptional likeness to early thymic precursors and best immunologically delineated poor prognosis group: Using gene expression profile of normal early thymic precursors to identify their leukemic counterparts and define their immunophenotype, Dario Campana's group in their study in children identified a novel poor prognosis group of T-ALL that was termed ETP-ALL, defined by a characteristic gene expression profile, increased genomic instability, and a distinct cell immunophenotype that made easy recognition possible: CD8$^-$ CD1a$^-$ defined by positivity in <5% blasts; negative or weak CD5 defined by positivity in <75% blasts; and positivity (>25% blasts) for one or more stem cell and myeloid markers CD34, CD117, HLA-DR, CD13, CD33, CD11b, CD65. ETP-ALL immunophenotype is the most validated prognostic

marker for identification of high-risk early immature T-ALL [45].

Biallelic deletion of TCRγ locus as a marker of immaturity: Using array comparative genomic hybridization and GEP, Guiterrez et al. [46] showed that absence of biallelic deletion (ABD) of TCRγ chain, a marker of developmental arrest at the earliest stages of thymocyte development, detected by QPCR, was a very good predictor of induction failure. ABD possibly represents early maturation arrest before the onset of T-cell receptor rearrangements [45, 46]. Given that *TCRγ* rearrangements occur early in normal T-cell development, it is not surprising that *TCR* loci deletions were found to be significantly less frequent in ETP T-ALL [38], and the majority of ABD patients possessed the ETP T-ALL gene expression signature. In marked contrast to this, however, only a minority of the ABD T-ALL patients [46] met the ETP T-ALL immunophenotype criteria, with most expressing CD5 on >75% of blasts. Because CD5 is expressed at low levels but is generally not absent on ETP-ALL blasts [38, 46] accurately distinguishing between the low (but not absent) CD5 expression characteristic of ETP-ALL lymphoblasts and the higher CD5 expression present in most T-ALL patient samples may be a problem. These discrepant results may thus very well reflect, at least in part, the challenge to accurately assess the ETP T-ALL immunophenotype across different laboratories. In fact many investigators studying immature T-ALL define it less narrowly than ETP-ALL and include CD5+ patients as well, thus defining an early immature group that is different from ETP-ALL, in that it includes CD5+ patients as well [39, 41].

Overlapping myeloid and T-ALL characteristics in early immature T-ALL—studies in adult-ALL: Investigating the possibility that early immature adult T-ALL (CD5$^{+/-}$) may be transcriptionally and genetically related to acute myeloid leukemias, based on the observation of marked enrichment in hematopoietic stem cell and granulocyte monocyte/macrophage precursor gene sets, Van Vlierberghe et al., 2011 [39], performed mutation analysis *of* AML oncogenes and tumor suppressor genes and found mutations in IDH1, IDH2, DNMT3A, FLT3, and NRAS *in 14/29 (48%)* of immature adult T-ALL cases. Prevalence of prototypical T-ALL genetic alterations such as activating mutations in the *IL7R* gene and in *NOTCH1* and *FBXW7* that activate the NOTCH-signaling pathway was low. These results suggested that early immature adult T-ALLs are a heterogeneous group with features of both myeloid and T-lymphoid genetic alterations. This analysis also revealed the presence of *ETV6* mutations, truncated forms of ETV6 with dominant negative activity, in approximately 25% early immature T-ALLs, but not in other groups, highlighting the potential role of ETV6 mutations in these tumors. A later reanalysis of the gene expression signatures associated with immunophenotypically defined pediatric ETP-ALLs also showed that the gene expression programs of these leukemias are most closely related to those of human hematopoietic stem cells and myeloid progenitors (Zhang et al. 2012).

MEF2C as a driving lesion in early immature T-ALL: The first indication of a specific genetic lesion possibly associated with the pathogenesis of early immature leukemias was the identification via 4C analysis of rare but recurrent rearrangements resulting in aberrantly high levels of expression of the *MEF2C* gene in this group. MEF2C encodes an important transcriptional regulator of lymphoid development which is expressed at high levels in very early pre-DN1 and DN1 thymocytes and whose expression dramatically drops beyond the DN2 stage of thymocyte development. Notably, and supporting a potential role as a master regulator of the early immature T-ALL transcriptional signature, MEF2C can directly induce the expression of *LYL1, LMO2, HHEX*, three oncogenic transcription factors expressed at high levels in early immature leukemias.

Early immature T-ALLs include ETP T-ALLs and related what are described as "close to ETP" leukemias: Cross examination of gene sets associated with the ETP T-ALL [38], the *LYL1* leukemias [35], and the immature T-ALL clusters [38, 39] has shown these to be closely related groups. Also, early immature T-ALLs identified

by gene expression signature encompass a broader patient group than the ETP T-ALLs defined on the basis of immunophenotype. The original report of Dario Campana's group [38], for example, showed that a few T-ALL cases that clustered together with ETP T-ALLs in an unsupervised gene expression analysis were CD5+ showing ETP-ALL to be a group larger than what would appear from its immunophenotypic definition. Conversely, in the study of Vlierberghe et al. (2011), the transcriptionally and immunophenotypically (positive for stem cell and myeloid-associated antigens) immature cluster was a mixture of CD5− as well as CD5+ cases, showing that only a fraction of these leukemias seem to strictly meet the immunophenotype criteria of ETP-ALL.

Genetics of ETP and early immature T-ALLs: Zhang et al. addressed the question of the absence of unifying genetic alteration by analyzing 12 ETP T-ALL cases using whole-genome sequencing and showed the presence of a high frequency of activating mutations in molecules mediating (1) cytokine receptor and RAS signaling—NRAS, KRAS, FLT3, IL7R, JAK3, JAK1, SH2B3, and BRAF; (2) inactivating mutations in genes encoding key transcription factors involved in hematopoietic development including GATA3, ETV6, RUNX1, IKZF1, and EP300; and (3) genes encoding histone modifiers such as EZH2, EED, SUZ12, SETD2, and EP300. Several ETP T-ALL cases showed multiple genomic rearrangements suggestive of genomic instability and deletions in the short arm of chromosome 9 encompassing the CDKN2A/B/B tumor suppressor genes were less prevalent in ETP T-ALLs compared with non-ETP leukemias.

11.5 Conclusion

Early immature T-ALLs encompass ETP-ALL and the related "close to" or "near" ETP-ALL and are defined by a gene expression signature that is most related to that of hematopoietic stem cells and myeloid progenitors. ETP T-ALL immunophenotype and the absence of biallelic deletion of the *TCRG* locus are associated with very poor prognosis in children. Though they harbor a distinct transcriptional signature, early immature T-ALLs seem to lack a distinct unifying genetic alteration and have a lower prevalence of NOTCH1 activating mutations, mutations in myeloid oncogenes and tumor suppressor genes, and genetic alterations disrupting key transcription factors involved in hematopoietic and lymphoid development.

Early immature T-ALLs encompassing ETP T-ALLs and related "close to" ETP tumors constitute a genetically heterogeneous group of leukemias characterized by a gene expression signature most related to that of hematopoietic stem cells and myeloid progenitors. Even though they harbor distinct transcriptional signature, early immature T-ALLs seem to lack a distinct unifying genetic alteration; they have a lower prevalence of NOTCH1 activating mutations, but have mutations in myeloid oncogenes and tumor suppressor genes, and genetic lesions that disrupt key transcription factors involved in hematopoietic and lymphoid development. Two recent studies have reported a possible worse prognosis for immature adult T-ALL leukemias harboring mutations in *RUNX1* and DNMT3A [14, 15]. Further evaluation of this heterogeneous leukemia group is needed to address the prognostic implications of specific immunophenotypes, transcriptional signatures, and genetic alterations. Therapeutically, drugs active in myeloid tumors, validated in relevant animal models may help in ETP T-ALLs. In addition, targeted therapies may help in those leukemias that have activating mutations in druggable factors and signaling pathways like FLT3, JAK1, JAK3, IL7R, and NOTCH1.

Early cortical/thymic T-ALL: This good prognosis CD1a+, CD4+, CD8+ favorable prognosis group corresponds to early stage of thymocyte maturation. These tumors are characterized by activation of TLX1, TLX3, NKX2.1, NKX2.2 homeobox genes and have the highest frequency of Notch 1 mutations, and CDNK2A is deleted in almost all cases.

Mature T-ALL: This third group has the mature T-ALL immuophenotype (sCD3+, CD4+, CD8+) and typically has activation of TAL1 gene.

References

1. Pui CH, Mullighan CG, Evans WE, Relling MV. Pediatric acute lymphoblastic leukemia: where are we going and how do we get there? Blood. 2012;120(6):1165–74.
2. Pui CH, Evans WE. Treatment of acute lymphoblastic leukemia. N Engl J Med. 2006;354(2):166–78.
3. Hunger SP, Mullighan CG. Redefining ALL classification: toward detecting high-risk ALL and implementing precision medicine. Blood. 2015;125: 3977–87.
4. Tasian SK, Loh ML, Hunger SP. Philadelphia chromosome-like acute lymphoblastic leukemia. Blood. 2017;130(19):2064–72.
5. Terwilliger T, Abdul-Hay M. Acute lymphoblastic leukemia: a comprehensive review and 2017 update. Blood Cancer J. 2017;7(6):e577.
6. Pui CH, et al. Acute lymphoblastic leukemia. N Engl J Med. 2004;350:1535–48.
7. Shuster JJ, et al. Identification of newly diagnosed children with acute lymphocytic leukemia at high risk for relapse. Cancer Res Ther Control. 1999;9:101–7.
8. Smith M, Arthur D, Camitta B, et al. Uniform approach to risk classification and treatment assignment for children with acute lymphoblastic leukemia. J Clin Oncol. 1996;14:18–24.
9. Schultz KR, Pullen DJ, Sather HN, et al. Risk-and response-based classification of childhood B precursor acute lymphoblastic leukemia: a combined analysis of prognostic markers from the Pediatric Oncology Group (POG) and Children's Cancer Group (CCG). Blood. 2007;109:926–35.
10. Hunger SP, Mullighan CG. Acute lymphoblastic leukemia in children. N Engl J Med. 2015;373: 1541–52.
11. Caye A, et al. Breakpoint-specific multiplex polymerase chain reaction allows the detection of IKZF1 intragenic deletions and minimal residual disease monitoring in B-cell precursor acute lymphoblastic leukemia. Haematologica. 2013;98:597–601.
12. Pui CH, et al. Immunologic, cytogenetic and clinical characterization of childhood acute lymphoblastic leukemia with the t(1;19)(q23;p13) or its derivative. J Clin Oncol. 1994;12:2601–6.
13. Den Boer ML, van Slegtenhorst M, De Menezes RX, et al. A subtype of childhood acute lymphoblastic leukaemia with poor treatmentoutcome: a genome-wide classification study. Lancet Oncol. 2009;10:125–34.
14. Moricke A, Reiter A, Zimmermann M, et al. Risk-adjusted therapy of acute lymphoblastic leukemia can decrease treatment burden and improve survival: treatment results of 2169 unselected pediatric and adolescent patients enrolled in the trial ALL-BFM 95. Blood. 2008;111:4477–89.
15. Bhojwani D, et al. Biology of childhood acute lymphoblastic leukemia. Pediatr Clin N Am. 2015;62(1):47–60.

16. Forghieri F, Luppi M, Potenza L. Philadelphia chromosome-positive acute lymphoblastic leukemia. Hematology. 2015;20(10):618–9.
17. Mullighan CG, et al. BCR-ABL1 lymphoblastic leukaemia is characterized by the deletion of Ikaros. Nature. 2008;453:110–4.
18. Mullighan CG, Downing JR. Genome-wide profiling of genetic alterations in acute lymphoblastic leukemia: recent insights and future directions. Leukemia. 2009 Jul;23(7):1209–18.
19. Kuiper RP, et al. High-resolution genomic profiling of childhood ALL reveals novel recurrent genetic lesions affecting pathways involved in lymphocyte differentiation and cell cycle progression. Leukemia. 2007;21:1258–66.
20. van der Veer A, Zaliova M, Mottadelli F, De Lorenzo P, Te Kronnie G, Harrison CJ, Cavé H, Trka J, Saha V, Schrappe M, Pieters R, Biondi A, Valsecchi MG, Stanulla M, den Boer ML, Cazzaniga G. IKZF1 status as a prognostic feature in BCR-ABL1-positive childhood ALL. Blood. 2014;123(11):1691–8.
21. Churchman ML, Evans K, Richmond J, Robbins A, Jones L, Shapiro IM, Pachter JA, Weaver DT, Houghton PJ, Smith MA, Lock RB, Mullighan CG. Synergism of FAK and tyrosine kinase inhibition in Ph+ B-ALL. JCI Insight. 2016;1(4):e86082.
22. Yeoh EJ, et al. Classification, subtype discovery, and prediction of outcome in pediatric acute lymphoblastic leukemia by gene expression profiling. Cancer Cell. 2002;1:133.
23. Mullighan CG, et al. Genome-wide analysis of genetic alterations in acute lymphoblastic leukaemia. Nature. 2007;446:758–64.
24. Clappier E, Auclerc MF, Rapion J, Bakkus M, Caye A, Khemiri A, Giroux C, Hernandez L, Kabongo E, Savola S, Leblanc T, Yakouben K, Plat G, Costa V, Ferster A, Girard S, Fenneteau O, Cayuela JM, Sigaux F, Dastugue N, Suciu S, Benoit Y, Bertrand Y, Soulier J, Cavé H. An intragenic ERG deletion is a marker of an oncogenic subtype of B-cell precursor acute lymphoblastic leukemia with a favorable outcome despite frequent IKZF1 deletions. Leukemia. 2014;28(1):70–7.
25. Zhang X, Rastogi P, Shah B, Zhang L. B lymphoblastic leukemia/lymphoma: new insights into genetics, molecular aberrations, subclassification and targeted therapy. Oncotarget. 2017;8:66728–41.
26. Rand V, Parker H, Russell LJ, Schwab C, Ensor H, Irving J, Jones L, Masic D, Minto L, Morrison H, Ryan S, Robinson H, Sinclair P, Moorman AV, Strefford JC, Harrison CJ. Genomic characterization implicates iAMP21 as a likely primary genetic event in childhood B-cell precursor acute lymphoblastic leukemia. Blood. 2011;117:6848–55.
27. Harrison CJ. Blood spotlight on iAMP21 acute lymphoblastic leukemia (ALL), a high-risk pediatric disease. Blood. 2015;125(9):1383–6.
28. Mullighan CG, Su X, Zhang J, et al. Deletion of IKZF1 and prognosis in acute lymphoblastic leukemia. N Engl J Med. 2009;360:470–80.
29. Roberts KG, Morin RD, Zhang J, et al. Genetic alterations activating kinase and cytokine receptor signaling in high-risk acute lymphoblastic leukemia. Cancer Cell. 2012;22:153–66.
30. Roberts KG, et al. Outcomes of children with BCR-ABL1–like acute lymphoblastic leukemia treated with risk-directed therapy based on the levels of minimal residual disease. J Clin Oncol. 2014;32: 3012–20.
31. Roberts KG, et al. Targetable kinase-activating lesions in Ph-like acute lymphoblastic leukemia. N Engl J Med. 2014;371:1005–15.
32. Pui CH, et al. Childhood acute lymphoblastic leukemia: progress through collaboration. J Clin Oncol. 2015;33:2938–48.
33. Van Vlierberghe P, Ferrando A. The molecular basis of T cell acute lymphoblastic leukemia. J Clin Invest. 2012;122(10):3398–406.
34. Girardi T, Vicente C, Cools J, De Keersmaecker K. The genetics and molecular biology of T-ALL. Blood. 2017;129(9):1113–23.
35. Ferrando AA, Neuberg DS, Staunton J, et al. Gene expression signatures define novel oncogenic pathways in T cell acute lymphoblastic leukemia. Cancer Cell. 2002;1:75–87.
36. Graux C, Cools J, Michaux L, Vandenberghe P, Hagemeijer A. Cytogenetics and molecular genetics of T-cell acute lymphoblastic leukemia: from thymocyte to lymphoblast. Leukemia. 2006;20: 1496–510.
37. Soulier J, et al. HOXA genes are included in genetic and biologic networks defining human acute T-cell leukemia (T-ALL). Blood. 2005;106(1): 274–86.
38. Coustan-Smith E, et al. Early T-cell precursor leukemia: a subtype of very high-risk acute lymphoblastic leukaemia. Lancet Oncol. 2009;10(2):147–56.
39. Homminga I, et al. Integrated transcript and genome analyses reveal NKX2-1 and MEF2C as potential oncogenes in T cell acute lymphoblastic leukemia. Cancer Cell. 2011;19(4):484–97.
40. Bene MC, Castoldi G, Knapp W, Ludwig WD, Matutes E, Orfao A, et al. Proposals for the immunological classification of acute leukemias. European Group for the Immunological Characterization of Leukemias (EGIL). Leukemia. 1995;9:1783–6.
41. Van Vlierberghe P, et al. ETV6 mutations in early immature human T cell leukemias. J Exp Med. 2011;208(13):2571–9.
42. van Grotel M, van den Heuvel-Eibrink MM, van Wering ER, van Noesel MM, Kamps WA, Veerman AJ, Pieters R, Meijerink JP. CD34 expression is associated with poor survival in pediatric T-cell acute lymphoblastic leukemia. Pediatr Blood Cancer. 2008;51(6):737–40.
43. Graux C, Cools J, Hagemeijer A. Fusion of NUP214 to ABL1 on amplified episomes in T-cell acute lymphoblastic leukemia. Nat Genet. 2004;36(10): 1084–9.

44. Belver L, Ferrando A. The genetics and mechanisms of T cell acute lymphoblastic leukaemia. Nat Rev Cancer. 2016;16(8):494–507.

45. Haydu JE, Ferrando AA. Early T-cell precursor acute lymphoblastic leukaemia. Curr Opin Hematol. 2013;20:369–73.

46. Gutierrez A, Dahlberg SE, Neuberg DS, et al. Absence of biallelic TCRgamma deletion predicts early treatment failure in pediatric T-cell acute lymphoblastic leukemia. J Clin Oncol. 2010;28:3816–23.

Minimal Residual Disease in Acute Lymphoblastic Leukemia

12

Richa Chauhan, Richa Juneja, Rahul Sharma, and Renu Saxena

12.1 Introduction

Acute lymphoblastic leukemia is now a treatable malignancy with cure achieved in more than 85% of patients and 5-year event-free survival (EFS) >94% in low and intermediate risk groups according to western literature [1]. With the current armamentarium of chemotherapeutic agents, target is to achieve more impressive results in terms of overall survival (OS) and progression-free survival (PFS). This requires stringent track of the disease burden; the most objective way of which is minimal residual disease (MRD) monitoring.

At the time of diagnosis of ALL, the overall burden of leukemic cells is 10^{12}. After induction therapy, cases that achieve complete remission (CR), defined as <5% blasts in normo-cellular marrow, still harbors residual 10^{10} leukemic cells [2]. Figure 12.1 depicts how greater log reduction in disease burden at end of induction reduces the risk of relapse. Moreover, there are limitations to morphology, i.e., its detection limit is only 1%. Therefore, more sensitive tools were needed to detect MRD. Patients with ALL are categorized into standard risk and high risk based on clinical characteristics (age and total leucocyte count) and biologic characteristics (immunophenotyping, ploidy, chromosomal structural anomaly, gene rearrangements). However, a proportion (20%) of standard risk ALL can relapse. Also some subset of standard risk cases might receive more intensive chemotherapy than is necessary. Multiple studies have demonstrated MRD as an important *independent* prognostic marker in B-ALL. So, in cases of achieving morphological remission, MRD assessment by multiparametric flow cytometry (MFC) or polymerase chain reaction (PCR) helps to prognosticate, decide treatment strategy and dynamic assessment of disease burden during sequential therapy.

12.2 Definition and Background

MRD is residual burden of leukemic cells that is below the limit of detection of conventional technique (morphology) during clinical remission.

Attempts to identify residual blasts in patients of ALL on treatment began in 1980s by detecting combination of CD3 and Tdt by immunofluorescence in T-ALL [3]. In the past three decades, various techniques utilized for this purpose with their respective sensitivities are enumerated below.

Technique	Blast per 100,000 cells	Sensitivity (%)
Morphology remission	5000	5
Karyotype analysis	5000	5
Expert microscopy	1000	1
MFC	10	0.01
Colony growth	1	0.001
PCR	0.1	0.0001

R. Chauhan · R. Juneja · R. Sharma · R. Saxena (✉)
Department of Hematology, All India Institute of Medical Sciences, New Delhi, India

© Springer Nature Singapore Pte Ltd. 2019
R. Saxena, H. P. Pati (eds.), *Hematopathology*, https://doi.org/10.1007/978-981-13-7713-6_12

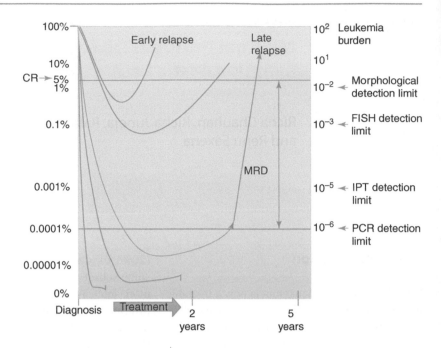

Fig. 12.1 Reduction in disease burden reduces the risk of relapse; chances of early relapse after cytomorphological remission and late relapse after deeper levels of MRD

As shown in the Fig. 12.1, MRD positivity by more sensitive technique is a better predictor of relapse. Therefore, optimal technique should have specificity (to discriminate malignant from normal cells), sensitivity (to detect at least 1 malignant cell in a background of $\geq 10,000$ normal cells), applicability (to be applicable in virtually every patient), reproducibility (standardized methods), and stability during the course of the disease, and allow timely output of the results [4].

Standard techniques for detection of MRD in the present time are following and will be discussed in the chapter:

1. Flow cytometry-based detection
2. Detection of target fusion gene by PCR
3. Detection of immunoglobulin (Ig) or T cell receptor (TCR) gene rearrangement by PCR

Basic principle of all MRD assays is that cellular changes induced by leukemogenic process are used to differentiate leukemic cells from normal. Differentially expressed molecules in leukemic cells form "*Leukemia associated phenotypes.*"

Before we go ahead with discussion of these individual techniques, some important aspects of MRD need to be addressed in detail.

12.2.1 Time Points to Do MRD

It is shown in various studies that MRD measurements at day 33 or end of induction and 3 months (day 78) provide the most important prognostic information [5, 6].

Early MRD measurements at day 15 in childhood ALL can provide additional information for identification of very early responders ($<10^{-3}$) and a small subgroup of poor responders ($\geq 10^{-2}$). However, so far there is no consensus about utilizing this early MRD detection in therapeutic decision-making [7].

12.2.2 Target Sensitivity

The cutoff for calling a particular case as MRD positive was different for different groups in various trials. Eventually, 10^{-4} came up as a target that could be achieved precisely with

Table 12.1 Summary of various studies on FCM-based MRD in B ALL

Study	Time point of MRD	Sensitivity (%)	Conclusion
A. *Pediatric ALL*			
Michael et al. (2015) (COG-AALL0232)	Post-induction day +33	≥0.01	• MRD as independent adverse prognostic factor • Treatment intensification cannot avert relapse, but prolongs timing of relapse
Borowitz et al. (2013) (COG)	Post-induction day +29	≥0.01	• 5 year DFS very low in day +29 MRD Neg (89 vs. 72%) • Day 14 BM morphologic evaluation can be omitted
Giuseppe et al. (2013)	Day +15	≥0.01	MRD as most powerful predictor of relapse
Coustan et al. (1998)	At week 14, 32, 56, and 120	≥0.01	MRD positivity at any time point : high risk of relapse
B. *Adult ALL*			
Ravandi et al. (2016)	Post-induction day 29	≥0.01	Independent predictor for DFS and OS
Samra et al. (2013)	Post-induction	≥0.01	Independent significant risk predictor for relapse
Vidriales et al. (2003)	Day +35	≥0.05	MRD as independent adverse prognostic factor
Mingming et al. (2016)	Post-induction	≥0.02	Independent predictor for low LFS and OS
Jerzy et al. (2008)	Post-induction	≥0.1	Independent predictor for low LFS and OS Combined post-induction and post-consolidation results same as for post-induction alone

Most accepted cutoff for MRD positivity in pediatric B-ALL is 0.01%, although time point of MRD assessment varies a lot. In adults, however, most MRD studies are on post-induction but cutoff varies a lot

technologies available and also provided prognostic information based on which therapeutic interventions are required. (Refer to Table 12.1 for various cutoffs used in different studies) With both FCM and PCR-based techniques 1 leukemic cell in 10^4 cells can be detected, i.e., 0.01% sensitivity [5, 8].

12.2.3 Ideal Sample for MRD Testing

Review of literature for comparison of peripheral blood (PB) MRD levels and marrow, revealed that though PB MRD in T-ALL patients were comparable or up to 1 log lower than in BM, in BCP-ALL patients, PB MRD levels were 1–3 logs lower than in BM, making PB MRD studies impossible in BCP-ALL patients. *Hence, BM sampling is a prerequisite*. The sample has to be the *first draw* from bone marrow. The storage of samples should not exceed 24 h after collection [5, 9].

Quantity of sample: Optimum quantity of sample to be collected is 2–5 mL of the *first* draw BM aspirate [9].

These basics of ALL MRD are applicable to MRD detection by any technique. We will be discussing standard available techniques in detail. First and widely available technique amongst these is multiparametric flow cytometry (MFC)-based detection of MRD.

12.3 Flow Cytometry-Based Detection of MRD

12.3.1 History and Evolution of FCM-Based MRD

History of MRD detection in ALL dates back to 1980s, when unique thymic immunophenotype of T blasts was detected in post-therapeutic bone marrow samples by immunofluorescence [3, 10]. However, same thing could not be easily replicated in B ALL cases because normal B cell progenitors/ hematogones are abundant in post-therapeutic bone marrow samples. Immunofluorescence technique offered two to three markers that were not sufficient to differentiate subtle difference in immunophenotype of B blasts and hematogones.

Flow cytometry technique allows assessment of multiple parameters on one cell and hence helps in identifying small population of interest (i.e., MRD) in milieu of millions of cells. So this problem was partly solved with availability of 4/6/8 or 10 color flow cytometers that helped in identifying residual B blasts with their aberrant immunophenotypic profile (Leukemia-associated immunophenotype—LAIP) [4]. However, inter-laboratory comparability of FCM-based MRD results continues to be a challenge to various groups working on standardization of this technique. Next step in evolution of FCM-based MRD in B ALL is Euro flow-based next-generation flow MRD, which offers standard panel of antibody-fluorochrome combinations with software-based analysis of cases [11].

Basic principle of above-mentioned techniques is detailed analysis of difference in phenotype of blasts versus normal counterpart. In T ALL cases, detection of residual blast is easier as bone marrow does not harbor any precursor T cell normally, their location being thymus. In more than 95%, B ALL cases leukemic cells can be distinguished from normal counterpart or hematogones by detailed phenotypic analysis. Thus, understanding normal maturation is essential to perform MRD testing.

12.3.2 Normal B Cell Maturation: Hematogones

Hematogones are normal B cell precursors that morphologically resemble blasts and are found predominantly in bone marrow. They can be seen in peripheral blood of neonates and in cord blood as well [12]. Hematogones can comprise 5–50% of BM cells. McKenna et al. demonstrated out of 662 BM, 79.8% showed hematogones. They occur across all ages and show significant decline with age and in cases of marrow involvement by blasts [13]. Hematogones are increased in normal healthy infants and young children, regenerating bone marrow (following chemotherapy and bone marrow transplant), autoimmune cytopenias (e.g., ITP), acquired immunodeficiency syndromes and lymphomas. Their characteristic maturation pattern defines normal maturation of

B cells. There are three stages of hematogone maturation.

The early hematogones (Stage 1) express dim CD45, Tdt, and CD34 positive and express bright CD10. Thereafter, the intensity of markers of immaturity diminishes and intensity of CD45, CD19, and CD20 increases. Note that CD20 is absent in early hematogones. Late hematogones (Stage 3) and mature B cells have polyclonal Kappa and Lambda expression [14].

In FCM, identification of hematogones can be done by using following clues (Fig. 12.2)

- On CD34/CD10 plot—Stage 1: CD34+/CD10 bright → Stage 2: CD34−/CD10+ → Stage3: CD34−/CD10-(plot H in Fig. 12.2).
- On CD45/SSC plot—shows the three stages with heterogeneous dim to higher expression of CD45 with very low side scatter (plot B in Fig. 12.2)
- CD10/CD20 plot—classical waterfall pattern (plot D in Fig. 12.2)
- CD19/CD10 plot—scattered events without a well-defined cluster
- They can also express CD38, CD58 and many other markers in variable intensities (plot G in Fig. 12.2)

Figure 12.3 summarizes the antigen expression pattern during maturation in normal B cells in marrow. After this brief introduction about hematogones and their phenotype, we go ahead with FCM-based detection of B ALL MRD. ALL blasts differ from normal precursors because of unique *Leukemia-associated immunophenotype* (LAIP). LAIP is defined by phenotype showing

- Maturation arrest
- Over or under expression of antigens
- Asynchronous expression of antigens
- Cross-lineage expression of antigens— "lineage infidelity"

So, quantitative abnormalities of antigen expression are seen in 30–50% cases of B ALL. Antigens that are commonly overexpressed on blasts are CD10, CD34, CD58, and CD20.

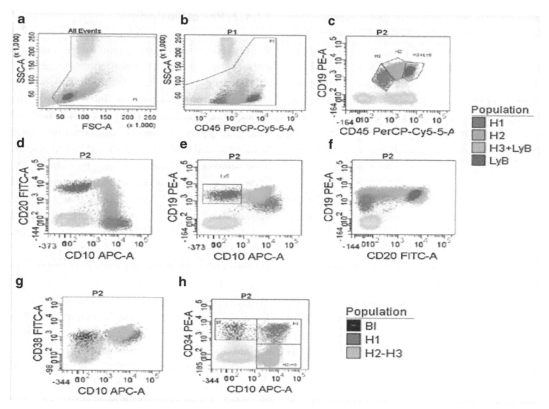

Fig. 12.2 FCM plots showing various patterns of hematogones. Population H1, H2 and H3 are stage 1, 2 & stage 3 hematogones and Bl denotes blast (Adapted from leukemia research article) [11]

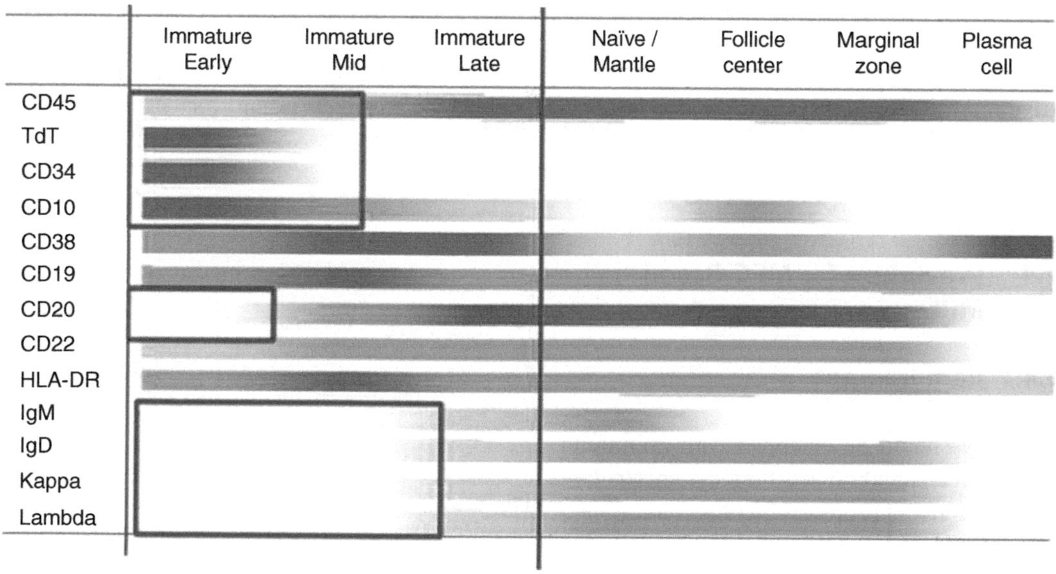

	Immature Early	Immature Mid	Immature Late	Naïve / Mantle	Follicle center	Marginal zone	Plasma cell
CD45							
TdT							
CD34							
CD10							
CD38							
CD19							
CD20							
CD22							
HLA-DR							
IgM							
IgD							
Kappa							
Lambda							

Fig. 12.3 Pattern of antigen expression in normally maturing B cells. (Adapted from Henry Todd Chapter by Brent Wood) [15]

Antigens that are commonly under expressed on blasts are CD45, CD38, CD10, CD20, and CD81.

Qualitative abnormalities are cross-lineage antigen expression (CD13/33, CD7, CD15, CD11a), antigens associated with fusion transcript (CD66c, CD15, NG2-Ab 7.1), ectopic phenotypes like Tdt+ cells in CSF, and maturational asynchrony (CD20 on CD19/CD34+ precursor B cells). With all these marker combinations, it is possible to detect MRD in 95% cases.

In diagnostic sample, LAIPs are defined for the blast of that particular case which is followed in subsequent MRD samples. However, there can be loss or change in expression (instability) of the LAIP marker that can affect MRD analysis. This can be due to therapy or can be part of disease process. Hence, most laboratories follow deviation from normal technique for LAIP detection in residual blasts.

MFC-based MRD detection in B-ALL is based on two strategies

– *Identification and following unique LAIP in their predefined gates*—Here regions are designed in different plots where blasts are expected to lie and residual blasts in posttherapeutic samples are tracked in predefined blast regions.
– *Deviation from normal maturation spectrum/ hematogones*—Here regions are designed where normal hematogones in multiple reactive marrows are expected to lie and residual blasts are detected as cluster of events outside these regions.

12.4 Procedure for MFC-Based MRD

12.4.1 Requirement

Laboratory should be equipped with (minimum of four color) standardized flow cytometer with correct setting. Appropriate quality control measures should be taken and both internal and external quality control and should be done regularly to keep system in place.

12.4.2 Panel Designing

With availability of more and more markers, appropriate choice of fluorochrome antibody combination is important task and depends on personalized approach of the lab. However, the basic concept remains same, i.e., one should have backbone gating markers to select the population of interest and other markers for detailed phenotypic analysis. These markers include cross-lineage markers, maturation markers, and markers associated with molecular lesions. Markers chosen should help hematopathologist to differentiate residual blast from normal precursors clearly. Few groups [16] recommend use of Syto16-a live cell permeant nucleated cell dye to monitor erythrocyte lysis efficiency and target live cells for further analysis. In case of precursor T cell ALL, presence of any immature T cell is indicator of residual disease as thymus is their normal location and not bone marrow [4, 9]. However, possibility of other cells like natural killer cells mimicking residual T blast should be excluded. Knowledge of antigen profile of acute leukemia blasts is continuously evolving with the help of gene expression profiling. Many markers are added to battery of conventional markers for MRD detection in ALL [17]. Figure 12.4 summarizes the panel of available markers that include both, gating backbone markers and LAIP markers for MRD.

Table 12.2 shows recommended four color panel by Brazilian group for B ALL MRD

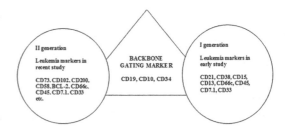

Fig. 12.4 Markers that can be used for MRD detection in B ALL. Triangle shows backbone gating marker showing immature lymphoid cells. Rest markers help to differentiate blast from hematogones. (Adapted from cytometry B) [4]

adapted from Brazilian Journal of Hematology and Hemotherapy [9]

Table 12.3 shows recommended four color panel by Brazilian group for T ALL MRD adapted from Brazilian Journal of Hematology and Hematotherapy [9]

Various groups [18, 19] are now suggesting single tube approach for MRD detection with optimum sensitivity. Following Table 12.4 addresses one such example.

12.4.3 Technique

Stain-lyse-wash is the routine technique to be used in sample preparation.

Fresh BM or PB samples containing 10^6 cells must be incubated for 15 min at room temperature in the dark, with pre-titrated saturating amounts of cocktail of fluorochrome conjugated monoclonal antibodies. Red cells are lysed, using commercial lysing solution following manufac-

Table 12.2 Four color panel for B ALL MRD

Mandatory panel	
Tube 1	CD20/CD10/CD19 and CD34
Tube 2	CD45/CD38/CD19 and CD34
Tube 3	nTdt/CD10/CD19 and CD34
Recommended panel	
	CD45/CD123/CD19 and CD34
	CD81/CD66c/CD19 and CD34
	CD15/CD65/NG2/CD45 and CD19
Optional marker	CD13 and or CD33/CD58/CD9/CD25, CD22

Table 12.3 Four color panel for T ALL MRD

Mandatory panel	
Tube 1	cCD3/mCD3/CD45 and CD7
Tube 2	nTdt/CD2/CD5 and CD7
Recommended panel	
Tube 3	CD1a/CD99/mCD3 and CD7
Optional marker	CD10, CD13, CD33, CD34, CD44, CD117

turer's instructions. The remaining cells are sequentially centrifuged (500 g) for 5 min, washed twice in phosphate buffered saline (PBS: pH 7.4) and resuspended in 300–500 μL in PBS for acquisition and analysis. Intracellular staining for various markers is performed after staining for cell surface/membrane markers using Fix & Perm solution [18].

12.4.4 Data Acquisition

Desired sensitivity of assay will decide minimum number of events that are to be acquired. After extensive research, it is found that MRD sensitivity of 10^{-4} is most informative and targeted by various laboratories. To attain this limit of detection with good reproducibility, cluster of 100 leukemic events should be formed. This target can be achieved by acquiring minimum 1,000,000 events [18]. Hence it is recommended that for each sample aliquot, a minimum of 500,000 and maximum of 1,000,000 events must be acquired [9].

12.4.5 Gating Strategy and Reporting

First step in data analysis is checking the quality of data and confirming that system is in place and working properly. In ideal setting, we assume that laser interrogates single cell and we collect its properties. However, this doesn't hold true when lacs of events are acquired with high speed and two cells may stick with each other and form "doublets." Their importance lies in the experiment like MRD, where we are trying to find small cluster of events (residual disease) with aberrant phenotype. These doublets may give erroneous positivity. Hence, it is very important to use height versus area/width plot for any parameter to segregate single events-"singlets" and include

Table 12.4 Single tube panel for B-ALL MRD

	PE	FITC	Per CP5.5	PC7	A594	APC	APC7
Tube 1	CD20	Syto16	CD10	CD19	CD38	CD58	CD45

these events only for further analysis [18, 20]. After we have excluded doublets from analysis, it is recommended to use Syto16 to target live cells for further analysis. "Gating marker" (most commonly CD 19 in B ALL MRD) will help us to segregate B-lineage cells and focus further analysis on these events. CD10 and CD34 will help to identify various stages of hematogones as described earlier. This forms the basis of using CD19, CD10, and CD34 as backbone gating markers. CD19 expression may be altered as part of disease or therapeutic modulation of antigen expression. In such cases, CD22 or CD24 will serve as better gating markers [21, 22]. After this, various marker combinations can be used to identify residual disease with its characteristic LAIP and differentiating it from hematogones. As discussed earlier, two strategies can be used for this purpose, namely tracking LAIP or deviation from normal. Each cluster of event recognized on dot plot should be recognized as normal population, artifact or residual disease. Presence of two or more LAIPs on residual disease population is required to report MRD positivity. Figure 12.5 summarizes the gating strategy of B ALL MRD showing analysis of both diagnostic and end of induction sample.

While reporting one must be aware of possibility of disease related or post-therapy alteration in antigen profile of blast (antigen modulation) and lineage switch. Few of these are enlisted in Table 12.5 below. Including newer markers which are differentially expressed in residual blast versus hematogones (e.g., CD24, CD44, CD49f, CD69, CD72, CD73, CD79b, CD86, CD97, CD99, CD102, CD123, CD130, CD164, CD200, CD300a, CD304, BCL2, HSPB1, PBX1, CTNNA1, and ITGB7) and stable markers associated with molecular lesion will help to improve the sensitivity of assay [9].

There is no consensus yet regarding minimum number of events required in cell cluster to ascertain it as residual disease. On 4/6 color FCM cluster of 20 events is taken as residual disease; however, the I-BFM-ALL-FLOW-MRD Network quantifies MRD in presence of cluster of 30 events which is confirmed by independent second tube. If the assay consists of several individual tubes, then the minimum requirements are the sum, not the average, of the individual tubes.

12.4.6 Reporting of Results

Final result of MRD should be reported as percentage of all viable cells.

$$\frac{\text{Maximum number of MRD events}}{\text{Total Syto16 positive events}} \times 100$$

If Syto16 is not added in all the tubes following correction formula should be applied. Correction of B cells due to variation in events acquired in different tubes

---

$$\text{Correction factor for B cells} \left(\text{CF}_\text{B} \right) = \frac{\% \text{of B cells in syto tube}}{\% \text{of B cells in low events tube}}$$

$$\text{Correction factor for singlets} \left(\text{CF}_\text{S} \right) = \frac{\% \text{of singlets in syto tube}}{\% \text{of singlets in low events tube}}$$

$$\text{Final correction factor} \left(\text{CF} \right) = \text{CF}_\text{B} \times \text{CF}_\text{S}$$

$$\text{MRD} = \% \text{of MRD in B cells of main tube} \times \text{CF}$$

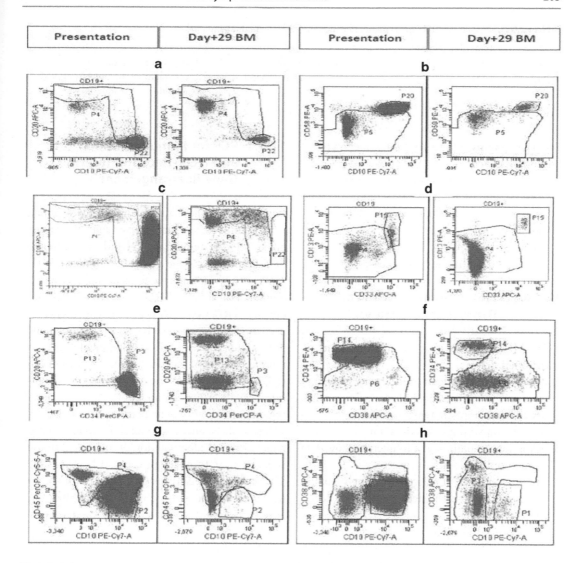

Fig. 12.5 Image depicts basic MRD assessment strategy. Only the CD19+ populations are displayed. Broad window in the dot plot delineates the area covered within normal B-cell maturation pattern whereas smaller window is anticipated leukemia window. (**a**) CD20$^{dim/-}$ CD10^{++} population screened at diagnosis could be seen persisting in MRD$^+$ day +29 BM. (**b**) CD58^{++} CD10^{++} bright population persists in MRD$^+$ case. (**c**) CD10^{++} CD20^{hetero} population present at diagnosis disappeared at post-induction in MRD$^-$ BM. (**d**) CD13^{++} CD33^{++} population screened at diagnosis could be seen persisting in MRD$^+$ day +29 BM. (**e**) CD34^{++} CD20$^{dim/-}$ population persists in MRD$^+$ case. (**f**) CD34^{++} CD38^{Neg} population persists in MRD$^+$ case. (**g**) A very small ($\geq$0.01%) CD45^{dim} CD10^{++} population persists in MRD$^+$ case. (**h**) CD38^{Neg} CD10^{++} population persists in MRD$^+$ case with marginal spill into narrow window

Table 12.5 Common post therapeutic antigenic modulation in acute leukemia [9]

	Induction therapy		At day 78 of induction
	Down modulation	Up modulation	
B ALL	CD10 and CD34	CD19, CD20, CD45 RA, and CD11a	Reversion of CD10 and 34 to initial expression
T ALL	Tdt, CD99, CD10, CD34		

The principal advantages of immunophenotyping-based MRD are:

1. Assessment of sample cellularity is possible.
2. Assessment of normal regeneration of bone marrow after immunosuppressive therapy is possible.
3. Rapid turnaround time.
4. It is applicable in most of the cases.

12.4.6.1 Flow Cytometry-Based MRD Reports in Pediatric vs. Adult ALL

FCM MRD has its own set of limitations as mentioned below:

1. At times, it is difficult to differentiate normal precursors from residual blast, due to similarity of immunophenotype.
2. Post-therapy antigen modulation.
3. Experienced pathologist to interpret flow data is required.
4. Inter-laboratory standardization and quality control is still a challenge.

To address few of these issues and enhance sensitivity of assay next-generation flow cytometry or Euroflow is emerging. However, whether it will actually solve challenges in path of FCM-based MRD detection in ALL is under study.

Second technique that is well standardized and described in literature to test for residual disease in B ALL is PCR-based techniques.

12.5 MRD by Molecular Techniques

Leukemic cells are unique because of acquisition and clonal proliferation of abnormal cells carrying mutations, fusion genes, and T-cell or immunoglobulin gene rearrangements. This monoclonality in ALL can be monitored using immunoglobulin or T cell receptor gene rearrangements.

12.5.1 PCR for Immunoglobulin and T-Cell Receptor (IG-TR) Gene Rearrangement

Since most B and T cell malignancies originate from immune cells that have already undergone physiologic gene rearrangement during differentiation, all cells of the malignant clone carry the same gene rearrangement as a unique clonal marker. For T cells, TRG, and TRD, TRB, and unusual TRD (Vδ2-Jα) gene rearrangements are used as PCR targets. The IG gene rearrangements during normal B cell development generate unique fusions of variable, diversity and joining (VDJ) segments, interspersed by random nucleotide (N) insertion and/or deletion. The junctional regions of clonal Ig gene rearrangements are fingerprint like sequences for each lymphoid malignancy. Precise identification of junctional region sequences of Ig genes in each ALL is feasible. The prerequisite is to design clone-specific oligonucleotide probes for each case and conduct sensitivity testing by serial dilution of diagnostic DNA sample.

The technique of real-time quantitative PCR (RT-qPCR) can be used for clone-specific MRD PCR targets. This reaches a sensitivity of 10^{-5}. At least 1×10^7 mononuclear cells should be available for evaluation. For follow-up samples, 1×10^6 cells should suffice [23].

EDTA sample is ideal for PCR analysis. DNA-based analysis should be done within 24 h. For primer designing and RQ-PCR, validated procedures should be followed [23].

Continuing rearrangements during disease course can cause false-negative MRD results. Therefore, at least two targets should be determined to account for leukemia heterogeneity and to take care of subclones [23].

False positivity due to massive regeneration of normal lymphoid progenitors might lead to very low level of nonspecific amplification. However, high degree of standardization is available, e.g., European Study Group on MRD detection in ALL (ESG-MRD-ALL) lays down protocols for standardization of techniques, interpretation, and reporting [23]. It conducts QC program every 6 months and also establishes quantitative range of an assay.

Newer PCR-based high-throughput sequencing Ig-TR gene rearrangements to quantify MRD employs multiplex PCR with V-, D-, J-primer sets to amplify all potential rearrangements. Consecutively, these can be sequenced to achieve a sensitivity of $>10^{-6}$ [23].

12.5.2 PCR Analysis of Fusion Transcripts

Quantitative PCR of target fusion genes for, e.g., BCR-ABL, MLL-AF4, TCF3-PBX1, WT-1 genes, achieves a sensitivity of 1 in 10^5 leukemic cells, hence is highly sensitive technique and is currently well standardized by different study groups.

In pediatric ALL, about 25% patients have cytogenetically cryptic TEL/AML1 transcripts. Genomic breakpoints in leukemia-specific translocations, e.g., MLL gene rearrangements are also DNA targets. Ph+ chromosome is seen in 25% adult ALL, 5% pediatric ALL and is associated with worse prognosis [24]. Most common

transcript of BCR-ABL associated with ALL is e1a2 (p190) seen in 70% cases. The second most common transcript is e13–14/a2 (p210) seen in 30% B-ALL [24, 25].

At diagnosis, RT-PCR is carried out for identification of fusion transcript. Thereafter, RQ-PCR can be done for follow-up MRD. Advantages of RQ-PCR for BCR-ABL include high sensitivity, ease, and rapidity of analysis and lower cost.

Disadvantages of PCR for BCR-ABL are that RNA is not so stable, and there is still lack of standardization of steps of RNA extraction and cDNA synthesis. The choice of control genes of variable amongst laboratories and different control genes lead to variability in sensitivity of the assay. There is a chance of false negativity due to poor RNA quality and also false positive due to cross contamination. Minimum requirements for interpretation and quantifiable range have not been developed [23].

Both FCM and PCR are highly sensitive technique to detect MRD; however, they have their pros and cons which are highlighted in Table 12.6 below [23].

Different groups across the globe have used either FCM-based/PCR-based MRD techniques or combination of both to assess MRD at various time points. Details of few of these studies are summarized in Table 12.7 below.

All the groups uniformly found MRD as good predictor of relapse and independent prognostic

Table 12.6 Comparison of different techniques available for B ALL MRD

Technique	Flow cytometry	PCR-IG-TCR	PCR fusion genes
Targets	LAIP	IG/TCR gene rearrangements	Fusion genes
Sensitivity	1 in 10^4	1 in 10^5	1 in 10^4
Applicability	90–95%—T cells 80–95%—B cells	90–95%	5% Ph+ pediatric 35% Ph+ adults
Advantages	– Widely applicable – Rapid – Additional information on benign and malignant cells	– Highly sensitive – Most standardized – Most evidence-based data published – DNA is stable	– Sensitive – Fast – Cheap – Stability of target DNA
Disadvantages	– Immunophenotype shift – Difference from regenerating B–precursors – Cellularity can be low after induction – Extensive standardization for $\geq$6 color MFC	– Time consuming – Clonal evolution: loss of target – Expensive expertise required	– Limited applicability – Instability of RNA – False positivity due to contamination

Table 12.7 Summary of the various studies showing utility of MRD in B ALL

Study	Protocol	Technique	Time point	Cutoff for MRD positivity	Outcome	Min events/ amount of DNA	Conclusion
Borowitz et al. (2008)	COG	FCM	– Day 8 PB – End of induction BM – End of consolidation BM	≥0.01	EFS	5,00,000	End of induction MRD best prognostic marker
Cave et al. (1998)	EORTC	IG/TCR	End of induction	≥0.1	Relapse-free interval	NA	MRD is robust prognostic marker to predict relapse
Flohr et al. (2008)	(AIEOP-BFMALL 2000)	IG/TCR	End of induction TP1 day 33 End of consolidation day 78	≥0.01	Relapse-free survival	≥5 µg of DNA (from 5×10^6 MNCs) ≥2 PCR targets	MRD used for risk stratification
Gaipa et al. (2012)	(AIEOP-BFMALL 2000)	MFC and IG/TCR	Day 15, 33, and 78	≥0.01	EFS	3,00,000	MRD-positive cases have poor EFS
Patkar et al. (India)	NM	MFC	Day +21 Day +33	≥0.01	NM	5,00,000	Cost-effective MRD panel useful in ≥90% pts

NM not mentioned

marker. Various studies and randomized control trial further consolidated the utility of MRD as an essential tool in treatment decision in patients of ALL on various drug regimens. In AIEOP-BFM-ALL 2000 study, MRD-based treatment strategies further improved outcomes [26]. UK-ALL 2003 RCT found that treatment can be tailored in MRD-based low risk patients and can be augmented in MRD-high risk patients [27]. Data from Indian literature is largely lacking. However, Patkar et al. have elaborated on standardization of the panel used for MRD [28].

To conclude potential role of MRD in current era is to evaluate efficacy of induction therapy, risk stratify, decide further therapeutic strategy, assess efficacy of treatment regimen in relation to that of its predecessor and determine leukemic burden before and after stem cell transplant [29]. MRD emerged as an important weapon in the battle against the occult leukemic burden. With euroflow and NGS, future of MRD technique has lot more to offer in terms of reliability, reproducibility, speed, and wider applicability.

References

1. Thomas A. How can we improve on the already impressive results in pediatric ALL? Hematology Am Soc Hematol Educ Program. 2015;2015(1):414–9.
2. Campana D, Coustan-Smith E. Detection of minimal residual disease in acute leukemia by flow cytometry. Cytometry. 1999;38(4):139–52.
3. Bradstock KF, Janossy G, Tidman N, Papageorgiou ES, Prentice HG, Willoughby M, et al. Immunological monitoring of residual disease in treated thymic acute lymphoblastic leukaemia. Leuk Res. 1981;5(4–5):301–9.
4. Gaipa G, Basso G, Biondi A, Campana D. Detection of minimal residual disease in pediatric acute lymphoblastic leukemia: MRD in pediatric ALL. Cytometry B Clin Cytom. 2013;84(6):359–69.
5. van Dongen JJM, van der Velden VHJ, Bruggemann M, Orfao A. Minimal residual disease diagnostics in acute lymphoblastic leukemia: need for sensitive, fast, and standardized technologies. Blood. 2015;125(26):3996–4009.
6. Borowitz MJ, Devidas M, Hunger SP, Bowman WP, Carroll AJ, Carroll WL, et al. Clinical significance of minimal residual disease in childhood acute lymphoblastic leukemia and its relationship to other prognostic factors: a Children's Oncology Group study. Blood. 2008;111(12):5477–85.

7. Sutton R, Venn NC, Tolisano J, Bahar AY, Giles JE, Ashton LJ, et al. Clinical significance of minimal residual disease at day 15 and at the end of therapy in childhood acute lymphoblastic leukaemia. Br J Haematol. 2009;146(3):292–9.

8. Borowitz MJ, Wood BL, Devidas M, Loh ML, Raetz EA, Salzer WL, et al. Prognostic significance of minimal residual disease in high risk B-ALL: a report from Children's Oncology Group study AALL0232. Blood. 2015;126(8):964–71.

9. Ikoma MRV, Beltrame MP, Ferreira SIACP, Souto EX, Malvezzi M, Yamamoto M. Proposal for the standardization of flow cytometry protocols to detect minimal residual disease in acute lymphoblastic leukemia. Rev Bras Hematol Hemoter. 2015;37(6):406–13.

10. Bradstock K, Papageorgiou ES, Janossy G, Hoffbrand AV, Willoughby M, Roberts P, et al. Detection of leukæmic lymphoblasts in CSF by immunofluorescence for terminal transferase. Lancet. 1980;315(8178):1144.

11. Pedreira CE, Costa ES, Lecrevisse Q, van Dongen JJM, Orfao A, EuroFlow Consortium. Overview of clinical flow cytometry data analysis: recent advances and future challenges. Trends Biotechnol. 2013;31(7):415–25.

12. Brady KA, Atwater SK, Lowell CA. Flow cytometric detection of CD10 (cALLA) on peripheral blood B lymphocytes of neonates. Br J Haematol. 1999;107(4):712–5.

13. McKenna RW, Washington LT, Aquino DB, Picker LJ, Kroft SH. Immunophenotypic analysis of hematogones (B-lymphocyte precursors) in 662 consecutive bone marrow specimens by 4-color flow cytometry. Blood. 2001;98(8):2498–507.

14. Chantepie SP, Cornet E, Salaün V, Reman O. Hematogones: an overview. Leuk Res. 2013;37(11):1404–11.

15. McPherson R, Pincus M. Henry's clinical diagnosis and management by laboratory methods E-book. Philadelphia: Elsevier Health Sciences; 2016.

16. Dworzak MN, Gaipa G, Ratei R, Veltroni M, Schumich A, Maglia O, et al. Standardization of flow cytometric minimal residual disease evaluation in acute lymphoblastic leukemia: multicentric assessment is feasible. Cytometry B Clin Cytom. 2008;74B(6):331–40.

17. Coustan-Smith E, Song G, Clark C, Key L, Liu P, Mehrpooya M, et al. New markers for minimal residual disease detection in acute lymphoblastic leukemia. Blood. 2011;117(23):6267–76.

18. Czader M. Hematological malignancies. Totowa: Humana Press; 2013.

19. Shaver AC, Greig BW, Mosse CA, Seegmiller AC. B-ALL minimal residual disease flow cytometry: an application of a novel method for optimization of a single-tube model. Am J Clin Pathol. 2015;143(5):716–24.

20. 6 flow cytometry gating tips that most scientists forget|expert cytometry|flow cytometry training [internet]. Expert cytometry. 2014 [cited 2017 Dec 18]. https://expertcytometry.com/6-flow-cytometry-gating-tips-that-most-scientists-forget/.

21. Ghodke K, Bibi A, Rabade N, Patkar N, Subramanian PG, Kadam PA, et al. CD19 negative precursor B acute lymphoblastic leukemia (B-ALL)-immunophenotypic challenges in diagnosis and monitoring: a study of three cases: CD19 negative precursor B-ALL-immunophenotypic challenges in diagnosis and monitoring. Cytometry B Clin Cytom. 2017;92(4): 315–8.

22. Theunissen P, Mejstrikova E, Sedek L, van der Sluijs-Gelling AJ, Gaipa G, Bartels M, et al. Standardized flow cytometry for highly sensitive MRD measurements in B-cell acute lymphoblastic leukemia. Blood. 2017;129(3):347–57.

23. Brüggemann M, Schrauder A, Raff T, Pfeifer H, Dworzak M, Ottmann OG, et al. Standardized MRD quantification in European ALL trials: proceedings of the Second International Symposium on MRD assessment in Kiel, Germany, 18–20 September 2008. Leukemia. 2010;24(3):521–35.

24. Gleissner B, Rieder H, Thiel E, Fonatsch C, Janssen LA, Heinze B, et al. Prospective BCR-ABL analysis by polymerase chain reaction (RT-PCR) in adult acute B-lineage lymphoblastic leukemia: reliability of RT-nested-PCR and comparison to cytogenetic data. Leukemia. 2001;15(12):1834–40.

25. Mitterbauer G, Nemeth P, Wacha S, Cross NC, Schwarzinger I, Jaeger U, et al. Quantification of minimal residual disease in patients with BCR-ABL-positive acute lymphoblastic leukaemia using quantitative competitive polymerase chain reaction. Br J Haematol. 1999 Sep;106(3):634–43.

26. Flohr T, Schrauder A, Cazzaniga G, Panzer-Grümayer R, van der Velden V, Fischer S, et al. Minimal residual disease-directed risk stratification using real-time quantitative PCR analysis of immunoglobulin and T-cell receptor gene rearrangements in the international multicenter trial AIEOP-BFM ALL 2000 for childhood acute lymphoblastic leukemia. Leukemia. 2008;22(4):771–82.

27. Vora AJ, Goulden N, Mitchell CD, Hough R, Rowntree C, Richards SM. UKALL 2003, a randomised trial investigating treatment intensification for children and young adults with minimal residual disease defined high risk acute lymphoblastic leukaemia. Blood. 2012;120(21):136.

28. Rambaldi A, Borleri G, Dotti G, Bellavita P, Amaru R, Biondi A, et al. Innovative two-step negative selection of granulocyte colony-stimulating factor–mobilized circulating progenitor cells: adequacy for autologous and allogeneic transplantation. Blood. 1998;91(6):2189–96.

29. Patkar N, Alex A, Bargavi B, Ahmed R, Abraham A, George B, Vishwabandya A, Srivastava A, Mathews V. Standardization minimal residual disease by flow cytometry for precursor B lineage acute lymphoblastic leukemia in a developing country. Cytometry B Clin Cytom. 2012;82B:252–8.

Diagnosis of Myeloproliferative Neoplasms: Current Perspectives from Recent Research

13

Prabhu Manivannan and Hema Subramanian

13.1 Introduction

The World Health Organization (WHO) classification of tumors of the hematopoietic and lymphoid tissues, 2017 revised edition, representing the most recent update of the customarily amended classification, last updated in 2008, has recently been published [1]. Since the last edition, there has been tremendous advancement in the basic understanding of disease pathobiology, leading to the discovery of newer biomarkers. This has impacted the diagnostic criteria in the myeloproliferative neoplasm (MPN) category significantly [1, 2]. Majority of the voluminous information has been obtained from research based on the gene expression analysis and next-generation sequencing (NGS) [3–8]. Nevertheless, this newer 2017 classification retains the basic approach hinged on clinical characteristics, morphological features, immunophenotype, and cytogenetics (CTG). This highlights a consensus of opinion and expertise recommendation from different hematopathologists, clinical hematologists and also from other branches related to hematology like oncologists and geneticists [1].

The myeloproliferative neoplasms (MPNs) are disorders of hematopoietic cells characterized by clonal expansion of a single somatically mutated hematopoietic stem cell. This genetic alteration leads to excessive proliferation of thoroughly functional, differentiated blood cells representing single or multilineage hyperplasia [9]. MPNs were primarily conceptualized in 1951 and included chronic myeloid leukemia (CML) in which the Philadelphia chromosome was discovered in 1960. This was followed by the landmark discovery of imatinib in 1996 which further led to the practical segregation of CML, defined by the presence of BCR-ABL1 positivity as a distinct entity [10]. The classical BCR-ABL negative MPNs include polycythemia vera (PV), essential thrombocythemia (ET), and primary myelofibrosis (PMF). Chronic neutrophilic leukemia (CNL) and chronic eosinophilic leukemia, not otherwise specified (CEL, NOS) were included under this category because of their close resemblance in the pathobiology [11]. Recently, mastocytosis has been excluded from this category owing to the discovery of newer pathways, unique pathobiology, and genetic distinction from MPNs [1, 8]. In this chapter, the main emphasis is on rationale for changes, revised diagnostic criteria, newer driver, other somatic mutations, and differentiation from reactive conditions, concluding with an algorithmic approach to MPNs with the updated knowledge of WHO 2017.

P. Manivannan (✉) · H. Subramanian
Department of Pathology, JIMPER, Puducherry, India
e-mail: prabhu.m@jipmer.edu.in

© Springer Nature Singapore Pte Ltd. 2019
R. Saxena, H. P. Pati (eds.), *Hematopathology*, https://doi.org/10.1007/978-981-13-7713-6_13

13.2 Rationale for Changes in Updated WHO 2017 Classification [1, 8, 12]

1. The groundbreaking revelation of calreticulin (CALR) apart from Janus kinase 2 (JAK2) and myeloproliferative leukemia (MPL) virus as a major driver mutation in ET and PMF, making it customary for this mutation to be included in standard diagnostic protocols with their possible prognostic implications.
2. Hemoglobin (Hb) cutoff for the diagnosis of PV has been lowered (16.5 g/dL for men and 16 g/dL for women from 18.5 g/dL for men and 16.5 g/dL for women) in recognition of entities such as "masked PV." This entity was invariably represented as under-recognized cases of "true PV."
3. The cardinal role of bone marrow (BM) morphology has been emphasized with respect to megakaryocyte number, their morphology, and without reticulin fibrosis. This has prognostic implications particularly in distinguishing true ET from pre-fibrotic PMF (grade 1 reticulin fibrosis) and in PV with borderline Hb.
4. Authentication of "pre-fibrotic PMF" as a distinct entity intermediate between ET and overt PMF is evidenced to have a higher tendency to develop overt MF and/or acute leukemia with lower overall survival (OS). The minor clinical criteria have now been precisely defined, which impact both the diagnosis and prognosis.
5. The colony stimulating factor 3 receptor (CSF3R) oncogenic mutation is strongly associated with CNL.
6. The entity "mastocytosis" is no longer a part of MPNs. High level of evidence obtained from various research suggests that there are novel pathways and recent recognition of newer mutations and that it follows a unique pathobiology distinct from the classic MPNs.

13.3 Revised WHO 2017 Classification and Diagnostic Criteria for MPNs

Table 13.1 lists the updated WHO 2017 classification for MPNs. The chronic phase (CP) of CML can be diagnosed in majority with peripheral blood (PB) morphological findings. This along with molecular techniques like polymerase chain reaction (PCR) or florescence in situ hybridization (FISH) is required for the detection of BCR-ABL1 positivity to confirm this disease entity [1, 2]. After much debate on the requirement of BM in all such cases, WHO 2017 has recommended BM aspiration and biopsy (Fig. 13.1) to be performed in all cases of CML-CP for the evaluation of morphology to confirm the phase of the disease and to ensure adequate material for karyotyping [1, 8]. In the era of targeted therapy with tyrosine kinase inhibitors (TKI), progression to the next higher stage of the disease, particularly accelerated phase (AP) is becoming less common. However, there are no universally accepted criteria for diagnosis. Table 13.2 summarizes the newer WHO 2017 criteria which included a conglomerate of hematologic, morphologic, and CTG parameters for diagnosing CML-AP (Fig. 13.2). Until supported by further studies, there is inclusion of "provisional entity" to look for "response to TKI therapy" [1, 8]. Diagnostic criteria of

Table 13.1 World Health Organization (WHO) 2017 classification of MPNs

Chronic myeloid leukemia (CML), BCR-ABL1-positive
Chronic neutrophilic leukemia (CNL)
Polycythemia vera (PV)
Primary myelofibrosis (PMF), early/pre-fibrotic stage
Primary myelofibrosis (PMF), overt fibrotic stage
Essential thrombocythemia (ET)
Chronic eosinophilic leukemia (CEL), NOS
Myeloproliferative neoplasm (MPN), unclassifiable

MPNs myeloproliferative neoplasms, *BCR-ABL1* breakpoint cluster region-Abelson1, *NOS* not otherwise specified

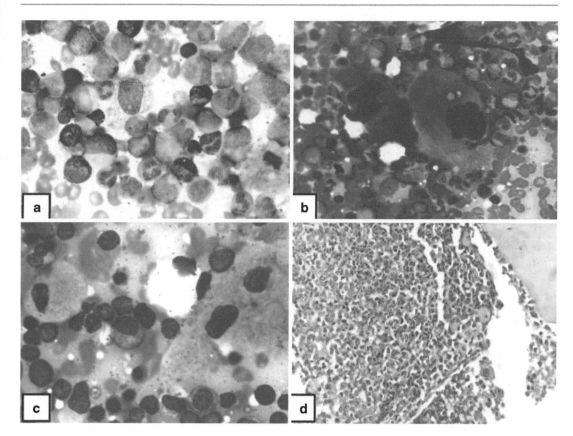

Fig. 13.1 Chronic myeloid leukemia in chronic phase (CML-CP). (**a**) Cellular BM aspirate with myeloid hyperplasia, basophilia, few blasts (<10%), and sea-blue histiocytes (Leishman stain, ×400); (**b**) Another case with dwarf megakaryocytes (Jenner-Giemsa stain, ×400); (**c**) Clusters of pseudo-Gaucher cells (Jenner-Giemsa stain, ×400); (**d**) Hypercellular BM biopsy showing myeloid hyperplasia with full range of maturation (H & E stain, ×100)

Table 13.2 WHO 2017 criteria for diagnosing CML-accelerated phase (AP)

Hematological criteria	Cytogenetics (CTG)	Response to TKI therapy
Persistent or increasing TLC >10 × 10^9/L unresponsive to therapy	Additional clonal chromosomal abnormalities that include major route abnormalities	Hematologic resistance to the first TKI
Persistent or increasing splenomegaly unresponsive to therapy	Second Ph chromosome	Failure to achieve a complete hematologic response[a] to the first TKI
Persistent thrombocytosis >1000 × 10^9/L unresponsive to therapy	Trisomy 8, 19 Isochromosome17q	Any hematological, CTG, or molecular indications of resistance to two sequential TKIs
Persistent thrombocytopenia <100 × 10^9/L unrelated to therapy	Complex karyotype	Occurrence of two or more mutations in BCR-ABL1 during TKI therapy
≥20% basophils in peripheral blood	New clonal chromosomal abnormality in Ph+ cells during therapy	
10–19% blasts in the peripheral blood and/or bone marrow	Abnormalities of 3q26.2	

Large clusters or sheets of small, abnormal megakaryocytes, associated with marked reticulin or collagen fibrosis in biopsy specimens may be considered as presumptive evidence of AP

CML chronic myeloid leukemia, *TLC* total leukocyte count, *Ph* Philadelphia, *TKI* tyrosine kinase inhibitor, *BCR-ABL1* breakpoint cluster region-Abelson1

[a]Complete hematologic response: TLC <10 × 10^9/L, platelet count <450 × 10^9/L, no immature granulocytes in the differential, and spleen non-palpable

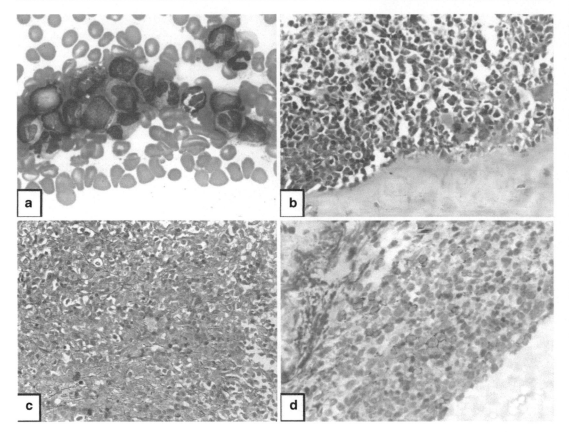

Fig. 13.2 Chronic myeloid leukemia in accelerated phase (CML-AP). (**a**) Peripheral smear showing hyperleukocytosis with myeloid bulge, increased blasts (10–20%), and basophilia (Jenner-Giemsa stain, ×400); (**b**) Hypercellular BM biopsy showing paratrabecular increase in blasts (H & E stain, ×400); (**c**) Reticulin stain (×400) showing WHO grade 2 myelofibrosis; (**d**) Immunohistochemistry (IHC) for CD34 (×400) highlighting increase in blasts

blast phase (BP) remain the same, which require either at least 20% blasts in the PB or BM or the presence of an extramedullary accumulation of blasts. It is emphasized that additional laboratory and genetic studies should be done in all cases. This is particularly important because of rapid onset of disease in an impending lymphoid BP (Fig. 13.3) whenever lymphoblasts are seen in PB or BM [8].

There have been major changes in BCR-ABL negative MPNs. Table 13.3 highlights the major and minor criteria for the diagnosis of PV, ET, pre-fibrotic, and overt stages of PMF. Tables 13.4 and 13.5 list the WHO grading for myelofibrosis (MF) and the diagnostic criteria for CNL, respectively [1, 8].

13.4 Driver Mutations and Their Clinical Significance

High-resolution genomic analysis using microarray and NGS determined the genetic framework of MPNs. There are three mutually exclusive MPN-restricted driver mutations, namely JAK2, CALR, and MPL located on chromosome 9p24, chromosome 19p13.2, and chromosome 1p34, respectively. They abnormally activate the cytokine receptor/JAK2 pathway, resulting in activation of downstream effectors including the signal transducers and activators of transcription (STATs), which lead to cellular proliferation [3, 7, 13, 14]. These driver mutations are discussed in detail in the following section.

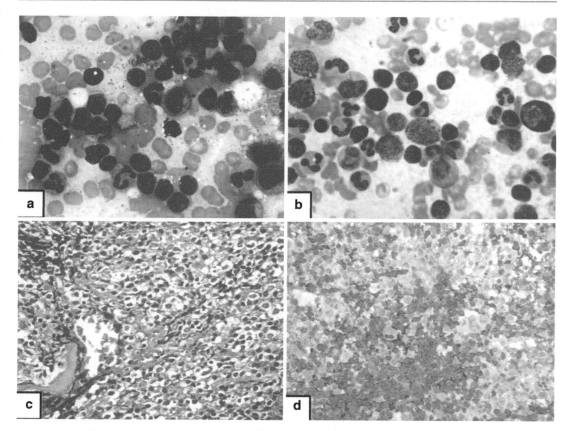

Fig. 13.3 Chronic myeloid leukemia in lymphoid blast crisis (CML-BC). (**a** and **b**) BM aspirate showing 30% lymphoblasts along with myeloid precursors (Jenner- Giemsa stain, ×400); (**c**) BM biopsy showing infiltration by immature cells (H & E stain, ×400); (**d**) These immature cells showed positivity for TdT (IHC stain, ×400)

13.4.1 CALR Mutations

A significant breakthrough occurred in 2013 when two independent group of researchers had identified a novel mutation that had completely revolutionized the basic concepts of MPNs and their pathobiology [3, 4]. They identified somatic mutation in *CALR* gene particularly in patients with ET or PMF who were negative for JAK2 V617F and MPL. This had laid down the foundation for the revised classification of MPNs. This gene produces a multifunctional CALR protein present in endoplasmic reticulum (ER). Its main function is that it acts as a molecular chaperone that ensures appropriate folding of newly synthesized glycoproteins and modulates calcium homeostasis. It has been implicated in cellular proliferation and apoptosis in other sites [7].

CALR has three main structural and functional domains. They are the lectin binding domain present in the N-terminus, a proline-rich P domain, and the most important acidic domain seen in the C-terminus. The nonmutant CALR C-terminal is largely negatively charged that contains multiple calcium-binding sites and also KDEL motif which are essential for binding to the ER. All mutant CALR proteins share a loss of 27 amino acid sequence and KDEL motif, resulting in positively charged amino acids in the C-terminus [3, 4, 15]. Consequently, they have impaired calcium binding function and altered subcellular localization [15].

This results in constitutive activation of receptor signaling through an abnormal interaction with MPL and subsequently causes dimerization and activation of JAK2 kinases [13]. Based on these findings, a potentially new approach using TPO-R (MPL) antagonists was tried in PMF patients [16].

Majority (84%) of the patients with CALR mutation possess either a 52-bp deletion (type 1)

Table 13.3 WHO 2017 diagnostic criteria for PV, ET, overt, and pre-fibrotic stage of PMF

		Polycythemia vera (PV)[a]	Essential thrombocythemia (ET)[b]	Overt primary myelofibrosis (PMF)[c]	Pre-fibrotic primary myelofibrosis (pre-PMF)[d]
Major criteria for diagnosis	1. Clinical criteria	Hemoglobin (Hb) >16.5 g/dL (men) >16 g/dL (women) (or) hematocrit (Hct) >49% (men) >48% (women) (or) 25% increase in RBC mass above mean normal predicted value	Platelet count 450 × 10⁹/L		
	2. BM morphology	Hypercellular BM with trilineage growth (panmyelosis) with pleomorphic and mature megakaryocytes	BM showing proliferation mainly of the megakaryocytic lineage with increased numbers of enlarged and mature megakaryocytes with hyperlobulated nuclei. No significant increase or left shift in granulopoiesis or erythropoiesis Minor (grade 1) increase in reticulin fibers	BM showing megakaryocytic proliferation and atypia accompanied by reticulin or collagen fibrosis $\geq$ grade 2	BM showing megakaryocytic proliferation and atypia accompanied by reticulin fibrosis < grade 1 Increased marrow cellularity and granulocytic proliferation with often decreased erythropoiesis
	3. Genetics	Presence of JAK2 mutation (or) exon 12 mutation	Presence of JAK2, CALR, or MPL mutation	Presence of JAK2, CALR, or MPL mutation (or) presence of another clonal marker (or) absence of evidence for reactive reticulin fibrosis	Presence of JAK2, CALR, or MPL mutation (or) presence of another clonal marker (or) absence of evidence for reactive reticulin fibrosis
	4. Others		Not meeting WHO criteria for CML, PV, PMF, MDS, or other myeloid neoplasm	Not meeting WHO criteria for CML, PV, PMF, MDS, or other myeloid neoplasm	Not meeting WHO criteria for CML, PV, PMF, MDS, or other myeloid neoplasm

Table 13.3 (continued)

		Polycythemia vera (PV)[a]	Essential thrombocythemia (ET)[b]	Overt primary myelofibrosis (PMF)[c]	Pre-fibrotic primary myelofibrosis (pre-PMF)[d]
Minor criteria	1	Subnormal serum EPO level	Presence of another clonal marker (or) absence of evidence for reactive thrombocytosis	Anemia	Anemia
	2			Leukocytosis >11 × 10⁹/L	Leukocytosis >11 × 10⁹/L
	3			Palpable splenomegaly	Palpable splenomegaly
	4			Increase in serum LDH	Increase in serum LDH
	5			LE blood picture	

BM bone marrow, *JAK2* Janus kinase 2, *CALR* calreticulin, *MPL* myeloproliferative leukemia, *CML* chronic myeloid leukemia, *MDS* myelodysplastic syndromes, *EPO* erythropoietin, *LDH* lactate dehydrogenase, *LE* leukoerythroblastosis

[a]Diagnosis of PV requires meeting all three major criteria or the first two major criteria and one minor criterion. Major criterion 2 (BM biopsy) may not be required in patients with sustained absolute erythrocytosis (Hb >18.5 g/dL in men or >16.5 g/dL in women and Hct >55.5% in men or >49.5% in women), if major criterion 3 and the minor criterion are present. However, BM biopsy is recommended because 20% of PV cases may show myelofibrosis at diagnosis, and this predicts rapid progression to overt PMF

[b]Diagnosis of ET requires meeting all four major criteria or first three major criteria and one minor criterion

[c]Diagnosis of PMF requires meeting all three major criteria and at least one minor criterion

[d]Diagnosis of pre-fibrotic PMF requires meeting all three major criteria and at least one minor criterion

Table 13.4 Semiquantitative grading of bone marrow fibrosis (WHO 2017)

Grading	Interpretation
MF-0	Scattered linear reticulin with no intersections (crossovers) corresponding to normal BM
MF-1	Loose network of reticulin with many intersections, especially in perivascular areas
MF-2	Diffuse and dense increase in reticulin with extensive intersections, occasionally with focal bundles of thick fibers mostly consistent with collagen, and/or focal osteosclerosis[a]
MF-3	Diffuse and dense increase in reticulin with extensive intersections and coarse bundles of thick fibers consistent with collagen, usually associated with osteosclerosis[a]

MF marrow fibrosis, fiber density should be assessed only in hematopoietic areas

[a]In grades MF-2 or MF-3, an additional trichrome stain is recommended

or a 5-bp deletion (type 2) residing in exon 9, while the rest are categorized into type-1-like and type-2-like mutations according to their molecular profile. CALR mutations are commonly heterozygous; however, homozygous mutations also occur [17]. In ET, CALR type 1 and 2 mutations account for 46% and 38%, respectively, whereas in PMF, they account for 25% and 35%, respectively [3, 4, 17–19]. The clinico-hematological presentation varies with the two types of mutations which are highlighted in Table 13.6 [17, 18].

13.4.2 JAK2 and MPL Mutations

The most common mutation JAK2 V617F (exon 14) activates all three major myeloid cytokine receptors namely erythropoietin (EPO) receptor, granulocyte-colony stimulating factor (G-CSF)

Table 13.5 WHO 2017 diagnostic criteria for chronic neutrophilic leukemia (CNL)

1. *Peripheral blood findings:*
   Peripheral blood WBC $\geq 25 \times 10^9/L$
   Segmented neutrophils plus band forms $\geq 80\%$ of white blood cells
   Neutrophil precursors (promyelocytes, myelocytes, and metamyelocytes) $<10\%$ of WBC
   Myeloblasts rarely observed
   Monocyte count $<1 \times 10^9/L$
   No dysgranulopoiesis

2. *Bone marrow findings:*
   Hypercellular bone marrow
   Neutrophil granulocytes increased in percentage and number
   Neutrophil maturation appears normal
   Myeloblasts $<5\%$ of nucleated cells

3. Not meeting WHO criteria for *BCR-ABL1*-positive CML, PV, ET, or PMF

4. No rearrangement of *PDGFRA*, *PDGFRB* or *FGFR1*, or *PCM1-JAK2*

5. Presence of *CSF3R* T618I or other activating *CSF3R* mutation or in the absence of a *CSFR3R* mutation, persistent neutrophilia defined by a duration of at least 3 months, splenomegaly, and no identifiable cause of reactive neutrophilia including absence of a plasma cell neoplasm or, if present, demonstration of clonality of myeloid cells by cytogenetic or molecular studies

PDGFRA and *PDGFRB* platelet-derived growth factor receptor A and B, *FGFR1* fibroblastic growth factor receptor 1, *CSF3R* colony-stimulating factor 3 receptor

receptor and MPL and hence leads to PV, ET or PMF. There is also evidence that negative regulators of JAK-STAT signaling pathway such as LNK, c-CBL, SOCS are somatically inactivated in MPNs [20]. Among the major driver mutations, JAK2 V617F mutations are recognized in 95–97% of PV, 50–60% of ET and 40–50% of PMF. In the remaining smaller proportion of PV cases, exon 12 mutation and very rarely CBL or LNK mutations are documented [1, 13, 17].

MPL gene encodes for the TPO-R MPL, when activated after binding with their ligand, downstream signaling pathway gets activated through JAK2 which is essential for megakaryopoiesis. Various gain-of-function mutations are documented, of which the most common is MPL W515L mutation, characteristically occurring in 4–5% of ET and 5–10% of PMF cases [21]. Novel mutations have been documented in both JAK2 and MPL genes to prove clonality through whole exome sequencing (WES); however their feasibility of application in routine clinical practice is yet to be determined [6]. The phenotypic correlation of CALR, JAK2 and MPL in prognostication and their therapeutic implications in MPNs [16–18, 21] are highlighted in Table 13.6.

13.4.3 Triple Negative MPNs

About 10–15% of ET and PMF do not carry any of these mutually exclusive CALR, JAK2, and MPL mutations and are referred to as "triple negative (TN)" MPNs. New somatic mutation variants (JAK2 and MPL) have been described in these patients [3–6, 22]. To document clonality as well as to prognosticate in such cases, one should look for other somatic mutations such as *ASXL1*, *EZH2*, *TET2*, *IDH 1/2*, *SRSF2*, and *SF3B1* genes. If all these markers are negative, strong possibilities of reactive conditions are to be kept in mind and a closer hematologic follow-up is warranted [23]. Also, myelodysplastic syndrome with fibrosis (MDS-F), considered as a close differential possibility for TN-PMF, usually presents with profound cytopenia, less commonly leukoerythroblastosis and splenomegaly, dysplasia in erythroid (90% vs. 34%) and myeloid (77% vs. 6%) series, and less circulating CD34 cells [24].

13.4.4 CSF3R Mutation

The clonal nature of CNL was confirmed in 2013 through the demonstration of novel mutations in

Table 13.6 Phenotypic and clinical correlates of driver mutations

Driver mutations	PV	ET	PMF
JAK2	Higher Hb, higher TLC, and lower platelet count Higher risk of thrombosis, lower thrombosis-free survival rate than in CALR	Higher Hb, higher TLC, and lower platelet count Higher risk of thrombosis, lower thrombosis-free survival rate than in CALR	Higher Hb, higher TLC, and lower platelet count Poor prognosis
MPL	Higher risk of thrombosis, lower thrombosis-free survival rate than in CALR	Higher risk of thrombosis, lower thrombosis-free survival rate than in CALR	
CALR type 1	Lower WBC count, higher platelet count than in JAK2 Longer OS than in JAK2/MPL (very rare)	Older male patients Significant thrombocytosis, an accelerated development into MF-like disease	Good prognosis
CALR type 2	Lower WBC count, higher platelet count than in JAK2 Longer OS than in JAK2/MPL (very rare)	Milder phenotype Less thrombocytosis, less likely to evolve	Higher TLC and higher circulating blasts Poorer prognosis
TN MPNs			Very poor prognosis

JAK2 Janus kinase 2, *MPL* myeloproliferative leukemia, *CALR* calreticulin, *PV* polycythemia vera, *ET* essential thrombocythemia, *PMF* primary myelofibrosis, *TN MPNs* triple negative myeloproliferative neoplasms, *Hb* hemoglobin, *TLC* total leukocyte count, *OS* overall survival

the *CSF3R* gene located on chromosome 1p34.3 which encodes for G-CSF. Two types of mutations occur: one in the extracellular domain and the other in the cytoplasmic domain, leading to truncation of the cytoplasmic domain. This eventually results in ligand-independent activation of CSF3R that further initiates downstream signaling through JAK2. The presence of CSF3R T618I or other membrane proximal CSF3R mutations are documented in variable frequency (59–100%) in CNL cases [25–27]. However, it is emphasized that in routine practice; CNL is extremely rare and one should be cautious in avoiding unnecessary molecular testing for these mutations in routine neutrophilia workup.

13.4.5 Other Somatic Mutations in MPNs

Various novel somatic mutations are being documented in MPNs which is now possible by simultaneous profiling of various genes by using NGS. These mutations can involve spliceosomes (SF3B1, U2AF1, and SRSF2), and genes involved in epigenetics modification (TET2, DNMT3A, EZH2, IDH1/2, and ASXL1) [10, 23]. These genes negatively regulate the JAK2 activation via the TPO receptor and are shown to be mutated in all MPNs at a low frequency (10–15%), predominantly found in PMF. These are also found in other myeloid malignancies and hence not specific for MPNs [23].

They are primarily background non-driver mutations; some are involved in early phase of MPNs (ASXL1) and others in disease progression (LNK, TET2, IDH1/2, and DNMT3A). By a higher frequency of some mutations in PMF and post-ET/PV MF, ASXL1 might predict disease progression in PV and ET patients. Mutations in DNMT3A and other transcription factors such as TP53, IKZF1, ETV6, and RUNX1 are associated with progression to acute myeloid leukemia (AML) [10, 23].

13.5   Approach to Integrated Clinicopathological Diagnosis of MPN (WHO 2017)

The holistic approach to the diagnosis of MPNs with revised WHO 2017 criteria requires integration of clinical features with careful exclusion of all reactive conditions, assessment of BM morphology, CTG, and other molecular techniques [1, 8]. These features are highlighted in the following sections.

13.5.1 Reactive Conditions Mimicking MPNs

In clinical practice, reactive conditions are far more common than MPNs particularly if patients presented with unilineage proliferation manifesting as isolated erythrocytosis, leukocytosis, or thrombocytosis. On the contrary, one can reasonably start with BM analysis or molecular tests if patient presented with multilineage proliferation where MPNs are more likely [28].

In patients with isolated erythrocytosis, secondary causes include smoking, high altitude, cardiorespiratory diseases (by spO_2, chest radiographs, electrocardiography, echocardiography, and pulmonary function tests), liver and renal disorders (by ultrasound), and sleep studies in selected patients by polysomnography. Following this, serum EPO level should be assessed which is usually elevated in secondary acquired causes and also in high affinity Hb and its variants. Very rarely, primary congenital familial erythrocytosis should be considered if low EPO level is detected, which occurs due to mutation in EPO receptor gene. The reason for inclusion of EPO level as minor criterion is that normal/elevated level does not rule out a few PV cases provided Hb level is above the cutoff with the presence of JAK2 muta-

tion and with consistent BM morphology [1, 8, 10, 28].

In patients with neutrophilia, infectious and inflammatory conditions should be ruled out before considering CNL (Table 13.5) [25–27]. Leukemoid reaction is considered in an appropriate clinical setting along with the presence of raised leukocyte alkaline phosphatase (LAP) score which helps to differentiate from CML [1, 2]. Similarly in cases with eosinophilia, infections particularly helminths and parasites (stool for ova and cyst), inflammatory conditions, skin diseases, paraneoplastic conditions, and other malignancies should be ruled out. In particular, mutation testing for PDGFRA and PDGFRB, FGFR1, and recently added PCM1-JAK2 should be considered before labeling these patients as CEL, NOS (Fig. 13.4) [1, 2, 8]. In monocytosis, after ruling out infection and inflammation-related causes, an approach to determine a neoplastic cause should be undertaken [1] as shown in Figs. 13.5 and 13.6. PB basophilia warrants an active workup for CML [1], and one should proceed further as shown in Figs. 13.5 and 13.6.

In patients with isolated thrombocytosis, secondary causes such as iron deficiency anemia, infections, inflammatory states, postsurgery bleeding, malignancies, and drug-induced thrombocytosis are to be ruled out [1, 2, 8]. Although extremely rare, aberrant megakaryocyte stimulation due to either mutation in TPO or its receptor MPL is documented in inherited thrombocythemia [29].

13.5.2 BM Morphology

BM biopsy has an indispensable role in MPNs that has been reemphasized in the WHO 2017 [1, 8]. The main morphologic criteria for MPN diagnosis are shown in Table 13.3 and Figs. 13.1, 13.2, 13.3, 13.4, 13.7, 13.8, 13.9,

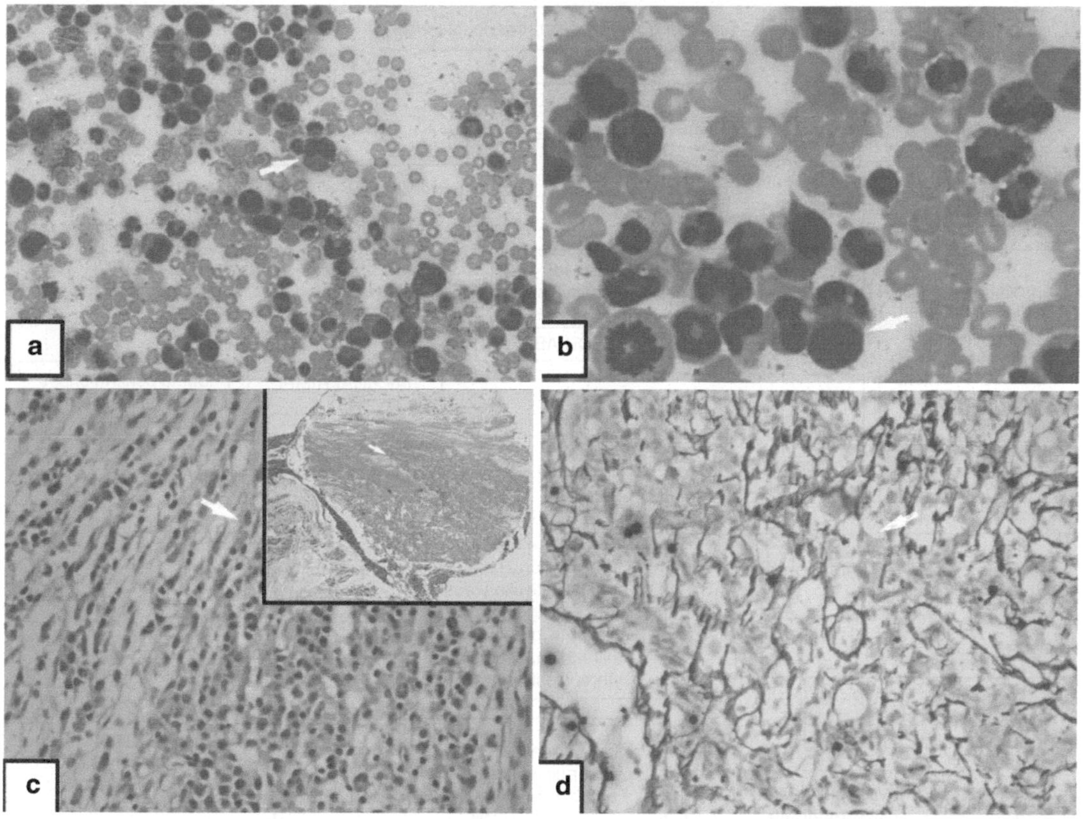

Fig. 13.4 Chronic eosinophilic leukemia, not otherwise specified (CEL, NOS). (**a**) Cellular BM aspirate from a patient who presented with sudden onset paraplegia showing myeloid hyperplasia with marrow eosinophilia (Jenner-Giemsa stain, ×100); (**b**) High-power view (Jenner-Giemsa stain, ×400) showing abnormal ring mitosis, increased eosinophils and arrow pointing a blast; (**c**) BM biopsy showed streaming of cells with marrow eosinophilia (H & E stain, ×400) with inset showing focal myelonecrosis; (**d**) Reticulin stain (×400) showing WHO grade 2 myelofibrosis

13.10, and 13.11. It has major role in (1) identification of "masked PV" with lower Hb levels; (2) distinguishing ET from pre-fibrotic PMF; (3) distinction between pre-fibrotic PMF and overt PMF based on grading of BM fibrosis (Table 13.4); and (4) diagnosing "TN" MPNs.

The "masked PV" is the terminology used for patients with Hb levels between 16 and 18.4 g/dL for males and 15 and 16.4 g/dL for females. These patients have BM morphology consistent with PV like hypercellular for age, panmyelosis, and mature megakaryocytes having pleomorphism, but Hb levels are below the defined threshold in WHO 2008 classification [2, 8]. In particular, if these patients have JAK2 negativity, they are at increased risk for progression to secondary MF and AML and also show inferior OS when compared to classical PV. It should also be noted that up to 20% of PV cases may have grade 1 fibrosis at diagnosis (Fig. 13.7); they are associated with higher risk of secondary MF [28, 30]. This underscores the

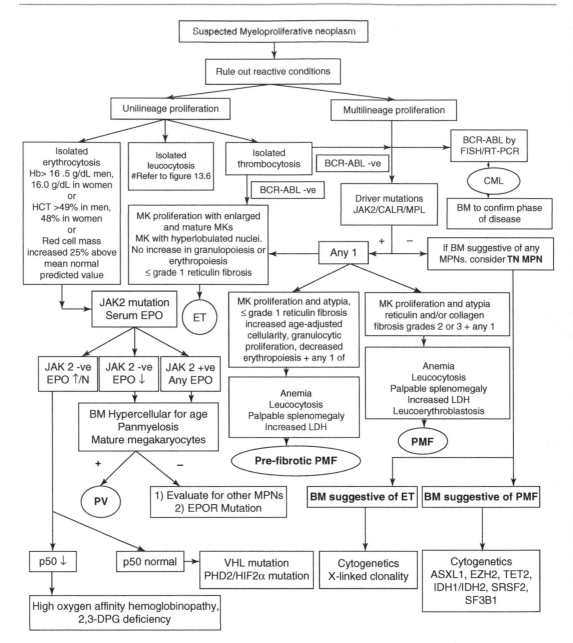

Fig. 13.5 Approach to an integrated clinicopathological diagnosis of suspected myeloproliferative neoplasms

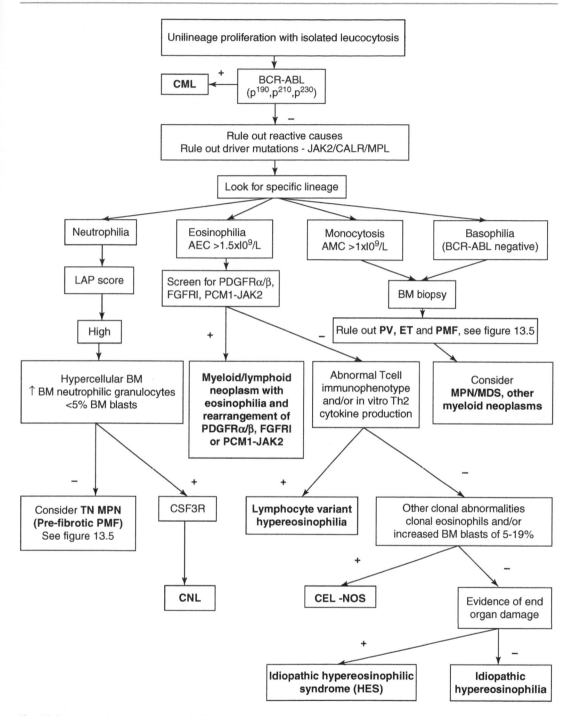

Fig. 13.6 Approach to an integrated clinicopathological diagnosis of patients having unilineage proliferation with isolated leukocytosis

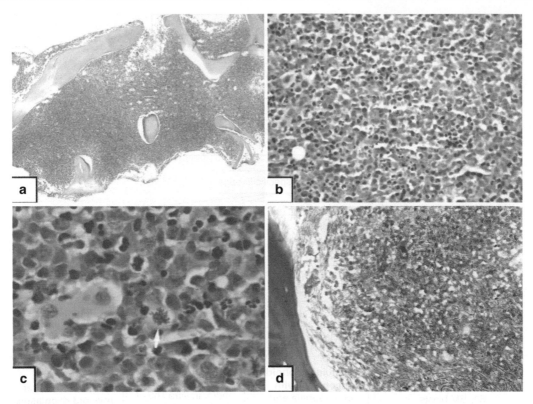

Fig. 13.7 Polycythemia vera. (**a**) BM is hypercellular for age (H & E stain, ×40); (**b**) Panmyelosis (H & E stain, ×100); (**c**) Mature megakaryocytes with arrow pointing typical mitosis (H & E stain, ×400); (**d**) Reticulin stain (×400) with WHO grade 1 myelofibrosis

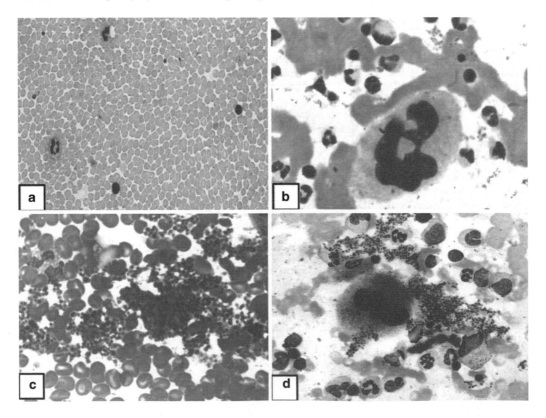

importance of bringing down the Hb threshold, so that these patients are given appropriate management.

Both ET (Figs. 13.8 and 13.9) and pre-fibrotic PMF are usually difficult to differentiate on clinical presentations because of overlapping features. Their distinction is very important not only because of increased risk of disease progression in the latter but also due to inferior OS. Table 13.7 highlights the features that are helpful in distinguishing these entities [1, 2, 8]. The semiquantitative grading of BM fibrosis becomes critical in WHO 2017 classification,

because grade 1 or less fibrosis is seen in ET and pre-fibrotic PMF, whereas grade 2 and 3 fibrosis along with megakaryocytic atypia is noted in overt PMF (Figs. 13.10 and 13.11) [1]. BM morphology gains its significance in yet another condition called as "TN" MPN, where cellularity may be increased showing proliferation of one or more lineages with or without megakaryocytic atypia and/or BM fibrosis. This condition warrants additional investigations like CTG and molecular techniques specifically to look for other somatic mutations to document the clonality [5, 6, 23].

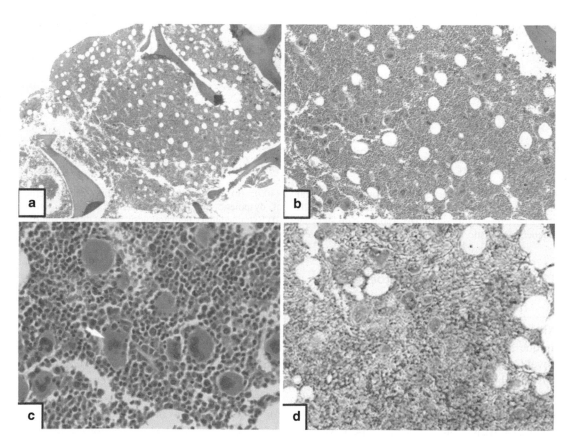

Fig. 13.9 Essential thrombocythemia. (**a**) Normocellular BM (H & E stain, ×40); (**b**) Prominence of megakaryocytes (H & E stain, ×100); (**c**) Mature megakaryocytes with hyperlobulated nuclei (arrow, H & E stain, ×400) and no significant increase in erythropoiesis or granulopoiesis; (**d**) Reticulin stain (×400) with WHO grade 0 myelofibrosis

Fig. 13.8 Polycythemia vera. (**a**) Peripheral smear (PS) is polycythemic with normal counts (Leishman stain, ×400); (**b**) BM aspirate showing increased marrow cellularity with normal marrow components, full range of maturation and mature megakaryocytes (Jenner-Giemsa stain, ×400); Essential thrombocythemia. (**c**) PS showing thrombocytosis with platelet anisocytosis and many clumps (Jenner-Giemsa stain, ×400); (**d**) BM aspirate showing increased mature megakaryocytes, many of which are caught up in platelet clumps (Jenner-Giemsa stain, ×400)

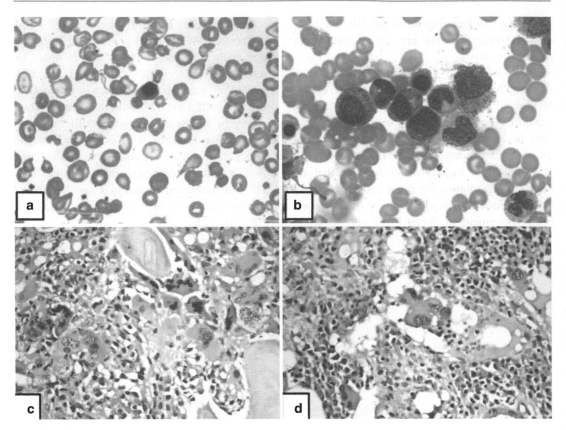

Fig. 13.10 Overt primary myelofibrosis. (**a**) Peripheral smear showing tear drop cells and nucleated red cells (Jenner-Giemsa stain, ×400); (**b**) Another case showing leukoerythroblastic blood picture (Jenner-Giemsa stain, ×400); (**c**) BM biopsy showing abnormal clustering of dyspoietic megakaryocytes (H & E stain, ×400); (**d**) Extramedullary hematopoiesis within dilated sinusoid (H & E stain, ×400)

13.5.3 Role of Immunohistochemistry (IHC)

All pathogenic CALR mutations produce a unique alternative reading frame, resulting in a novel C-terminus, against which antibody can be raised and used for IHC. Hence, whenever genotyping for CALR mutations is not possible, IHC with an antibody specifically directed against mutated CALR along with wild-type CALR as control can be used in clinical practice [31].

13.5.4 Molecular Testing

The National Comprehensive Cancer Network (NCCN) [32] and the European LeukemiaNet (ELN) [33] have come up with the recommendations and guidelines that incorporated the mandatory molecular testing not only for the diagnosis but also for appropriate treatment decisions especially when CML patients are treated with TKI. The qualitative techniques like FISH or reverse transcriptase (RT) PCR are recommended for diagnosis, whereas quantitative tests such as real-time quantitative (RQ) PCR are for monitoring. In order to have uniformity throughout the world as well as for standardization, the international reporting scale (IS) was introduced [34]. The time frame for molecular monitoring slightly differs between NCCN and ELN in order to achieve major molecular response. Mutation testing is also recommended if there is loss of previously achieved response or progression of the disease while patient is on TKI [32, 33].

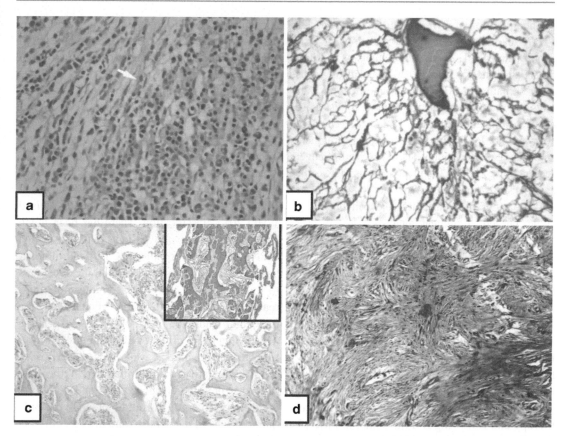

Fig. 13.11 Overt primary myelofibrosis. (**a**) Arrow showing streaming of hematopoietic cells (H & E stain, ×100); (**b**) Reticulin stain (×400) showing WHO grade 2 myelofibrosis; (**c**) Osteomyelosclerosis (H & E stain, ×400) in another case with inset showing reticulin grade 3 myelofibrosis; (**d**) Masson trichrome stain (×400) with WHO grade 3 myelofibrosis

Table 13.7 Differences between pre-fibrotic PMF and ET

Clinico-hematologic parameters	Pre-fibrotic PMF	ET
Clinical features	Higher incidence of palpable splenomegaly	Lower incidence of organomegaly
PB findings	Low Hb, leukocytosis, higher LDH, circulating CD34 cells	Higher Hb, polymorphous platelets with bizarre forms
BM morphology	1. Higher age-matched BM cellularity 2. Megakaryocytes show distinct nuclear features such as hypolobation, hyperchromatic, clumsy cloud-like, with maturation defects and aberrant nucleo-cytoplasmic ratio; seen in dense clusters and endosteal translocation of megakaryocytes (3) Granulocyte proliferation (4) Erythroid suppression with left shift	Predominantly large to giant mature megakaryocytes with hyperlobulated nuclei in a randomly arranged/loosely arranged clusters without significant dyspoiesis
Reticulin fibrosis	Nil or <5% grade 1 fibrosis	<5% grade 1 fibrosis
Complications and disease progression	Lower risk of bleeding complications	Survive up to 7 years longer than pre-fibrotic PMF, lower risk of progression to acute leukemia/high grade MF, superior overall survival

PMF primary myelofibrosis, *ET* essential thrombocythemia, *Hb* hemoglobin, *LDH* lactate dehydrogenase

Incorporation of driver mutations such as JAK2 V617F exon 14 and exon 12 mutations, CALR exon 9, and MPL exon 10 mutations as a major diagnostic criterion in WHO 2017 and also various other somatic mutations for prognostication warrants the use and knowledge of these robust diagnostic testing modalities [1, 2, 5, 7, 8]. They are conventional PCR-based assays, namely fragment analysis, gel electrophoresis, PCR with Sanger sequencing of which fragment analysis PCR is the easiest, least time consuming, and less expensive with considerable sensitivity, and can quantitate allele burden. Fragment analysis can however only detect indels and not point mutations. Pyrosequencing, allele-specific quantitative PCR (AS-qPCR) and digital droplet PCR not only detect target mutations but also are quantitative and highly sensitive. AS-PCR is recommended by ELN for JAK2 V617F testing and has been widely adopted.

The advantage of quantitating mutant allele burden would aid in predicting the risk of thrombosis in PV and ET. It also helps in assessing OS, monitoring treatment response, for detecting minimal residual disease during JAK2 inhibitor therapy and following BM transplant in PMF [5, 23]. Because of rarity of JAK2 exon 12 mutations and the variation of the mutant allele burden, it is difficult to choose an appropriate diagnostic test [35].

The maiden discovery of CALR exon 9 mutations was done through whole genome sequencing, a form of NGS technique, which is considered the most sensitive assay available at present. The length of the fragments in the wild-type, type 1, and type 2 CALR mutations are 357, 302, and 272 bp, respectively [3–5, 23]. But in routine molecular diagnosis, testing by fragment analysis yields comparable sensitivity as a screening test and should further be tested by Sanger sequencing in order to identify the exact nature of the mutation [5, 15]. Recently developed multiplex AS-PCR is available that detects four most common MPL exon 10 mutations (W515L, W515K, W515A, and S505N) with 100% specificity and 2.5% sensitivity. However, for allele burden and low-level mutation detection, AS-qPCR methods are required [5]. Finally to ensure the maximum

clinical utility and to maintain high performance of all testing laboratories, participation in external quality assurance program is recommended [5]. The integrated approach to the diagnosis of MPNs and especially in patients with leukocytosis are shown in Figs. 13.5 and 13.6, respectively.

13.6 Conclusion

The integrated approach to the diagnosis of MPNs is further validated and retained in revised WHO 2017 classification. There has been much emphasis given to the patients with suspected MPNs that BM morphology, CTG, and molecular studies are recommended in all these patients to look for driver and other somatic mutations, reaffirming the monumental changes in the molecular landscape of MPNs [1–10, 23]. These newer diagnostic criteria will be applied in routine clinical practice as well as in clinical trials, so as to identify their limitations in the near future. At present, advanced techniques like NGS are difficult to apply in routine practice not only due to issues in availability and affordability but also in standardization particularly in our country. Therefore, it is recommended to have continual education, training, and inter-laboratory participation in liaison with the regional referral laboratories, particularly for the standardization of BM morphology reporting patterns as well as molecular techniques in the era of targeted therapies, especially in MPNs [23, 28].

Conflict of Interest Nil.

References

1. Swerdlow SH, Campo E, Harris NL, Jaffe ES, Pileri SA, Stein H, Thiele J, Vardiman JW, editors. WHO classification of tumours of haematopoietic and lymphoid tissues. Lyon: International Agency for Research on Cancer; 2017.
2. Swerdlow SH, Campo E, Harris NL, Jaffe ES, Pileri SA, Stein H, Thiele J, Vardiman JW, editors. WHO classification of tumours of haematopoietic and lymphoid tissues. Lyon: International Agency for Research on Cancer; 2008.

3. Nangalia J, Massie CE, Baxter EJ, Nice FL, Gundem G, Wedge DC, et al. Somatic CALR mutations in myeloproliferative neoplasms with nonmutated JAK2. N Engl J Med. 2013;369:2391–405.

4. Klampfl T, Gisslinger H, Harutyunyan AS, Nivarthi H, Rumi E, Milosevic JD, et al. Somatic mutations of calreticulin in myeloproliferative neoplasms. N Engl J Med. 2013;369:2379–90.

5. Langabeer SE, Andrikovics H, Asp J, Bellosillo B, Carillo S, Haslam K, et al. Molecular diagnostics of myeloproliferative neoplasms. Eur J Haematol. 2015;95:270–9.

6. Milosevic Feenstra JD, Nivarthi H, Gisslinger H, Leroy E, Rumi E, Chachoua I, et al. Whole-exome sequencing identifies novel MPL and JAK2 mutations in triple-negative myeloproliferative neoplasms. Blood. 2016;127:325–32.

7. Kim Y, Park J, Jo I, Lee GD, Kim J, Kwon A, et al. Genetic–pathologic characterization of myeloproliferative neoplasms. Exp Mol Med. 2016;48:e247.

8. Arber DA, Orazi A, Hasserjian R, Thiele J, Borowitz MJ, Beau MML, et al. The 2016 revision to the World Health Organization classification of myeloid neoplasms and acute leukemia. Blood. 2016;127:2391–405.

9. Levine RL, Gilliland DG. Myeloproliferative disorders. Blood. 2008;112:2190–8.

10. Nangalia J, Green TR. The evolving genomic landscape of myeloproliferative neoplasms. Hematology Am Soc Hematol Educ Program. 2014;2014: 287–96.

11. Tefferi A, Vardiman JW. Classification and diagnosis of myeloproliferative neoplasms: the 2008 World Health Organization criteria and point-of-care diagnostic algorithms. Leukemia. 2008;22:14–22.

12. Barbui T, Thiele J, Vannucchi AM, Tefferi A. Rationale for revision and proposed changes of the WHO diagnostic criteria for polycythemia vera, essential thrombocythemia and primary myelofibrosis. Blood Cancer J. 2015;5:e337.

13. Skoda RC, Duek A, Grisouard J. Pathogenesis of myeloproliferative neoplasms. Exp Hematol. 2015;43:599–608.

14. Malherbe JAJ, Fuller KA, Arshad A, Nangalia J, Romeo G, Hall SL, et al. Megakaryocytic hyperplasia in myeloproliferative neoplasms is driven by disordered proliferative, apoptotic and epigenetic mechanisms. J Clin Pathol. 2016;69:155–63.

15. Ha J-S, Kim Y-K. Calreticulin exon 9 mutations in myeloproliferative neoplasms. Ann Lab Med. 2015;35:22–7.

16. Wang X, Haylock D, Hu CS, Kowalczyk W, Jiang T, Qiu J, et al. A thrombopoietin receptor antagonist is capable of depleting myelofibrosis hematopoietic stem and progenitor cells. Blood. 2016;127: 3398–409.

17. Tefferi A, Wassie EA, Guglielmelli P, Gangat N, Belachew AA, Lasho TL, et al. Type 1 versus type 2 calreticulin mutations in essential thrombocythemia: a collaborative study of 1027 patients: type 1 vs. type 2 CALR mutations in ET. Am J Hematol. 2014;89:E121–4.

18. Grinfeld J, Nangalia J, Green AR. Molecular determinants of pathogenesis and clinical phenotype in myeloproliferative neoplasms. Haematologica. 2017;102:7–17.

19. Tefferi A, Thiele J, Vannucchi AM, Barbui T. An overview on CALR and CSF3R mutations and a proposal for revision of WHO diagnostic criteria for myeloproliferative neoplasms. Leukemia. 2014;28: 1407–13.

20. De Freitas RM, da Costa Maranduba CM. Myeloproliferative neoplasms and the JAK/STAT signaling pathway: an overview. Rev Bras Hematol Hemoter. 2015;37:348–53.

21. Vannucchi AM, Antonioli E, Guglielmelli P, Pancrazzi A, Guerini V, Barosi G, et al. Characteristics and clinical correlates of MPL 515W>L/K mutation in essential thrombocythemia. Blood. 2008;112: 844–7.

22. Cabagnols X, Defour J-P, Ugo V, Ianotto JC, Mossuz P, Mondet J, et al. Differential association of calreticulin type 1 and type 2 mutations with myelofibrosis and essential thrombocytemia: relevance for disease evolution. Blood. 2014;124:1823.

23. Shammo JM, Stein BL. Mutations in MPNs: prognostic implications, window to biology, and impact on impact on treatment decisions. Hematology Am Soc Hematol Educ Program. 2016;2016(1):552–60.

24. Della Porta MG, Travaglino E, Boveri E, Ponzoni M, Malcovati L, Papaemmanuil E, et al. Minimal morphological criteria for defining bone marrow dysplasia: a basis for clinical implementation of WHO classification of myelodysplastic syndromes. Leukemia. 2015;29:66–75.

25. Pardanani A, Lasho T, Laborde R, Elliott M, Hanson C, Knudson R, et al. CSF3R T618I is a highly prevalent and specific mutation in chronic neutrophilic leukemia. Leukemia. 2013;27:1870–3.

26. Maxson JE, Gotlib J, Pollyea DA, Fleischman AG, Agarwal A, Eide CA, et al. Oncogenic CSF3R mutations in chronic neutrophilic leukemia and atypical CML. N Engl J Med. 2013;368:1781–90.

27. Ouyang Y, Qiao C, Chen Y, Zhang S-J. Clinical significance of CSF3R, SRSF2 and SETBP1 mutations in chronic neutrophilic leukemia and chronic myelomonocytic leukemia. Oncotarget. 2017;8:20834–41.

28. Passamonti F, Maffioli M. Update from the latest WHO classification of MPNs: a user's manual. Hematology Am Soc Hematol Educ Program. 2016;2016(1):534–42.

29. Plo I, Bellanné-Chantelot C, Mosca M, Mazzi S, Marty C, Vainchenker W. Genetic alterations of the thrombopoietin/MPL/JAK2 axis impacting megakaryopoiesis. Front Endocrinol. 2017;8:234. https://www.ncbi.nlm.nih.gov/pmc/articles/PMC5600916/.

30. Cerquozzi S, Tefferi A. Blast transformation and fibrotic progression in polycythemia vera and

essential thrombocythemia: a literature review of incidence and risk factors. Blood Cancer J. 2015;5:e366.

31. Vannucchi AM, Rotunno G, Bartalucci N, Raugei G, Carrai V, Balliu M, et al. Calreticulin mutation-specific immunostaining in myeloproliferative neoplasms: pathogenetic insight and diagnostic value. Leukemia. 2014;28:1811–8.

32. Mesa RA, Jamieson C, Bhatia R, Deininger MW, Fletcher CD, Gerds AT, et al. NCCN guidelines insights: myeloproliferative neoplasms, version 2.2018. J Natl Compr Cancer Netw. 2017;15:1193–207.

33. Baccarani M, Deininger MW, Rosti G, et al. European LeukemiaNet recommendations for the management of chronic myeloid leukemia: 2013. Blood. 2013;122:872–84.

34. Bauer S, Romvari E. Interpreting molecular monitoring results and international standardization in chronic myeloid Leukemia. J Adv Pract Oncol. 2012;3:151–60.

35. Shivarov V, Ivanova M, Yaneva S, Petkova N, Hadjiev E, Naumova E. Quantitative bead-based assay for detection of JAK2 exon 12 mutations. Leuk Lymphoma. 2013;54:1343–4.

Minimal Residual Disease Assessment in Myeloma

14

Jasmita Dass and Jyoti Kotwal

Multiple myeloma is a neoplastic proliferation of plasma cells that manifests as bone lesions, renal impairment, anaemia and hypercalcaemia [1]. Myeloma constitutes ~1% of all cancers diagnosed and ~13% of all haematological malignancies [2, 3]. Every year, ~86,000 new cases of myeloma are diagnosed [4]. The diagnostic criteria for myeloma were modified in 2017 by the International Myeloma Working Group (IMWG) to include asymptomatic patients with a high risk of progression to symptomatic myeloma within 2 years. These biomarkers were serum free light chain ratio abnormality with involved to uninvolved light chain ratio of >100, clonal plasma cells (PCs) $\geq$60% and presence of $\geq$1 lytic lesions on magnetic resonance imaging (MRI) of $\geq$5 mm in size [1]. The presence of these biomarkers was added to the classical 'CRAB' criteria that include hypercalcaemia, renal impairment, anaemia and bone lesions to form myeloma-defining events [1].

Nearly all myelomas come from a preceding monoclonal gammopathy of undetermined significance (MGUS) [5]. MGUS may be followed by an asymptomatic smouldering stage in which the clonal PC percentage is $\geq$30% and/or the monoclonal M band is $\geq$3 g/dL [1].

14.1 Why Assess Minimal Residual Disease (MRD) in Myeloma?

There has been a consistent improvement in survival in myelomas from <50% in 1980–1989 to ~75% in 2000–2009 [6]. The median overall survival (OS) has improved considerably in the last 15 years. In a series of >1000 myeloma patients diagnosed from 2001 to 2010, it was seen that median OS in patients treated from 2001 to 2005 was ~4.6 years while the median OS in patients treated from 2006 to 2010 was ~6.1 years [7]. The survival pre-2001 era was ~2.5 years [8]. This has been due to a marked improvement in the drug development and discovery with the advent of immunomodulatory agents like thalidomide [9], lenalidomide [10, 11] and bortezomib [3]. Further improvements in myeloma OS are expected with the flurry of new agents approved for treatment like pomalidomide [12], carfilzomib [13], daratumumab [14], elotuzumab [15] and ixazomib [16].

The improvements in OS also stem from higher rates of complete response (CR) and very good partial response (VGPR) [17, 18]. With the current anti-myeloma therapy, ~100% patients achieve an overall response with $\geq$VGPR seen in 80% patients [19–22]. This is in contrast to the

J. Dass ($\boxtimes$) · J. Kotwal
Department of Hematology, Sir Ganga Ram Hospital, New Delhi, India

© Springer Nature Singapore Pte Ltd. 2019
R. Saxena, H. P. Pati (eds.), *Hematopathology*, https://doi.org/10.1007/978-981-13-7713-6_14

earlier anti-myeloma agents which even when combined with autologous stem cell transplantation (ASCT) were able to achieve a ≥VGPR in <50% patients [23, 24]. These consistent improvements pave the need for better response assessment in myeloma to identify patients who do extremely well post ASCT and who will not.

14.2 Response Assessment in Myeloma

IMWG lays down the response assessment criteria for myeloma patients. The IMWG 2006 criteria were centred on the assessments of M bands in serum and urine by the use of serum and 24 h urine protein electrophoreses (SPE and UPE), serum and urine immunofixation electrophoresis (SIFE and UIFE) and bone marrow PC percentage. They divided patients into CR, VGPR, partial response (PR), stable disease (SD) and progressive disease. Patients in CR had a complete absence of M bands in SPE, UPE, SIFE and UIFE together with <5% PC in bone marrow. Patients in VGPR should have had ≥90% reduction in the amount of M band in all the serum and urine studies [25].

This definition will clearly be inadequate when assessing patients treated with immunomodulatory agents and proteasome inhibitors due to high numbers of patients in CR. To address this issue, the IMWG in 2011 gave a new set of response criteria to identify patients within the category of CR who would do better than the rest. The IMWG added serum free light chain ratio and bone marrow immunophenotyping using 2–4 colour flow cytometry to the response evaluation investigations. In addition, they included immunohistochemistry on bone marrow biopsy with an intent to identify clonal PCs. The category of stringent CR (sCR) was added, and this included absence of an abnormal free light chain ratio and ≤5% clonal PCs by either immunohisctochemistry on bone marrow biopsy or 2–4 colour flow cytometry in the bone marrow [26]. It has however been identified that immunohistochemistry may be relatively unreliable as the bone marrow post therapy generally shows regeneration of normal PCs, and this may lead to false-negative

assessment for clonal PCs [27, 28]. In addition, the IMWG 2011 criteria added the categories of immunophenotypic CR and molecular CR for those patients who are negative by 2–4 colour flow cytometry and using allele-specific oligonucleotide-polymerase chain reaction (ASO-PCR), respectively [26].

However, even these definitions were relatively inadequate for the continuing improvements in the OS rates and high rates of sCR achieved with modern anti-myeloma therapy. Minimal residual disease (MRD) in the myeloma patients may exist in the intramedullary location or the extramedullary locations. The last 8–10 years have witnessed a major surge in publications, addressing assessment of intramedullary minimal residual disease (MRD) in myeloma [29–40]. Most of these have used multiparameter flow cytometry (MFC) for MRD detection [29–36] while others have used molecular methods [37–40]. For the detection of extramedullary MRD in myeloma, imaging techniques like functional Magnetic resonance imaging (MRI) [41, 42] and 18-fluorodeoxyglucose positron emission tomography-computed tomography (PET/CT) scan [41, 43, 44] have been used.

14.3 Intramedullary MRD in Myeloma

MFC has been extensively applied to detect MRD in myeloma [29–36, 45–53]. Panels of monoclonal antibodies used by various studies on MRD are given in Table 14.1. As the years advance, the improvement in MFC techniques with the addition of more colours and better software leading to acquisition of more events and better analysis capabilities become visible with high sensitivities achievable with current methods of analysis.

14.3.1 Clinical Utility

Bruno Paiva's group at PETHEMA/GEM (Programa para el Estudio de la Terapéutica en Hemopatías Malignas/Grupo Español de Mieloma) [30, 33, 36, 47] and Andy Rawstron's

Table 14.1 Various panels used for MRD assessment in myeloma

Study (year)	Panel used	Sensitivity (%)
Rawstron et al. (2002) [29]	CD45-FITC/CD38-CECy5/CD138-PE CD45-FITC/CD38-CECy5/CD19-PE CD45-FITC/CD38-CECy5/CD56-PE	0.01
Sarasquete et al. (2005) [39]	CD38-FITC/CD56-PE/CD19-PerCP Cy5.5/CD45-APC CD138-FITC/CD28-PE/CD33-PerCP Cy5.5/CD38-APC CD20-FITC/CD117-PE/CD138-PerCP Cy5.5/CD38-APC	0.01
de Tute et al. (2007) [45]	CyIgλ-FITC/CD19-PE/CyIgκ-PE Cy5/CD38-PE Cy7/CD138-APC/ CD45-APC Cy7	0.01
Paiva et al. (2008) [30]	CD38-FITC/CD56-PE/CD19-PerCP Cy5.5/CD45-APC (only tube applied in 90% patients) CD38-FITC/CD27-PE/CD45-PerCP Cy5.5/CD28-APC β2 micro-FITC/CD81-PE/CD38-PerCP Cy5.5/CD117-APC	0.01
Gupta et al. (2009) [46]	CD19-FITC/CD56-PE/CD38-PerCP Cy5.5/CD138-APC CD45-FITC/CD52-PE/CD38-PerCP Cy5.5/CD138-APC CD20-FITC/CD117-PE/CD38-PerCP Cy5.5/CD138-APC	0.01
Paiva et al. (2011) [33], (2012) [35], (2014) [47]	CD38-FITC/CD56-PE/CD19-PerCP Cy5.5/CD45-APC CD38-FITC/CD27-PE/CD45-PerCP Cy5.5/CD28-APC β2 micro-FITC/CD81-PE/CD38-PerCP Cy5.5/CD117-APC	0.01–0.001
Puig et al. (2014) [40]	CD38-FITC/CD56-PE/CD19-PerCP Cy5.5/CD45-APC CD38-FITC/CD27-PE/CD45-PerCP Cy5.5/CD28-APC β2 micro-FITC/CD81-PE/CD38-PerCP Cy5.5/CD117-APC	0.01–0.001
Rawstron et al. (2013) [34]	CD27-FITC/CD56-PE/CD19-PerCPCy5.5/CD38-PE Cy7/ CD138-APC/CD45-APC Cy7 CD81-FITC/CD117-PE CD52-FITC/CD200-PE	0.01
Robillard et al. (2013) [48]; Rousel et al. (2014) [49]	CD38-HV450/CyIgλ-FITC/CD56+CD28-PE/CD138-PE Cy5/ CD19-PE Cy7/CyIgκ-APC/CD45-APC H7	0.001
Euroflow (2017) [50]	CD138-BV421/CD27-BV510/CD38-FITC/CD56-PE/CD45-PerCP Cy5.5/CD19-PE Cy7/CD117-APC/CD81-APC C750 CD138-BV421/CD27-BV510/CD38-FITC/CD56-PE/CD45-PerCP Cy5.5/CD19-PE Cy7/CyIgκ-APC/CyIgλ-APC C750	0.001
Euroflow (2010) [51]	CD138-BV421/CD27-BV510/CD117-BV605/CD38-FITC/ CD56-PE/CD45-PerCP Cy5.5/CD19-PE Cy7/CyIgλ-APC/ CyIgκ-APC A700/CD81-APC C750	NA
Roshal et al. (2017) [52]; Royston et al. (2017) [53]	CD81 PacBlue/CD38BV510/CD27 BV605/CD117 PerCPCy5.5/ CD19 PECy7/CD138 APC/CD56 APC-R700/CD45 APC-H7	0.001

group at Leeds [29, 34] have generated the most clinical data on MRD in myeloma. Only data from key papers is being presented here.

In the PETHEMA/GEM analysis of trials GEM2000 and GEM2005 >65 years, Paiva et al. showed that in 241 patients in CR at D100 post ASCT, the patients who did not sustain CR at 1 year post ASCT had a poor prognosis. The only two variables that could predict this unsustained CR were high-risk cytogenetic profile and presence of MRD-positive status at D100 post ASCT. Their data gave proof that patients who remain MRD positive at D100 post ASCT do poorly and should be enrolled in trials to intensify therapy or treat MRD-positive status [35]. In another analysis of GEM05 >65 years confined to elderly patients, 102/260 patients achieved at least a PR and were analysed using a serum free light chain assay, immunofixation, and MFC. After six cycles of induction therapy, CR was seen in 43%, sCR in 30% and MRD negative by MFC in 30% of the 102 patients. Patients in sCR when compared with patients in CR did not show any survival advantage while patients who were MRD negative by MFC had a longer progression-free survival (PFS) and time to progression. Seven patients were MRD negative by MFC but were positive on IFE studies, and all of them attained an IFE-negative status on follow-up. In contrast, patients who were MRD positive by MFC but were IFE negative showed early relapses on repeat IFE examinations [33]. In a subsequent series on relapsed myeloma patients, the prognostic impact on time to progression of attaining a MRD-negative status after salvage chemotherapy with or without ASCT could also be demonstrated. Importantly, in this series, MRD status was not useful for patients who underwent allogeneic stem cell transplantation as this was uniformly associated with a poor time to progression [47].

Rawstron in 2013 published the results from Medical Research Council Myeloma IX Study on >600 patients of myeloma who underwent MRD assessment by a six-colour MFC panel at the end of induction therapy with cyclophosphamide, vincristine, doxorubicin and dexamethasone (CVAD) or cyclophosphamide, thalidomide and dexamethasone (CTD) for intensive therapy followed by ASCT or attenuated CTD or melphalan and prednisolone (MP) for non-intensive treatment. The patients underwent bone marrow examination at diagnosis, end of induction and at day 100 (D100) of ASCT procedure, and MFC analysis was performed at all time points. For each tube, minimum 500,000 events were acquired and ≥50 cell cluster with an aberrant immunophenotype was considered abnormal. Of the 397 patients who received ASCT following intensive therapy (62.2%), an MRD-negative status at D100 post ASCT had a significantly longer PFS and OS. In the sub-analysis, patients who were MRD negative at the end of induction before undergoing ASCT had the best PFS, but this benefit was not translated to OS. The favourable impact of MRD negativity on PFS and OS was independent of cytogenetic risk groups with the benefit seen in both favourable and adverse risk groups. When they looked at patients achieving CR, an MRD-negative status was associated with a better OS. There were patients who were MRD negative but not in CR, and these patients were similar to MRD-positive cases. The MRD

negative but not in CR can be possibly explained by the longer half-life of M bands and possibly by patchy distribution of the disease. In a further analysis of patients randomized to receive thalidomide maintenance, it was seen that patients on maintenance thalidomide had higher chances of becoming MRD negative [34]. In a subsequent series from the same patient group, Rawstron et al. demonstrated that a reduction in MRD by each log predicted a better OS. Median OS achieved in ≥10% MRD group was 1 year while the corresponding figures for 1 to <10%, 0.1 to <1% and 0.01 to <0.1% groups were 5.9, 6.8 and >7.5 years, respectively. They concluded that 1-year OS benefit is achieved per log reduction of MRD [54].

Other studies have used molecular methods to assess MRD. Most published evidence is for ASO-PCR [37, 39, 40]. In the Spanish trials of myeloma, patients underwent both ASO-PCR and MFC to assess MRD. Of the 170 patients who achieved at least a PR, ASO-PCR could be successfully applied in only 42% patients as in many patients either clonality could not be demonstrated or sequencing analysis was unsuccessful or ASO performance was suboptimal. In patients who were assessable by both techniques, MRD could be demonstrated using MFC in 46% while ASO-PCR was positive in 52% patients. Overall, a good correlation was observed between both techniques. A better PFS and OS were reported for patients who were ASO-PCR negative versus those who were ASO-PCR positive [40]. Sarasquete et al. could identify an assessable ASO-PCR rearrangement in 24/32 patients of myeloma who achieved CR post ASCT and could predict improved PFS in MRD-negative group [39]. In an earlier analysis of patients who underwent either ASCT or allogeneic stem cell transplantation, MRD-negative patients by ASO-PCR were found to have a lower relapse rate and long-term relapse free survival than MRD-positive patients [38].

The benefit of attaining an MRD-negative status in myeloma has been the subject of two meta-analyses [55, 56]. In the first analysis by

Munshi et al., data from 21 eligible studies from January 1990 to January 2016 was pooled and impact on PFS and OS was examined. The meta-analysis showed that attaining an MRD-negative status was associated with a better PFS and OS. The median PFS was 54 months for MRD-negative patients while it was 26 months for MRD-positive patients. Interestingly, the benefit of MRD-negative status was seen in patients in CR also with patients who were in CR and MRD negative, having a better PFS and OS than patients who were MRD positive but in CR. They concluded that attaining MRD-negative status can be used as an end point in myeloma clinical trials [55]. This would mean that MRD-negative status could be used as a surrogate end point for studies on drug approval [57].

The second meta-analysis though started with 20 full texts, finally only included four studies—three using MFC and one using ASO-PCR. They also showed that MRD negativity was associated with a better PFS and OS. They also concluded that MRD can become a possible end point for regulatory drug approval in myeloma [56].

However, in all these papers, it was clear that MRD-negative status did not translate to cure. This clearly means that MRD-negative patients also possibly have a significant disease burden that is still present in the body. This could either be due to the fact that MRD techniques being used in pre-2015 era were possibly less sensitive than what is desirable or many patients have a patchy disease, and it might be that the site sampled for bone marrow may not contain MRD while other sites may have residual disease. A third possibility is that the relapses may originate from extramedullary sites.

14.3.2 Development of Next Generation Flow Cytometry for MRD Detection in Myeloma

To address the first issue, International Myeloma Foundation (IMF) initiated the Black Swan Research initiative who in concert with Euroflow Consortium tried to develop better methods and standardization of MFC technique. This was achieved with a two-tube eight-colour MFC approach with validated antibodies and bulk-lysis procedure to obtain ≥10 million events. This tube design was a result of five cycles of *design–evaluation–redesign*. The panel consists of two tubes: Tube 1 CD138 BV421/CD27 BV510/CD38 (multi-epitope) FITC/CD56 PE/CD45 PerCPCy5.5/CD19 PE-Cy7/CD117 APC/CD81 APC C750 and Tube 2 CD138 BV421/CD27 PE/CD38 (multi-epitope) FITC/CD56 PE/CD45 PerCPCy5.5/CD19 PE-Cy7/CyIgκ APC/CyIgλ APC C750. They also are validating a single-tube 10-colour panel version and are using the Infinicyt software, and automated identification of abnormal PCs is being explored. This method has been termed next generation flow cytometry (NGF) as it is capable of attaining sensitivity as high as next generation sequencing (NGS). NGF had a higher sensitivity of MRD detection than conventional MFC at 47% vs. 34%. This effectively meant that a quarter of patients who were MRD negative by conventional MFC were actually MRD positive by NGF, and this translated to an improvement in 75% PFS which was not reached in NGF-negative group compared to 75% PFS of 7 months in patients who were NGF positive. Interestingly this was regardless of the conventional response status of these patients. Interestingly, patients who were NGF positive but MRD negative by conventional MFC did worst. A small subset of patients also underwent NGS for the comparison of NGS and NGF, and they showed that NGF approach had higher applicability than NGS and higher sensitivity of MRD detection than NGS [50]. The validated panel is also being marketed through Cytognos (http://www.cytognos.com/index.php/euroflow/minimal-residual-disease-panels/1440-multiple-myeloma-mm-mrd-kits) [58]. There has been an attempt by other centres for the evaluation of a 10-colour panel that can give comparable results to the NGF using a two-tube eight-colour approach [52, 53].

14.3.3 Utility of Next Generation Sequencing for MRD Detection

Next generation sequencing (NGS) in the context of MRD in myeloma employs multiplex sequencing of the immunoglobulin heavy-chain regions (IgH) of plasma cells. It requires the diagnostic sample to identify the IgH rearrangements in the initial clone of neoplastic PCs, and in case of myeloma, multiple clones may be present at the time of diagnosis. All subsequent samples are also assessed using the same platform, and this technique can achieve a sensitivity of 10^{-6} or 0.0001%. Two studies have explored the use of a LymphoSIGHT™ (Sequenta, Inc., San Francisco, CA) high-throughput sequencing platform for immunoglobulin heavy-chain locus (IGH) complete (IGH-VDJH), IGH incomplete (IGH-DJH) and immunoglobulin κ locus (IGK) to assess MRD in myeloma [59, 60]. The first series from GEM trials included 133 patients whose diagnostic DNA was subjected to NGS followed by the analysis for MRD. Of 133 patients, an assessable clonotype was available in 121, and of these, 110 underwent MRD detection. Hence, NGS was applicable in 91% patients. MRD-positive status was present in 83% patients and MRD-negative patients by NGS had a higher time to tumour progression and OS. It was seen that patients who were in CR and MRD negative by NGS had the highest time to tumour progression. All patients had been assessed by MFC and ASO-PCR earlier. When MRD data by NGS was compared with MFC, 83% samples were concordant and for ASO-PCR, the corresponding figure was 85% [59].

The second study was a part of the IFM/DFCI 2009 Trial. Patients were assessed at pre-maintenance and post-maintenance time points. Patients who were MRD negative by NGS had a higher PFS than MRD-positive patients at both time points of assessments. The benefit of MRD negativity was also seen in patients in CR and was also seen in patients with t(4;14) cytogenetic abnormality [60].

Table 14.2 IMWG 2016 criteria pertaining to MRD [61]

Response category	Definition
Sustained MRD negative	MRD negativity in bone marrow by NGS, NGF or both and by imaging confirmed at least 1 year apart. There is a provision to identify further duration of MRD negativity
Flow MRD negative	Absence of aberrant clonal PCs by NGF on bone marrow samples using the standard operating procedure of the Euroflow consortium or a validated equivalent method; assay sensitivity of 0.001% or higher
Sequencing MRD negative	Absence of clonal PCs on bone marrow aspirate using the LymphoSIGHT platform or equivalent method at an assay sensitivity of 0.001% or higher
Imaging plus MRD negative	MRD negative as defined by NGF or NGS plus disappearance of every area of increased tracer uptake found at baseline or a preceding PET/CT or a matching uptake as mediastinal blood pool or less than surrounding normal tissue
Relapse from MRD negative	Loss of MRD-negative state (evidence of clonal plasma cells on NGF or NGS, or positive imaging study for recurrence of myeloma); or reappearance of M band or development of CRAB

With the exciting data from NGF and NGS, the two techniques were formally incorporated in the IMWG 2016 response and MRD assessment criteria for myeloma. The response criteria are mentioned in Table 14.2 [61].

14.4 Imaging to Detect Extramedullay MRD in Myeloma

In a series of 134 myeloma patients, an abnormal PET/CT was seen in 91% patients, and in ~32% of these patients, a normalization of PET/CT after three cycles of bortezomib/lenalidomide/dexamethasone therapy led to an improvement in progression free survival. RVD therapy was followed by ASCT. PET/CT normalization pre-maintenance was seen in 62% patients, and this was also associated with better PFS and OS. MRI in contrast was abnormal in 95% patients, but its normalization following three cycles of RVD therapy was not associated with an improved PFS [41].

In another abstract presented at American Society of Hematology (ASH) annual meeting at Atlanta in 2017, retrospective data of 87 patients treated from 2008 to 2017 and put on lenalidomide therapy was presented. Patients who were flow MRD negative and PET negative after lenalidomide maintenance therapy had a significantly higher PFS and a trend to better OS than all other groups [43]. In an earlier published study, it was seen that in 282 patients treated up front, PET-CT was positive in 70% at diagnosis, and after last cycle of first-line therapy, PET-CT was positive in 30% patients. A PET-negative status was associated with a better PFS and OS. Patients in CR with a PET-positive status did worse and PET-CT was an independent prognostic variable in patients with conventional CR [44].

In another abstract at ASH 2017, the authors specifically looked at 46 patients (35 newly diagnosed and 11 post relapse) who were in MRD-negative CR using eight-colour MFC from a total of 294 patients of myeloma treated with novel agents and ASCT but relapsed subsequently. The limit of detection (LOD) of the MFC assay was between 0.01% and 0.001%. The patients also underwent PET/CT and diffusion-weighted magnetic resonance imaging with background suppression (DWIBS). DWIBS could detect focal lesions in 12/46 patients while PET/CT could detect focal lesions in 3/46 patients. It was also seen that 9/14 patients presented with lesions in the contralateral side to the bone marrow assessment by MFC. This could explain the MRD-negative status using MFC [42].

The IMWG2016 criteria have incorporated MRD assessment by PET/CT in the response and MRD assessment in myeloma, Table 14.2 [61].

A comparison of the techniques used to detect myeloma MRD has been provided in Table 14.3.

Table 14.3 Comparison of the techniques used for MRD detection in myeloma [61, 62]

Criteria	MFC	NGF	ASO-PCR	NGS	PET/CT
Applicability	~100%	~100%	60–70%	90%	~100% for extramedullary disease
Sensitivity	10^{-4}	10^{-5} to 10^{-6}	10^{-5} to 10^{-6}	10^{-6}	High, even 4 mm lesions
Requirement of diagnostic sample	Preferable; not mandatory	Preferable; not mandatory	Mandatory	Mandatory	Preferable; not mandatory
Turnaround time	~2–3 h	~2–3 h	~1 week; ~4 weeks for first identification	≥1 week	2 h
Availability	Most labs worldwide	Most labs worldwide can apply	Intermediate	Low	Intermediate
Requirement of fresh sample	Yes; ≤36 h	Yes; ≤36 h	None	None	Not applicable
Impact from patchy disease	Yes	Yes	Yes	Yes	No
Assessment of sample quality	Possible	Easy	No	No	No
Cost	<350 USD	~350 USD	~500 USD (follow-up); ~1500 (diagnostic)	~700 USD	~2000 USD ~INR 12,000–14,000
Standardization	Poor	Ongoing	EuroMRD since 15 years	No	Ongoing

14.5 Nitty-Gritty of MFC to Assess MRD Using Conventional and NGF Approaches

The use of MFC has evolved from three- or four-colour panels [29, 30, 33–35, 39, 40, 46, 47] to 6–8 colours [45, 48, 49] and then the development of the NGF [50] and 10-colour panels [51–53]. The first guidelines for the determination of MRD by MFC were given in 2008 by European Myeloma Network [63]. These were followed after 7 years by a full issue on myeloma MRD published in *Cytometry B: Clinical Cytometry* [17, 64–73].

14.5.1 Specimen Requirement

The sample recommendations for MRD assessment are limited to bone marrow aspiration. The acceptable anticoagulants have been EDTA and sodium heparin, but since CD138 is a heparin sulphate, there might be some decrease in its intensity following heparin anticoagulation. Hence, some centres prefer EDTA as an anticoagulant [74]. Bone marrow can be transported at room temperature but should ideally be processed within 48 h of sample collection. It is however better if the sample is processed within 24 h of collection [66].

14.5.2 Sample Requirement

If MFC is being applied without NGF approach, 1–2 mL bone marrow sample is adequate, but if NGF approach is to be used, ~5 mL bone marrow sample should be taken. Ideally, the first pull sample should be taken for MFC/NGF unlike the usual scenario where first pull samples are used to prepare marrow films. To acquire 5 million events as recommended by NGF, it is required to start with 10–20 million events as ~50% cells may be lost during processing [50, 65]. However, this is only when the aim is to reach a sensitivity of 0.001%. A lower sensitivity threshold of 0.01% does not require these many cells to begin with and ~55% patients may have MRD higher than this threshold and would therefore not require NGF for detection. NGF processing can be applied to the rest 45% patients, and this approach has been tried at Leeds as they also send sample for molecular analysis as the first priority [65].

14.5.3 Processing Technique

The MFC sample should be processed using a lyse-wash-stain-wash approach. A pre-lysis step for NGF is a bulk-lysis approach with the addition of ~0.5% bovine serum albumin, and a FACS-lysing-fixation step is recommended (Protocol A1) [50]. If utilizing this approach, titration protocol should also follow the same method of processing. Ficoll-hypaque processing is not recommended as it may lead to PC loss. People have tried using higher amounts of sample volume with an appropriate increase in antibody cocktail, but this leads to increased cost and reduced limit of detection (LOD) as fewer cells are acquired when compared to bulk-lysis approach [66].

14.5.4 Panel Requirements

Gating markers: To identify PCs, the single most useful marker is CD38 as it is expressed at a high intensity on both normal and neoplastic PCs. However, it is also expressed by hematogones at an intensity intermediate between PCs and other cells, and this might create a problem when assessing neoplastic PCs which may show a slight downregulation of CD38 [67, 75]. Since CD38 is very brightly expressed, it is best tagged with a weak fluorochrome like FITC. CD138/syndecan is a specific marker for PCs in the context of bone marrow with bright expression seen only in PCs [76]. However, the NGF data has shown that this marker should be tagged with a bright fluorochrome to identify all neoplastic PCs in the context of MRD assessment [75]. The dye recommended by Euroflow in its diagnostic panel is V450, but in the myeloma panel, BV-421 is the recommended dye due to its exceptional brightness [50]. Other dyes like APC and PE can also be used [75].

In addition, CD45 should always be used as a gating marker to refine the PC gate and take care of contaminants. Forward and side scatter (FSC and SSC) are available with every acquisition and should be used to exclude debris and doublets that may contaminate the final gates [75].

With the advent of daratumumab therapy [14], which is an anti-CD38 monoclonal antibody, reductions in CD38 binding of some antibody clones may occur [50]. In addition, daratumumab may complicate IFE assessments as it comigrates with IgGκ bands and also complicates blood transfusion by interfering with serological cross-matches [77]. To circumvent its impact on MRD assessment, Euroflow has optimized a multi-epitope CD38 molecule that is capable of detecting MRD in patients treated with daratumumab [50, 58, 75].

There has also been an attempt to identify other potential gating markers for plasma cells. For this purpose, CD54, CD229 and CD319 were evaluated by the Euroflow group on 46 myeloma patients, 5 healthy controls, 3 extraosseous plasmacytomas and 2 uninvolved non-Hodgkin lymphoma (NHL) marrows. It was seen that all markers when combined with CD38 performed well, but if combined with CD138, only CD229 had a potential to identify all PCs [73]. However, in the final published manuscript and with detailed evaluation of the MRD panel, the group dropped CD229 also as it missed MRD in 8% myeloma cases and was also found at high levels in plasmacytoid dendritic cells and some lymphocytes [50].

Hence, the best approach is the use of a combination of CD138 tagged with a strong dye, CD38 tagged with a weak dye, and CD45 with FSC and SSC for plasma cell gating [63, 67]. In patients treated with daratumumab, a multi-epitope CD38 molecule should be used to identify neoplastic PCs.

Identification of neoplastic PCs: Identification of the abnormal always happens when we know what is normal. Normal PCs in the bone marrow express CD38 and CD138 but do not express the most mature B-cell markers like CD20, CD22

and surface immunoglobins. They however show cytoplasmic expression of light chains that can be used to assess clonality or lack thereof. Traditionally, it was thought that normal PCs show a dim expression of CD45, homogeneous expression of CD19 and lack CD56 [63, 78–80]. However, with modern MFC with acquisition of large number of events, small populations of PCs that could be considered abnormal or neoplastic could be identified in normal patients like CD19−, CD45−, CD56+, CD20+ and may complicate MRD analysis [81–84]. The immunophenotype of PCs shows a significant overlap between normal, neoplastic and reactive PC populations. After acquisition of 1 million events, populations like CD19−CD56/CD28+, CD19−CD56/CD28−, CD19+CD56/CD28+ could be discovered at less numbers [82]. CD81 is expressed at high intensity in normal plasma cells and hematogones and an underexpression is reported in neoplastic PCs [85], and this has not been observed in the normal PC compartment [81]. In contrast normal PCs do not express CD200, CD221 and CD117 [83].

Neoplastic PCs tend to be CD19 negative, and this is consistently seen in >90% myelomas [63, 67, 78–80]. Approximately 60–75% cases of myeloma are CD56 positive [63, 70, 78–80]. An incidence of aberrant patterns and the number of myelomas that show those patterns are given in Table 14.4. Some markers have been shown to have prognostic significance like CD28+CD117− myelomas were shown to have a high risk of

Table 14.4 Differently expressed markers between normal and neoplastic PCs

Marker	Incidence	Normal expression	Aberrancy
CD19	>90%	Positive	Negative
CD56	65–70%	Negative	Bright positive
CD81	55%	Bright positive	Negative or dimmer
CD117	30%	Negative	Positive
CD28	15–45%	Negative	Positive
CD27	40–68%	Positive	Negative or dim
CD45	73%	Dim positive	Negative
CD200	70%	Negative	Bright positive
CD38	80%	Bright	Dim
CD54	60–80%	Bright	Dim

progression [80]. Clonality assessment was not considered mandatory in the earlier published MRD literature [29, 30, 33–35, 39, 40, 46, 47], but the addition of cytoplasmic anti-κ and λ antibodies always adds utility for MRD assessment when a large number of events are acquired to establish clonality of small suspect populations and is included in most ≥8-colour combinations [48–53].

An abnormality in a few markers (one or two) should not be considered as evidence of neoplastic PCs. Multiple assessed markers must be considered when differentiating normal from neoplastic PCs [62, 70]. Addition of clonality assessment improves this distinction of minor populations of PCs. Increasing the number of markers assessed also adds utility to the analysis. Currently, the minimum recommended markers for MRD assessment in myeloma that can differentiate between normal and myelomatous PCs are CD38, CD19, CD45, CD56, CD27, CD81 and CD117. CD138 is required for gating PCs, and in addition, cytoplasmic light chain assessment adds utility when small suspicious PC subsets are present [70].

Acquisition of events: The number of acquired events determines the sensitivity of the assay. The EMN guidelines recommended a total of 1 million cells to be acquired with ~500,000 events per tube as a minimum guide [63]. However, as MFC and software capability have advanced, an acquisition of higher event numbers is achievable easily and is desirable to perform.

Most clinical data generated by MRD has used a threshold of 0.01% as a cut-off to differentiate MRD positive from negative [29, 30, 33, 35, 47]. However, relapses were seen in the MRD-negative group of patients also, and to circumvent that, NGF was developed [50]. This approach calls for an acquisition of a minimum of 3–5 million events to achieve a good limit of detection and lower limit of quantification (LOD and LLOQ, respectively).

Gating strategy: The gating strategy for neoplastic PCs should begin with refinement of data to exclude abnormal flow with CD38-time plot, doublet exclusion using FSC-area vs. FSC-height or SSC-area vs. SSC-height, exclusion of debris by FSC vs. SSC plot [67]. For the first identification of PCs from this refined data, CD38 vs. CD138 plot is used to generously gate all possible PC events. This can be further assessed on the CD38 vs. CD45 plot [67]. Further identification of neoplastic PCs and differentiating them from normal PCs uses a combination of multiple markers assessed in the panel [63, 67, 70]. Normal PCs most often are CD19+/CD45 dim/CD38 bright/CD138 bright/CD27+/CD81+/CD56−/CD117−/CD200− with a polyclonal light chain expression. In contrast most neoplastic PCs exhibit a combination of abnormalities including CD19−/CD45−/CD38 dim/CD138 bright/CD27− or dim/CD81− or dim/CD56+/CD117+/CD200+ [63, 67, 70]. An example of a case is shown in Fig. 14.1.

LOD and LLOQ: LOD and LLOQ are functions of total acquired events, the size of the cluster considered as neoplastic, number of events required to attain reproducibility of detection and quantification. LOD is estimated as having a cluster of at least 30 cells as a percentage from total cells while LLOQ is calculated using a cluster of 50 cells as a percentage of the total cells. This automatically means that in an analysis of 100,000 cells, LOD is 0.03% while LLOQ is ~0.05%. This increases to 0.003% and 0.005% when 1 million cells are analysed and increases further to 0.001% and 0.0017%, respectively, when 3 million cells are interrogated. If 5 million events are analysed, the LOD of 0.0006% and LLOQ of 0.001% are achievable.

How to report MRD: As described earlier, MRD was initially reported at a 0.01% cut-off at EMN recommendations [63]. Some studies reported MRD as aberrant to total PC number ratio [46] and some as neoplastic PC percentage from all leucocytes [34] while others from all events acquired [35, 40]. The current recommendations state that neoplastic PCs be determined as a percentage of total assessed PCs but MRD to be reported as percentage of all nucleated cells [67, 70]. This makes sense as MRD reported by molecular methods also utilizes the entire genomic DNA with no selection of populations [67].

Assessment of sample quality: Concerns pertaining to a representative marrow sample have

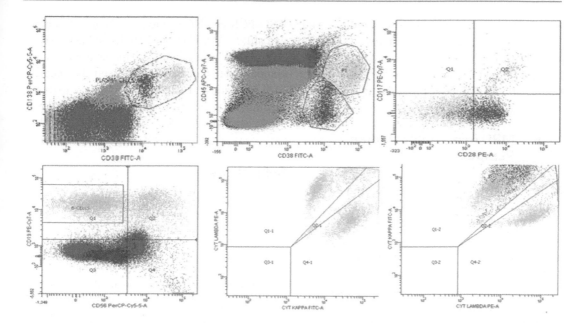

Fig. 14.1 Detection of MRD in myeloma: a gating approach. Plasma cells after exclusion of doublets and debris were gated on the CD38 vs. CD138 plot. From these, two populations were separated on the CD45 vs. CD38 plot into CD45–CD38 dim dark blue PCs and aqua CD38+ bright CD45+ PCs. These two populations exhibited a different immunophenotype. The dark blue is the neoplastic PC population that constituted ~0.1% of all events and was CD38 dim/CD45–/CD2+/CD117–/ CD19–/CD56– and exhibited clonality for kappa. In contrast, the aqua population was CD38 bright/CD45+/ CD28–/CD117–/CD19+/CD56+ and was polyclonal. Clearly the dark blue population is neoplastic while aqua population is normal PCs. This case highlights a variable immunophenotype within the normal PCs with enrichment of the CD19+/CD56+ subpopulation and shows that a single marker should never be relied upon while assessing for MRD

always been raised for MRD in myeloma. The EMN guidelines in 2008 stated that if polyclonal PCs are present within an MRD sample, it should be considered as representative. If they were undetectable, a recommendation was made to look for erythroid or normal myeloid blasts and hematogones. In a situation where MRD was present but sample lacked all these, a comment stating that sample is positive but unsuitable for MRD quantification was recommended [63]. There have been attempts to identify normal ranges for multiple normal populations that can be assessed using markers used for MRD assessment. In the paper on NGF [50], the authors have published ranges for mast cells, erythroid cells, %CD27+ B-cell precursors, %CD27– B-cell precursors, % mature B cells, % myeloid precursors and % endothelial and mesenchymal cells which can serve as a potential guide to validation of sample quality. In their analysis, they could

demonstrate that the two patients who progressed despite being NGF MRD negative could be explained by a suboptimal sample submitted for NGF. However, this finding will require confirmation in other large series of patients to be considered as the only reason for progression while being NGF MRD negative. Other investigators have used normal PCs, mononuclear cells, erythroid cells, granulocytes, CD117+CD27– myeloid progenitors, CD27+CD117– lymphoid cells, B cells, NK cells and hematogones [69].

Final report of MRD by flow cytometry: In addition to the sample time point and patient demographic data, it is recommended that results be reported as event number of neoplastic PCs along with total events analysed as well as the LOD and LLOQ values. If the results are between LOD and LLOQ values, then MRD should not be reported as a percentage but as a range between LOD and LLOQ. Total events in this context represents the denominator after doublets and debris have been excluded for refining the data acquired [67]. A comment on sample adequacy by reporting on normal cell types assessed in the sample should also be a part of the final report.

14.6 MRD in Myeloma: Indian Perspective

Myeloma MRD has lagged behind in India with published data only from AIIMS Gupta et al. [46]. They had reported their data in 2009 using a four-colour panel (given in Table 14.1) and targeted a threshold of 0.01% neoplastic plasma cells. They managed to detect aberrancies in at least two antigens in 90.7% cases and observed a change in immunophenotype at the time of MRD assessment with that from the diagnostic time point in 78% cases. Their initial work highlighted that neoplastic PCs may upregulate or downregulate antigens after therapy and stressed the need to evaluate multiple antigens. In their assessment, they did not assess clonality of PCs due to a limited four-colour panel, but this has been subsequently assayed and is now a part of the myeloma MRD detection.

We have used a six-colour and subsequently an eight-colour panel to detect MRD in myeloma. Using a six-colour approach also, it is feasible to detect MRD and determine clonality of neoplastic PCs.

Hopefully with the incorporation of MRD assessment in IMWG response criteria [61], there would be an increase in the centres evaluating it in India.

Take Home Message
MRD in myeloma has undergone a drastic progress in the past 10 years and has kept pace with the novel agent discovery that led to improved survivals in myeloma. The most utilized approach is multiparameter flow cytometry and is capable of detecting MRD at $\geq 0.01\%$ threshold. This can be further improved by utilizing next generation flow cytometry and standardized approach to MRD, and increased sensitivity of 0.001% is achievable. Most molecular methods used like

ASO-PCR and NGS require a diagnostic sample and still have limited availability and are expensive. MRD assessments in the extramedullary compartment require PET/CT, and the data on both intramedullary and extramedullary MRD in myeloma has been incorporated in the IMWG 2016 response criteria.

References

1. Rajkumar SV, Dimopoulos MA, Palumbo A, et al. International Myeloma Working Group updated criteria for the diagnosis of multiple myeloma. Lancet Oncol. 2014;15:e538–48.
2. Moreau P, Attal M, Facon T. Frontline therapy of multiple myeloma. Blood. 2015;125:3076–84.
3. Rajkumar SV. Multiple myeloma: 2014 update on diagnosis, risk-stratification, and management. Am J Hematol. 2014;89:998–1009.
4. Howlader N, Noone A, Krapcho M, et al. Seer Cancer Statistics Review, 1975–2009 (Vintage 2009 populations). Bethesda: National Cancer Institute; 2012.
5. Landgren O, Weiss BM. Patterns of monoclonal gammopathy of undetermined significance and multiple myeloma in various ethnic/racial groups: support for genetic factors in pathogenesis. Leukemia. 2009;23:1691–7.
6. Kristinsson SY, Anderson WF, Landgren O. Improved long-term survival in multiple myeloma up to the age of 80 years. Leukemia. 2014;28:1346–8.
7. Kumar SK, Dispenzieri A, Lacy MQ, et al. Continued improvement in survival in multiple myeloma: changes in early mortality and outcomes in older patients. Leukemia. 2014;28:1122–8.
8. Kumar SK, Rajkumar SV, Dispenzieri A, et al. Improved survival in multiple myeloma and the impact of novel therapies. Blood. 2008;111:2516–20.
9. Singhal S, Mehta J, Desikan R, et al. Antitumor activity of thalidomide in refractory multiple myeloma [see comments]. N Engl J Med. 1999;341:1565–71.
10. Richardson PG, Blood E, Mitsiades CS, et al. A randomized phase 2 study of lenalidomide therapy for patients with relapsed or relapsed and refractory multiple myeloma. Blood. 2006;108:3458–64.
11. Rajkumar SV, Hayman SR, Lacy MQ, et al. Combination therapy with lenalidomide plus dexamethasone (Rev/Dex) for newly diagnosed myeloma. Blood. 2005;106:4050–3.
12. Richardson PG, Sonneveld P, Schuster MW, et al. Bortezomib or high-dose dexamethasone for relapsed multiple myeloma. N Engl J Med. 2005;352:2487–98.
13. Siegel DS, Martin T, Wang M, et al. A phase 2 study of single-agent carfilzomib (PX-171-003-A1) in patients with relapsed and refractory multiple myeloma. Blood. 2012;120(14):2817–25. https://doi.org/10.1182/blood-2012-05-425934.

14. Lonial S, Brendan M, Usmani SZ, et al. Single-agent daratumumab in heavily pretreated patients with multiple myeloma (Sirius): an open-label, international, multicentre phase 2 trial. Lancet. 2016;387:1551–60.

15. Lonial S, Dimopoulos M, Palumbo A, et al. elotuzumab therapy for relapsed or refractory multiple myeloma. N Engl J Med. 2015;373:621–31.

16. Moreau P, Masszi T, Grzasko N, et al. Ixazomib, an investigational oral proteasome inhibitor (PI), in combination with lenalidomide and dexamethasone (IRd), significantly extends progression-free survival (PFS) for patients (Pts) with relapsed and/or refractory multiple myeloma (RRMM): the phase 3 tourmaline-MM1 study (NCT01564537). Blood. 2015;126. Abstract 727.

17. Landgren O, Owen RG. Better therapy requires better response evaluation: paving the way for minimal residual disease testing for every myeloma patient. Cytometry B Clin Cytom. 2016;90:14–20.

18. Mailankody S, Korde N, Lesokhin AM, et al. Minimal residual disease in multiple myeloma: bringing the bench to the bedside. Nat Rev ClinOncol. 2015;12:286–95.

19. Attal M, Lauwers-Cances V, Marit G, et al. Lenalidomide maintenance after stem-cell transplantation for multiple myeloma. N Engl J Med. 2012;366:1782–91.

20. McCarthy PL, Owzar K, Hofmeister CC, et al. Lenalidomide after stem-cell transplantation for multiple myeloma. N Engl J Med. 2012;366:1770–81.

21. Jakubowiak AJ, Dytfeld D, Griffith KA, et al. A phase 1/2 study of carfilzomib in combination with lenalidomide and low-dose dexamethasone as a frontline treatment for multiple myeloma. Blood. 2012;120:1801–9.

22. Kumar S, Flinn I, Richardson PG, et al. Randomized, multicenter, phase 2 study (EVOLUTION) of combinations of bortezomib, dexamethasone, cyclophosphamide, and lenalidomide in previously untreated multiple myeloma. Blood. 2012;119:4375–82.

23. Attal M, Harousseau JL, Stoppa AM, et al. A prospective, randomized trial of autologous bone marrow transplantation and chemotherapy in multiple myeloma. Intergroupe Francais du Myelome. N Engl J Med. 1996;335:91–7.

24. Child JA, Morgan GJ, Davies FE, et al. High-dose chemotherapy with hematopoietic stem-cell rescue for multiple myeloma. N Engl J Med. 2003;348:1875–83.

25. Durie BG, Harousseau JL, Miguel JS, et al. International uniform response criteria for multiple myeloma. Leukemia. 2006;20:1467–73.

26. Rajkumar SV, Harousseau JL, Durie B, et al. Consensus recommendations for the uniform reporting of clinical trials: report of the International Myeloma Workshop Consensus Panel 1. Blood. 2011;117:4691–5.

27. Tatsas AD, Jagasia MH, Chen H, McCurley TL. Monitoring residual myeloma: high-resolution serum/urine electrophoresis or marrow biopsy with immunohistochemical analysis? Am J ClinPathol. 2010;134:139–44.

28. Chee CE, Kumar S, Larson DR, et al. The importance of bone marrow examination in determining complete response to therapy in patients with multiple myeloma. Blood. 2009;114:2617–8.

29. Rawstron AC, Davies FE, DasGupta R, et al. Flow cytometric disease monitoring in multiple myeloma: the relationship between normal and neoplastic plasma cells predicts outcome after transplantation. Blood. 2002;100:3095–100.

30. Paiva B, Vidriales MB, Cervero J, et al. Multiparameter flow cytometric remission is the most relevant prognostic factor for multiple myeloma patients who undergo autologous stem cell transplantation. Blood. 2008;112:4017–23.

31. Korde N, Roschewski M, Zingone A, et al. Treatment with carfilzomib-lenalidomide-dexamethasone with lenalidomide extension in patients with smoldering or newly diagnosed multiple myeloma. JAMA Oncol. 2015;1:746–54.

32. Mateos MV, Oriol A, Martinez-Lopez J, et al. GEM2005 trial update comparing VMP/VTP as induction in elderly multiple myeloma patients: do we still need alkylators? Blood. 2014;124:1887–93.

33. Paiva B, Martinez-Lopez J, Vidriales MB, et al. Comparison of immunofixation, serum free light chain, and immunophenotyping for response evaluation and prognostication in multiple myeloma. J ClinOncol. 2011;29:1627–33.

34. Rawstron AC, Child JA, de Tute RM, et al. Minimal residual disease assessed by multiparameter flow cytometry in multiple myeloma: impact on outcome in the Medical Research Council Myeloma IX Study. J ClinOncol. 2013;31:2540–7.

35. Paiva B, Gutiérrez NC, Rosiñol L, et al. High-risk cytogenetics and persistent minimal residual disease by multiparameter flow cytometry predict unsustained complete response after autologous stem cell transplantation in multiple myeloma. Blood. 2012;119:687–91.

36. Mathis S, Chapuis N, Borgeot J, et al. Comparison of cross-platform flow cytometry minima residual disease evaluation in multiple myeloma using a common antibody combination and analysis strategy. Cytometry B Clin Cytom. 2015;88:101–9.

37. Silvennoinen R, Kairisto V, Pelliniemi TT, et al. Assessment of molecular remission rate after bortezomib plus dexamethasone induction treatment and autologous stem cell transplantation in newly diagnosed multiple myeloma patients. Br J Haematol. 2013;160:561–4.

38. Martinelli G, Terragna C, Zamagni E, et al. Molecular remission after allogeneic or autologous transplantation of hematopoietic stem cells for multiple myeloma. J Clin Oncol. 2000;18:2273–81.

39. Sarasquete ME, García-Sanz R, Gonzalez D, et al. Minimal residual disease monitoring in multiple myeloma: a comparison between allelic-specific oligonucleotide real-time quantitative polymerase

chain reaction and flow cytometry. Haematologica. 2005;90:1365–72.

40. Puig N, Sarasquete ME, Balanzategui A, et al. Critical evaluation of ASORQ-PCR for minimal residual disease evaluation in multiple myeloma. A comparative analysis with flow cytometry. Leukemia. 2014;28:391–7.

41. Moreau P, Attal M, Caillot D, et al. Prospective evaluation of magnetic resonance imaging and [18F] fluorodeoxyglucose positron emission tomography-computed tomography at diagnosis and before maintenance therapy in symptomatic patients with multiple myeloma included in the IFM/DFCI 2009 trial: results of the IMAJEM study. J Clin Oncol. 2017;35:2911–8.

42. Rasche L, Schinke C, Alapat D, et al. Functional imaging detects residual disease in MRD-negative multiple myeloma patients who subsequently relapse. Blood. 2017;130:4510.

43. Fernandez RA, Cedena MT, Rios R, et al. Maintenance treatment with lenalidomide for multiple myeloma increases the proportion of MRD negative (flow-/PET-CT-) patients. Blood. 2017;130:3098.

44. Zamagni E, Nanni C, Mancuso K, et al. PET/CT improves the definition of complete response and allows to detect otherwise unidentifiable skeletal progression in multiple myeloma. Clin Cancer Res. 2015;21(19):4384–90.

45. de Tute RM, Jack AS, Child J, et al. A single-tube six-colour flow cytometry screening assay for the detection of minimal residual disease in myeloma. Leukemia. 2007;21:2046–9.

46. Gupta R, Bhaskar A, Kumar L, Sharma A, Jain P. Flow cytometric immunophenotyping and minimal residual disease analysis in multiple myeloma. Am J Clin Pathol. 2009;132:728–32.

47. Paiva B, Chandia M, Puig N, et al. The prognostic value of multiparameter flow cytometry minimal residual disease assessment in relapse multiple myeloma. Haematologica. 2015;100:e53–5.

48. Robillard N, Bene MC, Moreau P, Wuilleme S. A single-tube multi-parameter seven-colour flow cytometry strategy for the detection of malignant plasma cells in multiple myeloma. Blood Cancer J. 2013;3:e134.

49. Roussel M, Lauwers-Cances V, Robillard N, et al. Front-line transplantation program with lenalidomide, bortezomib, and dexamethasone combination as induction and consolidation followed by lenalidomide maintenance in patients with multiple myeloma: a phase II study by the Intergroupe Francophone du Myelome. J Clin Oncol. 2014;32:2712–7.

50. Flores-Montero J, Sanoja-Flores L, Paiva B, et al. Next generation flow for highly sensitive and standardized detection of minimal residual disease in multiple myeloma. Leukemia. 2017;31:2094–103.

51. Domingo E, Moreno C, Sanchez-Ibarrola A, et al. Enhanced sensitivity of flow cytometry for routine assessment of minimal residual disease. Haematologica. 2010;95:691–2.

52. Roshal R, Flores-Montero JA, Gao Q, et al. MRD detection in multiple myeloma: comparison between MSKCC 10-color single-tube and EuroFlow 8-color 2-tube methods. Blood Adv. 2017;1(12):728–32.

53. Royston DY, Gao Q, Nguyen N, et al. Single-tube 10-fluorochrome analysis for efficient flow cytometric evaluation of minimal residual disease in plasma cell myeloma. Am J Clin Pathol. 2016;146:41–9.

54. Rawstron A, Gregory WM, de Tute RM, et al. Minimal residual disease in myeloma by flow cytometry: independent prediction of survival benefit per log reduction. Blood. 2015;125:1932–5.

55. Munshi NC, Avet-Loiseau H, Rawstron A, et al. Association of minimal residual disease with superior survival outcomes in patients with multiple myeloma a meta-analysis. JAMA Oncol. 2017;3:28–35.

56. Landgren O, Devlin S, Boulad M, Mailankody S. Role of MRD status in relation to clinical outcomes in newly diagnosed multiple myeloma patients: a meta-analysis. Bone Marrow Transplant. 2016;51:1565–8.

57. Gromley NJ, Farrell AT, Pazdur R. Minimal residual disease as a potential surrogate end point—lingering questions. JAMA Oncol. 2017;3:18–20.

58. http://www.cytognos.com/index.php/euroflow/minimal-residual-disease-panels/1440-multiple-myeloma-mm-mrd-kits. Accessed 26 Dec 2017.

59. Martinez-Lopez J, Lahuerta JJ, Pepin F, et al. Prognostic value of deep sequencing method for minimal residual disease detection in multiple myeloma. Blood. 2014;123:3073–9.

60. Avet-Loiseau H. Minimal residual disease by next-generation sequencing: pros and cons. Am Soc Clin Oncol Educ Book. 2016;35:e425–30.

61. Kumar S, Paiva B, Anderson KC, et al. International Myeloma Working Group consensus criteria for response and minimal residual disease assessment in multiple myeloma. Lancet Oncol. 2016;17: e328–46.

62. Paiva B, van Dongen JJ, Orfao A. New criteria for response assessment role of minimal residual disease in multiple myeloma. Blood. 2015;125:3059–68.

63. Rawstron AC, Orfao A, Beksac M, et al. Report of the European Myeloma Network on multiparametric flow-cytometry in multiple myeloma and related disorders. Haematologica. 2008;93:431–8.

64. Wood BL. Principles of minimal residual disease detection for hematopoietic neoplasms by flow cytometry. Cytometry B Clin Cytom. 2016;90B:47–53.

65. Rawstron AC, Pavia B, Stetler-Stevenson M. Assessment of minimal residual disease in myeloma and the need for a consensus approach. Cytometry B Clin Cytom. 2016;90B:21–5.

66. Stetler-Stevenson M, Paiva B, Stoolman L, et al. Consensus guidelines for myeloma minimal residual disease sample staining and data acquisition. Cytometry B Clin Cytom. 2016;90B:26–30.

67. Arroz M, Came N, Lin P, et al. Consensus guidelines on plasma cell myeloma minimal residual disease analysis and reporting. Cytometry B Clin Cytom. 2016;90B:31–9.

68. Oldaker TA, Wallace PK, Barnett D. Flow cytometry quality requirements for monitoring of minimal disease in plasma cell myeloma. Cytometry B Clin Cytom. 2016;90B:40–6.

69. Rawstron AC, de Tute RM, Haughton J, Owen RG. Measuring disease levels in myeloma using flow cytometry in combination with other laboratory techniques: lessons from the past 20 years at the Leeds Haematological Malignancy Diagnostic Service. Cytometry B Clin Cytom. 2016;90B:54–60.

70. Flores-Montero J, de Tute R, Paiva B, et al. Immunophenotype of normal vs. myeloma plasma cells: toward antibody panel specifications for MRD detection in multiple myeloma. Cytometry B Clin Cytom. 2016;90B:61–72.

71. Gormley NJ, Turley DM, Dickey JS, et al. Regulatory perspective on minimal residual disease flow cytometry testing in multiple myeloma. Cytometry B Clin Cytom. 2016;90B:73–80.

72. Vittorio Emanuele M, Elona S, Milena G, et al. Multiple myeloma: new surface antigens for the characterization of plasma cells in the era of novel agents. Cytometry B Clin Cytom. 2016;90B:81–90.

73. Pojero F, Flores-Montero J, Sanoja L, et al. Utility of CD54, CD229, and CD319 for the identification of plasma cells in patients with clonal plasma cell diseases. Cytometry B Clin Cytom. 2016;90B:91–100.

74. Barnett DSI, Wilson GA, Granger V, Reilly JT. Determination of leucocyte antibody binding capacity (ABC): the need for standardization. Clin Lab Haematol. 1998;20:155–64.

75. Terstappen LW, Johnsen S, Segers-Nolten IM, Loken MR. Identification and characterization of plasma cells in normal human bone marrow by high-resolution flow cytometry. Blood. 1990;76:1739–47.

76. Wijdenes J, Vooijs WC, Clement C, et al. A plasmocyte selective monoclonal antibody (B-B4) recognizes syndecan-1. Br J Haematol. 1996;94:318–23.

77. Darzalex (daratumumab) injection [prescribing information]. Horsham: Janssen Biotech, Inc; 2015.

78. Lin P, Owens R, Tricot G, Wilson CS. Flow cytometric immunophenotypic analysis of 306 cases of multiple myeloma. Am J Clin Pathol. 2004;121:482–8.

79. Almeida J, Orfao A, Ocqueteau M, et al. High-sensitive immunophenotyping and DNA ploidy studies for the investigation of minimal residual disease in multiple myeloma. Br J Haematol. 1999;107:121–31.

80. Mateo G, Montalban MA, Vidriales M, et al. Prognostic value of immunophenotyping in multiple myeloma: a study by the PETHEMA/GEM cooperative study groups on patients uniformly treated with high-dose therapy. J Clin Oncol. 2008;26:2737–44.

81. Tembhare P, Yuan CM, Venzon D, et al. Flow cytometric differentiation of abnormal and normal plasma cells in the bone marrow in patients with multiple myeloma and its precursor diseases. Leuk Res. 2014;38:371–6.

82. Robillard N, Wuilleme S, Moreau P, Bene MC. Immunophenotype o fnormal and myelomatous plasma-cell subsets. Front Immunol. 2014;5:137.

83. Cannizzo E, Bellio E, Sohani AR, et al. Multiparameter immuno-phenotyping by flow cytometry in multiple myeloma: the diagnostic utility of defining ranges of normal antigenic expression in comparison to histology. Cytometry B Clin Cytom. 2010;78:231–8.

84. vanDongen JJM, Lhermitte L, Bottcher S, et al. EuroFlow antibody panels for standardized n-dimensional flow cytometric immunophenotyping of normal, reactive and malignant leukocytes. Leukemia. 2012;26:1908–75.

85. Paiva B, Gutierrez NC, Chen X, et al. Clinical significance of CD81 expression by clonal plasma cells in high-risk smoldering and symptomatic multiple myeloma patients. Leukemia. 2012;26:1862–9.

Hodgkin Lymphoma: Revisited

15

Brig Tathagata Chatterjee and Ankur Ahuja

15.1 Introduction and Epidemiology

Hodgkin lymphoma (HL), which in the past was called Hodgkin disease, has always been one of the front runners of research in lymphomas. It usually arises from germinal centre or post-germinal centre B cells. Composition of HL is commonly defined as having predominantly inflammatory cells having minor population of neoplastic cells which were named as Reed–Sternberg cells.

Age Spectrum: It comprises approximately 10% of entire lymphomas and 0.6% of all cancers [1]. In the USA, 8500 new cases and about 1120 deaths are reported due to HL [1]. In the developed countries, there are usually two peaks, one in young adults which are in the majority (approximately age 20 years) and other in adults of older age (approximately age 65 years) [2]. While in developing countries, the initial peak is in childhood for boys, there is relative low rate in young adults, and a late peak in older adults [3]. In economically underdeveloped countries, the overall incidence of HL is lower than in developed countries, with the exception of children under the age of 15, where a higher incidence is seen.

Histological spectrum: Developed countries have nodular sclerosis HL (NSHL) as the predominant histological subtype and majority of them are seen in young adults, while in developing countries, mixed cellularity HL (MCHL) is more frequent in children and older adults. Countries having transitional economies have roughly equal frequencies of the MCHL and NSHL subtypes [3–5].

15.2 Etiopathogenesis

(a) **Role of EBV**: Epstein–Barr virus (EBV) is a herpes virus. Its role has been proven in the development of HL.

Evidence of EBV Role

1. Increased EBV antibody titres in HL and these antibodies actually preceded the disease [6].
2. EBV in the tumour cells of patients suffering from HL [7].
3. While the risk of developing EBV-negative HL after infectious mononucleosis was not increased (relative risk 1.5, 95% CI 0.9–2.5), the risk of developing EBV-positive HL was increased (relative risk 4.0, 95% CI 3.4–4.5) [8].

HL in immunodeficient populations is almost universally EBV associated [9], and the HL is

B. T. Chatterjee (✉)
Department of Lab Sciences and Molecular Medicine, AH (R&R), New Delhi, India

A. Ahuja
Army Hospital (R&R), New Delhi, India

© Springer Nature Singapore Pte Ltd. 2019
R. Saxena, H. P. Pati (eds.), *Hematopathology*, https://doi.org/10.1007/978-981-13-7713-6_15

Fig. 15.1 Pathophysiology of EBV in Hodgkin lymphoma

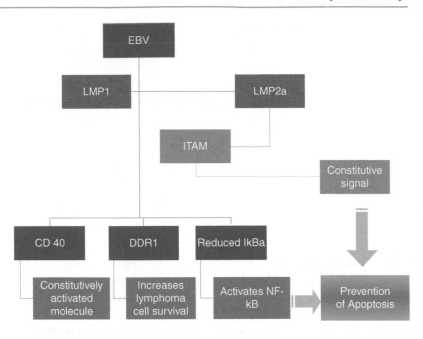

usually of the mixed cellularity subtype [10, 11]. EBV is most commonly associated with the mixed cellularity and lymphocyte-depleted HL subtypes while nodular sclerosis HL is affected less commonly. Nodular lymphocyte predominant HL is almost always EBV negative [12].

EBV DNA that is detected in Reed–Sternberg cells is clonal, which indicates that the origin of virus-infected population is from a single infected cell [13]. Figure 15.1 summarises pathophysiology of EBV in HL.

Regarding prognostic influence pre-treatment serum EBV level had no prognostic significance, but post treatment 8 day persistence of serum EBV DNA is correlated with an unfavourable outcome.

EBNA1 expression is required for the replication and maintenance of the viral genome in proliferating cells [14]. B cells that lack functional immunoglobulin would die by apoptosis. Expression of LMP1 or LMP2a helps in escaping apoptosis. Latent membrane protein 1 (LMP1) encodes transmembrane protein resembling tumour necrosis factor receptor CD40 [15]. Since signalling through CD40 can delay apoptosis, LMP-1 through CD40 therefore can function like a constitutively activated molecule, providing a mechanism by which the expression of EBV genes could facilitate the escape of Reed–

Sternberg cells, or their precursors, from destruction in the germinal centres [16]. In addition, it has been shown that LMP-1 increases inhibitor of kB activator (IkBa) turnover, thus activating nuclear factor kappa B (NF-kB) [17]. The constitutive activation of NF-kB leads to growth and survival of classical Reed–Sternberg cells. A third mechanism by which LMP-1 may promote the survival of Reed–Sternberg cells is through discoidin domain receptor 1 (DDR1) which is a tyrosine kinase receptor which, when binds with collagen, increases lymphoma cell survival [18]. Latent membrane protein 2a (LMP2a) co-localises with LMP1 in the plasma membrane of EBV-infected lymphocytes [19]. LMP2a contains an immunoreceptor tyrosine-based activation motif (ITAM) which resembles motifs on immunoglobulin molecules. Expression of LMP2a produces a constitutive signal, which prevents apoptosis of pre-B cells which failed to express immunoglobulin molecule [19].

15.3   Cellular Origin

The most morphological characteristic of classical Hodgkin lymphoma (CHL) is binuclear Reed–Sternberg cell (the malignant cells in HD) which results from incomplete cytokinesis of mononuclear Hodgkin cells [20, 21]. Another interesting but confusing aspect is that cells of classical HL don't exhibit phenotypes typical of any normal cell, for example they are negative for leukocyte common antigen (LCA), T cell, and B-cell markers except PAX5, a B-cell marker which is weakly positive in RS cells; CD20 can also be detected on RS cells in a few cases [22]. CD15 which is known to be a marker of granulocytes is characteristically positive in classical RS cells. CD30 is also positive in classical Hodgkin lymphoma [23]; this entire observation has questioned the ontogeny of RS cells.

Evidence related to origin of cells from germinal centre has emerged in the past. Analysis of rearranged antigen receptor genes isolated from single cells has been done and has shown some clues which are:

(a) Rearrangement and mutation of the immunoglobulin (Ig) genes are restricted to germinal centre B cells.
(b) Another well-known aspect is that patients with nodular sclerosis HL have shown to have clonal rearrangement of the V, D, and J segments of the (Ig) heavy chain locus with somatic mutations in the RS cells, thus resulting in non-functional Ig variable regions [24–26].

Despite of these evidences of a germinal centre B-cell origin, why RS cells lose the phenotypic features of germinal centre B cells like BCL6 has been suggested by various theories:

1. Impaired function of Ig gene promoters and enhancers [25–27]
   (a) Downregulation of known B-cell transcription factors such as OCT2, BOB-1, early B-cell factor 1 (EBF1), and PU.1 [28, 29]
   (b) Acquisition of epigenetic changes that result in silencing of IgH promoters, receptors BLNK [30–32]
2. Aberrant expression of regulators of other haematopoietic cell lineages

(a) Possibly hypoxia-induced upregulation of NOTCH1 and Id2—antagonising E2A and PAX5 [33, 34]
3. Over-activation of the transcription factors STAT5A and STAT5B [35]

15.4 Mechanisms of Tumorigenesis

1. Activation of the nuclear factor kappa B (NF-kB) transcription factor-signalling pathway
   (a) Association of NF-kB has been seen in many neoplasms and is associated with oncoproteins.
   (b) Two types of NF-kB heterodimers are found in normal mature B cell which are NF-kB1/c-REL and anothr is NF-kB/REL-A. NF-kB/c-REL is associated with lymphocytic transformation and its nuclear accumulation thus leading to RS cell transformation [36].
   (c) Inhibitor of kB (IkB) normally regulates the activity of NF-kB.
   (d) Constitutive activity of NF-kB leads to neoplasia which may be because of:
      • Mutation or loss of IkB.
      • Modification of NF-kB thus leading to insensitivity to inhibition by IkB.
      • Amplification of the REL oncogene secondary to chromosomal gains
      • LMP-1 expressed by EBV activates NF-kB by promoting IkBa turnover.
      • CD30 activates TRAF2- and TRAF5-dependent signals, thus leading to NF-kB activation [37, 38].
   (e) Constitutive NF-kB activation leads to
      • Targeting genes intercellular adhesion molecule (ICAM-1), granulocyte macrophage colony-stimulating factor (GM-CSF), interleukin (IL)-6, and TNF which have been related to effects on the surrounding characteristic background of classical HL [39]
      • The well-established role of antiapoptotic effects of NF-kB [40, 41]

- DDR-1
  - A receptor tyrosine kinase which is upregulated by LMP-1
  - Related to enhance resistance to apoptosis
2. Interleukin-13 signalling pathway
   (a) IL-13 and IL-4 activate JAK kinases, thus leading to stimulate the transcription factor, STAT6 [42, 43], which upregulates NF-kB promoters.
3. NOTCH signalling pathway
   (a) Regulator of normal T-cell development has been implicated in the role of RS cells.
4. Interferon regulatory factors
   (a) IRF5
   - Protect RS cells from cell death
   - Increased expression of proinflammatory genes
   - Downregulation of genes which are required for initiation and maintenance of the B-cell lineage differentiation programme
   - Upregulation of their transcriptional antagonists [44]
   - Transcriptional activation of the activator protein-1 (AP-1) complex, resulting in increased CD30 expression
5. Genomic alterations affecting HRS cell survival and immunoevasion
6. T-cell response
   (a) RS cell secretes lymphotoxin-alpha, which stimulates endothelial cells, thus upregulating adhesion molecules such as ICAM-1, VCAM-1, and E-selectin which recruits T cell [45].
   (b) Activated CD4+ TH2 cells lead to eosinophilia, plasmacytosis, and fibrosis.
   (c) IL-13 produced by RS cells promotes T helper cell differentiation to the TH2 phenotype.

15.5 Classification of HD

Table 15.1 shows the various classifications used in various literatures. Among all, WHO 2008 classification gains the most popularity and has been in use frequently.

15.5.1 WHO 2008 Classification

Classical HL—This group comprises neoplastic cells which are originated from germinal centre B cells, but failed to express the genes and its products that defines its derivation site. Based on morphological appearance of the tumour cells and the composition of the background which classically is reactive, this particular group is further subdivided into the following subtypes:

- Nodular sclerosis classical HL (NSHL)
- Mixed cellularity classical HL (MCHL)
- Lymphocyte-rich classical HL (LRHL)
- Lymphocyte-depleted classical HL (LDHL)

Table 15.1 Various classification systems for HL

Jackson and Parker	Lukes and Butler	Rye Conference	R.E.A.L. Classification	World Health Organization (WHO) Classification
Paragranuloma	Lymphocytic and/or histiocytic, nodular	Lymphocyte predominance	Nodular lymphocyte predominance	Nodular lymphocyte predominant HL
	Lymphocytic and/or histiocytic, diffuse		Classical lymphocyte-rich HL	Lymphocyte-rich classical HL
Granuloma	Nodular sclerosis	Nodular sclerosis	Classical nodular sclerosis HL	Nodular sclerosis classical HL
Mixed cellularity	Mixed cellularity	Classical mixed cellularity HL	Mixed cellularity classical HL	Mixed cellularity
Sarcoma	Diffuse fibrosis	Lymphocyte depletion	Classical lymphocyte depletion HL	Lymphocyte-depleted classical HL
	Reticular			

Nodular lymphocyte predominant HL— The neoplastic cells in this subtype have the immune-phenotypic features suggesting derivation from germinal centre B cells.

15.5.2 WHO 2016 Updated Classification

Some minor changes are there. NLPHL is known to have transformation phase which includes diffuse large cells which are rich in T cells, T-cell histiocyte-rich large B-cell lymphoma (THRLBCL). The update revision of WHO classification in 2016 [46] recommends that this transformation can be renamed as THRLBCL-like transformation of NLPHL which has aggressive behaviour and therefore requires more intensive treatment [46].

15.6 Clinical Features

Classic Hodgkin lymphoma commonly presents as an overt disease, with an asymptomatic enlarged lymph node mass, nonspecific symptoms which may be present since weeks to months. Mediastinal masses (involved in 60–70%) are only noticed symptomatically when they become large enough (>1/3rd of greatest intrathoracic diameter of chest wall or >10 cm in transverse diameter) which is considered as an adverse prognostic factor. Among the sites of lymph nodes involvement, axillary lymph nodes are present in 10–20% of patients while inguinal lymphadenopathy is seen in 6–12% [47, 48]. Retroperitoneal lymph nodes are seen in 25% and can present as pain in loin regions at supine position. Infra-diaphragmatic lymphadenopathy (<10% of patients) in HL as an isolated presentation is uncommon. Many a time systemic symptoms arise prior to lymphadenopathy and these symptoms which are commonly called as B symptoms include fever of more than 100.4 °F, drenching night sweats, and unexplained weight loss (>10% in 6 months). These B symptoms are not common in stage I/II HL (<20%) but as the stage advances they become common and are seen in 50%. Fever is more common in the evening and with time it progresses. Though Pel–Ebstein fever which has tendency to recur at variable intervals for many weeks is very characteristic, it is relatively uncommon [49]. Pruritus is another important symptom which precedes the diagnosis of HL by several months [50] and when it is severe it is considered as a poor prognostic sign [50]. Occasionally patients may complain of localised pain at involved sites after alcohol ingestion which is very specific for HL [51, 52]. In one study it was found Nodular sclerosis to have the most common histology [51]. The mechanism of this pain is not known. Skin lesions are also common in HL and include erythema multiforme, erythema nodosum, ichthyosis, acrokeratosis, urticaria, necrotizing lesions, hyperpigmentation, and sometimes skin infiltration [53, 54]. Among paraneoplastic syndrome, nephrotic syndrome can occur as a consequence of lymphokines, such as IL-13. Among the neoplastic syndrome, minimal change disease, focal segmental glomerulosclerosis, are common [55, 56]. Another paraneoplastic syndrome is hypercalcemia, which is commonly due to increased production of calcitriol [57, 58]. Association of HL with eosinophilia is a well-known entity which may be due to chemokines, such as interleukin-5 and eotaxin [59, 60].

Patterns of Disease Presentation—While in the initial stage of HL contiguous spread is common, bone marrow involvement is uncommon [61–63], but in the recurrent cases non-contiguous spread and bone marrow infiltration are common.

Variation by histology—Various morphological subtypes have peculiar pattern of disease involvement as has been shown in one large study [47]. It was evident from the study that patients having nodular lymphocyte predominant HL presented commonly with localised involvement which was common in the upper neck, while abdominal lymph nodal and extranodal disease was common in patients with the lymphocyte-depleted subtype. Patients with nodular sclerosis often had lymphadenopathy above the diaphragm as well as mediastinal involvement. The study also showed that patients diagnosed with mixed cellularity subtype had disease in the liver. Lymphocyte-depleted patients were presented frequently with advanced stage disease, liver involvement, and systemic B symptoms [64].

15.7   Diagnosis

Diagnosis of any disease starts from detailed history and proper examination. Thorough physical examination should be done to look for lymph nodes, organomegaly, tonsil area, and base of the tongue. Performance status should always be done at the time of presentation and better before every cycle. Karnofsky performance status and

the Eastern Cooperative Oncology Group (ECOG) performance status are two methods for assessment.

Workup of HL is extensive for the diagnosis but also in the follow-up of HL. This is summarised in Table 15.2 [65].

No diagnosis starts without clinical details. The clinical details are summarised in Table 15.3. Diagnosis of HL is best made by a biopsy. Fine-needle aspiration or core needle biopsies though are simple procedures but generally couldn't able to finalise the diagnosis because of several reasons common being lack of presence of

Table 15.2 Diagnostic workup pre-chemotherapy

Diagnosis	Workup pre-chemotherapy
• Excision biopsy and IHC evaluation (recommended)	• Performance status
• Core needle biopsy only if diagnostic HPE and IHC	• CBC, platelets, differentials
	• ESR, LDH, LFT
	• Child bearing woman—pregnancy test
	• Contrast CT scan, PET scan
	• Counselling—smoking cessation, fertility, psychosocial
	• Fertility preservation (semen preservation, IVF)
	• Vaccines—pneumococcal, meningococcal, H-flu if splenic RT contemplated
	• HIV, Hep B
	• Chest X-ray for mediastinal mass
	• CT neck if RT neck contemplated
	• Pulmonary function test—ABCD/BEACOPP therapy
	• Cardiac evaluation—doxorubicin
	• Bone marrow biopsy if cytopenias, ≥3 lesions by PET/CT

Table 15.3 Clinical and epidemiological differences between various subtypes of HL

Nodular lymphocyte predominance	Nodular sclerosis	Mixed cellularity	Lymphocyte depletion	Lymphocyte-rich
• Common in adult males	• Common in adolescents and young adults	• Common in adults	• Common in elderly patients	• Older age common
• Localised at diagnosis	• Females > Males	• Males > Females	• Abdominal lymphadenopathy is common	• Less aggressive
• Stage-IV disease is rare	• Mediastinal involvement is common	• Advance stage is common	• Advance stage at diagnosis is common	• Early stage at diagnosis
• Cervical or inguinal	• Upper thoracic movement		• Treatment response is worst	• Subdiaphragmatic sites common
• Nodes commonly involved	• Localised in lymph nodes			• Systemic symptoms are less

Table 15.4 Histopathology differences between various subtypes of HL

Nodular lymphocyte predominance	• Effaced lymph node architecture • Nodular growth pattern which are B-cell areas • Nearby progressive transformation of germinal centres • The neoplastic cells known as lymphocytic and histiocytic (L&H cells)/popcorn cells are large cell with an abundant cytoplasm with vesicular chromatin, irregular and polylobated nuclei with small nucleoli and are present as scattered cells in minority • The non-neoplastic cells which are present in majority are predominantly small lymphocytes with rare presence of plasma cells, eosinophils • Variable histiocytes with non-necrotising granulomas • Differential diagnosis T-cell-rich large B-cell lymphoma
Nodular sclerosis	• Varied sized nodules with dense collagenous fibrous bands showing green birefringence in polarised light • Coagulative necrosis • Reed–Sternberg (R–S) cell in minority—Large, polynucleated, prominent, basophilic nucleoli • R–S like cells—mononuclear cells including lacunar cells • Background comprised of small lymphocytes, plasma cells, eosinophils, neutrophils, and histiocytes
Mixed cellularity	• Diffuse infiltrate to vaguely nodular • Fine interstitial fibrosis • R–S cells
Lymphocyte depletion	• Completely effaced lymph node architecture • Diffuse and dense fibrosis which is non birefringent collagen • Residual cells are predominantly R–S cells forming confluent sheets • Non-neoplastic elements in the background are uncommon • Close mimicker is anaplastic large cell lymphoma—ALK protein can differentiate
Lymphocyte-rich	• Diffuse or focal disease • May have interfollicular involvement with frequent presence of nodules with germinal centres • Focal areas of fibrosis • Reactive cellular background comprising small lymphocytes predominantly • Sparse population of neutrophils, eosinophils, and plasma cells • R–S and lacunar cells are present, infrequently

architecture, insufficient or probable lack of characteristic morphology cells as they are present in minority among large reactive population, and difficulty in IHC interpretation. Biopsy actually can subtype based upon architecture of lymph node and morphology, architecture as seen in Table 15.4. IHC can further help in subtyping of various subtypes of HL as summarised in Table 15.5. Figures 15.2, 15.3, 15.4, 15.5, and 15.6 depict HPE and IHC of lymph node biopsy in HL.

Imaging studies—Positron emission tomography/computed tomography (PET/CT) scan of the chest, abdomen, and pelvis [67] are required before the treatment for the staging purpose. HL

Table 15.5 Differences between various subtypes of HL on basis of IHCs

NLPHL	• Positive markers—CD45+, CD19, CD20, CD22, CD79a, Bcl-6, PAX-5, Oct-2, PU.1, BOB.1 a, HGAL, AID, and centerin [66, 67] • Negative or partial positivity—EMA, CD15, CD30
Classical HL	• R–S cells • Positive—Strong CD30 (membrane and/or dotlike), PAX-5 (Less strong nuclear signal in comparison to small B lymphocytes), CD15, CD20 in 30–40%, MUM-1 • Negative—CD45, Oct-2, BOB.1

Fig. 15.2 Classical Hodgkin lymphoma in lymph node H&E 20×—Section from lymph node shows effaced lymph node architecture with RS and mononuclear RS cells surrounded by reactive inflammatory cells with sclerosis in background

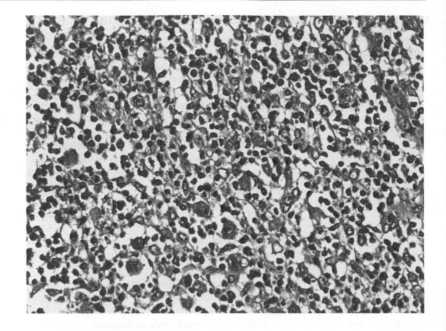

Fig. 15.3 Classical Hodgkin lymphoma in lymph node H&E 40×—High power shows classical RS cells surrounded by mononuclear inflammatory cells

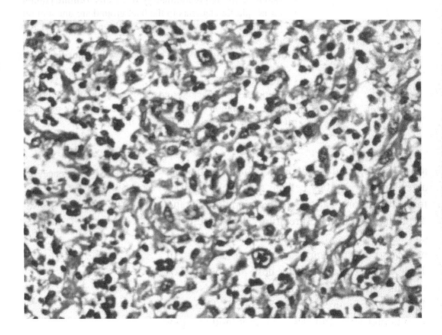

Fig. 15.4 Classical
Hodgkin lymphoma in
lymph node H&E
CD15—Section from
lymph node shows
positivity for CD15 in
malignant cells

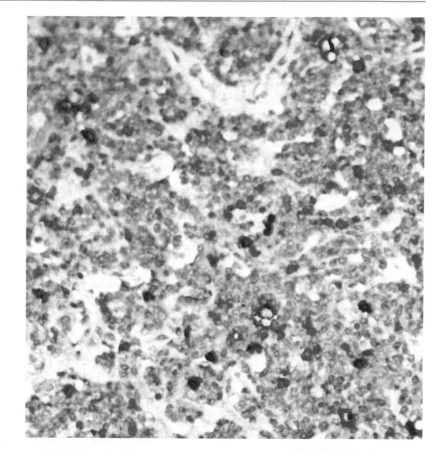

Fig. 15.5 Classical
Hodgkin lymphoma in
lymph node H&E
CD30—Section from
lymph node shows
positivity for CD30 in
malignant cells

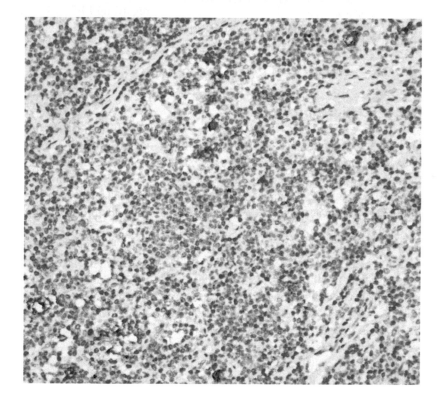

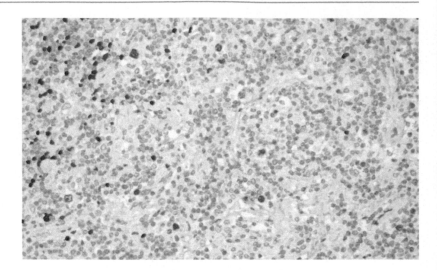

Fig. 15.6 Classical Hodgkin lymphoma in lymph node PAX 5—Section from lymph node shows dim positivity for PAX 5 in malignant cells

being FDG avid tumour and hence PET scan provides information pertaining to tumour burden.

Score PET/CT result (Deauville score) [68]

Score	PET/CT result
1	No uptake above background
2	Uptake ≤mediastinum
3	Uptake >mediastinum but ≤liver
4	Uptake moderately increased compared to the liver at any site
5	Uptake markedly increased compared to the liver at any site
X	New areas of uptake unlikely to be related to lymphoma

15.8 Staging and Prognosis

Ann Arbor staging system with modified Cotswolds is in use in HL [69, 70]. Recently some revisions known as Lugano classification were proposed for staging of lymphomas though still they are not widely accepted [68, 71] [Table 15.6].

Recently imaging modality in the form of PET/CT scan has superseded others. With the inclusion of PET scan there was change of stage in approximately 20% of patients and thus have led to change of management [72–75] and in many situations has replaced pathological staging [76, 77]. In lieu of PET, a contrast-enhanced CT can be used for staging though it may not be the better option except where PET scan doesn't provide complete information especially neck area.

Various studies have stated risk factors on the basis of age, ESR, B symptoms and nodal, extranodal sites, bulky mass as well as mediastinal mass as mentioned in Table 15.7.

International prognostic system for an advanced disease has been for management of HL and has been shown in Fig. 15.7.

IPS score in a modern ERA of newer chemotherapy has been studied extensively [78] and following inferences have been made regarding FFP, OS, and prevalence as shown in Table 15.8.

15.9 Primary Hodgkin Lymphoma of Bone

Definition—This entity is defined as presence of confirmed HL in the bone marrow and absence of extra-osseous involvement. Absence of disease has to be confirmed by PET/CT, biopsy and clinically.

Epidemiology—Extranodal lesions in HD are rare and commonly involve lung, liver, bone, and bone marrow [79]. Primary extranodal presentation of HL involving bone and bone marrow involvement is very uncommon (0.25%) [80–83]. The presence of limited literatures of primary HL bone marrow with approximately 30 cases itself shows the rarity of the disease.

Importance—It is very important that primary HL should be distinguished from systemic HL involving bone marrow (Stage IV) as both prog-

Table 15.6 Lugano classification (derived from Ann Arbor staging with modified Cotswolds) [adapted from [70, 71]]

Stage	
I	Involvement of a single lymph node region (e.g. cervical, axillary, inguinal, mediastinal) or lymphoid structure such as spleen, thymus, or Waldeyer's ring
II	Involvement of two or more lymph node regions or lymph node structures on the same side of the diaphragm. Hilar nodes should be considered to be "lateralized" and when involved on both sides, constitute stage II disease. For the purpose of defining the number of anatomic regions, all nodal disease within the mediastinum is considered to be a single lymph node region, and hilar involvement constitutes an additional site of involvement. The number of anatomic regions should be indicated by a subscript (For e.g. II-3 means 3 anatomical regions)
III	Involvement of lymph node regions or lymphoid structures on both sides of the diaphragm. This may be subdivided into stage III-1 or III-2: stage III-1 is used for patients with involvement of the spleen or splenic hilar, celiac, or portal nodes; and stage III-2 is used for patients with involvement of the paraaortic, iliac, inguinal, or mesenteric nodes
IV	Diffuse or disseminated involvement of one or more extranodal organs or tissue beyond that designated E, with or without associated lymph node involvement.
Special points	All cases are subclassified to indicate the absence (A) or presence (B) of the systemic symptoms of significant unexplained fever, night sweats, or unexplained weight loss exceeding 10% of body weight during the 6 months prior to diagnosis
	The designation "E" refers to extranodal contiguous extension (i.e. proximal or contiguous extranodal disease) that can be encompassed within an irradiation field appropriate for nodal disease of the same anatomic extent. More extensive extranodal disease is designated stage IV.
	Bulky disease: A single nodal mass, in contrast to multiple smaller nodes, of 10 cm or $\geq 1/3$ of the transthoracic diameter at any level of thoracic vertebrae as determined by CT; record the longest measurement by CT scan. The term "X" (used in the Ann Arbor staging system) is no longer necessary
	The subscript "RS" is used to designate the stage at the time of relapse.

Table 15.7 Unfavourable risk factors for stage I–II HL for ≥ 18 years

Risk factor	GHSG	EORTC	NCCN
Age	–	≥ 50 years	–
ESR and B symptoms	>50 if A, >30 if B	>50 if A, >30 if B	>50 if A, any B symptoms
Nodal sites	>2	>3	>3
Mediastinal mass	MMR > 0.33	MTR > 0.35	MMR > 0.33
Bulky mass	–	–	>10 cm
Extranodal lesion	Any	–	–

GHSG German Hodgkin Study Group, *EORTC* European Organisation for Research and Treatment Centre, *NCCN* National Comprehensive Cancer Network, *MTR* ratio of max mediastinal mass to intrathoracic diameter at T5–T6, *MMR* ratio of max mediastinal mass to max intrathoracic diameter

nosis and treatment modalities vary as the former has much better prognosis.

C/F—Many a time symptoms are either not there or very nonspecific in the form of bony pains. Hence its diagnosis becomes difficult and therefore on an average it takes 6–8 months to diagnose from the time when they first presented. While systemic HL with bone marrow involvement is painless, primary HL bone marrow is quite painful [84]. Because of the symptoms, they are frequently confused with osteomyelitis. Bony lesions can be osteolytic with ill defined borders, sclerotic to mixed though former is most common [80, 81, 84]. The common bony sites involved are dorsolumbar spine > pelvis > ribs, femur > sternum [80]. It can present as both solitary and multi focal lesion [84].

D/D

- Osteomyelitis
- Osseous tumour with fibrous stroma (e.g. malignant fibrous histiocytoma)
- Primary bone tumour specific or common to that particular site

Fig. 15.7 International prognostic score for advanced disease [85]

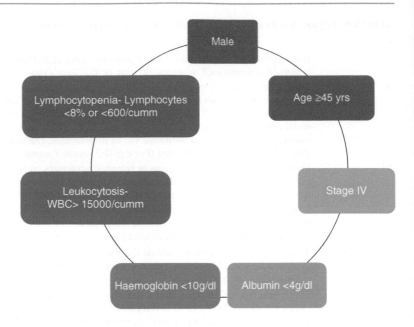

Table 15.8 Association of various IPS scores with FFP, OS, and prevalence

	Freedom from progression (%)	Overall survival (%)	Prevalence (%)
No factors	88	98	8
One factor	84	97	26
Two factors	80	91	26
Three factors	74	88	21
Four factors	67	85	12
Five factors	62	67	7

15.10 Management

15.10.1 Risk-Adapted Initial Therapy

Before initiation of treatment, risk factors which were mentioned previously have to be considered. While prior to chemotherapy there should be extensive evaluation of risk factors, one has to continuously monitor the parameters especially by means of PET scan during the course of treatment because it may help in to add or omit chemotherapy. For example, if PET scan is positive after two cycles of chemotherapy, then intensification of chemotherapy is desired. If there is positivity by PET scan at the end of treatment, then addition of consolidation radiotherapy at positive sites is required to be done. Positive PET scan may require repeating biopsy for confirmation [86]. PET is a better tool for progression-free survival and overall survival than staging of lymphoma and other prognostic factors if done after two cycles of chemotherapy as it can predict progression-free survival [87, 88].

In general, patients presented with an early stage HL have to be treated by courses of combination chemotherapy followed by involved-field radiation therapy (IFRT), while patient who are presented at an advanced stage of HL should receive longer cycles of chemotherapy without radiation therapy. Management of HL as followed by most of the groups considering the stage and prognostic factors has been summarised (Figs. 15.8 and 15.9).

15.10.2 Management of Relapsed/ Refractory Disease

It has been seen in various studies that 5–10% of HL patients don't respond to initial treatment and there were 10–30% patients who had disease relapse after achieving complete remission [89,

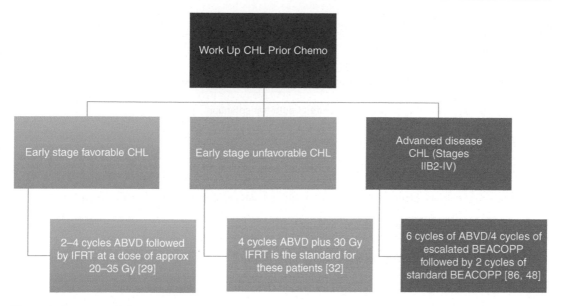

Fig. 15.8 Treatment of classical Hodgkin lymphoma

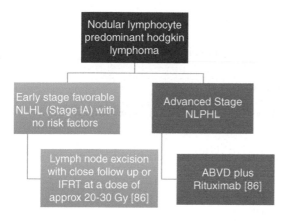

Fig. 15.9 Treatment of nodular lymphocyte predominant Hodgkin lymphoma

90]. Various newer modalities have been tried, some being successful in achieving remission in these resistant groups.

Primary refractory disease—It is defined as progression of the disease or disease showing no response during induction treatment/within 90 days of completion of treatment. There is a low response rate by second-line chemotherapy in HL showing long-term disease-free survival (DFS) in 5–10% of patients [91, 92]. In view of it, other alternatives in the form of high dose chemotherapy (HDCT) with autologous stem cell transplantation (ASCT) are currently the favourite treatment modality [93, 94].

Relapsed disease—Various studies have reported better outcome in relapsed HL treated with HDCT followed by ASCT in comparison to conventional salvage chemotherapeutic regimens [95, 96].

Therapeutic options following relapse after HDCT and ASCT—Generally these patients have worst outcome with median time to progression after the next high dose chemotherapy to be only of 3.8 months and the median survival after ASCT failure to be around 26 months [97]. Patients who failed with both HDCT and ASCT had hardly any treatment options in the past. However with new drugs like vinorelbine [98] and gemcitabine [99] availability hopes have arisen as they have shown some good results. We know that neoplastic cells of CHL are CD 30 positive and therfore use of anti-CD 30 is being thought of in relapsed and refractory cases of CHL. Brentuximab vedotin which acts against CD30 and is being conjugated to an antitubulin agent auristatin has shown a promising response [100, 101]. There are agents which block interactions between the cell surface receptor programmed cell death 1 (PD-1) and its ligands PD-L1 and PD-L2, thus resulting in good clinical response rates. These agents are pembrolizumab

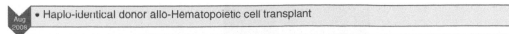

Aug 2008 • Haplo-identical donor allo-Hematopoietic cell transplant

Aug 2009 • Deauville scale for Interim PET

Aug 2010 • Reduced Intensity chemo-radiotherapy in early stage favourable classical HL

Aug 2011 • Brentuximab Vedotin approved after failure of auto-transplantion

Dec 2012 • PET/CT made bone marrow biopsy redunant

Aug 2015 • Brentuximab Vedotin approved for high risk post-Auto consolidation

2015 • P13 kinase delta inhibitorin combination with a selective JAK1 inhibitor has shown promising results in HL

May 2016 • Nivolumab approved for relapsed/refractory classical HL

June 2016 • PET-CT response adapted therapy in advanced classical HL

Aug 2016 • Programmed Death-1 genetic alterations defined classical HL and predicted outcomes

Mar 2017 • Pembrolizumab approved for relapsed/refractory classical HL

Fig. 15.10 Landmarks in treatment of Hodgkin lymphoma

Consensus of the imaging subcommittee of international harmonisation project in lymphoma [110]

Response of disease	Definition
Complete remission	1. Disappearance of all evidence of disease. 2. PET negative residual mass of any size. 3. No evidence of lymphoma deposit in bone marrow biopsy if the bone marrow was involved before treatment.
Unconfirmed CR	Complete elimination of disease
Partial response	1. ≥50% decrease of the sum of the products of the diameters of up to six largest dominant masses. 2. No increase should be observed in the size of other nodes, spleen, or liver. 3. Post-treatment 18FDG-PET should be positive in at least one previously involved site. 4. Bone marrow assessment is not relevant.
Stable disease	1. Absence of criteria defining CR, PR, and progressive disease. 2. No new positive areas of involvement in 18FDG-PET besides the old ones.
Progressive disease	1. Appearance of a new lesion >1.5 cm in any axis after confirmation with other modality as PET is not only the sufficient evidence. 2. More than 50% increase of the sum of the product of the diameters of >1 node. 3. More than 50% increase in longest diameter of a previously identified node >1 cm in short axis by 18FDG-PET.

and nivolumab which have shown good overall response rate of 65% and 88%, respectively, in patients previously treated by stem cell transplantation and brentuximab [102–104]. Other newer agents who have shown positive results are histone deacetylase (HDAC) inhibitors (panobinostat, mocetinostat) [105, 106], mTOR inhibitors (everolimus) [107], and immunomodulator agents. These drugs in relapsed HL have shown reduction of tumour in 60% of patients and partial remissions in 24% patients [108]. Another promising drug idelalisib which is an oral PI3K-d-selective inhibitor has shown promising effects in relapsed HL [109].

Summarised form of landmarks of management of HL has been depicted in Fig. 15.10.

15.11 Response of Disease

15.12 Summary

Hodgkin lymphoma has gone into various historical landmarks. Clinical features have been varied but common symptoms in majority of patients remained present. Its pathophysiology now is well understood better and hence has led to better management and discovery of effective newer drugs. Till a few years back ABVD came up with supreme results but as time passed cases of refractory and relapse also increased and this led to discovery of newer monoclonal conjugate drugs.

References

1. Siegel RL, Miller KD, Jemal A. Cancer statistics, 2017. CA Cancer J Clin. 2017;67:7.
2. Ries LA, Kosary CL, Hankey BF, et al., editors. SEER cancer statistics review: 1973-1994, NIH publ no. 97-2 789. Bethesda: National Cancer Institute; 1997.
3. Correa P, O'Conor GT. Epidemiologic patterns of Hodgkin's disease. Int J Cancer. 1971;8:192.
4. Correa P, O'Conor GT. Geographic pathology of lymphoreticular tumours: summary of survey from the geographic pathology committee of the international union against cancer. J Natl Cancer Inst. 1973;50:1609.
5. Gutensohn N, Cole P. Childhood social environment and Hodgkin's disease. N Engl J Med. 1981;304:135.
6. Alexander FE, Jarrett RF, Lawrence D, et al. Risk factors for Hodgkin's disease by Epstein-Barr virus (EBV) status: prior infection by EBV and other agents. Br J Cancer. 2000;82:1117.
7. Chang KL, Albújar PF, Chen YY, et al. High prevalence of Epstein-Barr virus in the Reed-Sternberg cells of Hodgkin's disease occurring in Peru. Blood. 1993;81:496.
8. Hjalgrim H, Askling J, Rostgaard K, et al. Characteristics of Hodgkin's lymphoma after infectious mononucleosis. N Engl J Med. 2003;349:1324.
9. Tinguely M, Vonlanthen R, Müller E, et al. Hodgkin's disease-like lymphoproliferative disorders in patients with different underlying immunodeficiency states. Mod Pathol. 1998;11:307.
10. Carbone A, Gloghini A, Larocca LM, et al. Human immunodeficiency virus-associated Hodgkin's disease derives from post-germinal center B cells. Blood. 1999;93:2319.
11. Levine AM. HIV-associated Hodgkin's disease. Biologic and clinical aspects. Hematol Oncol Clin North Am. 1996;10:1135.
12. Weiss LM, Chen YY, Liu XF, Shibata D. Epstein-Barr virus and Hodgkin's disease. A correlative in situ hybridization and polymerase chain reaction study. Am J Pathol. 1991;139:1259.
13. Gledhill S, Gallagher A, Jones DB, et al. Viral involvement in Hodgkin's disease: detection of clonal type A Epstein-Barr virus genomes in tumour samples. Br J Cancer. 1991;64:227.
14. Gahn TA, Schildkraut CL. The Epstein-Barr virus origin of plasmid replication, oriP, contains both the initiation and termination sites of DNA replication. Cell. 1989;58:527.
15. Kilger E, Kieser A, Baumann M, Hammerschmidt W. Epstein-Barr virus-mediated B-cell proliferation is dependent upon latent membrane protein 1, which simulates an activated CD40 receptor. EMBO J. 1998;17:1700.
16. Jarrett RF, MacKenzie J. Epstein-Barr virus and other candidate viruses in the pathogenesis of Hodgkin's disease. Semin Hematol. 1999;36:260.
17. Sylla BS, Hung SC, Davidson DM, et al. Epstein-Barr virus-transforming protein latent infection membrane protein 1 activates transcription factor NF-kappaB through a pathway that includes the NF-kappaB-inducing kinase and the IkappaB kinases IKKalpha and IKKbeta. Proc Natl Acad Sci U S A. 1998;95:10106.
18. Cader FZ, Vockerodt M, Bose S, et al. The EBV oncogene LMP1 protects lymphoma cells from cell death through the collagen-mediated activation of DDR1. Blood. 2013;122:4237.
19. Mancao C, Hammerschmidt W. Epstein Barr virus latent membrane protein 2A is a B-cell receptor mimic and essential for B-cell survival. Blood. 2007;110:3715.
20. Rengstl B, Newrzela S, Heinrich T, et al. Incomplete cytokinesis and re-fusion of small mononucleated Hodgkin cells lead to giant multinucleated Reed-Sternberg cells. Proc Natl Acad Sci U S A. 2013;110:20729.
21. Xavier de Carvalho A, Maiato H, Maia AF, et al. Reed-Sternberg cells form by abscission failure in the presence of functional Aurora B kinase. PLoS One. 2015;10:e0124629.
22. Tzankov A, Zimpfer A, Pehrs AC, et al. Expression of B-cell markers in classical Hodgkin lymphoma: a tissue microarray analysis of 330 cases. Mod Pathol. 2003;16:1141.
23. Kadin ME, Muramoto L, Said J. Expression of T-cell antigens on Reed-Sternberg cells in a subset of patients with nodular sclerosing and mixed cellularity Hodgkin's disease. Am J Pathol. 1988;130:345.
24. Liso A, Capello D, Marafioti T, et al. Aberrant somatic hypermutation in tumor cells of nodular-lymphocyte predominant and classic Hodgkin lymphoma. Blood. 2006;108:1013.
25. Marafioti T, Hummel M, Foss HD, et al. Hodgkin and Reed-Sternberg cells represent an expansion of

a single clone originating from a germinal center B-cell with functional immunoglobulin gene rearrangements but defective immunoglobulin transcription. Blood. 2000;95:1443.

26. Kanzler H, Küppers R, Hansmann ML, Rajewsky K. Hodgkin and Reed-Sternberg cells in Hodgkin's disease represent the outgrowth of a dominant tumor clone derived from (crippled) germinal center B cells. J Exp Med. 1996;184:1495.

27. Theil J, Laumen H, Marafioti T, et al. Defective octamer-dependent transcription is responsible for silenced immunoglobulin transcription in Reed-Sternberg cells. Blood. 2001;97:3191.

28. Stein H, Marafioti T, Foss HD, et al. Down-regulation of BOB.1/OBF.1 and Oct2 in classical Hodgkin disease but not in lymphocyte predominant Hodgkin disease correlates with immunoglobulin transcription. Blood. 2001;97:496.

29. Jundt F, Kley K, Anagnostopoulos I, et al. Loss of PU.1 expression is associated with defective immunoglobulin transcription in Hodgkin and Reed-Sternberg cells of classical Hodgkin disease. Blood. 2002;99:3060.

30. Ushmorov A, Ritz O, Hummel M, et al. Epigenetic silencing of the immunoglobulin heavy-chain gene in classical Hodgkin lymphoma-derived cell lines contributes to the loss of immunoglobulin expression. Blood. 2004;104:3326.

31. Marafioti T, Pozzobon M, Hansmann ML, et al. Expression of intracellular signaling molecules in classical and lymphocyte predominance Hodgkin disease. Blood. 2004;103:188.

32. Ushmorov A, Leithäuser F, Sakk O, et al. Epigenetic processes play a major role in B-cell-specific gene silencing in classical Hodgkin lymphoma. Blood. 2006;107:2493.

33. Mathas S, Janz M, Hummel F, et al. Intrinsic inhibition of transcription factor E2A by HLH proteins ABF-1 and Id2 mediates reprogramming of neoplastic B cells in Hodgkin lymphoma. Nat Immunol. 2006;7:207.

34. Renné C, Martin-Subero JI, Eickernjäger M, et al. Aberrant expression of ID2, a suppressor of B-cell specific gene expression, in Hodgkin's lymphoma. Am J Pathol. 2006;169:655.

35. Scheeren FA, Diehl SA, Smit LA, et al. IL-21 is expressed in Hodgkin lymphoma and activates STAT5: evidence that activated STAT5 is required for Hodgkin lymphomagenesis. Blood. 2008;111:4706.

36. Gilmore TD, Kalaitzidis D, Liang MC, Starczynowski DT. The c-Rel transcription factor and B-cell proliferation: a deal with the devil. Oncogene. 2004;23:2275.

37. Horie R, Watanabe T, Morishita Y, et al. Ligand-independent signaling by overexpressed CD30 drives NFkappaB activation in Hodgkin-Reed-Sternberg cells. Oncogene. 2002;21:2493.

38. Horie R, Watanabe T, Ito K, et al. Cytoplasmic aggregation of TRAF2 and TRAF5 proteins in

the Hodgkin- Reed-Sternberg cells. Am J Pathol. 2002;160:1647.

39. Buri C, Körner M, Schärli P, et al. CC chemokines and the receptors CCR3 and CCR5 are differentially expressed in the nonneoplastic leukocytic infiltrates of Hodgkin disease. Blood. 2001;97:1543.

40. Ghosh S, May MJ, Kopp EB. NF-kappa B and Rel proteins: evolutionarily conserved mediators of immune responses. Annu Rev Immunol. 1998;16:225.

41. Wu M, Lee H, Bellas RE, et al. Inhibition of NF-kappaB/Rel induces apoptosis of murine B cells. EMBO J. 1996;15:4682.

42. Takeda K, Kamanaka M, Tanaka T, et al. Impaired IL-13-mediated functions of macrophages in STAT6- deficient mice. J Immunol. 1996;157:3220.

43. Skinnider BF, Elia AJ, Gascoyne RD, et al. Signal transducer and activator of transcription 6 is frequently activated in Hodgkin and Reed-Sternberg cells of Hodgkin lymphoma. Blood. 2002;99:618.

44. Kreher S, Bouhlel MA, Cauchy P, et al. Mapping of transcription factor motifs in active chromatin identifies IRF5 as key regulator in classical Hodgkin lymphoma. Proc Natl Acad Sci U S A. 2014;111:E4513.

45. Fhu CW, Graham AM, Yap CT, et al. Reed-Sternberg cell-derived lymphotoxin-α activates endothelial cells to enhance T-cell recruitment in classical Hodgkin lymphoma. Blood. 2014;124:2973.

46. Swerdlow SH, Campo E, Pileri SA, Harris NL, Stein H, Siebert R, Advani R, Ghielmini M, Salles GA, Zelenetz AD, Jaffe ES. The 2016 revision of the World Health Organization classification of lymphoid neoplasms. Blood. 2016;127:2375–90.

47. Mauch PM, Kalish LA, Kadin M, et al. Patterns of presentation of Hodgkin disease. Implications for etiology and pathogenesis. Cancer. 1993;71:2062.

48. Kaplan HS. Hodgkin's disease. 2nd ed. Cambridge: Harvard University Press; 1980.

49. Good GR, DiNubile MJ. Images in clinical medicine. Cyclic fever in Hodgkin's disease (Pel-Ebstein fever). N Engl J Med. 1995;332:436.

50. Gobbi PG, Cavalli C, Gendarini A, et al. Reevaluation of prognostic significance of symptoms in Hodgkin's disease. Cancer. 1985;56:2874.

51. Atkinson K, Austin DE, McElwain TJ, Peckham MJ. Alcohol pain in Hodgkin's disease. Cancer. 1976;37:895.

52. Cavalli F. Rare syndromes in Hodgkin's disease. Ann Oncol. 1998;9(Suppl 5):S109.

53. Lucker GP, Steijlen PM. Acrokeratosis paraneoplastica (Bazex syndrome) occurring with acquired ichthyosis in Hodgkin's disease. Br J Dermatol. 1995;133:322.

54. Perifanis V, Sfikas G, Tziomalos K, et al. Skin involvement in Hodgkin's disease. Cancer Investig. 2006;24:401.

55. Dabbs DJ, Striker LM, Mignon F, Striker G. Glomerular lesions in lymphomas and leukemias. Am J Med. 1986;80:63.

56. Case records of the Massachusetts General Hospital. Weekly clinicopathological exercises. Case 15-1983. A 24-year-old man with cervical lymphadenopathy and the nephrotic syndrome. N Engl J Med. 1983;308:888.

57. Seymour JF, Gagel RF. Calcitriol: the major humoral mediator of hypercalcemia in Hodgkin's disease and non-Hodgkin's lymphomas. Blood. 1993;82:1383.

58. Rieke JW, Donaldson SS, Horning SJ. Hypercalcemia and vitamin D metabolism in Hodgkin's disease. Is there an underlying immunoregulatory relationship? Cancer. 1989;63:1700.

59. Di Biagio E, Sánchez-Borges M, Desenne JJ, et al. Eosinophilia in Hodgkin's disease: a role for interleukin 5. Int Arch Allergy Immunol. 1996;110:244.

60. Teruya-Feldstein J, Jaffe ES, Burd PR, et al. Differential chemokine expression in tissues involved by Hodgkin's disease: direct correlation of eotaxin expression and tissue eosinophilia. Blood. 1999;93:2463.

61. Peters MV, Alison RE, Bush RS. Natural history of Hodgkin's disease as related to staging. Cancer. 1966;19:308.

62. Kaplan HS. The radical radiotherapy of regionally localized Hodgkin's disease. Radiology. 1962;78:553.

63. Rosenberg SA, Kaplan HS. Evidence for an orderly progression in the spread of Hodgkin's disease. Cancer Res. 1966;26:1225.

64. Klimm B, Franklin J, Stein H, et al. Lymphocyte-depleted classical Hodgkin's lymphoma: a comprehensive analysis from the German Hodgkin study group. J Clin Oncol. 2011;29:3914.

65. NCCN guidelines version 2; 2016.

66. Gaulard P, Jaffe E, Krenacs L, Macon WR. Hepatosplenic T-cell lymphoma. In: Swerdlow SH, et al., editors. WHO classification of tumours of hematopoietic and lymphoid tissues. Lyon: IARC; 2008. p. 292–3.

67. Martelli M, Ferreri AJ, Johnson P. Primary mediastinal large B cell lymphoma. Crit Rev Oncol Hematol. 2008;68(3):256–63.

68. Barrington SF, Mikhaael NG, et al. Role of imaging in the staging and response assessment of lymphoma: consensus of International conference on Malignant lymphoma Imaging work group. J Clin Oncol. 2014;32(27):3048–58.

69. Carbone PP, Kaplan HS, Musshoff K, et al. Report of the Committee on Hodgkin's Disease Staging Classification. Cancer Res. 1971;31:1860.

70. Lister TA, Crowther D, Sutcliffe SB, et al. Report of a committee convened to discuss the evaluation and staging of patients with Hodgkin's disease: Cotswolds meeting. J Clin Oncol. 1989; 7:1630.

71. Cheson BD, Fisher RI, Barrington SF, et al. Recommendations for initial evaluation, staging, and response assessment of Hodgkin and non-Hodgkin lymphoma: the Lugano classification. J Clin Oncol. 2014;32:3059.

72. Barrington SF, Mikhaeel NG. When should FDG-PET be used in the modern management of lymphoma? Br J Haematol. 2014;164:315.

73. Hutchings M, Loft A, Hansen M, et al. Position emission tomography with or without computed tomography in the primary staging of Hodgkin's lymphoma. Haematologica. 2006;91:482.

74. Naumann R, Beuthien-Baumann B, Reiss A, et al. Substantial impact of FDG PET imaging on the therapy decision in patients with early-stage Hodgkin's lymphoma. Br J Cancer. 2004;90:620.

75. Barrington SF, Kirkwood AA, Franceschetto A, et al. PET-CT for staging and early response: results from the Response-Adapted Therapy in Advanced Hodgkin Lymphoma study. Blood. 2016;127: 1531.

76. Advani RH, Horning SJ. Treatment of early-stage Hodgkin's disease. Semin Hematol. 1999; 36:270.

77. Ng AK, Weeks JC, Mauch PM, Kuntz KM. Decision analysis on alternative treatment strategies for favorable-prognosis, early-stage Hodgkin's disease. J Clin Oncol. 1999;17:3577.

78. Moccia AA, Donaldson J, Chhanabhai M, Hoskins PJ, Klasa RJ, Savage KJ, Shenkier TN, Slack GW, Skinnider B, Gascoyne RD, Connors JM, Sehn LH. International Prognostic Score in advanced-stage Hodgkin's lymphoma: altered utility in the modern era. J Clin Oncol. 2012;30(27):3383. Epub 2012 Aug 6.

79. Stein RS. Hodgkin's disease. In: Lee GR, Foerester J, Lukens J, editors. Wintrobe's clinical hematology. 10th ed. Baltimore: Williams and Wilkins; 1999. p. 2530–71.

80. Guermazi A, Brice P, de Kerviler EE, Fermé C, Hennequin C, Meignin V, et al. Extranodal Hodgkin disease: spectrum of disease. Radiographics. 2001;21:161–79.

81. Eustace S, O'Regan R, Graham D, Carney D. Primary multifocal skeletal Hodgkin's disease confined to bone. Skelet Radiol. 1995;24: 61–3.

82. Fried G, Ben Arieh Y, Haim N, Dale J, Stein M. Primary Hodgkin's disease of the bone. Med Pediatr Oncol. 1995;24:204–7.

83. Munker R, Harenclever D, Brosteanu O. Bone marrow involvement in Hodgkin's disease: an analysis of 135 consecutive cases. German Hodgkin's lymphoma study group. J Clin Oncol. 1996;14: 682–3.

84. Ostrowski ML, Inwards CY, Strickler JG, Witzig TE, Wenger DE, Unni KK. Osseous Hodgkin disease. Cancer. 1999;85:1166–78.

85. Hasenclever D, Diehl V. A prognostic score for advanced disease—international prognostic factors on advanced Hodgkin disease. NEJM. 1998;339:1506–14.

86. Ansell SM. Hodgkin lymphoma: 2016 update on diagnosis, risk-stratification, and management. Am J Hematol. 2016;91(4):434–42.

87. Hutchings M, Loft A, Hansen M, et al. FDGPET after two cycles of chemotherapy predicts treatment failure and progression-free survival in Hodgkin lymphoma. Blood. 2006;107:52–9.

88. Gallamini A, Hutchings M, Rigacci L, et al. Early interim 2-[18F]fluoro-2-deoxy-D-glucose positron emission tomography is prognostically superior to international prognostic score in advanced-stage Hodgkin's lymphoma: a report from a joint Italian-Danish study. J Clin Oncol. 2007;25:3746–52.

89. Horning S. Hodgkin's disease. In: Kaye S, editor. Textbook of medical oncology. 2nd ed. London: Martin Dunitz Publishers; 2000. p. 461–74.

90. Diehl V, Mauch PM, Harris NL. Hodgkin's disease. In: De Vita VT, Hellman S, Rosenberg SA, editors. Principles and practice of oncology, vol. 2. 6th ed. Philadelphia: Lippincott Williams & Wilkins; 2001. p. 2339–86.

91. Longo DL, Duffey PL, Young RC, et al. Conventional- dose salvage combination chemotherapy in patients relapsing with Hodgkin's disease after combination chemotherapy: the low probability for cure. J Clin Oncol. 1992;10:210–8.

92. Bonfante V, Santoro A, Viviani S, et al. Outcome of patients with Hodgkin's disease failing after primary MOPP-ABVD. J Clin Oncol. 1997;15:528–34.

93. Andre M, Henry-Amar M, Pico JL, et al. Comparison of high-dose therapy and autologous stem-cell transplantation with conventional therapy for Hodgkin's disease induction failure: a case-control study. Societe Francaise de Greffe de Moelle. J Clin Oncol. 1999;17:222–9.

94. Reece DE, Barnett MJ, Shepherd JD, et al. High dose cyclophosphamide, carmustine (BCNU), and etoposide (VP16-213) with or without cisplatin (CBV 1/2 P) and autologous transplantation for patients with Hodgkin's disease who fail to enter a complete remission after combination chemotherapy. Blood. 1995;86:451–6.

95. Linch DC, Winfield D, Goldstone AH, et al. Dose intensification with autologous bone marrow transplantation in relapsed and resistant Hodgkin's disease: results of a BNLI randomised trial. Lancet. 1993;341:1051–4.

96. Schmitz N, Pfistner B, Sextro M, et al. Aggressive conventional chemotherapy compared with high-dose chemotherapy with autologous haemopoietic stem-cell transplantation for relapsed chemosensitive Hodgkin's disease: a randomised trial. Lancet. 2002;359:2065–71.

97. Kewalramani T, Nimer SD, Zelenetz AD, et al. Progressive disease following autologous transplantation in patients with chemosensitive relapsed or primary refractory Hodgkin's disease or aggressive non-Hodgkin's lymphoma. Bone Marrow Transplant. 2003;32:673–9.

98. Devizzi L, Santoro A, Bonfante V, et al. Vinorelbine: a new promising drug in Hodgkin's disease. Leuk Lymphoma. 1996;22:409–14.

99. Santoro A, Bredenfeld H, Devizzi L, et al. Gemcitabinen in the treatment of refractory Hodgkin's disease: results of a multicenter phase II study. J Clin Oncol. 2000;18:2615–9.

100. Younes A, Bartlett NL, Leonard JP, et al. Brentuximab vedotin (SGN-35) for relapsed CD30- positive lymphomas. N Engl J Med. 2010;363:1812–21.

101. Younes A, Gopal AK, Smith SE, et al. Results of a pivotal phase II study of brentuximab vedotin for patients with relapsed or refractory Hodgkin's lymphoma. J Clin Oncol. 2012;30:2183–9.

102. Ansell SM, Lesokhin AM, Borrello I, et al. PD-1 blockade with nivolumab in relapsed or refractory Hodgkin's lymphoma. N Engl J Med. 2015;372:311–9.

103. Armand P, Shipp MA, Ribrag V, et al. PD-1 blockade with pembrolizumab in patients with classical Hodgkin lymphoma after brentuximab vedotin failure: safety, efficacy, and biomarker assessment. In: 57th ASH annual meeting 2015; abstract 584.

104. Herbaux C, Gauthier J, Brice P, et al. Nivolumab is effective and reasonably safe in relapsed or refractory Hodgkin's lymphoma after allogeneic hematopoietic cell transplantation: a study from the Lysa and SFGM-TC. In: 57th ASH annual meeting 2015; abstract 3979.

105. Zhou N, Moradei O, Raeppel S, et al. Discovery of N-(2-aminophenyl)24-[(4-pyridin-3-ylpyrimidin-2-ylamino)methyl]benzamide (MGCD0103), an orally active histone deacetylase inhibitor. J Med Chem. 2008;51:4072–5.

106. Fournel M, Bonfils C, Hou Y, et al. MGCD0103, a novel isotype-selective histone deacetylase inhibitor, has broad spectrum antitumor activity in vitro and in vivo. Mol Cancer Ther. 2008;7:759–68.

107. Johnston PB, Pinter-Brown L, Rogerio J, et al. Everolimus for relapsed/refractory classical Hodgkin lymphoma: multicenter, open-label, single-arm, phase 2 study. In: 54th ASH annual meeting 2012; abstract 2740.

108. Younes A, Oki Y, Bociek RG, et al. Mocetinostat for relapsed classical Hodgkin's lymphoma: an open-label, single-arm, phase 2 trial. Lancet Oncol. 2011;12:1222–8.

109. Meadows SA, Vega F, Kashishian A, et al. PI3Kdelta inhibitor, GS-1101 (CAL-101), attenuates pathway signaling, induces apoptosis, and overcomes signals from the microenvironment in cellular models of Hodgkin lymphoma. Blood. 2012;119: 1897–900.

110. Juweid ME, Stroobants S, Hoekstra OS, et al. Use of positron emission tomography for response assessment of lymphoma: consensus of the imaging subcommittee of International Harmonization Project in Lymphoma. J Clin Oncol. 2007;25:571–8.

Pathology of Lymphoreticular Tissues

Sumeet Gujral

16.1 Introduction and Scope of This Chapter

Hematopathology is a discipline in which the routine methods of clinical and morphologic analysis are interwoven with routine laboratory as well various ancillary techniques for diagnosis and management of hematolymphoid lesions. Such lesions broadly may be divided into non-neoplastic (like viral, tubercular, autoimmune, drug induced) and neoplastic. Neoplastic lesions involving nodes could be hematolymphoid or non-hematolymphoid neoplasms. Scope of this chapter is hematolymphoid neoplasms (HLN) as defined by the WHO 2017 Classification of HLN and others [1–3]. Here we discuss the morphology of normal lymphoreticular tissues (primarily lymph nodes, bone marrow trephine biopsy, spleen, and thymus) followed by an approach to diagnosis and subtyping of HLN based on morphology and various ancillary techniques, primarily immunohistochemistry (IHC) (Figs. 16.1, 16.2, 16.3, and 16.4). Bone marrow aspirate is not a part of the scope of this chapter.

Diagnostic hematopathology has been a nemesis for pathologists. Contributing factors to the difficulty of diagnosing HLN include lack of trained hematopathologist and lack of widespread use of various ancillary techniques. To be

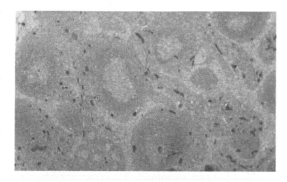

Fig. 16.1 Normal LN showing secondary follicles with outer marginal zone, middle mantle zone, and inner germinal center

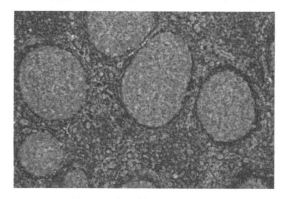

Fig. 16.2 Normal LN showing bcl2 stain—IHC

an expert in hematopathology, a pathologist needs to see an adequate number of cases of such lesions on a daily basis along with various ancillary techniques. It is desirable to have a trained hematopathologist who has expertise in both his-

S. Gujral (✉)
Department of Pathology, Tata Memorial Hospital, Mumbai, India
e-mail: gujrals@tmc.gov.in

© Springer Nature Singapore Pte Ltd. 2019
R. Saxena, H. P. Pati (eds.), *Hematopathology*, https://doi.org/10.1007/978-981-13-7713-6_16

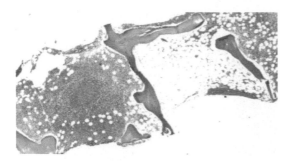

Fig. 16.3 BM biopsy showing secondary follicles in intertrabecular location

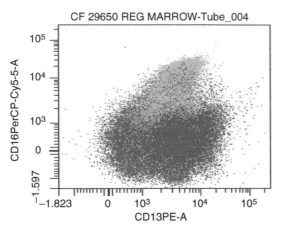

Fig. 16.4 Multicolor immunophenotyping of bone marrow aspirate showing myeloid maturation patterns

topathology (LN, extranodal lymphoid lesions, BM biopsy) and liquid hematology (peripheral blood smear and BM aspirate) with training in various ancillary techniques. Such kind of training programs are available in the USA where they have fellowship programs in hematopathology which encompasses both liquid and solid hematolymphoid tissues with an exposure in various ancillary techniques. In India, most of the hematopathology training programs (post residency fellowship or a DM program) are tilted toward liquid hematology (peripheral blood and bone marrow) and a very little exposure to solid tissue hematopathology (including lymph nodes). Similarly, body fluids may be seen and reported in another division (cytopathology) in most centers. Though IHC is available in many centers, flow cytometry, cytogenetics, and molecular diagnostics are available in few selected centers.

Very few residency programs in India encompass exposure in all these areas including various ancillary techniques.

HLN range from the most indolent to highly aggressive neoplasms. They arise from cells of immune system at different stages of differentiation. Various hematolymphoid tissues include peripheral blood, bone marrow, lymph nodes, thymus, spleen, Waldeyer's ring, and lymphoid tissue at mucosal and other sites. Some of these HLN present as leukemia (primary involvement of peripheral blood and bone marrow), some as lymphomas (primarily involving lymph nodes, spleen, thymus, and other solid organs), and some as combined. Clinical course can change over the course of the disease. Therefore, the terms leukemia and lymphoma may be used interchangeably. HLN constitute approximately 8–10% of all neoplasms in our practice at Tata Memorial Hospital, Mumbai with equal contribution from both solid and liquid HLN. Recent years have brought an explosion of new diagnostic tools to the pathology of HLN, which have permitted more precise disease definition and recognition of factors that can predict prognosis and response to treatment with targeted therapies. Thus, it is imperative for a hematopathologist to have an updated clinical knowledge and also various modalities to reach a final impression. Standard protocols should be followed for various procedures, and it starts with sampling, grossing, processing of tissues so as to finally obtain a good-quality well-stained thin H&E section.

16.2   Brief About HLN

Older classification systems of lymphoid and myeloid neoplasm were separate; however, these have come under one umbrella, latest one being the WHO 2017 Classification of HLN. It has been broadly divided into tumors of precursor lymphoid neoplasms, mature B-cell neoplasms, mature T- and NK-cell neoplasms, Hodgkin lymphoma, immunodeficiency-associated LPD, histiocytic and dendritic cell neoplasms, and myeloid neoplasms, each having further subtypes (Table 16.1).

Table 16.1 Broad subtypes of hematolymphoid tumors [1]

Classification of hematolymphoid neoplasm	Subclassification
Myeloid neoplasms	(a) Myeloproliferative neoplasms (b) Mastocytosis (c) Myeloid/lymphoid neoplasm with eosinophilia and gene rearrangement abnormalities of PDGFRA, PDGFRB, FGFR1, or PCM1-JAK2 (d) Myelodysplastic/myeloproliferative neoplasms (e) Myelodysplastic syndromes (f) Myeloid neoplasms with germline predisposition (g) AML and related precursor neoplasms (h) Blastic plasmacytoid dendritic cell neoplasm (i) Acute leukemia of ambiguous lineage
Lymphoid neoplasms	(a) Precursor lymphoid neoplasms (B, T, and NK lymphoblastic lymphoma/leukemia) (b) Mature B-cell neoplasms (c) Mature T- and NK-cell neoplasms
Hodgkin lymphoma	(a) Nodular lymphocyte predominant Hodgkin lymphoma (NLPHL) (b) Classical HL • Nodular sclerosis • Mixed cellularity • Lymphocyte rich • Lymphocyte depleted
Immunodeficiency-associated lymphoproliferative disorders (LD)	(a) LD with primary immune disorder (b) Lymphoma associated with HIV infection (c) Post-transplant lymphoproliferative disorders (d) Other iatrogenic immunodeficiency-associated LD
Histiocytic and dendritic cell neoplasms	(a) Histiocytic sarcoma (b) Tumors derived from Langerhans cells (c) Indeterminate dendritic cell tumor (d) Interdigitating dendritic cell sarcoma (e) Follicular dendritic cell sarcoma (f) Fibroblastic reticular cell tumor (g) Disseminated juvenile xanthogranuloma (h) Erdheim–Chester disease

Lymphoid neoplasms can occur anywhere as lymphoid cells exist all over. Nodal lymphomas include lymph node, Waldeyer's ring, bone marrow aspirate and biopsy, thymus, and spleen. Remaining may be considered as extranodal. In the following sections, we discuss HLN as per primary organ involved. There is a huge list of lymphoma subtypes; hence, to simplify, we may study it under various headings such as low-grade and high-grade types, pediatric and adult types, and nodal and extranodal types. Common HLN subtypes in adults include diffuse large B-cell lymphoma, chronic myeloid leukemia (CML), chronic lymphocytic leukemia/small lymphocytic lymphoma (CLL/SLL), acute myeloid leukemia (AML), Hodgkin lymphoma (HL), follicular lymphoma (FL), T-cell lymphoblastic lymphoma (T-LL), anaplastic large cell lymphoma (ALCL), Burkitt lymphoma (BL), etc. (as seen in our practice). Common HLN subtypes in children include precursor B-cell lymphoblastic lymphoma/leukemia (B-LL), T-LL, HL, ALCL, and BL. Kindly refer WHO 2017 Classification of HLN for its detailed classification for myeloid neoplasms and WHO-EORTC 2005 classification for cutaneous lymphomas [1, 4, 5].

16.3 Investigations Required

Workup of a case of HLN needs multimodality approach. Routine investigations include complete blood counts, serum proteins (globulin and albumin), erythrocyte sedimentation rate (ESR), serum uric acid, serum calcium, creatinine, lactate dehydrogenase (LDH), beta 2 microglobulin, etc. Morphological evaluation of the tissue like peripheral blood smear, bone marrow aspirate/biopsy, lymph node and extranodal biopsy specimen (including spleen) is of utmost importance. Various ancillary techniques can detect proteins [immunophenotyping by immunohistochemistry (IHC) and flow cytometric immunophenotyping (FCI)], messenger RNA (in situ hybridization), or changes in DNA [Southern blot, PCR, fluorescence in situ hybridization (FISH), and gene expression profile]. Next-generation sequencing (NGS) has joined the long list of the investigative tools in workup of hematolymphoid neoplasms (still at very few centers in west). Ann Arbor staging system is used to stage these lymphomas [6, 7]. Thus, common diagnostic modalities include morphology, cytochemistry (e.g., myeloperoxidase, nonspecific esterase, Perls' Prussian blue), immunophenotyping (IHC and FCM), cytogenetics (both conventional cytogenetics and FISH), and molecular diagnostics (including NGS). Consent for all laboratory procedures as well as investigations are essential for diagnosis, starting from fine needle aspirate to DNA/RNA studies, and it should be a part of the initial consultation with the patient. In all cases, adequate clinical information is essential to assess the risk of the specimen and plan the investigations accordingly. Request forms must include relevant clinical as well as laboratory information including complete blood counts, biochemical investigations, and results of any preceding investigations such as peripheral blood FCI. Findings of radiological investigations like ultrasound abdomen, CT scan, and PET/CT scan are useful.

16.4 Lymph Node: Interpretation and Lymphomas

16.4.1 Introduction and Indication for Biopsy

In adults, under normal conditions, only the inguinal nodes are palpable as 0.5–2.0 cm nodules. Similarly, in children, small 0.5–1.0 cm cervical nodes may be palpable. It may be difficult to define absolute indications for LN biopsy as tuberculosis is one of the commonest causes of lymphadenopathy, which can be diagnosed on FNAC with special stains for mycobacteria and other microorganisms (AFB, GMS, PAS) and culture. FNAC may be a screening test for any lump, and it will help decide if a biopsy is required. However, any lymphadenopathy (solitary or generalized) which is of size >1.5 cm, long-standing (4–6 weeks), firm to hard, movable, non-tender, and suggestive of lymphoma/neoplasm must be biopsied. It is advisable to do a whole node excision biopsy of the largest palpable node. Other indications may include persistent lymphadenopathy, mediastinal mass, abdominal mass or any other extranodal mass, and unexplained fever. History of persistent B symptoms, hepatosplenomegaly, etc. further indicates the need of a biopsy of any palpable mass. Frozen section diagnosis is avoided as it might lead to loss of tissue and also cause freezing artifacts, thereby limiting morphological interpretations with paraffin sections. Needle core biopsy (NCB) is getting popular these days, and role of FNAC is diminishing in many areas. It is done primarily when the lesion is in inaccessible sites (retroperitoneal, mediastinal) or else in incapacitated sick patients. But number of NCB has increased in past, and we get to see larger number of core biopsies even from palpable nodes where a whole node biopsy would have given much more information.

Histopathological examination is the primary mode of diagnosis for any patient with a clinical diagnosis of lymphoma. However, before invasive procedures are attempted, a complete blood count with a manual differential count should be performed as the presence of cytopenia or increased leukocyte counts may suggest bone marrow involvement. In such cases, peripheral blood smear with FCI may provide a lead and also the diagnosis in many cases. FCI has its limitations, as it does not provide morphology (architecture and cytology) of the lesion, and also difficult to diagnose lesions like Hodgkin lymphoma (owing to number and nature of tumor cells). FCI provides invaluable information of background cells. In addition, many lymphomas are easily diagnosed based on FCI like hepatosplenic gamma-delta T-cell lymphoma, hairy cell leukemia, etc. FCI may obviate the need for invasive tests and risks of anesthesia in a significant number of cases. In patients who present with acute severe respiratory distress due to airway obstruction (superior vena cava syndrome due to a mediastinal mass), every attempt should be made to make a diagnosis before starting steroids or chemotherapy; otherwise, it may be difficult to diagnose. A diagnostic tap of pleural fluid or ascites may reveal tumor cells in T-lymphoblastic and Burkitt lymphoma, respectively (similarly precursor B-cell lymphoblastic lymphoma in cerebrospinal fluid). Laparotomy and resection of the bowel may be indicated in patients who present with intussusception or intestinal obstruction, the cause being a lymphomatous process.

Few patients being referred to tertiary care centers for further management might have already received some preliminary treatment in the form of steroids, heavy metals, local herbs, or blood transfusion. This might cause a temporary decrease in tumor load leading to a delayed diagnosis. In such situations, a trephine biopsy done upfront at the primary center is crucial, as this paraffin block may be used to perform IHC to further classify the acute leukemia. Thus, it is suggested that a BM biopsy can be done upfront in all cases of HLN along with BM aspirate, especially in acute leukemias. Such paraffin blocks are invaluable material, as IHC can be performed at a later stage even if there are no blasts seen on peripheral blood or repeat BM aspirate. BM biopsy is also useful in evaluating metastatic deposits, fibrosis, granulomas, etc. Bone marrow aspirates in partially treated acute leukemias may help in detecting minimal residual disease (MRD) in acute leukemias, extremely important in country like ours where most patients get steroids before they reach a tertiary care cancer center. MRD detection may help in picking up scanty cancer cells and hence a definitive diagnosis for further management.

16.4.2 Procedure, Collection, and Transport of Lymph Node Biopsy Material

Lymph node biopsy should be performed by a surgeon (likewise endoscopic biopsy by a gastroenterologist and skin biopsy by a dermatologist). A pediatric surgeon should preferably perform LN biopsy in a child. Whole node biopsy of the largest palpable node should be done. (do not cut the lymph node and send it to two or more laboratories at one time). NCB may be done for non-palpable lesions (inaccessible sites). Multiple cores may be obtained from deep-seated lesions such as abdominal, mediastinal, and retroperitoneal nodes. Tissue should be handled gently to avoid crushing artifacts. Do not use blunt needles or forceps, so as to avoid crushing of nodal tissue. Many surgeons practice NCB even on the large-sized palpable nodes for want of time and ease, and this should be discouraged unless otherwise indicated. Whole node biopsy of the largest palpable node is the mantra. If lymph node biopsy cannot be transported to the histopathology laboratory immediately, lymph node should be sliced serially (3–4 mm thin) perpendicular to its long axis and fixed in optimum quantity of buffered formalin (10 times the volume of the tissue biopsied). This will ensure optimal preservation of morphology and good results on IHC. In hospital-based laboratories, LN may be immediately submitted fresh to the laboratory for grossing and other ancillary tests. Specimens should reach the laboratory immediately after collection since cytogenetic analysis requires live cells for culture and RNA degrades rapidly. This requires close liaison with the operating theater staff because lymph node biopsies are frequently done by junior surgeons/trainees and are added to the end of operation theater list and thus reach laboratory late in the day. In cases where a specialized test like FCI or cytogenetic analysis is to be carried out at a remote location, transport or appropriate tissue culture media should be used. A part of the sample may be sent for snap freezing for the preservation of sample for ancillary molecular investigations. If the clinical impression is of an infective lesion, a fresh sample should be sent directly to the microbiology laboratory for culture and sensitivity testing. For histopathology, the sample should be immersed in buffered formalin for 24–48 h for adequate fixation. Mention the number of lymph nodes and the size of the largest node. The lymph node may be sectioned perpendicular to the long axis of the node. This orientation provides the greatest assessment of the architecture. Majority of the tissue is put in formalin for histopathology laboratory. The bisected LN tissue should be fixed in formalin for 24–48 h; less than this might lead to poor preservation of cytological detail and can make the tissue difficult to interpret. Standardization of fixation makes IHC more reliable. Prolonged fixation makes IHC more difficult and recovery of DNA from paraffin blocks unreliable. In case of a small lymph node and needle-core biopsies, there may be material just enough for histopathology processing, and no additional investigations may be possible. However, if the specimen received is a whole fresh lymph node, which has sufficient volume, the specimen can be divided. Major chunk of the tissue specimen is sent for histological sections (in formalin or other fixative) and a part may be divided for DNA/RNA or FCI studies. Most labs in India prepare paraffin blocks only, which is still the gold standard for lymphoma diagnosis. Flow cytometry immunophenotyping has picked up in the last decade and so.

16.4.3 Histopathology and Ancillary Techniques: Lymph Node and Extranodal Tissues

Morphology: LN (and extranodal) biopsy sections should always be stained with Hematoxylin and Eosin. Scanner view (2×) is the most important, followed by low-power examination. Scanner reveals extranodal fat, capsule, and above all architectural patterns within the node. Abnormal patterns, infiltrates, and then cytological interpretation are picked up in the scanner view (using less light and lowering the condenser). *IHC* is required in almost all suspected cases of HLN for diagnosis and further subtyping. Cases like classical HL may

be diagnosed based on morphology; however, IHC is required in most cases to exclude a wide range of morphological differential diagnoses from viral infections to a high-grade B- or T-cell lymphoma. IHC may be performed by manual or automated methods. *For FCM*, fresh lymph node samples are best analyzed as early as possible, preferably within 6–8 h. If sample has to be transported to a reference laboratory, a laboratory should have standard operating procedures (SOPs) for disaggregating and fixation of the sample in a transport media. *For cytogenetics*, a fresh sample of the specimen (BM aspirate and lymph node) that you want to specify in tissue culture medium should be sent for cytogenetic analysis. Cytogenetic analysis should be performed only once the morphological impression is made. This will help in saving costs in unnecessary screening. FISH may be done on imprint smears as well as on tissue sections. If fresh samples are processed for metaphases, these should be stored, and analysis is attempted after morphological assessment of the sample indicates a need for cytogenetics. The cytogenetic laboratory may store cell suspensions. EDTA may be used as an anticoagulant for molecular tests such as RT-PCR. A sample of fresh tissue may be rapidly frozen and stored for subsequent analysis if required.

16.4.4 Normal Histology and Immunophenotypic Profile

Normal lymph nodes are small, about 1 cm in size, but the size can vary depending upon the site and activity. It is important to understand normal histology along with IHC patterns of normal lymph nodes biopsied from various sites to understand different compartments and dynamic nature of the lymph node. Though it is a dynamic structure and no two normal nodes look similar; broadly, a lymph node may be divided into different compartments mainly capsule, cortex, paracortex, sinuses, and medulla. The understanding of physiology including normal architectural and functional compartment of lymph node is essential to make a diagnosis of pathology of node including nodal lymphoma. Lymph node is a dynamic structure where lot of immunological responses occur to various stimuli like bacterial, viral, or parasitic infections, autoimmune disorders, drug-induced reactions, etc. The lymph node reacts to each of these stimuli differently, and accordingly its histology varies. There may be slight variation in its histology depending upon anatomical site of node. For example, the thoracic nodes show anthracotic pigment, inguinal and pelvic nodes show de novo sclerosis, mesenteric nodes have significant sinus histiocytosis, and spleen and its nodes may show a prominent marginal zone. Multiple reactive (non-metastatic) axillary nodes dissected in a case of mastectomy might show different morphological patterns (dynamic nature of the nodes). Varying morphological features on a scanner view in different nodes may include follicular hyperplasia, prominent T zone with features of dermatopathic lymphadenitis, and sinus histiocytosis, and an occasional node might show distended medullary cords rich in plasma cells. Various nodules can be seen in a low-power examination of the node. These may be B-cell nodules (common) or T-cell nodules. Among B nodules, it might be a primary follicle or a secondary follicle (has a germinal center). Section from an edge of a secondary follicle will appear as a nodule without germinal center (like section from an edge of a boiled egg).

These nodules (rich in mature looking small lymphoid cells) from an edge of a secondary follicle may mimic a primary B follicle or a low-grade B-cell lymphoma. The lymphoid cells in these nodules will diffusely express CD20 and bcl2 (with a low MIb1 and hardly any CD23) and may be diagnosed as low-grade B-cell lymphoma/marginal zone lymphoma on tiny/needle core biopsies of abdominal/retroperitoneal nodes. Bcl2 is a tricky stain. It is positive in most lymphoid cells in a normal node including marginal and mantle zone cells. It is negative primarily in centrocytes and centroblasts of the secondary follicle. CD4+ T follicular helper cells within germinal center will also express bcl2, and excess of these bcl2+ T cells may lead to misdiagnosis of follicular lymphomas in some situations. Sinuses

are common sites of deposits of carcinomas, ALCL, etc. Paracortical T zone is rich in small lymphoid cells in a background of high endothelial capillaries. It may show a mottling pattern rich in interdigitating reticulum cells, which may weakly express cytokeratin called as cytokeratin-positive interdigitating reticulum cells (CIRCs). Pigment-laden macrophages are found here in cases of dermatopathic lymphadenitis (with a prominent T zone). Such conditions and also viral infections may lead to an increase in large-sized mononuclear cells (immunoblasts) in the T zone and may mimic RS cells. Immunoblasts express CD20 and Pax5 (strongly) and CD30; however, classic RS cells (morphology is important) express CD30, CD15, and EBV and weakly express Pax5 (generally CD20−). Nodes with granuloma are classically seen in infective conditions, and common microorganisms must be excluded starting from *Mycobacterium tuberculosis* (caseating granulomatous inflammation). Special stains like AFB, GMS, and PAS for microorganisms must be performed in such cases. Granulomas may also be seen in toxoplasmosis and in lymphomas like HL and Lennert's T-cell lymphoma. Nodes with patches of necrosis with increased apoptosis (karyorrhexis) may be seen in Kikuchi Fujimoto disease (mimic high-grade lymphoma). Here crescentic histiocytes within the necrotic patches express AMPO and plasmacytoid dendritic cells express CD123.

16.4.5 Immunophenotypic Profile of Normal Reactive Lymph Node

Normal lymph nodes reveal a spectrum of histological features. Immunophenotyping of lymphomas as B- or T-cell type is not straightforward as many of the lymphomas exhibit a polymorphous population, and majority of the cells in the background may be non-neoplastic, as seen in T-cell histiocyte-rich B-cell lymphoma (TCHRBCL), nodular lymphocyte predominant HL (NLPHL), and cHL (tumor cells are very scanty). High-grade lymphomas like angioimmunoblastic T-cell lymphomas may mimic cHL, TCHRBCL, and even a reactive node.

Pathologist has to decide on which are the cells of interest (tumor cells) because they may be small size and innocuous looking (like PTCL-NOS) or else may be scanty in nature (like HL, TCHRBCL, etc). Small size of lymphoblastic lymphomas may mimic small size of small lymphocytic lymphoma (SLL) cells. Thus, identifying cells of interest is the key. Morphology followed by extensive IHC panel for T, B, NK cells will help. Deciding on cells of interest may depend on morphology and sometimes on IHCs. Similarly, interpretations of IHC stains may be tricky and not be straightforward. CD5 expression in tumor cells in mantle cell lymphoma may be weaker than the background CD5/CD3-positive T cells (strongly positive). Similarly, Pax5 expression in RS cells in cHL is weak in comparison with brightly lit reactive B cells in the background. Internal control is as important as is external control (Table 16.2). Plasma cells and immunoblasts are the internal control for CD30, while histiocytes and eosinophils are for CD15. CD34, and cyclinD1 may highlight endothelial cells. CD10 and bcl6 will light up the germinal centers. MIB-1 is almost 100% seen within the germinal centers of secondary follicles, where bcl2 is negative. BCL2 may highlight scanty CD4+ T helper cells within the germinal center. Similarly, CD21, CD23, and CD35 are good markers to highlight compact germinal centers, where they stain follicular dendritic cells.

Table 16.2 IHC expression pattern of normal lymph nodal cells

Germinal center (GC) cells: CD10+, BCL6+, and BCL2−
Germinal center B cells: CD20+, CD79a+, Pax5
Germinal center T cells: CD3+, CD4+, CD57+, PD-1 (programmed death-1)+
Follicular dendritic cells: CD21+, CD23+, CD35+
Proliferation index (Ki67 or MIB-1 labeling index): high in GC (almost 100%)
Mantle zone cells: CD20+, CD79a+, CD5+, IgD+, IgM+, BCL2+
Marginal zone cells: CD20+, CD79a+, IgM+, IgD−/+, BCL2+
Paracortical T cells: CD3+, CD4+ or CD8+, CD43+, CD7, CD5, CD2
Histiocytes: CD68+, CD163, CD43+, S100−, CD1a− (S100 and CD1a will be positive in Langerhans cells)
Plasma cells: CD138+, CD38+, CD19+, Ig+, kappa or lambda light chains, EMA+/−, CD20−

16.4.6 Lymphoma Diagnosis

Lymphoma can have a wide range of clinical, morphological, and immunological findings. In our practice, the commonest subtypes of lymphoma are DLBCL and HL. Diagnosis of lymphoma requires multidisciplinary approach. Regardless of the type of lymphoma, initial evaluation of patient should include careful history and physical examination. Important clinical information includes age and sex of the patient, duration of symptoms, presence of B symptoms (like fever, weight loss, night sweats), lymphadenopathy, hepatosplenomegaly, and skin lesions. The baseline radiological investigations (CT scan, PET scan) help in staging and follow-up of the disease response evaluation. The biochemical parameters like albumin and globulin levels, ß2 microglobulin levels, serology for HIV, HBV, HCV, and hematological parameters like hemoglobin, platelet count, and lymphocyte percentage (absolute) are important baseline investigations. All these investigations are complementary to each other. All these parameters help to confirm the diagnosis and identify those manifestations of the lymphoma that might require prompt attention and also aid in the selection of further ancillary investigations, if required, for optimal characterization of lymphoma and to allow the best choice of therapy. Though it is a combined diagnostic approach, for convenience sake the approach to lymphoma diagnosis has been divided into four parts:

1. Morphological/histopathological approach
2. Immunophenotypic analysis
3. Cytogenetic studies
4. Molecular studies

16.4.6.1 Morphological/ Histopathological Approach to Lymphoma Diagnosis

Optimal fixation and processing of lymph node is important for morphological as well as immunohistochemical interpretation. A good quality H&E section is a key to lymphoma diagnosis. It is important to have a low-power lens in the microscope, preferably 1× (most expensive) or else a 2× lens.

For a pathologist, once the H&E-stained slide of suspected hematolymphoid lesion is on the microscope, the dilemma of lymphoma verses non-lymphoma starts. Common non-neoplastic lymphoid proliferations at these sites may be further subdivided into various categories based on etiology and morphological patterns. To take an example of a benign nodal lesion, we may have the following common patterns:

1. Follicular/nodular patterns are commonly seen in reactive follicular hyperplasia, viral infections, autoimmune disorders like rheumatoid arthritis lymphadenitis, hyaline vascular Castleman disease, progressive transformation of germinal centers, mantle and marginal zone hyperplasia.
2. Predominantly sinusoidal pattern is seen in reactive sinus histiocytosis, Rosai Dorfman disease, and hemophagocytic syndrome.
3. Paracortical T-zone expansion may be seen in dermatopathic lymphadenitis, granulomatous lymphadenitis (tubercular and others), Kimura's disease, toxoplasmosis, systemic lupus erythematosus, Kikuchi lymphadenitis, Kawasaki disease, and inflammatory pseudo tumor (IgG4-related diseases).
4. Diffuse patterns are commonly seen in viral infections such as infectious mononucleosis, cytomegalovirus infection, herpes simplex lymphadenitis, and also because of drugs.

The above benign lesions may mimic a lymphoma. Though morphology remains the cornerstone in diagnostic approach, a detailed history with various ancillary techniques including clonality studies may be required to reach a final diagnosis.

First question is whether we are dealing with a lymphoma or a reactive/infective/autoimmune disorder leading to lymphadenopathy. Many drug-related adenopathies (phenytoin, isoniazid, iodides, tetracycline, sulfonamides, allopurinol, etc.) may give rise to an abnormal pattern mimicking lymphoma. Dilantin-associated lymphadenopathy may mimic a high-grade lymphoma, and drugs like thiomercazol may lead to increase in hematogones like cells in the bone marrow,

thus mimicking acute leukemia. Clinical history, along with ancillary techniques like IHCs and FCI (flow cytometric immunophenotyping), helps confirm reactive lymphoid cell patterns including hematogones. Many viral infections like EBV- and HIV-associated adenopathy may mimic cHL, T-cell histiocyte-rich B-cell lymphoma and PTCL-NOS, plasmablastic lymphomas, etc. Tubercular nodes on histology may resemble Hodgkin lymphoma or Lennert's lymphoma, a variant of peripheral T-cell lymphoma. Many patients diagnosed and treated as tuberculosis on the basis of fine needle aspirate might have a hematolymphoid neoplasm. This must be confirmed on a biopsy examination. Kikuchi Fujimoto disease (necrotizing lymphadenitis) with abundant karyorrhexis and plasmacytoid dendritic cells (which express CD123) may resemble high-grade NHL. Such cases require a thorough workup to exclude a possibility of an autoimmune disease and tuberculosis. Thus, a detailed history, thorough examination, complete autoimmune workup, and also special stains for fungus and mycobacteria may be mandatory in such situations. Castleman disease may mimic plasmacytoma and cHL. Light chain clonality and markers like CD15 and CD30 might help differentiate. All these are made complicated sometimes by IHC stains; to give an example, CD30+ B-immunoblasts are seen scattered all over in EBV adenopathy. They also express EBVLMP1 by IHC or else EBER by ISH. These may be confused as RS cells of cHL. However, these are generally mononuclear cells in morphology and also express LCA, CD20, and Pax5 strongly while may be negative for CD15. Thus, IHC alone will not help in differentiating these benign lymphoid proliferations from neoplastic ones. It is important to rule out the possibility of related benign entities and obtain adequate history. Toxoplasmosis commonly occurs in posterior cervical and occipital nodes (with a classical triad of follicular hyperplasia, microgranulomas, and monocytoid B-cell hyperplasia). A large-sized axillary or inguinal node of long duration in an otherwise asymptomatic patient suggests a Nodular Lymphocyte Predominant Hodgkin lymphoma (NLPHL). Patent sinuses, mottled T zone, and preserved secondary follicles favor a benign node and, however, may be preserved in many lymphomas like AITL. Nodal architecture is well preserved in ALCL and metastatic carcinomas where scanty tumor cells might be seen in sub-capsular sinuses.

The second question is whether it is a hematolymphoid neoplasm or some other tumor. Common differential diagnoses include round cell tumors, carcinoma, melanoma, germ cell tumors, etc. depending upon the architecture and cytology of the tumor cells. Large cell lymphomas (like DLBCL, ALCL) may mimic deposits of carcinoma, germ cell tumor, and even malignant melanoma. Small cell hematolymphoid neoplasms (like blastic hematolymphoid neoplasms and extramedullary myeloid tumor) may resemble small cell carcinoma, rhabdomyosarcoma, Ewing sarcoma, etc. Plasmacytoma in the head and neck region may resemble neuroendocrine tumors. Thus, a meticulous morphological examination and an adequate immunohistochemistry (IHC) workup may be required. IHC markers may include LCA, CD20, CD3, CD7, Pax5, CD10, Tdt, CD34, AMPO, c-kit (for blastic hematolymphoid neoplasms), CK and EMA (for epithelial carcinoma), S100, HMB45, Melan-A (for melanoma), c-kit, CD30, PLAP, AFP (for germ cell tumors), Desmin, Myogenin, Myo-D1 (for myogenic tumors), Mic-2, EWS-FLI1 (for PNET/ES), others like CD56, synaptophysin, and chromogranin (for neuroendocrine tumors), etc. Be aware that CD99 is expressed in round cell tumors such as PNET/ES and also in blastic lymphomas. Round cell tumors which are negative for LCA, CD3, and CD20 (initial panels employed in most histopathology lab) and express CD99 have been labeled as PNET/Ewing sarcoma. Such cases may be mislabeled as ES/PNET, if additional markers (like Pax5, CD79a, CD10, Tdt, CD34) are not done. Moreover, new entities like early T precursor ALL might be weakly positive or negative for CD3, highlighting the importance of CD7 in such cases for identifying T-cell lineage of these blastic lymphomas (author's experience). One has to be aware of rare

spindle cell lesions in nodes like myofibroblastoma, IgG4-related diseases, etc.

The third question may be to differentiate HL from NHL and also further subtyping of HL and/or NHL. Few subtypes of NHL like PTCL-NOS, Lennert's lymphoma, and AITL may resemble classic HL. Granulomas as previously mentioned may be seen in infective conditions like tuberculosis and also in lymphomas such as cHL and PTCL. Occasionally, both HL and NHL may mimic a reactive node. cHL may even mimic NLPHL. More than 95% of HL is of classical subtype, and NLPHL constitutes approximately 5% in our practice, as reported elsewhere [1]. Further subtyping of a hematolymphoid neoplasm is important for the management and prognostication of the patient. The pathological diagnosis of lymphoma is based on morphological interpretation aided by immunophenotypic analysis (either immunohistochemistry or flow cytometry). The ancillary techniques like cytogenetic and molecular analysis provide diagnostic and prognostic information in lymphoma diagnosis and may be important in certain unresolved cases. Many large cell lymphomas have an immune profile of classical HL. These may be labeled as large cell lymphoma with Hodgkin phenotype or else may belong to the category of classical HL—lymphocyte depleted. HL is the common lymphoma subtype seen in practice. It is easily diagnosed based on RS-like cells in a polymorphous background. However, it is one of the most commonly misdiagnosed diseases as differentials vary from a reactive node to other B-cell lymphomas like TCRBCL, NLPHL diffuse variant, and Gray zone lymphoma to T-cell lymphomas like ALCL and PTCL-NOS. Thus, HL is another big waste basket like DLBCL and PTCL-NOS.

Low magnification or scanning objective lens for patterns: Either 1× (expensive lens) or a 2× objective lens is preferred in the diagnosis of HLN. Low magnification gives information about the architecture of the lymph node, different compartments of the node, their size and relationship with each other. The whole mount view of lymph node is best seen under scanner view with optimum increase in contrast obtained by altering the intensity of light (low) and moving the condenser up and down. Pathologist must spend maximum time on scanner or a low-power view. Most of the times, the diagnosis is established on a scanner view of the whole node. At least it gives a lead and direction, whether one is dealing with reactive lymphoid proliferations or a lymphoma or a metastatic carcinoma. Identifying the pathologic process, that is, focal, multifocal, or predominantly diffuse is very important for the formation of a differential diagnosis of lymphoma. It is good practice to evaluate various componants of lymph node sequentially at scanning magnification namely the capsule, sub-capsular and medullary sinuses, follicles, mantle and marginal zones, interfollicular areas, and medullary cords for abnormalities. There are specific abnormalities that occur in specific compartments, and their recognition permits formulation of a differential diagnosis. Examine all nodes of a given case as one may observe different patterns in different sections. Most lymphomas have a diffuse involvement; however, few may have focal involvement.

Scanner view gives an impression on cellularity, architecture, and color of the node. Architecture is effaced loosely (and commonly). We know nodes have a dynamic structure and hence different nodes as in a case of axillary dissection in carcinoma breast reveal different architecture. Some have a prominent follicular pattern, other might have prominent T zone, and some may have sinus histiocytosis. It does not imply that the architecture is effaced. Absence of secondary follicles does not mean the architecture is effaced. Architecture is effaced as in when nodes reveal something which should not belong there like necrosis, granulomas, metastatic deposits, fibrotic bands, etc. Appearance of nodularity (pseudo-follicular structure or spherical structure), diffuse nature, sclerotic bands, and proliferation centers are best appreciated at scanner and low power. Blue looking node means that the lesion is composed of monomorphic small cells with scanty cytoplasm. Likewise, a pink appearing node means that the lesion is composed of a polymorphous infiltrate of hematopoietic cells and may include neutrophils, eosinophils, histiocytes, immunoblasts, and plasma cells, apart from the atypical lymphoid cells containing more cytoplasm. Blue appearing nodes are classically blastic lymphomas (LL and myeloid sarcomas) and also small cell lymphomas like mantle cell lymphoma, follicular lymphoma, and small lymphocytic lymphoma. Pink looking nodes (polymorphous background and tumor cells with more cytoplasm) include cHL, PTCL, AITL, ALCL, MZL, etc. Nodular looking lymphomas include cHL, NLPHL, FL, MCL, MZL, SLL, etc. while diffuse looking lymphomas include DLBCL, ALCL, cHL, PTCL, MCL, SLL, MZL, plasmacytoma, blastic lymphoma, etc. Tumors with a thick capsule include cHL. Tumors with granulomas include PTCL (Lennert's lymphoma) and cHL. Lymphomas with a rich vasoformative background and high endothelial venules include PTCL and AITL. Tumor cells in PTCL may be small size admixed with large-sized background immunoblasts. Such cases can only be diagnosed with comprehensive T-cell panels including CD2, CD3, CD4, CD5, CD7, CD8 and also PD1, CD23, bcl6, and CD10 (for AITL). T/NK-cell lymphomas need extra markers including CD56, CD57, granzyme, perforin, and TIA-1.

Various patterns in lymphomas: Various patterns like follicular, nodular, mantle, marginal, sinusoidal, Indian file, interfollicular, and starry sky have been described. Different lymphomas have different patterns and similar pattern can be seen in different lymphomas (Table 16.3).

High-power lens for determining the cell size and other cellular features (40× objective lens): Different types of cells occur in compact groups and can be recognized (with higher power of objective lens) on the basis of their color or their locations (e.g., follicles, mantle or marginal zones, interfollicular areas, sinuses, and medulla). The size of tumor cells is usually compared to that of nucleus of endothe-

Table 16.3 Differential diagnosis of various patterns

Pattern seen in lymph node	Differential diagnosis
Nodular/follicular pattern: ball-like structure of one or two layers with follicular center cells	It is seen in follicular lymphoma grade I, II, and IIIA Follicular pattern can be seen due to follicular colonization by mantle cells in MCL or by marginal zone B cells in marginal zone B-cell lymphoma
Pseudofollicular pattern/proliferation centers: pale staining, hypodense, vague nodular structures without color of mantle zone cells, with or without mitotic activity, and tingible body macrophages	Commonly seen in SLL and rarely in lymphoplasmacytoid lymphomas, pseudofollicles being rich in prolymphocytes
Mantle/marginal zone pattern	Mantle cell lymphoma and marginal zone lymphoma, respectively
Nodules with intermingling of layers	Seen in NLPHL; single to multiple large-sized, closely packed spherical structures, also called as progressive transformation of germinal centers (PTGC), with preponderance of small, dark blue lymphocytes (mostly CD20+ small B cells) containing scattered L&H type RS cells (CD20+ large B cells)
Fibrous nodular pattern	Classical HL—nodular sclerosis and, rarely, ALCL may show this pattern
Starry sky pattern: presence of numerous benign histiocytes with abundant clear cytoplasm and phagocytosis	BL and blastic lymphomas (also seen in Kikuchi Fujimoto disease)
Sinus pattern	ALCL, mycosis fungoides, Langerhans cell histiocytosis, marginal zone B-cell lymphoma, etc. Metastasis of carcinoma may show sinus pattern. Subtle sinusoidal pattern in BM trephine is commonly seen in hepatosplenic gamma-delta T-cell lymphoma (CD3+) and SMZL (CD20+) and intravascular large B-cell lymphoma
Interfollicular pattern	PTCL, leukemia, interfollicular-type cHL, etc.
Vascular pattern	Angioimmunoblastic T-cell lymphoma and PTCL-NOS

lial cells or reactive histiocytes. Small-, medium-, and large-sized cells refer to the nuclei, respectively, smaller than, approximately the same size as, or larger than those of the reactive endothelial cell or the reactive histiocyte. Fine cellular details like nuclear configuration (e.g., cleaved cells), features of nucleoli, and cytoplasmic characteristics are visualized best at high magnification. Small-cleaved cell lymphomas include follicular lymphoma (FL) and mantle cell lymphoma (MCL) while large cell lymphomas commonly are diffuse large B-cell lymphoma (DLBCL), anaplastic large cell lymphoma (ALCL), plasmablastic lymphoma (PBL), etc. BL are classically composed of monomorphic intermediate-sized cells with numerous tingible body macrophages and mitoses in the background:

The cellular microenvironment also contributes to differential diagnosis of lymphoma. The background of plasma cells, eosinophils, neutrophils, and histiocytes is mostly seen in cHL, PTCL-NOS, AITL, etc. Increased histiocytic cells in the background are seen in classical HL, T-cell histiocyte-rich B-cell lymphoma, PTCL, or AITL. For mantle cell lymphoma, scattered pink histiocytes between sheets of monomorphic small-cleaved lymphocytes may be a helpful diagnostic clue (with the absence of nucleolated cells). Clusters of epithelioid histiocytes may be seen in T-cell lymphomas (Lennert's lymphoma) and cHL. Tingible body macrophages containing cellular debris give a starry sky pattern in BL and in lymphoblastic lymphoma (not to confuse with normal T zone mottling seen in reactive nodes or in dermatopathic lymphadenitis).

Benign Versus Malignant Lymphoid Proliferations

Diagnosis of lymphoma is mostly based on the examination of a H&E stain slide. IHC stains can further substantiate morphological findings (and help it further subtype). Many benign diseases of lymph node like bacterial and viral infections including HIV, toxoplasmosis, Kikuchi Fujimoto disease, dermatopathic lymphadenitis, sinus histiocytosis, lymphadenopathy related to collagen vascular diseases, and drugs and also immune reactions (like autoimmune lymphoproliferative syndrome) might mimic a hematolymphoid neoplasm. These nodes may be small to large in size and have a partial effacement of architecture with a prominent follicular hyperplasia and/or paracortical T-zone expansion. Immunoblasts may be prominent in the follicular and paracortical zones and may be confused with RS cells and may express CD45, CD20, and CD30. Kimura disease, Castleman disease, and dermatopathic lymphadenitis may resemble HL while Kikuchi Fujimoto disease may resemble DLBCL/BL. Another common diagnostic dilemma is differentiating reactive follicular hyperplasia from follicular lymphoma. Reactive follicular hyperplasia has classical morphological features. It shows preservation of nodal architecture and low density of follicles, which are variable in size and shape with interfollicular zone. The follicles have sharp demarcation of germinal center from that of mantle zone. Germinal centers will show polarization, brisk mitosis, and tingible body macrophages. Many a times reactive follicular hyperplasia may mimic with follicular lymphoma and IHC with BCL2 may or may not help solve this issue. BCL2 staining within the germinal centers favors a diagnosis of follicular lymphoma, though the FL grade 3 may be negative for bcl2 expression (as seen in cutaneous FL). In reactive germinal center, bcl2 is negative in centrocytes and centroblasts (B cells); however, CD4+ T-helper cells within germinal centers may express bcl2. In situations where CD4+ T cells (bcl2+) predominate within the germinal center, it may mislead to a diagnosis of follicular lymphoma. These CD4+ T-helper cells within germinal centers may give rise to AITL (in addition to T-cell markers, they express CD4, CD10, bcl6, PDI) and CD21/CD23 highlights an extra germinal center follicular dendritic cell proliferations.

Common infectious agents associated with various lymphomas include Epstein–Barr virus (Burkitt lymphoma, cHL, extranodal T/NK-cell lymphoma, angioimmunoblastic T-cell lymphoma, primary CNS large B-cell lymphoma, EBV-positive DLBCL, post organ transplant lymphomas), HTLV-1 (adult T-cell leukemia lymphoma), HIV (DLBCL, BL, plasmablastic lymphoma), hepatitis C virus (lymphoplasmacytic lymphoma), human herpes virus 8 (primary effusion lymphoma, multicentric Castleman disease).

IgG4-related disease is a newly recognized fibro-inflammatory condition characterized by several features: a tendency to form tumefactive lesions in multiple sites; a characteristic histopathological appearance; and often-elevated serum IgG4 concentrations [8]. Such patients may present to any of the following specialties including pathology, rheumatology, gastroenterology, allergy, immunology, nephrology, pulmonary medicine, oncology, ophthalmology, and surgery. Diagnosis of IgG4-related disease is based on the combined presence of the characteristic histology (triad of dense lymphoplasmacytic infiltrate, a storiform pattern of fibrosis, and obliterative phlebitis) and increased numbers of IgG4+ plasma cells. In tissues, dense diffuse infiltrates of IgG4+ plasma cells that number >50/hpf are reportedly highly specific. IgG4+/IgG+ plasma cell ratio of >40% as a comprehensive cutoff value in any organ is also very specific of IgG4RD.

16.4.6.2 Immunophenotyping and Lymphoma

The different methods of immunophenotyping that yield similar information are IHC, FCM, and immunofluorescence, with the former two being mandatory for any laboratory reporting HLN. It may be expensive to do both IHC and FCM in each case of lymphoma. FCM is best done for blood/bone marrow/fluids, while IHC is optimal for lymph nodal and extranodal lesions. Both the techniques are complementary. FCI may also be done on FNAC of lymph nodes or tissue homogenate from lymph node. Few centers use both FCI and IHC in the diagnosis of lymphomas. FCI is performed as a panel rather than an individual marker. Furthermore, understanding of the normal staining pattern and cross-reactions of an antibody is crucial for the correct interpretation and diagnosis. There are markers that work better on IHC like cyclinD1 and other markers that are more popular on FCI like CD200, etc. All labs doing IHC and FCI must have a stringent internal quality control program and also participate in a proficiency-testing (external quality assurance) program. Each new lot of antibody needs to be verified, as required, before it is put in to the diagnostics. All laboratories should preferably be accredited and conform to international quality standards (ISO:15189:2012).

Immunohistochemistry

Of all the available ancillary techniques, IHC is a more widely available tool for diagnosing HLN. FCI of lymphomas as B-, T-, or T/NK-cell type is not straightforward as many of them have a polymorphous population in the background. There are more than 250 CD markers available today and approximately 40–45 being routinely used in IHC labs for the diagnosis of HLN (Figs. 16.5, 16.6, 16.7, 16.8 and Tables 16.4, 16.5, 16.6, 16.7, 16.8, 16.9, 16.10, 16.11, 16.12). It is important to understand the reactions of these markers with respect to different normal

Fig. 16.5 Hans algorithm

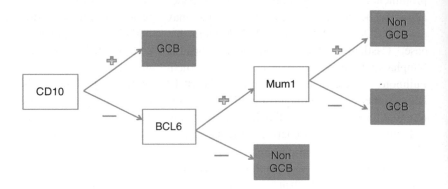

Fig. 16.6 Differentials in mature B-cell neoplasms based on bright CD45 and CD19 positivity

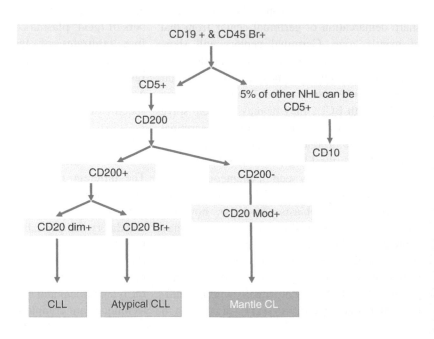

Fig. 16.7 Mature B-cell neoplasms based on bright CD45 and CD19 positivity

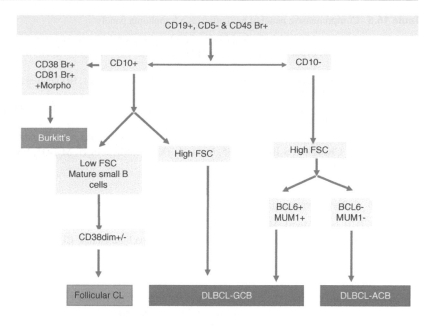

Fig. 16.8 Mature B-cell neoplasms based on bright CD45 and CD19 positivity

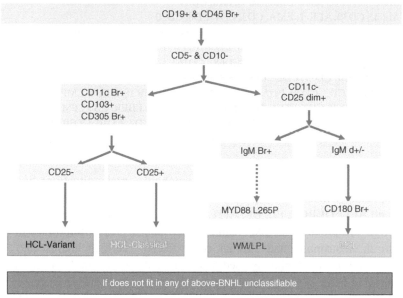

Table 16.4 Essential markers for a hematopathology laboratory

LCA, CD20, CD3, CD5, CD23, cyclinD1, Mib1, CD10, bcl6, bcl2, CD43, CD15, CD30, Alk1, Pax5, Tdt, CD34, CD138, MPO, Mum1, EBVLMP1/EBER (ISH)

cells in the lymphoid and non-lymphoid organs. An example is of bcl2 reaction in a normal lymph node. Bcl2 is commonly used in the differential diagnosis of follicular lymphoma from follicular hyperplasia. In a normal node, bcl2 is expressed by mantle cells, marginal zone cells, interfollicular T cells, and in T cells (CD4+) present within the germinal centers. Similarly, Pax5 is a B-cell marker with the strongest expression in mantle zone cells, weak to moderate in germinal center C cells, weak in RS cells (in CHL), and negative in marginal zone B cells, plasma cells, and T cells. CD138 is a marker for plasma cells and is also expressed in epithelial

Table 16.5 Comprehensive panel of antibodies as a lymphoma panel

B-cell lymphoma panels: CD20, CD79a, CD19, CD23, CD10, MYC, CD5, BCL2, BCL6, Ki67, IRF4/Mum1, CD21, CD23, CD35, cyclin D1, Pax5, Tdt, CD138, kappa and lambda light chains, CD43, p21, Annexin A1, CD123
Hodgkin lymphoma panel: LCA, CD3, CD20, CD15, CD30, Pax5, ALK1, IRF4/Mum1, EBV-LMP1, EBE-EBER (ISH), Oct2, Bob1, EMA, CD57
T/NK-cell lymphoma panel: CD2, CD3, CD4, CD5, CD7, CD8, CD56, Ki67, CD23, CD10, CD25, CD30, Alk1, Tdt, CD56, CD57, Perforin, Granzyme, TIA-1, PD1, CD123
Miscellaneous: C-kit, MPO, CD33, HLADR, CD1a, CD163, CD61/CD41, CD235, CD71, etc.
Other markers: CK, EMA, S-100, HMB45, Melan A, Desmin, Mic2, FLI1, MyoD1, Myogenin, Synaptophysin, Chromogranin, ER, PR, Cerb b2

Table 16.6 Different lymphoma subtypes and panels

DLBCL: CD10, bcl6, Mum1, Mib1, bcl2, MYC
Plasma cell neoplasms: CD79a, CD38, CD138, kappa/lambda light chains, CD56, EMA, Mum1, cyclinD1, CD19, C-kit
Small cell lymphomas: CD5, CD23, cyclinD1, bcl6, CD10, CD43, bcl2
Burkitt lymphoma: bcl2, MiB1, CD10
Lymphoblastic lymphoma: CD3, CD99, TdT, Pax5, CD79a, CD10, CD4, CD8 (for B-LL, CD79a and CD19 are better markers as the blasts might be negative for LCA and CD20)
Granulocytic sarcoma: CD43, MPO, cKit, CD34
ALCL: CD30, ALK-1, EMA, CD3, CD4, CD8, CD20
PTCL/AITL: CD3, CD2, CD5, CD7, CD56, CD30, ALK1, CD23, CD10, CD4, CD8, PD1, Tdt
Suspected NK cell lymphoma: CD3, CD56, CD57, EBER (others: CD8, TIA-1, granzyme B)
Histiocytic differentiation: PGM1 (CD68), CD163, CD1a
Dendritic cell: CD21, CD23, CD35, S-100
cHL: LCA, CD3, CD20, Pax5, CD15, CD30, Alk1, EBER ISH, EBV LMP1
NLPHL: CD20, CD3, CD56, Oct2, Bob1, CD23. CD30, EBER, EBVLPM1
Cutaneous lymphomas: CD3, CD20, CD4, CD8, CD5, CD7, CD10, CD30, BCL2
EBV-related lymphomas: EBER by in situ hybridization

cells. CD10 is a marker used in hematolymphoid neoplasms where it is expressed in precursor B-cell ALL, DLBCL, FL, BL, AITL, and also in benign lymphoid cells like hematogones and also in neutrophils and stromal cells. CD10 expression in neutrophils is used as an internal control in FCI.

Large list of CD markers is available, and newer ones are added on a regular basis. Histopathologist shall decide the panel based on morphology and his/her expertise. Most of the time, a provisional diagnosis for the lesion is established on morphological examination. Accordingly, a panel of antibodies is applied to confirm this and further subtype the neoplasm. The panel also helps in identifying predictive markers (CD20+ B-cell lymphoma may receive rituximab therapy) and prognostic markers (CD38 and Zap 70 in CLL). IHC may also help in

tricky situations like in differentiating a benign from a malignant proliferation (follicular hyperplasia versus follicular lymphoma).

It is important to select and understand the cells of interest and interpret the IHC patterns accordingly. There are neoplasms where tumor cells are very scanty (may be <1% tumor cells), as seen in classical HL. Here the tumor cells are RS cells while the majority of the cells in the background (lymphocytes, plasma cells, histiocytes, neutrophils, and eosinophils) are believed to be a response to the tumor. Thus, IHC is evaluated accordingly. HL has overlapping morphological features with T-cell histiocyte-rich B-cell lymphoma and peripheral T-cell lymphoma (NOS). Selection and interpretation of cells of interest is crucial and may be based on morphological and/or immunophenotypic evaluation.

Table 16.7 Differential diagnosis of HL and NHL resembling Hodgkin lymphoma

Lymphoma	Principle site of involvement	Histology	Tumor cell immunophenotype
cHL	Peripheral lymphadenopathy, mediastinal mass, spleen, Para-aortic LN	RS cell is a constant feature. Sinus infiltration usually absent. Sheets of RS cells can surround area of necrosis in syncytial variant of HL	CD45−, CD30+, CD15+/−, PAX5+, ALK−. EMA−, EBV+/−,BOB1,OCT2−/+,CD20+/− Background is T cell (CD3) rich
NLPHL	Peripheral lymphadenopathy, mediastinal mass, spleen, and bone marrow involvement are rare	Usually a nodular or a diffuse infiltrate with small lymphocytes, histiocytes with scattered tumor cells (RS like, popcorn, L&H cells etc)	CD45+, CD30, CD15−, CD20+, BCL6+, OCT2+, BOB1+, EMA+/−, ALK1−. EBER negative. PTGC nodules rich in CD20+ small B cells admixed with CD20+ L&H cells T-cell rosetting around L&H cells: CD3+, CD4+, CD57+, PD1+
ALCL	Peripheral lymph node, extranodal sites (skin, gastrointestinal tract, bone)	Hallmark cells having eccentric, horseshoe, kidney, or embryo shaped nuclei with eosinophilic region near nuclei seen in sheets. Sinus infiltration is common. RS cells are rare	CD45+/−, CD30+, ALK+/−, CD15-,CD3+/−,CD4+,EMA+/−
PTCL-U	Generalized lymphadenopathy, spleen, skin	Some cases have numerous large cells, which mimic RS cells. Surrounding cells show spectrum of medium and small atypical cells	CD45+, T-cell markers+ however may show loss of any of T-cell antigens (CD7, CD5, CD3, or CD2). Ratio of CD4/ CD8 is altered. CD30 may be focally positive while Tdt is negative B-cell markers negative (rarely CD20+ PTCLs have been described)
T-cell/ histiocytic-rich B-cell lymphoma (T/ HRBCL)	Peripheral lymphadenopathy, but bone marrow, liver, and spleen are frequently involved at the time of diagnosis	A small number of large cells (around 10% neoplastic B cells) seen surrounded by bland-looking histiocytes and small lymphocytes (T type). Tumor cells do not form aggregates or sheets	CD45+, CD20+, BCL6+, BCL2+/−, EBV+, EMA+/− and CD30−, CD15−, CD138− and T−. Background T cells CD3+ along with histiocytes. The T cellsareCD3+,CD57−,andPD1−
Primary mediastinal large B cell lymphoma	Mediastinal mass (thymus), spread to kidneys, adrenals, liver; common in young females	Tumor cells are medium-sized to large cells with abundant pale cytoplasm. Pleomorphic and/or multilobated nuclei may resemble RS cells. Bands of collagen surround the individual and small groups of cells (alveolar fibrosis)	CD45+, CD20+, CD23+/−, CD30+ (+ in about 80% cases), MUM1+,BCL6+/−,BCL2+/−,CD10−

Lymphoma Diagnostic Panels for IHC

Subtle diagnoses that are easily missed on the basis of standard H&E-stained sections include interfollicular HL, sinusoidal infiltration by ALCL, partial nodal involvement by follicular lymphoma or in situ lymphomas, etc. MCL has many morphological variants like in situ type, classical lymphocytic type, blastoid type, and rare polymorphous type. Thus, MCL may have a morphological differential with FL Grade 1 (or SLL) and also a blastic lymphoma. These should be recognized by careful analysis at light micros-

Table 16.8 IHC and genetic features of common mature B-cell NHL

Mature B-cell NHL	CD5	CD23	CD10	CD43	BCL2	Annexin A1	CyclinD1	Genetic abnormality
CLL/SLL	+	+	−	+	+	−	−/+	13q deletion (commonest), trisomy12, deletion of 11q22–23(ATM), and 17p13(p53)
MCL	+	−/+	−/+ in blastoid variant	+	+	−	+	t(11;14)(q13;q32) between IGH@ and/ cyclinD1(CCND1) gene
LPL (IgM+)	−	−	−	+	−	+	−	No specific abnormalities, del6q on BM and rarely t(9;14)(IGH/PAX5)
FL	−	−	+ with BCL6+	−	+	−	−	t(14;18)(q32;q21) between IGH@/BCL2
DLBCL (germinal center/ GC type) and (activated B cell/ ABC type)	−/+	−	+(with BCL6+ in GC)/− (with BCL6− in ABC)	−/+	+	−	−	t(14;18)/IGH@/BCL2, abnormality of 3q27(BCL6 gene), gain of 9p and 12q12
Burkitt lymphoma (Mib-1-100%)	−	−	+	−	−	−	−	t(8;14), t(2;8), and t(8;22):Detection by MYC break-apart by FISH
HCL (CD11c, CD25, CD123, CD103)	−	−	−	+	+	+	+	No specific abnormality
SMZL (IgM+, IgD+)	−	−/+	−	−	+	−	−	Allelic loss of 7q31–32
Mucosa-associated lymphoid tissue lymphoma	−	−/+	−	−/+	+	−	−	t(11;18)(q21;q21) (API2/MALT1) t(1;14), t(14;18), and t(3;14) deregulation of BCL10, MALT1, and FOXP1, respectively

copy, but a small panel of antibodies will be required to correctly subtype these lymphomas. Though there is no defined list for minimal markers, a laboratory must have adequate B, T, myeloid, and other common markers for subtyping of HLN. Attached are the tables with suggested list of the common antibodies used in lymphoma diagnosis (Figs. 16.5, 16.6, 16.7, 16.8 and Tables 16.4, 16.5, 16.6, 16.7, 16.8, 16.9, 16.10, 16.11, 16.12). It is important to mention

here that many carcinomas or round cell tumors might mimic a HLN and hence smaller panels can be misleading.

Specialized centers should aim to perform a comprehensive diagnostic workup as per WHO 2017 Classification of HLN. Smaller labs might have lesser markers in their armamentarium (Table 16.4) and, however, can refer cases to specialized centers for additional IHC markers, as and when need arises. Though there is no list of

Table 16.9 IHC and genetic features of common mature T-cell lymphoma (TCL)

T-cell neoplasm	CD3	CD5	CD4	CD8	CD30	TCR	NK (CD16, CD56)	Viral infection	Genetic abnormalities
T-PLL	+	−	+/−	−/+	−	αβ	−/+	−	inv(14), trisomy 8q
T-LGL	+	−	−	+	−	αβ	+/−	−	No specific abnormality
NK LGL	−	−	−	+	−	−	+	EBV+	No specific abnormality
ATLL	+	+	+	−/+	−/+	αβ	−	HTLV1	No specific abnormality
Extranodal NK/TCL, nasal type	−/+	−	−	−	−	−	+	EBV++	Deletion (6) (q21;q25) commonest abnormality
Hepatosplenic γδ TCL	+	−	−	−/+	−	γδ	+/−	−	iso(7q) abnormality
Enteropathic type TCL	+	+	−	−/+	+/−	−	−	−	No specific abnormality
Subcutaneous panniculitis like TCL	+	+	−	+	−	αβ	−	−	TCR gene rearrangement
Primary cutaneous γδ TCL	+,+/−					γδ	+	−	No specific abnormality
Mycosis fungoides	+	+	+	−	−	αβ	−	−	No specific abnormality
PTCL-NOS	+/−	+/−	+/−	−/+	−/+	αβ > γδ	−/+	EBV−/+	Complex karyotype
Angioimmunoblastic	+	+	+/−	−	−	αβ	−	EBV+/−	No specific abnormality
Primary systemic ALCL (ALK+/−)	+/−	−/+	+/−	−/+	+	αβ	−	−	t(2;5) NPM/ALK
Cutaneous ALCL (ALK−)	+/−	−	+	−	+	αβ	−	−	No translocation involving ALK gene

minimal markers for the diagnosis of lymphomas, two levels (based on number of antibodies used) of antibodies may be suggested (Tables 16.4 and 16.5): first level of best laboratory practice where all available markers are available and second level where bare essential markers are available to make a diagnosis in the vast majority of cases.

Various lymphoma subtypes may look similar on morphology and may also mimic non-neoplastic lesions or other tumors like a carcinoma, melanoma, germ cell tumor, or even a round cell tumor. Moreover, a pathologist will not know what is going to be on his/her reporting table next. Few common morphological mimics include HL and ALCL or a T-cell histiocyte-rich B-cell lymphoma, nasopharyngeal carcinoma, and DLBCL, plasmablastic lymphoma and malignant melanoma, and lymphoblastic lymphoma and any other round cell tumor. Many of B-cell lymphomas like plasmablastic lymphomas might not express CD20, thereby highlighting the requirements of more extensive panels like CD138, Mum1, and CD79A. Moreover, ALK1, which is classically expressed in ALCL, may also be expressed in large B-cell lymphomas, and cyclinD1 may be expressed in hairy cell leukemia and plasma cell neoplasm, apart from mantle cell lymphoma. Few MCL might not express cyclinD1 where we need additional stains including Sox11.

Small-cleaved cell lymphomas (monomorphic cells) include differential diagnoses of MCL and FL (grade 1). MCL generally has a

Table 16.10 Differentials considered for mature B-cell neoplasms based on the following groups

CD5/CD10	Differential diagnosis
CD5+ CD10−	1. CLL: CD23, CD19+, FMC7−, CD22, CD20, and CD79b are weak positive 2. MCL: CD23− or only weak positive, CD19+, FMC7+, CD22, CD20, and CD79b are positive but confirmation is by either cyclinD1 positivity by IHC or t(11;14)(q13;q32) by cytogenetic studies 3. B-PLL: In comparison with CLL, prolymphocytic transformation shows decreased staining for CD5 and increased staining for CD20 and acquisition of FMC7 4. Marginal zone lymphoma (MZL): 5% MZL may be CD5+ and difficult to differentiate from CLL 5. Lymphoplasmacytic lymphoma (LPL): Approximately 5% of LPL are CD5+ and need to be distinguished from MZL and other B-cell lymphoma with plasmacytoid differentiation 6. DLBCL: A subset of DLBCL is CD5+ and it is difficult to differentiate between de novo DLBCL and Richter transformation in CLL
CD5− CD10+	FL and DLBCL represent the most frequent CD10+ and CD5− mature B-cell NHL, followed by Burkitt lymphoma. The lymph node biopsy and cytogenetic study for t(14;18) and c-myc gene rearrangement (BL) may solve the dilemma. It is known to be present in B-ALL Uncommonly, CD10 can be seen in hairy cell leukemia, MCL (CD5+ and blastic variant), and MZL. Very rarely CD10 is also present in T lymphoma like precursor T-cell lymphoblastic lymphoma and angioimmunoblastic lymphoma
CD5− CD10−	The common group involved under this group is DLBCL (may be activated cell type), SMZL, HCL, and LPL. Very rarely CD5− MCL and CD10− FL should be considered Additional marker like CD25, CD103, CD11c, and CD123 by flow cytometry helps in differential diagnosis of SMZL, HCL, and HCL variant HCL: CD25, CD103, CD11c, and CD123+ with annexin a1, DBA.44. and cyclinD1+ (maybe) on trephine biopsy HCL-variant: CD25−CD123− with CD103+ CD11c+ with annexin a1− and DBA.44+ on trephine biopsy SMZL: CD180 bright, CD25dim, CD103− and CD11c+/−, cyclinD1−, and DBA.44+/− on trephine biopsy
CD5+ CD10+	Very rarely this pattern is seen in MCL, DLBCL, and FL

Table 16.11 Differentials considered for mature T-cell neoplasms based on the following groups

CD4/CD8	Differential diagnosis
CD4+ CD8−	Sézary syndrome/cutaneous T-cell lymphoma, T-cell PLL, adult T-cell leukemia/lymphoma (ATLL), ALCL (rarely present as leukemic phase), angioimmunoblastic T-cell lymphoma, PTCL-U, and rarely CD4+ T large granular leukemia (LGL)
CD4− CD8+	T-cell LGL is the most frequent CD8+ T-cell neoplasm. Other T-cell lymphomas with CD8 positivity are hepatosplenic T-cell lymphoma, NK cell LGL, CD8+ PTCL-U. and rarely T-cell PLL
CD4+ CD8+	Dual expression of CD4 and CD8 is usual in T-ALL (TdT or CD34+) and unusual in mature T-cell lymphoma. Though, double positivity for CD4 and CD8 can be seen in T-PLL with surface CD3 positivity and lack of TdT and CD34. Very rarely, ATLL and LGL may show this co-positivity
CD4− CD8−	Enteropathic T-cell lymphoma, hepatosplenic gamma-delta T-cell lymphoma, PTCL-U, and rarely NK/T-cell lymphoma nasal type with T-cell type lymphoma

classical monomorphic pattern of involvement by small-cleaved cells admixed with pink histiocytes and hyalinized capillaries, and absence of nucleolated cells. MCL and MZL can have various patterns including nodular, diffuse, and also mantle/marginal zone growth pattern. Mantle cell lymphoma blastic variant may resemble lymphoblastic lymphoma. Here additional stains like Tdt, CD34, CD5, cyclinD1, and Sox11 are helpful. NLPHL classically presents as single or multiple large-sized nodules (progressive transformation of germinal centers) with the presence of L&H cells expressing LCA and CD20 strongly.

Table 16.12 Useful markers (reagents) for acute leukemia panel

Backbone marker	CD45 (leucocyte common antigen)
Markers of immaturity	CD34, dim CD45, TdT
Myeloid lineage	Cytoplasmic MPO, CD117, CD13, CD33, CD15, CD11b
Monocytic lineage	CD4, CD14, CD11b, CD11c, CD36, CD64, CD65, CD66, HLADR
Megakaryocytic	CD41, CD61, CD36
B lymphoid	CD10, CD19, CD22, cytoCD79a, CD20
T lymphoid	Cytoplasmic CD3, surface CD3, CD1a, CD2, CD4, CD5, CD7, CD8
Plasmacytoid dendritic	CD123, CD302, 303 (CCD4, CD56, CD43)
Erythroid	CD235a, CD71, CD36
Leukemia-associated immunophenotypes (LAIPs)	
AML	CD7, CD19, CD56
B/T-ALL	CD13, CD15, CD33, CD117
Markers for B-cell chronic lymphoproliferative disorder (lymphoma) panel	
General	CD19, CD20, CD22, cyto79a, CD79b, CD23, FMC7, kappa, lambda
Markers useful for further subclassification in B NHL	
CLL/MCL	CD5, CD23, CD43, CD200, CD38, Zap70, light chain restriction
FCL/BL/DLBCL	CD10
HCL	CD11c, CD25, CD103, CD123
Markers for T-cell chronic lymphoproliferative disorder (lymphoma) panel	
General	CD2, CD3, CD4, CD5, CD7, CD8, TCRαβ, TCRγδ
Markers useful for further subclassification in T NHL	
ATLL/CTCL	CD25, CD26
AITL	CD10
ALCL	CD30
LGL	CD56, CD57
EATCL	CD103
NK cells	CD16, CD56, CD57, CD94, CD158
Markers for plasma cell dyscrasia panel	
General	CD138, CD38, CD19, and cytoplasmic kappa and lambda
Abnormality associated	CD56, CD20, CD28, CD117; also loss of CD27 and CD81

Small non-cleaved cell lymphomas (monomorphic small- to intermediate-sized cells) with high mitoses and apoptosis is a classical morphology of BL. BL has a common differential with DLBCL, and there is an entity with overlapping features labeled as high-grade NHL, with features intermediate between BL and DLBCL (an entity deleted in new WHO 2017 Classification of HLN). Similarly, mediastinum, which is a common site of HL (nodular sclerosis pattern), primary mediastinal large B-cell lymphomas (PMLBCL) and DLBCLs, also has a neoplasm with overlapping features between HL and DLBCL labeled as high-grade B-cell lymphoma with features intermediate between HL and DLBCL (a type of gray zone lymphoma). PMBCL is commonly seen in middle-aged to elderly women and has a classical morphology and immunophenotypic pattern.

PTCL is a common subtype of T-cell lymphomas and should be differentiated from ALCLs, AITL, and T-lymphoblastic lymphomas. T-LL must be differentiated from extramedullary myeloid tumors, biphenotypic acute leukemias and also from early T-precursor ALL. ALCL need to be differentiated from Alk-negative ALCL, classical HL, mastocytosis, deposits of carcinoma, and a germ cell tumor (all may express CD30).

DLBCL is the commonest subtype of lymphoma and is considered a wastebasket. They are aggressive lymphomas with considerable clinical, biologic, and pathologic diversity and reflect the functional diversity of the B-cell system and multiple pathways of transformation. Using a multi-modality approach, the updated WHO 2017 Classification has defined some new subgroups, including DLBCLs associated with age groups or anatomic sites. Thus, DLBCLs have broadly been divided into various subtypes like DLBCL, NOS (primary DLBCL of the CNS, primary cutaneous DLBCL, leg type, intravascular large B-cell lymphoma), TCHRBCL, EBV-positive DLBCL, DLBCL associated with chronic inflammation, PMLBCL, ALK-positive large B-cell lymphoma, PBL, PEL, MCD, and B-cell unclassifiable between cHL and DLBCL. Entity B-cell unclassifiable between BL and DLBCL (gray zone lymphomas) has been deleted in new WHO 2016 Classification of HLN. Although DLBCL is curable with standard chemoimmunotherapy (R-CHOP), over 30% of patients with advanced stage disease experience refractory disease or progression. To differentiate the good DLBCL from the bad DLBCLs, gene expression studies were conducted, and they indicated that DLBCL is a heterogeneous disease entity, as cell-of-origin studies reveal at least three distinct subtypes: primary mediastinal, activated B-cell (ABC), and germinal center B-cell (GCB) types [9]. Genomic profiling has been translated to IHC and by using different algorithms, most commonly Hans algorithm (Fig. 16.5), we can differentiate ABC from GCB subtype [10]. Both subtypes express CD10. GCB express BCL6, while any tumor expressing MUM1 is of ABC subtype. Thus, MUM1 is a bad prognostic marker in DLBCLs.

Laboratory Approach in Case of Large Cell Lymphoma

Most labs have a policy to use a smaller primary panel based on morphology and do a more elaborate secondary panel depending on the findings of primary panel. Others might prefer doing a comprehensive panel upfront, saving turnaround time. Most of these large cell lymphomas are of B-cell type; however, a few of these may be ALCL (T/Null-cell type) or other subtypes. To

begin with, three most important markers are (a small primary panel) LCA, CD3, and CD20 in a case suspected to be a large cell lymphoma. In case the tumor cells express CD20, the lab may do secondary panel (depending upon morphology), which may include at least Mib1, CD10, and bcl2 to differentiate DLBCL from BL, and cyclinD1 may be used to differentiate mantle cell lymphoma (pleomorphic variant). Likewise, additional markers like CD10, bcl6, and Mum1 may be required to differentiate good subtype GCB from bad subtype ABC of DLBCL [10]. Newer entities like double-expressor lymphoma (DEL) and double-hit lymphoma (DHL) have been identified in the recent WHO 2017 Classification of HLN [2]. MYC (traditionally a FISH marker) protein has been introduced as an IHC stain. Approximately 30–50% of cases of DLBCL express MYC protein (by IHC) in >40% tumor cells and show BCL2 mutations in >50% cells (in 20–35% such cases) and are labeled as DEL. These are generally ABC subtype and have a bad prognosis. These cases of DEL may be further taken up for FISH studies for MYC/BCL2/BCL6 mutations. Cases of DLBCL expressing MYC by FISH are approximately 5–15%, and these are generally associated with BCL2/BCL6 mutations and are labeled as DHL or Triple Hit Lymphomas (THL) [2]. Thus, in a new case of DLBCL, one may do IHC (MYC, BCL2, BCL6) and follow Hans algorithm. FISH (MYC, BLC2, and BCL6) is not mandatory in all cases of DLBCL and, however, may be attempted in situations like DLBCL with GCB subtype, DLBCL with high-grade morphology and DLBCL with >40% MYC on IHC. Entity of BCLU (intermediate between BL and DLBCL) has been eliminated in new WHO 2017 Classification. High-grade B-cell lymphoma, NOS (HGBL, NOS), is a new entity in WHO 2017 Classification, and it encompasses high-grade B-cell lymphoma with BCLU-like morphology and IHC or high-grade B-cell lymphoma with blastoid morphology but lacks MYC and BCL2, and/or BCL6 rearrangements. Thus, in order of severity, HGBL with MYC, BCL2, and BCL6 rearrangement are the worst subtype followed by DHL/THL (by FISH) and DEL (by IHC). To sum up how to workup a case of DLBCL, one may do only two stains CD3 and CD20, or else an extensive IHC panel including CD3, CD20, MIB1, BCL6, MUM1, CD10, MYC, BCL2, CD30, CD5, cyclinD1, Alk1, CD138, EBER and also FISH for MYC, BCL2, and BCL6.

Similarly, WHO 2017 Classification classifies mantle cell lymphoma into three subtypes. Classical MCL is unmutated subtype, expresses SOX11, is a lymph nodal disease, may involve extranodal sites too, may be blastoid and pleomorphic in morphology, and may have mantle cell zone growth pattern. Another subtype is leukemic non-nodal MCL which is a mutated subtype, SOX11 negative, involves peripheral blood, bone marrow, and spleen, is indolent, is rarely associated with TP53 mutations, and can behave aggressively. The third rare subtype is in situ MC neoplasia where we find cyclinD1-positive cells in inner MC zone [2].

Similarly, dendritic, interdigitating, and histiocytic cells and immunodeficiency-related neoplasms are not uncommon and need an immunomorphological approach. Classical HL needs Pax5 (weak cytoplasmic positivity), EBER (or EBVLMP1) (almost all cases express EBV) in addition to LCA, CD30, CD15, CD3, and CD20. Other situations where NLPHL is close differential, additional markers CD23, CD4, CD8, CD56, Oct2, Bob1, GATA3, etc. may be employed.

Basic IHC panel for lymphoma diagnosis includes LCA, CD20, and CD3. For subtyping, additional markers are required as shown in the tables. Additional panel for other circumstances (based on morphological impression):

Variation in IHC Expression May Help in Interpretation of Hematolymphoid Neoplasms

Aberrant expression by B cells: Co-expression of CD20 (B-cell marker) with CD5 (T-cell marker) may suggest a neoplastic proliferation, though a tiny population of CD5 expressing B-cells has been described in the peripheral blood of normal healthy adults. Expression of cyclinD1 is always abnormal and suggests mantle cell lymphoma, though it can be expressed in hairy cell leukemia and plasma cell neoplasm also.

Aberrant expression by T cells: One can identify abnormal T/NK cells on IHC or FCI if there is

1. Lack of expression of pan T-cell markers like CD7, CD5, CD3, or CD2 (normal NK cells are CD5−).
2. Abnormal intensity of expression of antigen as compared to normal T/NK cells.
3. Aberrant expression of non-T/NK-cell-associated antigen.
4. Abnormal CD4/CD8 ratio or CD4 and CD8 double-positive or negative T cells.
5. Predominance of gamma-delta T cells (double-negative T cells). Normally these are less than 2% of all T cells.
6. The presence of CD1a and Tdt indicates the precursor lymphoblastic lymphoma. CD10 expression can be seen aberrantly in T-cell lymphoma either in T-LL or angioimmunoblastic T-cell lymphoma.

It is important to note that LCA may be negative in few of the HLN like T-LL, B-LL, plasmablastic lymphoma, classical HL, plasma cell neoplasms, etc. BCL2 has a limited role in lymphoma diagnosis. Its expression is seen in normal T cells, marginal zone B cells, mantle zone B cells. Its main use is in differentiating Burkitt lymphoma (BCL2−) from DLBCL (BCL2+) and also in differentiating follicular lymphoma (Bcl2+) from follicular hyperplasia (BCL2−) (best done on morphology).

IHC has an advantage that the histologically abnormal cells can be seen on microscopy to express or lack a particular marker. It may supplement the information generated by FCM and may be the only investigation when FCI is not available. Representative paraffin blocks may be selected for IHC staining. When selecting panels for IHC, it is important to include antibodies that are expected to give negative as well as positive results.

Indian data shows [11, 12] distribution of various NHL subtypes in India. Follicular lymphoma and mantle-cell lymphoma are less common in India compared to Europe and the USA. Peripheral T-cell lymphomas and T/NK-cell lymphomas of nasal type, which are common in many other Asian countries, are also less prevalent. T-cell lymphoblastic lymphoma and anaplastic large T/null-cell lymphoma are more prevalent in India. In this study, B-cell lymphomas formed 79.1% of the NHLs, whereas T-cell lymphomas formed 16.2% of the NHLs. DLBCL was the most common subtype (34% of all NHLs). FL, B-cell SLL, MCL, and MZL (including MALT lymphomas) amounted to 12.6%, 5.7%, 3.4%, and 8.2%, respectively. Among the T-cell lymphomas, T-cell LL, ALCL of T/null-cell type, and other nodal peripheral T-cell lymphomas accounted for 6%, 4.3%, and 2.9% of all cases, respectively.

Flow Cytometric Immunophenotyping (FCI)

FCI is useful in diagnosing and subtyping chronic lymphoproliferative disorders (CLPDs) in peripheral blood, BM, other body fluids, and in FNAC of lymph nodes [13–18]. Most labs do 3–4 color FCI, a few do 6 colors and a selective few do 8–10 color FCI. The data generated by FCM are not limited to the percentage of cells positive with a marker, but extend to simultaneous expression of markers, pattern evaluation, and the intensity of staining. FCI has its own limitations. Evaluation of possible T-cell-rich B-cell lymphoma or a HL can be problematic because of scanty tumor cells and also nodal fibrosis, which might prevent recovery of Reed–Sternberg cells. Similarly, necrotic tumors can give negative results if the small sample used in the flow analysis for FCI does not contain any viable tumor cells.

Most lymphomas are substantially defined by their immunoprofile. When there is a discrepancy between morphology and FCI (technical failure, incorrect diagnosis, or a genuinely aberrant result), further investigations are needed to clarify the results. The final report must highlight discrepancies and should suggest an explanation for abnormal or conflicting immunophenotypic findings.

FCI is the most reliable and robust test for the diagnosis of CLPDs in peripheral blood (Figs. 16.6, 16.7, 16.8 and Tables 16.10 and 16.11). It is performed virtually in all cases with lymphocytosis to confirm the diagnosis (suspected by PBS morphology) and to further subtype the disorders [5]. Mostly these are B-cell phenotype; common subtypes include chronic lymphocytic leukemia followed by follicular lymphoma, mantle cell lymphoma, hairy cell leukemia, Waldenstrom macroglobulinemia, splenic marginal zone lymphoma, and the rarer T-cell CLPDs which may include T/NK large granular cell leukemia, T-cell prolymphocytic leukemia, Sézary syndrome, adult T-cell leukemia/lymphoma, etc. Thus, immunological markers will allow the separation of B- from T-cell-derived diseases and, within the B-cell conditions, will establish the clonal nature of the lymphocytes by showing Ig light chain restriction and subtype CLPDs based on morphology and immunoprofile. Documentation of B-cell clonality (by doing light chain restriction) in cases with borderline lymphocytosis is important to differentiate neoplastic, clonal B-cell disorders from benign conditions. It is important to note that clonality is not equivalent to malignancy. Multicolor nature of FCI helps do an extensive panel B/T/NK/plasma cell marker to reach a diagnosis. FCI of mature B-cell non-Hodgkin lymphoma involving the bone marrow and peripheral blood by flow cytometry showed CLL (68.5%) is the commonest followed by follicular lymphoma (30 cases, 8.5%), mantle cell lymphoma (20 cases, 5.5%), splenic marginal zone lymphoma (18 cases, 5%), hairy cell leukemia (18 cases, 5%) [15].

FCI can also be performed on body fluids (like pleural fluid, ascitic fluid, and CSF) and lymph node aspirate samples with low cell yield. Being a rapid diagnostic method, it is helpful in the diagnosis of oncological emergencies like superior vena cava syndrome (SVCS). FCI performed on the lymph node aspirate may solve the diagnostic dilemma especially when poor fixation or processing of the tissue hampers the interpretation of IHC markers. These two techniques of biopsy with IHC and aspirate with FCI are complementary.

Lymphoma Diagnostic Panels

Bone marrow aspirate with subtle involvement is difficult to comment for involvement by NHL. Usually a cutoff of 30% lymphocytes or 5% of large atypical cells on differential count is considered suspicious of involvement. However, FCI may be required to confirm the nature of lymphoid cells. The focal clustering on imprint smear gives better idea of marrow involvement. Circulating lymphoma cells in peripheral blood smear (PBS) are seen in 40–50% of cases with bone marrow involvement. Incidence of circulating lymphoma cells is highest for low-grade lymphomas like CLL, MCL, FL, SMZL, HCL, ATLL, mycosis fungoides, etc. Cytological features of lymphoma cells are best appreciated on PBS. FCI (combination of various antibodies) assists in the diagnosis (determining the clonality of B/plasma cells) and classification of B/T/NK/plasma cell lymphoid neoplasm. Also, it gives simultaneous co-expression of various B/T/NK/plasma cell markers and even aberrant expression on these cells. Also, it can provide additional prognostic information such as CD38 and ZAP-70 expression in CLL. With increasing sensitivity and specificity, it is becoming an established method for the evaluation of minimal residual disease. Correlation of aspirate and trephine findings are mandatory.

Approach of Lymphoma Diagnosis on Flow Cytometry

Approximately 95% of low-grade lymphomas presenting as leukemia are of B-cell phenotype [15]. The commonest approach in mature B-cell lymphoproliferative disorders is shown below (Figs. 16.6, 16.7, 16.8 and Table 16.10) like CD11c, CD25, CD103, and CD123 may be employed (along with B-RAF mutation studies). SMZL becomes diagnosis of exclusion (IgM+, IgD+).

16.4.6.3 Cytogenetics in Hematolymphoid Neoplasms

Cytogenetics has an important diagnostic and prognostic role in various lymphomas. Interphase fluorescent in situ hybridization (FISH) is mainly performed in lymphomas as it is difficult to get adequate mitoses in lymphoma cells. FISH analysis can be performed on peripheral blood, bone marrow aspirate, fluids or cytology smears, lymph node paraffin sections, etc. The panel for FISH is mainly dependent on the final tissue · diagnosis. In B-cell lymphoma, IgH gene rearrangement and TCR gene rearrangement by FISH do the screening role to define the presence of lymphoma or not. Specific chromosome abnormalities are strongly associated with particular subtypes, for example, t(8;14) or variants in Burkitt lymphoma and t(11;14) in Mantle cell lymphoma. Refer to Table 16.9 for common cytogenetic abnormalities seen in HLN.

16.4.6.4 Diagnostic Panels for Molecular Tests

T and B lymphoid cells are involved in immune function for the recognition of foreign antigens by the specificity of their surface T-cell receptor (TCR) and immunoglobulin, produced by gene rearrangement. Each T and B lymphocyte carries a unique arrangement of TCR or immunoglobulin genes, which helps in the identification of clonality of mature T- and B-cell proliferations. IGH and TCR gene rearrangement by polymerase chain reaction (PCR) can be performed on any sample, that is, peripheral blood, bone marrow aspirate, or paraffin-embedded tissues (lymph node or bone marrow biopsy). Molecular studies are important for diagnosis as well as detection of minimal residual disease. While the use of PCR for specific translocations such as t(14:18), and for detection of T-cell and B-cell clonality based on TCR and Ig heavy and light chain gene rearrangement studies, is an important diagnostic test, false positives and negatives are not uncommon; therefore, PCR results should not form the sole basis for diagnosis.

Conventional karyotyping and FISH for specific translocations are more useful at the time of diagnosis than during disease monitoring, as they are sensitive in lymph node/spleen and relatively insensitive in blood and bone marrow. Molecular monitoring of a known detectable translocation is much more sensitive, although FISH will pick up a higher proportion of cases with standard translocations at diagnosis.

Take Home Message: Lymph Node/ Extranodal Sites

1. Avoid making a definitive diagnosis on FNAC except in suspected cases of relapse of HLN. FNAC may be performed to obtain tissue for flow and molecular studies.

2. Avoid frozen section if tissue is scanty. It may lead to freezing artifacts and depletion of the tissue.

3. Biopsy is mandatory (largest palpable node, needle core). Pediatric surgeon should preferably do a pediatric node biopsy.

4. Quality fixation and processing are extremely important so as to obtain a good quality H&E section (2–3 μm thick).

5. An accurate diagnosis of HLN requires multidisciplinary approach which includes clinical, biochemical, radiological, hematological parameters with morphological and immunophenotyping analysis by IHC and/or FCI.

6. Clinical history is extremely important including age of the patient, complete blood counts, peripheral blood smear, and BM aspirate findings.

7. Spend adequate time on scanner/low magnification as it gives vital information about the architecture and contents of the node/tissue biopsy, cellularity, fibrosis, monomorphous/polymorphous nature of the lesion, focal involvement, any abnormal infiltrates, etc.

8. Higher magnification addresses the cytological features in detail.

9. Common IHC markers include CD20, CD3, CD10, MIB-1, and CD23. These will briefly outline the architecture of the node. CD23, CD21, and CD35 are markers for follicular dendritic cells. FDCs are naked looking cells and may rarely be binucleate.

10. Lymphoma may show diffuse, nodular, or mixed pattern of involvement. It may even show sinusoidal (ALCL, HSGDTCL, MZL) or an Indian file pattern (EMMT).

11. Scanty CD4+ Th cells may be seen within the germinal center. These are cells of origin of AITL. Rarely, they are increased and may be confused with follicular lymphoma as they express CD10 and bcl2.

12. Sheets of CD20+ cells favor a lymphoma; however, this needs to be substantiated with other factors.

13. Mimics of lymphomas include viral infections, granulomatous infections, drugs (phenytoin, etc.), and autoimmune diseases. Other common mimics include Kikuchi Fujimoto disease, Kawasaki disease, Castleman disease, Kimura disease, and toxoplasmosis. Toxoplasmosis classically involves posterior cervical nodes and shows a triad of microgranulomas, follicular hyperplasia, and monocytoid B-cell hyperplasia. Kikuchi Fujimoto disease classically involves young Asian women, shows geographical necrosis on low power and abundant karyorrhectic debris on high power. Burkitt lymphoma shows highest number of apoptotic bodies and karyorrhectic debris. Viral infections might show increase in CD20 and CD30+ immunoblasts.

14. Thoracic nodes might show abundant anthracotic pigment, and pelvic nodes show hyalinization.

15. Infidelity of IHC stains is well known. CyclinD1 may also be expressed in a plasma cell neoplasm and hairy cell leukemia, in addition to mantle cell lymphoma. CyclinD1-negative MCL are also known. Sox11 is another marker for MCL. Bcl2 stain has a limited role and is primarily used in differentiating BL from DLBCL.

16. Follicular lymphoma grade 1 is a common differential diagnosis of MCL, while FL grade 3 is a differential diagnosis of follicular hyperplasia.

17. A lab must possess adequate IHC panels (including those for non-hematolymphoid tumors, like Pan-cytokeratin, S-100, round cell tumor panel, etc.).

18. Diagnosis is a multidisciplinary approach and includes clinical, morphological, phenotypical, and molecular data so as to categorize lymphomas into germinal center (GC) and extracentric subgroups. GC entities include NLPHL, follicular, BL, AITL, and DLBCL with (GC profile), and they express bcl6, CD10, and/or the GC-homing chemokine CXCL13. Post-GC entities like classical HL, MZL, and LPLs, half of CLL/small lymphocytic lymphoma, DLBCL with "activated" or post-GC profile, primary effusion lymphoma, plasmacytoma, and myeloma express MUM.1 and/or CD138, harbor static

rather than ongoing SHM, and may harbor EBV in higher latency states.

19. Cotswold Modification of Ann Arbor Staging System is used in staging of lymphomas.

16.5 Bone Marrow Biopsy Interpretation

16.5.1 Introduction

Bone marrow (BM) is encased by cortical bone and traversed by trabecular bone and consists of hematopoietic cells, capillary venous sinuses (basic structural unit of BM), and extracellular matrix within the bony trabeculae. Microenvironment consists of stromal cells consisting of fibroblasts, macrophages, adipocytes, and endothelial cells. Extracellular matrix consists of collagen, fibronectin, laminin, thrombospondin, and proteoglycans. Fat cells are admixed with hematopoietic cells. Approximately 0.01–0.05% of BM mononuclear cells are hematopoietic stem cells [19, 20]. Major hematopoietic cells belong to any of the three lineages, namely myeloid/monocytic, erythroid and megakaryocytic apart from lymphocyte, natural killer cells, and plasma cells. Myeloid/monocytic lineage includes neutrophils, eosinophils, basophils, monocytes/macrophages, dendritic cells, and mast cells (and their precursors).

BM biopsy reporting has been a difficult area for pathologists for various reasons. Most importantly, there is lack of training and experience in hematopathology, followed by suboptimal tissue processing protocols and unavailability of immunohistochemistry (IHC) stains. Few centers in India do trephine biopsy on a regular basis. Trephine biopsy specimen is immediately transferred into a suitable fixative and decalcified, and further embedded in paraffin wax [21]. Section is stained with hematoxylin and eosin (H&E), with or without a reticulin, iron, and Giemsa stain. Need for other histochemical stains (like AFB, etc.) or IHC is determined by the clinical and the morphological features. BM biopsy reporting is done in a systematic manner, starting from structure of bone (cortical as well as trabecular)

to various marrow elements (which include the vessels, stroma, and the hematopoietic or other tissue).

Aspirate versus biopsy: BM aspirate and biopsy are complementary and have their own advantages. Though morphology is best studied in an aspirate smear stained by a Romanowsky stain, trephine in addition helps in the assessment of bony structure, architecture, cellularity, patterns, and deposits, if any. The combined information becomes critical in management of many cases.

16.5.2 Indications for a Trephine Biopsy

1. Investigation of a peripheral blood abnormality if cause cannot be ascertained by other means.
2. Pyrexia of unknown origin for granulomatous disease or parasites like leishmaniasis, etc.
3. Assessment of cellularity as in aplastic anemia.
4. Inadequate or failed aspirate/dry tap as in hairy cell leukemia.
5. Suspected bone marrow fibrosis (myelofibrosis).
6. Staging purposes as in lymphomas and round cell tumors.
7. Suspected focal lesions/nodular deposits (as in suspected granulomatous disease, myeloma, Hodgkin or non-Hodgkin lymphoma).
8. Unexplained pancytopenia and leucoerythroblastic picture.
9. Diagnosis of hematolymphoid neoplasm (HLN) especially in myelodysplastic syndrome (MDS).
10. Study BM architecture or bone structure.
11. IHC in cases of minimal residual disease.

Site and technique of biopsy: Patients are informed about the procedure in advance and a written consent is obtained if the procedure is to be carried out under general anesthesia (consent taken from parent/guardian in pediatric patients).

Verbal consent is usually considered sufficient if the patient will be fully conscious during the biopsy; however, local hospital/laboratory policy should be followed in this regard. Thrombocytopenia is, as such, not a contraindication for doing a trephine biopsy. Adequate clinical data, peripheral blood smear, CBC findings, and any other necessary details must accompany the BM biopsy requisition form. It is a painful procedure and should be performed only when there is a clear-cut clinical indication and should be done under adequate local anesthesia in adults and a suitable anesthesia in pediatric patients. A trephine biopsy is usually most easily carried out on the posterior superior iliac spine, with the patient in the left or right lateral position and with the knees drawn up. Adequate local anesthesia must be given with particular attention being paid to infiltrating an adequate area of the periosteum. The biopsy needle should be firmly fixed in the cortex of the bone before the trocar is removed, to avoid including extraneous tissues in the biopsy specimen. Only appropriately trained personnel, usually consultant hematologist, hematopathologist, or a trainee in these disciplines should carry out trephine biopsies. It is preferable to use disposable needles to avoid the risks associated with cleaning reusable needles including Jamshidi and Islam needles. Do not use blunt needles so as to avoid crushing artifacts. A trephine biopsy and aspiration biopsy can be carried out through the same skin incision but different tracts to avoid a hemorrhagic BM trephine, a common artifact [19]. All biopsy samples are considered a potential biohazard. Thus, a possibility of tuberculosis, HIV, or hepatitis B needs to be carefully considered in each case. If tuberculosis is suspected, a fresh sample should be sent directly to the microbiology laboratory. Tissues may be collected upfront in different fixatives for ancillary studies including DNA/RNA and flow cytometry.

BM aspirates as well as touch imprint smears should be prepared immediately, using wedge slide method (similar to peripheral blood smear preparation). Imprint smears should be prepared by rolling of trephine biopsy core on glass slides. Imprint smears from the biopsy are also made, and these are more important in cases where aspiration is difficult (dry tap, fibrotic BM). Imprint smears give invaluable information in addition to BM aspirate smears, as seen in hairy cell leukemia. If trephine sample is clotted, the sample may be fixed (formalin) and sent for histopathological examination. Trephine biopsy should be immediately transferred to appropriate fixative. Keep fixative away from the aspirate smears to avoid staining artifacts.

Adequacy of biopsy: Biopsy size after processing should be at least 1.6 cm, and the biopsy on microscopy should show to contain at least five to six intertrabecular spaces. Amount of assessable marrow elements within the trephine is of more importance than the total length of the biopsy [19, 20, 22]. A pediatrician should be aware of the fact that BM biopsy in a child might contain a majority component of cartilage limiting interpretations owing to inadequacy of marrow component. Cartilage can be grossly identified as a glistening blue core. Single BM biopsy is enough for obvious reasons. A higher pickup rate seen in bilateral biopsies done in staging purposes do not really affect the disease management.

Processing of biopsy specimens and staining of sections: After making touch imprints, the biopsy specimen is subsequently put in a suitable fixative and later decalcified and processed further. There are many protocols for BM processing. We follow Hammersmith protocol [21], which recommends aceto-zinc formalin (AZF) as a fixative. Addition of zinc, to stabilize nucleic acids, can protect against hydrolysis in the presence of a weak acid and hence AZF preparations can effectively speed up decalcification without detriment to morphology or antigen preservation. Later, tissue is transferred to a decalcification solution (10% FA and 5% formaldehyde). The process of fixation and decalcification takes less than a day. Plastic embedding of trephine biopsy specimens is practiced at very few centers. Its main advantages include obtaining very thin sections, which stain well with Giemsa leading to good morphological details. It also obviates the need of any decalcification. However, it is a cumbersome, technically demanding, and expensive procedure. Moreover, good quality 2–3 μm thin sections can be obtained from paraffin wax-embedded biopsy specimens; hence, plastic embedding of BM biopsy has lost its popularity. All biopsy specimens should have sections stained with hematoxylin and eosin (H&E). Stains like reticulin, iron, Giemsa may be performed as they might provide additional valuable information. Giemsa stain also helps in highlighting mast cells. An iron stain is unreliable as it may be lost during decalcification and, however, may be useful in few cases. Most laboratories cut a single section (H&E stain), while others obtain 2–3 or more deeper sections at different levels in each case. Few centers do iron and reticulocyte stains as a routine in every case. Special stain for microorganisms (AFB, GMS, PAS) and IHC should be applied as and when required.

16.5.3 Different Samples and Ancillary Techniques Required

16.5.3.1 Peripheral Blood and BM Aspirate Specimens

Apart from morphological assessment after Romanowsky staining, it is used for cytochemistry, FCM, PCR, FISH, and conventional cytogenetic studies. It should be collected in an appropriate anticoagulant (EDTA, etc.), and the sample is best studied within 24 h of collection. Heparin is preferred if a delay is anticipated (up to 72 h).

Flow Cytometry: Samples for analysis by FCM should be kept at room temperature and received within 24 h of collection, as there can be sample degeneration, reduction in antigen strength, or complete loss of antigen with time (maximum within 2 days of collection). *Cytogenetics:* Heparin is the preferred anticoagulant for peripheral blood and BM. Unfixed blood films made using silane-coated slides can be used for FISH. Such films must be made fresh, but can give adequate results even after years if stored at room temperature. They have the advantage that morphology can be seen alongside FISH. *Molecular Tests:* EDTA may be used as an anticoagulant for molecular tests such as

RT-PCR. A sample of fresh tissue may be rapidly frozen and stored for subsequent analysis such as DNA analysis, if required.

16.5.3.2 BM Trephine Biopsy: Collection and Preparation

Lab needs to follow standard published protocols for processing of BM biopsy specimen [21]. Fixatives should be available in the BM operation theaters. *Morphology:* Obtain good quality thin sections (<3 μm thick). BM trephine sections are stained with hematoxylin and eosin. Additional stains include reticulin, Giemsa, and an iron stain. Each slide should be examined initially for cellularity and trilineage hematopoiesis. Any abnormal infiltrate should be identified and described in terms of cellular morphology and type/pattern of infiltration. Lymphoma infiltration can be in the form of one or a combination of the four categories including interstitial, paratrabecular, nodular, and diffuse pattern. Subtle BM infiltrates may be seen in ALCL, SMZL (intrasinusoidal infiltrates), etc. and are picked up by IHC.

16.5.3.3 Body Fluid Samples

Body fluids like CSF and pleural fluid are best examined within 4–6 h of collection. As quantity of CSF is small, selection of IPT panel becomes crucial so as not to miss the cells of interest. Pleural fluids in adolescents are generally involved by T-lymphoblastic lymphomas, so it is important to accordingly do cytoplasmic CD3 and Tdt apart from routine stains. Similarly, ascitic fluid may show the presence of Burkitt lymphoma or DLBCL. Cytomorphology along with FCI is helpful in such situations.

16.5.4 BM Biopsy (Trephine)

BM biopsy (trephine) are studied under the following subheadings.

16.5.4.1 Morphological Approach to a Normal BM

Important components are quality of processing, adequacy of BM, bony architecture, architecture and cellularity of BM, trilineage hematopoiesis, any abnormal cells or aggregates, and background stroma. H&E-stained sections are best examined systematically at scanner view (1X or 2X objective), followed by a low-power (10X) and high-power (40X objective) examination. Oil immersion examination is best done for peripheral blood and BM aspirate smears (100X). Scanner/low-power examination is important for the evaluation of the adequacy of the biopsy specimen, assessment of cellularity (uniform or patchy), patent sinuses, adequacy of megakaryocytes, and detection of focal lesions or any deposits. It also helps in selecting areas for further high-power evaluation. Any abnormality in the trabecular bone is also best assessed in scanner/low power. Focal lesions that may be noted at low power include granulomas and focal infiltrates of mast cells, lymphoma cells, or other tumors.

Trephine is the best modality to judge BM cellularity, done at the scanner view. Cellularity is based on the proportion of hematopoietic cells and adipocytes (fat cells). Cellularity is maximum in neonates and in young children (100% hematopoietic cells and negligible fat cells) and declines with age (Table 16.13) [19, 20, 22]. An arbitrary rule of 100 minus age gives a rough estimate of cellularity. Infants have packed cellularity, and this should not be called as a hypercellular marrow and appears blue on morphology as it has an increased number of lymphoid cells and hematogones [19, 20, 22]. Likewise, old age individuals will reveal a less cellular marrow with increased adipocytes and lesser hematopoietic cells, normal for their age. It is difficult to comment on cellularity, if the biopsy is small, hemorrhagic, or contains subcortical bone only. However, in our experience, a significant number of trephine done in infants as in staging of round cell tumors reveal cellularity less than what is

defined in literature. A tiny biopsy containing only subcortical bone marrow may be inadequate for assessment because it normally shows hypocellular marrow and may mislead a pathologist in overdiagnosing hypocellular BM. It is difficult to comment on cellularity of BM in a fibrotic marrow, and also in edematous stromal background, which may be due to treatment-related changes. There are various systems of grading of fibrosis and popularly followed is the European consensus [23] as shown in Table 16.14.

At low and high power, the location of cells of erythroid and granulocytic lineages and their relative proportions can be assessed, the nature of any focal lesions can be determined, and sinuses/blood vessels are examined. Examination at high power is important for finer morphological details. Dyspoiesis and other finer details including microorganisms and parasites (cryptococci, histoplasmosis, leishmania donovani bodies) are best detected in high power/oil immersion (these are best appreciated in aspirate). After examination of the H&E-stained sections, a reticulin and iron stain may be examined. The reticulin should be graded, according to a standardized published system, and any focal increase in reticulin deposition should be noted (Table 16.14). The presence of focal reticulin deposition is an indication to re-examine the H&E-stained sections to exclude any possibility of a focal infiltrate like lymphoma or mast cell lesion or a granuloma. This may demand deeper sections of trephine biopsy. Specialized cytochemical stains (such as Congo red stain or Ziehl–Neelsen stain) or IHC may be performed as and when needed.

Trilineage Hematopoiesis and Other Cells

Hematopoiesis is best studied on low- and high-power examination. It is the next most important feature (after cellularity) where pathologist

Table 16.13 Age related BM cellularity

Age	% Cellularity	% Granulocytes	% Erythroid	% Lymphocytes
Newborn	80–100	50	40	10
1–3 months	80–100	50–60	5–10	30–50
Child	60–80	50–60	20	20–30
Adult	40–70	50–70	20–25	10–15
Old age >70 years	20–40	50–70	20–25	10–20

Table 16.14 European consensus on the grading of bone marrow fibrosis [23]

Grade 0: Scattered linear reticulin with no intersection (crossovers) corresponding to normal bone marrow
Grade 1: Loose network of reticulin with many intersections, especially in perivascular areas
Grade 2: Diffuse and dense increase in reticulin with extensive intersections, occasionally with only focal bundles of collagen and/or focal osteosclerosis
Grade 3: Diffuse and dense increase in reticulin with extensive intersections with coarse bundles of collagen, often associated with significant osteosclerosis

Table 16.15 Normal adult values for BM differential cell counts

Cell type	Normal range (%)
Myeloblasts	0–3
Promyelocytes	2–8
Myelocytes	10–13
Metamyelocytes	10–15
Neutrophils plus band	25–40
Eosinophils and precursors	1–3
Basophils and precursors	0–1
Monocytes	0–1
Erythroblasts (early)	0–2
Other erythroid elements (late)	15–25
Lymphocytes	10–15
Plasma cells	0–1
Megakaryocytes	1%
Mast cell	0–1

should look for trilineage hematopoiesis (myeloid, erythroid, and megakaryocytic lineages), in amount, proportions, and morphology and other cells including lymphoid cells (Table 16.15). Lymphocytes may mimic erythroid precursors and it can be tricky to differentiate them.

1. *Erythroid series cells*:

    Normal M:E ratio is 2:1 to 4:1. Erythroid cells may occur singly interspersed with myeloid cells or else come in clusters/colonies. They have a uniformly round nuclear contour, prominent cell membranes, perinuclear halo, and a dense homogeneous chromatin (ink dot). The nucleus appears very dark, and chromatin character is difficult to ascertain. Erythroid colonies are small and intertrabecular in location and are commonly

seen in anemia, myelodysplastic syndrome (MDS), and regenerating BM post induction. Megaloblasts are larger round to polygonal cells and have moderate cytoplasm, round nuclei with vesicular chromatin, and a crisp nuclear membrane with 2–3 nucleoli. CD36, CD235, and CD71 highlight erythroid cells. C-kit (CD117) may weakly highlight both megaloblasts and myeloblasts and, however, is strongly expressed in mast cells.

2. *Myeloid series cells*:

    It is the most prominent series in an adult BM and accounts for 50–70% of all nucleated cells. These are granular cells with pinkish granular cytoplasm. Granules of mast cells and basophils get washed off and are not seen on H&E stain. The most immature myeloid cells are myeloblasts and promyelocytes, which are located in paratrabecular and perivascular location, while mature cells like neutrophils and metamyelocytes are located intertrabecularly. These might be confused with megaloblasts and histiocytes (agranular). MPO highlights myeloid series cells on IHC. Myeloid proliferation is seen in infections and also in neoplasms, like myeloid neoplasms, etc. Promyelocytes are large-sized myeloid precursors and have pinkish granular cytoplasm.

3. *Megakaryocytic series cells*:

    Megakaryocytes are largest hematopoietic cells, smaller only to fat cells in BM trephine, and are easily picked up on the scanner view. They constitute less than 1% of all nucleated BM cells. BM biopsy is the best mode of examining megakaryocytes in number, morphology, and distribution. They are distributed all over, mostly adjacent to sinusoids. There are approximately 2–4 megakaryocytes per high-power field on a trephine. They might show emperipolesis, where normal hematopoietic cells are seen within the cytoplasm of the megakaryocytes. They are multilobated (nuclear lobulations) and have a granular cytoplasm, and should not be confused with multinucleated giant osteoclasts.

    A megakaryocytosis may be congenital or acquired and, however, is extremely rare.

Megakaryocytes may be increased in BM in megakaryocytic thrombocytopenia, lupus-associated thrombocytopenia, AIDS, MDS, chronic myeloproliferative disorders (may be associated with myelofibrosis), etc. [19]. Morphology of megakaryocytes is an important factor in differentiating early premyelofibrosis from essential thrombocytosis. CD36, CD41, and CD61 are stains to highlight megakaryocyte and AML-M7.

4. *Lymphoid series cells and lymphoid aggregates*:

Larger number of lymphoid cells is seen in pediatric BM, where they may reach up to 60% of all nucleated BM cells. Morphologically, these are singly scattered, darkly stained, small-sized cells. They might have angulated nuclear contours with appreciable chromatin (in comparison with erythroid cells which have a black round dot like nucleus with a clear halo). Hematogones and benign lymphoid aggregates are seen in benign reactive conditions and need a special mention.

(a) *Hematogones*: BM may show immature lymphoid precursors called hematogones, seen normally in larger numbers in normal infant/pediatric BM. They are increased following viral infections, post chemotherapy, post-transplant, and in association with round cell tumors, lymphomas, etc. On morphology, they are small to medium sized, with scant cytoplasm, round to irregular nuclei with dense homogeneous bland-looking chromatin, and inconspicuous nucleoli. They appear as diffuse subtle infiltrates, singly scattered cells, and rarely as small aggregates. Hematogones are a spectrum of B cells (CD19+) and express a range of markers with variable intensity depending upon its stage of maturity. CD20 is the strongest in mature hematogones (stage 3) while CD34, CD10, and Tdt are the strongest in immature hematogones (stage 1). Thus, hematogones show a variable expression of CD20, CD10, CD38, CD56, CD34, and Tdt. They are best studied on FCI and have a classical pattern of lymphoid maturation (dot plots of CD20 and CD10, and of CD34 and CD38). They may be confused with lymphoblasts, and few cases continue to be misdiagnosed as B-cell acute lymphoblastic leukemia. Hematogones are important to understand as they mimic tumor cells during minimal residual disease (MRD) detection of B-ALL. In such cases, morphological examination of peripheral blood smear may help as it reveals an otherwise normal differential count with near normal complete blood counts. Hematogones are normally not seen in peripheral blood; however, precursor B cells may be seen in neonates. BM aspirate morphology also reveals trilineage hematopoiesis in cases with increased hematogones.

(b) *Benign lymphoid aggregates*: Lymphocytes appear singly scattered and rarely form lymphoid aggregates. Cytology of lymphoid aggregates is best seen on aspirate while patterns and extent of involvement are best picked up on trephine. Paratrabecular aggregates are those which are adjacent to trabecular bone, almost kissing the bone, while intertrabecular aggregates are within two bony trabeculae, far away from bony surface. Most paratrabecular lymphoid aggregates are neoplastic, commonly seen in follicular lymphomas (and mantle cell lymphoma). Thus, benign lymphoid aggregates are usually small, few in number, perivascular, and commonly intertrabecular in location. They are mostly well circumscribed (except in HIV patients where they may be poorly demarcated). These aggregates are polymorphous and composed of mature lymphoid cells may also include plasma cells, histiocytes, and mast cells and occasionally show germinal centers. These are commonly seen in old age, autoimmune disease, and MDS. IHC may be helpful in differentiating benign from malignant lymphoid aggregates. On IHC, most of the lymphoid cells are CD3+ T cells admixed with a few CD20+ B cells. Other important markers include CD10, CD5, CD23, and cyclinD1. Look for RS or RS-like cells and appropriate IHC (CD15, CD30, etc.) may be done in a known case of HL to confirm infiltration. To rule out a T-cell lymphoma infiltration, an extensive T-cell panel is required including CD2, CD3, CD4, CD5, CD7, and CD8, along with CD10, Tdt, CD56, and CD30. T-cell clonality is best studied by T-cell receptor gene rearrangement studies by polymerase chain reaction.

5. *Plasma cells*:

Plasma cells constitute less than 1% of all nucleated BM cells. They may be increased in neoplastic conditions like plasma cell neoplasm, Hodgkin lymphoma, peripheral T-cell lymphoma, AITL, etc. and also in infectious diseases like leishmaniasis, tuberculosis, HIV, etc. Plasma cells may be seen scattered singly or in clusters, nodules, and sheets, as seen in plasma cell neoplasm. They are medium to large sized, egg-shaped cells with abundant blue cytoplasm, and a round eccentric nucleus, which may show a cartwheel nuclear pattern. Plasma cells and lymphocytes are the only remaining hematopoietic cells in the BM of patients of aplastic anemia where rest of the normal hematopoietic cells including megakaryocytes is depleted. These cases have been sometimes mislabeled as plasma cell neoplasm. Plasma cells are highlighted with CD138 (and Mum1), and their clonality is demonstrated by kappa and lambda light chain restriction studied by IHC and FCM (along with loss of CD19 and/or gain of CD56 and cyclinD1) and gain of CD28 and loss of CD27 and CD81.

6. *Other cells* include mast cells, histiocytes, stromal cells, fat cells, osteoblasts, osteoclasts, etc. Mast cells are best appreciated on aspirate smears (Romanowsky stained). They are singly scattered cells in trephine and have a nucleus like a lymphocyte with moderately abundant cytoplasm, seen adjacent to blood vessels, and express tryptase and CD117. Abnormal mast cells are spindle shaped, come in clusters, may look like focal fibrosis, and express CD2 and CD25. Macrophages and hemophagocytosis are best appreciated on aspirate smears. IHC stains for CD68 highlight histiocytes. Scattered or clusters of histiocytes may also be seen in other disorders as histiocytic sarcomas, Langerhans cell histiocytosis, hemophagocytic syndrome, Gaucher disease, Niemann–Pick disease, etc. Microorganisms like LD bodies, *histoplasma capsulatum* can be identified on high-power examination. Granulomas can be identified on trephine only, not on aspirate. AFB, GMS, and PAS stains are performed for mycobacteria and fungus.

Bone and BM Stroma: Any structural abnormalities in the trabecular bone may be observed at scanner power. BM stroma is very inconspicuous in a normal marrow. Reticulin in a normal BM is very thin and can be seen only with special reticulin stain. Stroma in post-chemotherapy BM might show edema, microvascular adipocytes, etc. in a marrow with variable cellularity (normo to hypo to hypercellular marrow). It is also prominent in chronic myeloid disorders like CML, myelofibrosis, and in rare conditions like serous atrophy. Blood vessels may be highlighted by CD34 stains (stain for endothelial cells and blasts). The eosinophilic trabecular bone is thicker in children and thinner in adults and contains osteocytes. Osteoclasts and osteoblasts are more prominent in children.

Common BM Trephine Artifacts: Poor-quality techniques of BM processing produce many artifacts, thereby limiting morphological interpretations. These may include inadequate or excessive fixation, excessive decalcification, etc. These are the most common causes of error in BM biopsy interpretation. Use of blunt needles might cause crushing artifacts. Hemorrhagic BM biopsy is another major artifact caused by aspiration of the marrow from the same site where the biopsy is taken. Other sampling artifacts include a falsely hypocellular BM as seen in subcortical BM, which are normally hypocellular and may be misinterpreted as an aplastic marrow (more so in old age).

BM Infiltration

1. *BM Biopsy and Lymphoma Infiltration*: There
   are certain histological features which help in
   differentiating benign from malignant lymphoid aggregates. Features favoring malignancy include topography, that is, localization
   of the lymphoid aggregates within the bone
   marrow space (paratrabecular aggregates are
   highly abnormal), relation to the surrounding
   tissue (margination or interstitial spillage of
   lymphoid cells), and increase in reticulin
   fibers [1]. Lymphomas are best diagnosed by
   a lymph node (LN) biopsy, with morphology
   substantiated with various ancillary techniques, mainly IHC. However, there are lymphomas, which initially present as
   lymphocytosis (chronic leukemias) and fall
   in a broad category of chronic lymphoproliferative disorders (CLPDs). Morphologically,
   these are more like mature lymphoid cells.
   CLPDs are best diagnosed on peripheral
   blood smear examination and immunophenotyping by FCM. BM biopsy in lymphomas is
   done mainly for staging purposes, except in
   few cases where it may help in diagnosis, as
   in hairy cell leukemia (HCL) which commonly presents as pancytopenia and reveals a
   dry bone marrow tap due to myelofibrosis.
   HCL reveals interstitial to diffuse interstitial
   increase in atypical lymphoid cells (substantiated with IHC like CD20, CD11c, CD25,
   CD103, CD123, etc.). BM biopsy is also
   helpful in follow-up of lymphoma cases to
   detect residual focal disease when a BM aspirate is normal. HL is difficult to diagnose on
   aspirate and, however, can easily be detected
   on trephine biopsy histology where classical
   RS cells, mononuclear RS-like cells, fibrosis,
   granulomas, etc. may be seen. CD20 also
   highlights small clusters of intrasinusoidal
   infiltration in BM as seen in SMZL. CD3 will
   also pick up intrasinusoidal spread of tumor
   T cells in cases of hepatosplenic gamma-
   delta T-cell lymphoma (which otherwise
   might be missed on H&E stain).

   Trephine and aspirate are complementary
   techniques in lymphoma evaluation because
   either may reveal infiltration when the alternative procedure fails to do so. A trephine
   biopsy performed for staging sometimes
   shows discordant morphology (grade) where
   a nodal high-grade large cell lymphoma
   might look like a low-grade small cell lymphoma on BM biopsy.

   BM biopsy in cases of lymphoma might
   show various patterns of infiltration. It may
   show diffuse involvement as seen in chronic
   lymphocytic leukemia (CLL) and patchy or
   partial involvement as seen in HL. IHC has
   an important role mainly in the detection of
   lymphoma involvement by singly scattered
   lymphoma cells, as in ALCL. Common patterns of marrow involvement in trephine
   biopsy in lymphoma are:

   (a) *Diffuse pattern*: Infiltrates that efface mar-
       row architecture, for example, ALL and
       CLL. Hairy cell leukemia (HCL) has a
       diffuse or interstitial involvement.
   (b) *Interstitial pattern*: Tumor cells infiltrate
       the BM without disruption of overall mar-
       row architecture, commonest example
       being hairy cell leukemia (HCL) and oth-
       ers like BL, ALL, PTCL, etc. Normal
       hematopoietic cells are intermingled with
       the tumor cells.
   (c) *Paratrabecular pattern*: Lymphoid cell
       aggregates extend along the bony trabecu-
       lae, internally along the bony surface and
       extend away from trabeculae. It might
       show a rough wedge-shaped infiltrate
       (with broad base toward the trabecular
       bone) or a wavy infiltrate kissing the tra-
       becular bone. It is classically seen in FL,
       and also in MCL, splenic marginal zone
       lymphoma (SMZL), and PTCL. Poorly
       delineated paratrabecular aggregates may
       be seen in T-cell-rich B-cell lymphomas.
   (d) *Intertrabecular pattern*: This may be
       focal and random. It is a common pattern
       seen in benign lymphoid aggregates, may
       come as nodular form, and is commonly
       seen in SMZL, CLL, and MCL. Patchy
       intertrabecular infiltrates with fibrosis and
       polymorphous background along with
       RS-like cells are commonly seen in
       HL. Patchy or nodular deposits may be

seen in myeloma. Patchy, poorly circumscribed lymphoid infiltrates may be seen in AITL, with fibrosis and vascular proliferation in the background (morphological features similar to those in lymph node).

(e) *Sinusoidal or intravascular*: Commonly seen in T-cell lymphomas like ALCL and hepatosplenic T-cell lymphoma (HSTCL) and B-cell lymphomas like SMZL and intravascular lymphoma and also seen in deposits of metastatic carcinomas or a round cell tumor.

HL may have different patterns, patchy focal involvement to extensive sclerotic involvement. It may consist of polymorphous cellular populations of lymphocytes, eosinophils, plasma cells, histiocytes, neutrophils with/without RS-like cells (or mononuclear RS-like cells) in a fibrotic background and may be associated with granulomas and focal necrosis. IHC stains (LCA, CD3, CD20, Pax5, CD15, CD30) are helpful. Megakaryocytes may mimic RS cells. Morphologic features of PTCL and HL may overlap in BM biopsy as RS-like cells may be seen in both and in other conditions such as viral infections, CLL, ALCL, and AITL. BM involvement may be suspected even in the absence of classical RS cells, if characteristic milieu of fibrosis (focal to diffuse) containing eosinophils, histiocytes, plasma cells with mononuclear RS-like cells is noted. CD30 will highlight RS-like cells.

2. *Plasma cell neoplasms*: Myeloma diagnosis requires a multidisciplinary approach, from clinical to laboratory to radiological investigations. It might be difficult to obtain a BM biopsy in myeloma cases, as the bones are brittle, thus highlighting the importance of processing the clot like a trephine. However, it might be essential for diagnosis in some cases. Myeloma can be in the form of nodular deposits in the trephine, apart from other patterns like interstitial, diffuse, or mixed types. Aspirates in such cases might reveal a falsely low count of plasma cells where the plasma cell percentage could vary anywhere from 1% to more than 10%. Thus, nodular deposits, clusters, or sheets of plasma cells in a BM biopsy highly suggest a plasma cell neoplasm.

Plasma cells can morphologically mimic any other hematopoietic cell, namely blast, promyelocyte, histiocyte, erythroid cell, lymphocyte, etc. Normal plasma cells tend to arrange in perivascular areas; however, clonal plasma cells infiltrate adipocytes and form clusters, nodules, or sheets. Morphological variants include mature, immature, and plasmablastic subtypes. Plasmablasts have high nucleocytoplasmic ratio, fine chromatin, a prominent nuclei, and blue cytoplasm. Plasma cells get highlighted with CD138. CD138 also helps in quantitation of plasma cells, especially when they are interstitially interspersed. CD138 also stains epithelial cells apart from plasma cells. BM biopsy is also important as a baseline for comparison with repeat (sequential) biopsies during follow-up of myeloma. Immunophenotyping by FCM or IHC on trephine can be useful in establishing the presence of a relatively small plasma cell clone. Clonal plasma cells might express CD56, cyclinD1, CD117, CD28, and loss of expression of CD19 and CD27 (expressed in normal plasma cells). Neuroendocrine carcinoma cells also stain with CD138 and CD56, a common morphological differential of myeloma/plasmacytoma. Additional markers should be done for light chain restriction, etc. BM biopsy is also helpful in detecting small deposits of amyloid in suspected cases of amyloidosis (perivascular deposits of extracellular amorphous eosinophilic material). Congo red stain may be performed to look for apple green birefringence under polarizing microscopy.

Waldenstrom macroglobulinemia may also have similar patterns of involvement as myeloma and shows a mixture of plasma cells, lymphocytes, and hybrid lymphoplasmacytic cells. Plasma cells may also be increased in chronic infections as tuberculosis, leishmaniasis, etc., in other neoplasms as HL, AITL, PTCL, etc., and also in leukemias as AML-M5. BM biopsy in cases of aplastic anemia and post induction BM might show only plasma cells and lymphocytes in an otherwise hypocellular marrow. Cases of aplastic anemia and AITL have been misdiagnosed as plasma cell neoplasm on aspirate smears. Thus, it is important to correlate with cellularity on trephine and with other clinical and radiological findings.

3. *Acute leukemia*: A trephine biopsy is not required for the diagnosis/subtyping of acute leukemia, as long as there are adequate tumor cells in the peripheral blood or a cellular aspirate is available. However, paraffin block is an archival material and additional studies like IHC can be performed for subtyping of HLN even at a later stage. Thus, trephine biopsy becomes extremely important in a country like ours where many a time patients are given blood transfusion and/or steroids/heavy metals at the primary health center after/before a diagnosis of acute leukemia. Such patients when referred to a cancer center have no circulating tumor cells, causing a delay in diagnosis. Stained peripheral blood smears or bone marrow (BM) aspirates, if available, might not help further subtype the leukemia. Paraffin block if available at this stage is an invaluable material. BM biopsies in cases of acute leukemias are hypercellular, except for rare hypoplastic AMLs and hypoplastic MDS. BM is packed with similar looking blasts (CD34, Tdt). Rarely, normal or differentiating cells may be seen in the background as in AML-M2, etc. Blasts vary in size from small to large. Lymphoblasts (CD19, CD79a, CD10, Tdt, CD3) are smaller in size with coarse nuclear chromatin. Myeloblasts (CD34, MPO, c-kit) are larger in size and have distinct cytoplasm and vesicular nuclear chromatin. Monoblasts (CD34, MPO, and CD64) are large, with fine nuclear chromatin, and may have a convoluted nuclear membrane. It is important to rule out associated dysplasia in any of the three lineages. CD19 and CD79a are better stains for B-cell ALL as CD20 might be weakly positive or negative in majority of B-cell ALLs. Plasmacytosis is commonly seen associated with AML-M5 and AML-M2 with t(8;21). CD19 is a more popular stain with FCI. Differential diagnosis of acute leukemia in BM may include hematogones, Ewing sarcoma, rhabdomyosarcoma, neuroblastoma, anaplastic large cell lymphoma, and multiple myeloma.

4. *Chronic myeloid neoplasms including chronic myeloid leukemia (CML)*: BM biopsy is markedly hypercellular in CML and shows myeloid and megakaryocytic preponderance. Blasts are not increased in the chronic phase. There is a relative paucity of erythroid series cells. Fibrosis may be seen in CML and other chronic myeloproliferative disorders and shall be graded and reticulin stain may be used. Clusters of megakaryocytes and micromegakaryocytes may be seen. Stains for CD34 and C-kit may be helpful in highlighting blasts. Cellularity and morphology of megakaryocytes may help in distinguishing essential thrombocytosis from early prefibrotic myelofibrosis. In early/prefibrotic myelofibrosis, it is a hypercellular marrow with a prominent granulocytic and megakaryocytic proliferation with a concomitant reduction of red cell precursors with absence of reticulin MF (MF-0 and MF-1). Abnormalities in the megakaryocytopoietic cell lineage include extensive and dense clustering and translocation of megakaryocytes toward the endosteal borders. There is a high variability in size ranging from small to giant megakaryocytes along with prominent aberrations of the nuclei (marked hypolobulation, condensed chromatin, and irregular foldings creating a bulbous, cloud-like aspect) and marked elevation of the nuclear-cytoplasmic ratio, as well as an increased frequency of bare (denuded) nuclei. While in essential thrombocytosis, it reveals an age-matched cellular BM with a predominant megakaryopoiesis, but without a significant erythroid or neutrophilic myeloproliferation. Here the megakaryocytes reveal a more or less random distribution or very loose groupings within the BM space. Megakaryocytes are large to giant cell forms with extensively folded (hyperlobulated) nuclei, surrounded by

well-differentiated cytoplasm. An increase in reticulin is not compatible with early stages of ET.

5. *Myelodysplastic syndrome (MDS) and megaloblastic anemia*: Diagnosis of MDS requires integration of various peripheral blood and BM parameters along with clinical and cytogenetic findings. MDS has various subtypes. Morphological dysplasia is best appreciated on an aspirate smear. Trephine is important in commenting on architecture, cellularity (hypercellular BM), megakaryocyte morphology including dyspoietic forms like micromegakaryocytes, multinucleated megakaryocytes, and also monolobated megakaryocytes (as seen in 5q- syndrome), presence of megaloblasts, abnormal localization of immature myeloid precursors (ALIP), and CD34+ blasts. Fibrosis may be seen in secondary MDS (post-alkylating agent therapy). Epstein–Barr virus infection might produce morphological changes that might mimic MDS features in BM. Common differential diagnoses of MDS in pediatric BM trephine include chronic viral infections, juvenile rheumatoid arthritis, megaloblastic anemia, heavy metal toxicity, chronic myeloproliferative disorders, acute leukemia, etc. Common differential diagnoses of MDS in adult BM trephine include congenital dyserythropoietic anemia, aplastic anemia, hypocellular AML, chronic viral infections, megaloblastic anemia, heavy metal toxicity, AIDS, autoimmune disorders, chronic myeloproliferative disorders, acute leukemia, etc. Micromegakaryocytes are smaller sized cells, have darkly stained nuclei, and scant cytoplasm (bare nuclei). These are commonly seen singly scattered or in clusters in chronic myeloid leukemia, accelerated phase (CML-AP), and MDS. IHC (CD41, CD61, factor VIIIRA) may be done to highlight megakaryoblast and micromegakaryocytes. Small blast-like cells with one or more distinct nucleoli located away from the endosteal surface (paratrabecular) correspond to immature precursors/blasts. Cases with at least three clusters (groups of three to five immature myeloid precursors) or aggregates (more than five myeloid precursors) distributed in the intertrabecular region are defined as being ALIP positive (abnormal localization of immature myeloid precursors). ALIP islands might express CD34 and CD117. These may also be seen in regenerating BM, post chemotherapy, and in CML. BM is hypercellular in megaloblastic anemia, with erythroid hyperplasia. M:E ratio is reversed. Nucleo-cytoplasmic dissociation is most evident in erythroid lineage. Megaloblasts are large round to polygonal cells with large round nuclei, vesicular chromatin, 1–2 small nucleoli, a crisp nuclear membrane, and moderately abundant basophilic/amphophilic cytoplasm. Megaloblasts may be seen as singly scattered cells or else seen in clusters with a background of erythroid hyperplasia. These features may also be seen in MDS. These may be highlighted with CD71 on IHC. Myeloid series also shows giant forms.

6. *Mast cell disease*: Mast cells are best seen in a Romanowsky stained smear. It may show different patterns of involvement in BM mainly paratrabecular, perivascular, parafollicular, and diffuse. Granules are washed off during processing. Mast cells are oval shaped with abundant clear cytoplasm, no mitotic activity, and are associated with fibrosis and admixed eosinophils, histiocytes, and lymphocytes. They may be associated with other myeloproliferative neoplasms like systemic mastocytosis with associated clonal hematological non-mast cell lineage disease. Mast cell disorders are more commonly seen in the Western population. Mast cells are strongly positive for CD117, while CD2 and CD25 highlight clonal mast cells.

7. *BM biopsy and minimal residual disease (MRD)*: MRD detection is best done by multicolor FCM or molecular methods. Best methods to detect MRD in B-ALL, T-ALL, and AML is by FCI, while in case of CML-CP and APML, it is done by molecular methods. CD34 and CD117 stains may be performed to detect scanty myeloblasts in

the BM biopsy. Hematogones may be confused with blasts in post induction BM of B-cell ALL. Clusters of CD34/Tdt-positive cells herald an early relapse of ALL. Hematogones might express CD20, CD10, and Tdt in different stages of their maturation (as stated earlier). We have seen 10–15% Tdt expressing lymphoid cells in post induction regenerating bone marrows (cases of B-cell ALL). Likewise we have seen up to 20% normal myeloblasts (CD34+) in post induction marrow in a case of AML. FCM is a superior technique to differentiate cancer lymphoblasts from hematogones and also cancer myeloblasts from normal myeloblasts, as it gives more flexibility in the form of multicolor immunophenotyping and patterns analysis, using principles of leukemia-associated immunophenotype and concepts of away from normal. One should avoid commenting on the presence of MRD on trephine interpretations.

8. *BM biopsy and metastatic tumors*: BM biopsy is essential if BM examination is being carried out for metastatic workup. Clusters of megakaryocytes may rarely mimic metastatic carcinoma. Though the aspirate is helpful, BM biopsy has better chances of picking up scanty tumor cells. IHC can also be performed for evaluation of unknown primary (like breast, GIT, lungs, prostate, etc.), where common markers include CK, EMA, CK7, CK20, TTF1, PSA, CDX2, etc. Aspirates might show degenerating tumor cells that can easily be missed; however, BM biopsy reveals viable tumor cells in a desmoplastic background. Trephine and aspiration are complementary investigations because either may show tumor cells when the other procedure fails to do so. In rare instances, round cell tumor deposits are seen as clusters in the aspirate and missed in the trephine. This is likely when the aspirate is done at a different angle from where the trephine is done. BM biopsy is done for staging of round cell tumors such as neuroblastoma, rhabdomyosarcoma, and primitive neuroectodermal

tumor. Common IHC markers include Mic2, FLI1, desmin, myogenin, MyoD1, synaptophysin, chromogranin, CD56, etc. (along with hematolymphoid markers). Rarely, round cell tumors may mimic acute leukemia on aspirate smears, and immunophenotyping by FCM reveals negative markers (since all markers used are hematolymphoid specific). Trephine is helpful in these cases where a battery of hematolymphoid as well as non-hematolymphoid markers may be done. Sarcomas, melanomas, and germ cell tumors also rarely metastasize to BM.

9. *BM biopsy and granulomatous diseases*: BM biopsy is a part and parcel of investigation for pyrexia of unknown origin. Other specific indications in this context include pancytopenia, fever, and lymphadenopathy. Common causes of granulomatous diseases include tuberculosis, leishmaniasis, sarcoidosis, cryptococcosis, aspergillosis, and histoplasmosis. Granulomas may be seen in trephine sections (but not in a BM aspirate). BM biopsy has an important role in human immunodeficiency virus-positive patients, where granulomas, necrosis, and stain for AFB and other microorganisms should be done. Granulomas in BM may also be seen in various neoplastic conditions such as HL, PTCL, mycosis fungoides, carcinomas, and MDS. Relevant cultures are to be sent after discussion with the clinicians.

10. *BM biopsy and AIDS*: BM may be near normal or show significant morphological changes. Morphologic features may be divided into specific and nonspecific categories. Nonspecific category includes reactive plasmacytosis, megaloblastosis, multilineage dysplasia, poorly circumscribed lymphoid aggregates, diffuse interstitial histiocytic proliferation, hypo-, hyper- to normocellular BM, fibrosis, etc. Specific categories include infiltration by NHL (plasmablastic lymphomas, BL, HL, etc.), Kaposi sarcoma, and opportunistic infections (bacterial, fungal, or protozoal), absence of storage iron, red cell aplasia, etc.

Other Common Findings

(a) *BM Necrosis*: Causes of BM necrosis vary from neoplastic (ALL, AML, myeloma, HL, NHL, carcinomas, PNET, neuroblastoma, etc.) to non-neoplastic (sickle cell anemia, infections, DIC, acute GVHD, etc.) and to treatment related (e.g., post steroids in ALL, post bone marrow transplantation). It should be differentiated from fibrinoid necrosis or stromal edema as seen post chemotherapy or after bone marrow radiation.

(b) *BM biopsy changes post chemotherapy*: Morphologic features of BM in patients undergoing myeloablative chemotherapy may be immediate effects like cell ablation and late effects like bone marrow regeneration (1–2 weeks after the ablative therapy). Immediate effects include apoptosis, followed by fibrinoid necrosis, stromal edema, prominent and dilated sinuses, increased macrophages, and large number of multiloculated adipocytes. Scanty normal hemopoietic cells may be seen, predominantly comprising of lymphocytes and plasma cells. Bone marrow regeneration occurs 1–2 weeks later and may show the appearance of paratrabecular immature myeloid cells, followed by the appearance of neutrophils and erythroid colonies. Megakaryocytes appear late and come in clusters, which is followed by resolution of fibrinoid necrosis (which may stay for a longer duration in some cases). Intra-nuclear parvovirus inclusions may be evident in large-sized proerythroblasts in post induction chemotherapy patients of ALL. These cells resemble RS-like mononuclear cells. These patients may have a delayed recovery of peripheral blood counts. It is a common practice to confuse interstitial edema (commonly seen in post induction marrows) with marrow fibrosis and one has to be careful.

(c) *BM biopsy in post BM transplantation period*: Earliest features (days 1–14) are of cell death, and include fat necrosis, proteinaceous debris, stromal edema, and negligible normal hematopoietic cells. Regeneration starts from day 7 to 14 post-transplant and reveal non-paratrabecular erythroid colonies, myeloid precursors followed by megakaryocytic clusters. Any presence of blasts post day 7 of transplant indicates the presence of residual disease. At the end of a month (day 28), complete engraftment occurs, that is, all cell lines are engrafted. BM may show variable cellularity. Morphologic features of rejection (post day 28) include declining peripheral blood cell counts and features of BM microenvironment damage like fat necrosis, stromal edema, plasmacytosis, histiocytic proliferations, or lymphocytosis.

(d) *BM post growth factor therapy*: Growth factors like GM-CSF lead to interstitial foci of immature myeloid cells in a hypercellular marrow. Myeloid cells show prominent granules and may mimic acute or chronic myeloid neoplasm, and rarely may look like acute promyelocytic leukemia.

16.5.4.2 Immunohistochemistry

Similar to lymph node biopsy, IHC is an important tool in interpretation of HLN in BM biopsies. Use of FCM on peripheral blood/aspirated marrow cells along with IHC provides complementary information, and the two sets of data should be considered together. If FCM data is available from peripheral blood or aspirated bone marrow, it should be taken into account when assessing the trephine morphology. They can aid selection of appropriate antibodies for IHC and, in some cases, reduce or remove completely the need for complex and expensive IHC assessment, avoiding unnecessary duplication. Panels for markers including non-hematolymphoid tumors have been suggested; however, it is at the discretion of the hematopathologist to decide on IHC panel on a case-by-case basis. Tumors like round cell tumors/carcinomas/melanomas may mimic lymphoma, thus it becomes essential to have corresponding markers for these tumors. Minimal suggested basic panel for any hematolymphoid lesion include three markers, namely LCA (CD45), CD20 (B-cell marker), and CD3 (T-cell marker). For blastic lymphoid cell proliferations, CD79a and CD19 are markers of choice in B-ALL (CD20 may be negative). CD20 is a predictive marker in B-cell lymphomas, as these patients can be given anti-CD20 targeted therapy (rituximab). Additional panels may be suggested based on morphological impression. Common markers in a case of acute leukemia include CD3, CD7, CD20, CD10, CD56, CD4, CD33, CD41, CD61, Pax5, CD79a, CD19, CD34, Tdt, Ckit, AMPO.

16.5.4.3 Cytogenetics/FISH and Molecular Diagnostics

Unfixed BM aspirate sample is a better sample than extracted nuclei from fixed trephine biopsy specimens for conventional karyotyping and interphase fluorescence in situ hybridization (FISH) analysis. However, with newer protocols, good FISH results can also be obtained from trephine cores (fixed tissues). Thin sections offer an advantage of retained architecture and cytology of cells of interest. Trephine FISH may be critical in demonstration of MYC abnormalities in suspected Burkitt lymphoma and in confirmation of t(11;14) in mantle cell lymphomas. PCR may be done to detect IGH and TCR rearrangements using sections from decalcified BM cores.

Reporting of a trephine biopsy: Trephine report shall contain both gross and microscopic descriptions. It should mention the number of BM fragments and length of the longest fragment. The report may begin with a statement on the adequacy of specimen for diagnosis and should then comment systematically on cellularity, bone structure, trilineage hematopoiesis, M:E ratio, dyspoietic features, and stroma and abnormal infiltrates, if any. It should include a comment on special stains including IHC, if any performed. Clinical, peripheral blood smear, and BM aspirate findings should be correlated before the final report is issued. Ancillary techniques like IHC/FCM, cytogenetics, FISH, and PCR reports should be included after correlation to give a comprehensive report based on the current WHO classification of HLN [2]. The report should finish with a final impression of all findings and its clinical significance. Advice on further workup may be given, if required. Provisional report may be sent if deeper sections or special stains are pending or if a second opinion is being

sought. This is followed by a final report. Provisional as well as final report must contain the name and signatures of the authorized signatory or by a secured computer authorization.

Who should report a trephine biopsy? Ideally, an experienced pathologist or a hematopathologist who has been trained adequately in both laboratory hematology and histopathology should do this. He/she should also be competent to assess blood films and BM aspirates and evaluate FCM results. It is preferable that all hematopoietic tissues including peripheral blood, BM aspirate, BM biopsy along with lymph node, spleen, and extranodal lymphoid lesions, are reported by a trained hematopathologist, who shall compile the results of various ancillary techniques. The other option is close cooperation between various disciplines. In any case, a pathologist should not release a trephine biopsy report without ascertaining the opinion on the blood film and BM aspirate (done by him/herself or by another pathologist). If there is any apparent discrepancy between the findings, this should be resolved by a joint examination of the slides of the case or, at the very least, by a telephone conversation between those responsible for reporting the specimens.

Conclusion: Trephine biopsy is an essential technique for the assessment and treatment of patients with a wide range of hematological conditions as well as some other disorders that involve BM. BM trephine is an integral component of diagnosis, staging, and follow-up of HLN. Biopsy is a painful procedure, and due care should be taken by all professionals involved in collection, processing, and reporting of trephine specimens. Trephine should be of adequate volume and integrity, fixed promptly, decalcified fully before being processed, sectioned thinly (2–3 μm), and stained. Routine stains (H&E staining and other special stains) and IHCs must be well standardized with adequate panels. Trephine is used in morphological interpretation and also in the application of various ancillary techniques, including immunohistochemistry, DNA/RNA in situ hybridization, and polymerase chain reaction. It is mandatory to have standard operating procedures for performing a trephine biopsy, processing of the biopsy specimen, various ancillary techniques, and reporting of the histological sections. In most institutes or hospital settings, BM biopsy and aspirate are mostly reported in different departments, where histopathologists take primary responsibility for bone marrow trephine reporting and hematologists/pathologists report BM aspirates. In few places, both are done by a hematopathologist, which is an ideal situation. There is dire need of qualified hematopathologists who can report benign as well as malignant (bone marrow, nodal, and extranodal) hematopathology. The BM trephine biopsy provides just one piece in this diagnostic jigsaw. Appropriate IHCs are used to detect subtle infiltrates (e.g., intrasinusoidal infiltration as seen in splenic marginal zone B-cell lymphoma and in ALCL). Consideration should be given to take a second opinion from a specialist hematopathologist without wasting time. Who reports the trephine is not important, whether it is a liquid pathologist, surgical pathologist, or a hematopathologist. What is important is to have sufficient expertise available among pathologists reporting trephine specimens in order to ensure that a full range of appropriate investigations is applied in each case, with available detailed clinical and hematological data, and ready access to further specialist advice. Communication and dialog between the hematologist/oncologist and the pathologist is crucial. Ideally, such dialog should occur as the specimen is being reported and generally before multidisciplinary joint clinic (at this time, diagnostic uncertainties should have been resolved). World Health Organization 2008 Classification of HLN [1] requires integration of clinical information, peripheral blood findings, BM aspirate, and trephine morphology, other tissue diagnosis, and data from various ancillary techniques (IHC/FCM, cytogenetic/molecular diagnostics), still a distant reality in India.

Take Home Message: Trephine

1. Aspirate and biopsy are complementary.
2. Good quality fixation, decalcification, and processing are extremely important so as to obtain a good quality H&E section (2–3 μm thick).
3. An accurate diagnosis of HLN requires multidisciplinary approach which includes clinical, biochemical, radiological, hematological parameters with morphological and immunophenotyping analysis.
4. Spend adequate time on scanner/low magnification as it gives vital information about the architecture of BM biopsy, BM cellularity, adequacy of megakaryocytes, any abnormal infiltrates, etc. Cellularity is best commented upon on BM biopsy examination.
5. Higher magnification addresses the cytological features in detail and the presence of parasites, if any.
6. Erythroid cells resemble lymphoid cells, and megaloblasts may resemble blasts. IHC for CD3, CD20, and CD71/CD235 may be performed. LCA (CD45) is strongest in lymphoid cells and may be negative or weakly expressed in erythroid cells. Megaloblasts (as well as mast cells, myeloblasts, plasma cells) might express CD117.
7. Lymphoma and myeloma may present as a nodular deposit. BM aspirate in a few of such cases might reveal a normal marrow differential count. Stain and examine all aspirate smears. Serial deeper cuts on trephine always help.
8. Lymphoid cells constitute approximately 10–20% in a normal healthy adult BM aspirate and biopsy. CD20+ B cells are scanty and singly scattered. CD3+ T cells are also singly scattered and, however, are more in number.
9. Scanty hidden lymphoid infiltrates on trephine may be picked up by CD20 and CD3 stains (for B and T cell, respectively). BM might reveal "missing" B cells (CD20−) in patients of DLBCL (post rituximab). CD19, CD79a, Pax5 are useful B-cell markers in these situations. Overall, CD20 is an extremely important marker. Subtle intrasinusoidal lymphoid infiltrates are well highlighted by IHCs, as the tumor cells in hepatosplenic gamma-delta T-cell lymphoma are picked up by CD3 (double-negative T cells) and tumor cells in splenic marginal zone lymphoma by CD20. These can be eas-

ily missed on H&E images. It is a good idea to do CD3 and CD20 in BM biopsy in cases suspected of hematolymphoid neoplasm.

10. Mimics of lymphomas in BM biopsy are many, from hematogones to benign lymphoid aggregates. Hematogones generally are scattered as single cells in trephine and may express CD10, CD34 and Tdt. It is important to correlate with CBC findings and a meticulous BM aspirate morphology examination followed by flow cytometric immunophnotyping for pattern evaluation. This helps in differentiating hematogones from minimal residual disease in cases of precursor B cell lymphoblastic leukemia (post induction).

11. Plasma cells can mimic morphologically anything under the sun. Minimal or atypical plasma cell infiltrates may be interpreted as either reactive or may be missed. IHC for CD138, cyclinD1, and CD56 may be helpful. Refer text for morphological differences. Plasma cells may be increased in leishmaniasis, aplastic anemia, HL, and angioimmunoblastic T-cell lymphoma apart from plasma cell neoplasm.

12. Bilateral BM biopsies may be performed in staging of neuroblastoma.

13. Aspirate smears may be diluted due to poor technique; hypocellular marrow or else a fibrotic marrow (exclude a possibility of chronic myeloproliferative neoplasm, hairy cell leukemia, CML, HL, and metastatic carcinomas).

14. Granulomas (commonly an infective etiology) may be associated with mast cell lesions or HL.

15. Acute leukemias are best subtyped based on FCI. Blast counts are also best done on aspirate smears. Trephines are best for architecture, cellularity, focal nodular deposits (and tumor deposits), granulomas, fibrosis, interstitial edema, etc.

16. Hypocellular marrow might contain blasts, which can be missed (post treatment, hypocellular AML, and hypocellular MDS). Stains for CD34, glycophorin, and CD117 are helpful.

17. Edematous background may be seen as a treatment-related change.

18. Infidelity of IHC stains is well known. For example, CD56 is expressed by natural killer (NK) cells and their neoplastic counterparts, in AMLs, myeloma plasma cells, small cell carcinomas, and also in cells of other neuroendocrine tumors. CyclinD1 may also be expressed in a plasma cell neoplasm and hairy cell leukemia, in addition to mantle cell lymphoma.

19. Lab must possess adequate IHC panels (including for non-hematolymphoid tumors).

20. Turnaround time should not exceed 3 working days, and 5–7 days where IHC is required. Second opinion may be sought in difficult cases.

21. To err is human, and the pathologist must admit any mistake if it happens.

22. There are gray areas in pathology. Communication between the pathologist and the treating hematologist/oncologist is important.

23. Request for a re-biopsy in case of inadequate/crushed or poorly processed biopsy.

24. A formal/informal training in a busy hematopathology laboratory is highly desirable.

25. Stakeholders for good laboratory practice include physician doing the biopsy (and the anesthetist), OT nurse, medical laboratory technologist and scientists, pathologist, hematologist, administrator, vendor supplying the reagents/equipment to the patient him/herself.

26. Trephine is a painful procedure for the patient and carries some risks; therefore, it should be performed only when there is a clear clinical indication (megaloblastic anemias are best diagnosed based on serum B12/FA levels). Clinical details and the results of relevant laboratory tests including the blood count and blood film features must be known before this procedure is done. It can be performed safely on patients with severe thrombocytopenia, but prolonged pressure may be applied to achieve primary hemostasis.

16.6 Spleen: Interpretation and Lymphomas

Splenomegaly is a common feature in hematolymphoid neoplasms. Mostly spleen is involved by lymphoma elsewhere during its dissemination process. Rarely it may represent the exclusive site of the lymphomatous burden. Thus the designation "primary splenic lymphomas" (PSLs) may be classically restricted to neoplasms fulfilling this latter condition and constitute approximately 6% of all lymphoid neoplasms. However, it must be noted that PSLs commonly involve bone marrow and peripheral blood at presentation.

16.6.1 Normal Spleen

Careful gross evaluation of the specimen and optimal tissue fixation are most important. Because of the high vascularity of the spleen, thin sections are particularly important. Look out for additional lymph nodes with the main splenectomy specimen. The spleen is primarily composed of two distinct regions. The lymphoid tissue of the spleen is called the white pulp (nodules of lymphoid cells) and is associated with the splenic arterial circulation. The central arteries, which arise from trabecular arteries within the fibrous trabeculae, are surrounded by cylindrical cuffs of lymphocytes called periarteriolar lymphoid sheaths (PALS), containing an admixture of B and T cells, with a predominance of CD4+ T cells. Splenic lymphoid follicles (malpighian corpuscles) occur as outgrowths of the periarteriolar lymphoid sheaths. The germinal center is similar to germinal centers seen in lymph nodes. It is surrounded by a mantle zone that is further encased by marginal zone, a cellular layer at the interface between the white and red pulp. The marginal zone is composed of both B and T cells. The red pulp is composed of splenic vascular sinuses and the cords of Billroth, which are made up of splenic macrophages, scattered cord capillaries, venules, and stromal cells. B cells in mantle zone bear surface immunoglobulin, with co-expression of immunoglobulin IgM and IgD. Marginal zone B cells express predominantly IgM, with only a small minority expressing IgD. IgG expression is lacking in these areas and is limited to scattered cells in the red pulp, where rare IgA-containing cells are also found.

16.6.2 Procedure, Collection, and Transport of Specimens: Extranodal Biopsies and Spleen

Measure the weight and describe the gross appearance, including the presence of any focal lesions (e.g., infarcts, nodules, hemorrhage) and gross abnormalities of red or white pulp. The spleen must be sectioned at 3–5 mm intervals, to look for grossly identifiable lesions. Fixation, grossing, and tissue processing are extremely important so as to avoid autolysis of spleen. Splenic FNAC is not used as a diagnostic test. Biopsies from other sites like skin, GIT, etc. are immediately transferred into a suitable fixative (e.g., formalin).

Lymphomas commonly presenting as PSLs are SMZL, splenic lymphomas-unclassifiable (SL-u) [which include splenic diffuse red pulp small B-cell lymphoma (SDRPSBCL) and HCL variant], HCL, LL, B-PLL, T-LGL, and hepatosplenic T-cell lymphoma. Primary splenic presentations of nodal lymphomas are commonly seen in MCL, FL, DLBCL, not otherwise specified, micronodular T-cell/histiocyte-rich large B-cell lymphoma, HL, and PTCL. The commonest PSL is SMZL, and this is a close differential diagnosis of other B-cell lymphomas, namely SL-u, and LPL (waste-basket). All these subtypes belong to low-grade lymphoma category with a wait–and-watch policy for management.

Patterns with involvement of the spleen by lymphoma can be broadly studied in categories of "predominantly red pulp based" and "predominantly white pulp based," both having diffuse and nodular subtypes. Predominantly red pulp involvement is commonly seen with diffuse patterns in HCL, HCL variant, SDRPSBCL, hepatosplenic T-cell lymphoma, acute leukemias, hemolytic anemias, nonspecific congestion, extramedullary hematopoiesis, etc. It may show a focal or nodular/variable pattern as seen in HL, DLBCL, T-PLL, etc. Similarly, predominantly white pulp involvement may be seen in small B-cell lymphomas (CLL, LPL, SMZL, PTCL, etc.) and may show focal involvement in inflammatory pseudotumor, hamartomas, etc.

Diagnostic Workup in Case of Primary Splenic Lymphomas

1. Complete blood count.
2. Peripheral blood smear and/or bone marrow aspirate examination with FCI.
3. Bone marrow biopsy examination with IHC (CD3, CD4, CD8, CD7, CD5, CD2, CD19, CD20, CD5, CD23, CD10, bcl6, cyclinD1, CD15, CD30, Pax5, EBER, Tdt, CD34) (similar to that for nodal tissues).
4. Cytogenetics and molecular studies (similar to that for nodal tissues).
5. Splenectomy is the last resort (similar IHC panel as above).

Splenic marginal zone lymphoma, the commonest subtype, commonly presents with leukocytosis and splenomegaly. PBS/BM morphology reveals a low-grade B-cell lymphoma that may be labeled as SMZL after excluding other common B-cell lymphomas, namely CLL/SLL, MCL, FL, HCL, LPL (WM), etc. Splenectomy is rarely indicated and reveals a nodular pattern of involvement with a similar IHC profile. SMZL (as per WHO classification) is a B-cell neoplasm comprising small lymphocytes that surround and may replace the splenic white pulp germinal centers, may efface the follicle mantle, and merge with a peripheral (marginal) zone of larger cells, including scattered transformed blasts/immunoblasts; both small and large cells infiltrate the red pulp. Most cases have prominent splenomegaly, and bone marrow and peripheral blood infiltration. Cells in peripheral blood can frequently be recognized morphologically as mature looking lymphoid cells with or without villous projections. SMZL and splenic lymphoma with villous lymphocytes are same entities. SMZL is a diagnosis of exclusion. Tumor cells express pan B-cell markers like CD19 and CD20, however are negative for CD5, CD10, and cyclinD1, and have a low MIB-1 proliferation index. SDRPSBCL reveals a diffuse pattern of involvement with similar morphology of lymphoid cells and IHC profile.

HCL is another common splenic lymphoma, which has a classical morphology on peripheral blood smear, bone marrow aspirate, trephine, and also on splenectomy specimen (widened red lakes). Tumor cells express B-cell markers, show light chain restriction, also express CD11c, CD25, CD103, and CD123, and show BRAFV600E mutation on molecular studies.

16.7 Thymus: Interpretation and Lymphomas

The thymus is located in the anterior mediastinum, where immature T-cell precursors (prothymocytes) that migrate from the bone marrow undergo maturation and selection to become mature, naïve T cells that are capable of responding to antigenic stimuli. It is the site of development of a normal T cell.

Thymus is broadly divided into a cortex and a medulla. The cortex contains cortical epithelial cells and macrophages. Cortical thymocytes (lymphocytes) range in morphology from medium-sized blastic cells with dispersed chromatin and nucleoli located in the outer cortex, to somewhat smaller, more mature-appearing, round lymphocytes located in the inner cortex. Occasional apoptotic bodies and phagocytosis by histiocytes may be seen. The immunophenotype of most cortical thymocytes is that of precursor T cells (TdT+, CD1a+, CD4+, CD8+). The medulla (and perivascular spaces) contains medullary epithelial cells with Hassall corpuscles and dendritic cells. Medullary thymocytes (lymphocytes) are small, morphologically mature-appearing lymphocytes and have immunophenotype of mature T cells (TdT−, CD1a−, CD3+, CD4+, or CD8+). Medulla also contains a particular population of B cells (asteroid cells) with dendritic morphology that expresses mature B-cell markers CD23, CD37, CD72, CD76, immunoglobulin IgM, and

IgD. These cells form rosettes with non-B cells and are cells of origin of primary mediastinal large B-cell lymphoma. Common lymphomas arising in the thymus include T-lymphoblastic lymphoma (T-LL), HL (nodular sclerosis), PMLBCL, and gray zone lymphoma (GZL). Other tumors at this site include thymoma and germ cell tumors. Hodgkin lymphoma has to be differentiated from GZL (intermediate between HL and DLBCL), while T-LL has to be differentiated from normal thymus, thymic cyst, thymoma, etc. Lymphoid cells in normal thymus may contain double-positive T cells, double-negative T cells, and also express Tdt. This may cause an erroneous labeling as blastic lymphoma even in a normal thymic tissue, benign cyst, or thymoma. T-LL presents as a mediastinal mass in a young patient complaining of severe dyspnea as an emergency. On a needle core biopsy, it does not show any neoplastic epithelial component on histopathology and even on IHC will reveal scanty epithelial cells (expressing cytokeratin). T-LL lacks a thick fibrous capsule, lobularity of normal thymus, and also medullary foci. It is seen in young adolescent age group, may show blasts in peripheral blood or bone marrow, and usually shows a uniform immunophenotype among the lymphoid population.

16.8 Extranodal Lymphomas: Interpretation

Although 25–40% of NHL patients present with a primary extranodal lymphoma, in almost every organ in the body, however, common extranodal sites are skin and GIT. Lymphomas arising in extranodal sites vary widely from one extranodal site to another. Some are associated with an underlying immunodeficiency syndrome, autoimmune disease, infection, or other immunologic disorder, or a predilection to affect patients of certain ethnic origins. Common extranodal lymphomas are extranodal marginal zone B-cell lymphoma, mediastinal large B-cell lymphoma, intravascular large B-cell lymphoma, primary effusion lymphoma, plasmablastic lymphoma, DLBCL leg cell type, mantle cell lymphoma,

follicular lymphoma, extranodal natural killer/T-cell lymphoma: nasal-type, enteropathy-type intestinal T-cell lymphoma, etc. [24].

16.9 Cutaneous Lymphomas

Most cutaneous lymphomas are of T-cell subtype and show a top heavy infiltrate of atypical lymphoid cells in the upper dermis. Cutaneous T-cell lymphoma (CTCL) is the most common type of cutaneous lymphoma that typically presents with red, scaly patches or thickened plaques that often mimic eczema or chronic dermatitis. CTCL is a group of lymphoproliferative disorders characterized by localization of neoplastic T lymphocytes to the skin. CTCLs are of indolent or aggressive subtypes. The commonest subtype is mycosis fungoides (non-sun-exposed areas).

CTCLs with indolent clinical behavior include the following:

- Mycosis fungoides
- Mycosis fungoide variants and subtypes (e.g., folliculotropic mycosis fungoides, pagetoid reticulosis, granulomatous slack skin)
- Primary cutaneous CD30+ lymphoproliferative disorder (e.g., primary cutaneous ALCL, lymphomatoid papulosis)
- Subcutaneous panniculitis-like T-cell lymphoma (provisional)
- Primary cutaneous CD4+ small/medium-sized pleomorphic T-cell lymphoma (provisional)

CTCLs with aggressive clinical behavior include the following:

- Sézary syndrome
- Adult T-cell leukemia/lymphoma
- Extranodal NK/T-cell lymphoma, nasal type
- Primary cutaneous peripheral T-cell lymphoma, unspecified
- Primary cutaneous aggressive epidermotropic CD8+ T-cell lymphoma (provisional)
- Cutaneous gamma/delta-positive T-cell lymphoma (provisional)

Cutaneous B-cell lymphomas (CBCLs) are a less common version of cutaneous lymphomas, making up about 20–25% of all cutaneous lymphomas. The most common forms of CBCL are slow growing or indolent variations and respond well to mild treatments.

Newer subtypes have been defined in past few years as cutaneous T-cell lymphomas (two subtypes—CD4 small and medium; CD8 ear type), indolent GI T-cell lymphoma (CD8 equivalent of ear type), mucocutaneous ulcer [25, 26]. Similarly, indolent lymphomas at other sites have been defined as indolent B-cell lymphoproliferations in the blood and bone marrow, indolent B-cell lymphomas (duodenal, pediatric follicular lymphoma, marginal zone that do not progress), early (in situ) lymphomas [2].

16.10 Multidisciplinary Meetings

Data generated from all modes of investigation need to be collated and interpreted in a clinical context. Not every case of lymphoma will have a classical clinical presentation, morphology, immunophenotype, or genetic profile. The reporting pathologist remains responsible for diagnosis and for ensuring appropriate additional investigations are instituted to resolve discrepancies. An individual's experience of all the different investigations, the staining patterns of IPT, the interpretation of FISH, and cytogenetic analysis is useful in weighing up the contribution each investigation makes to the final diagnosis. All diagnoses of hematological malignancy should be discussed in multidisciplinary meetings/boards which include medical, pediatric, and radiation oncologists along with a hematopathologist. Both the diagnosis and clinical management decisions should be recorded in the case file at the meeting. Diagnosis of lymphomas cannot be made without understanding of the clinical background and such multispecialty group meetings help pathologists reach there.

16.11 Reporting

Lymphoma diagnosis on tissue biopsy (nodal, splenic, trephine, as well as extranodal tissue) is done in histopathology department, which may be in a different location from where peripheral blood/BM aspirate is reported (hematology laboratory). It is preferable that both these (tissues and liquid hematopathology) are reported under one roof, so that a final comprehensive report may be generated based on current WHO classification systems. Few clinical hematologists also report BM aspirate smears. The best person to do reporting is a trained and/or experienced pathologist who will report both biopsy and aspirate and should be responsible for integrating the results with ancillary techniques.

The final report should include prognostic and/or predictive markers, if any. These may be assessed by IHC, cytogenetics, or molecular diagnostic methods. For example, CD20 is a predictive marker for B-cell lymphomas. CD38 and Zap70 are prognostic markers in CLL. DLBCL has been further subclassified based on IPT (germinal center or non-germinal center phenotype), based on the site of origin (DLBCL, leg cell type, etc.), based on age (DLBCL of elderly), association with low-grade disease, presence of t(14;18), and expression of BCL2. Though the treatment protocol of all such subtypes of DLBCL is very similar at this moment, it may be a good idea to subtype these for future studies.

The provisional report may be released at first, followed by a final impression along with IHC findings. Supplementary report should follow in case molecular studies/FISH is performed. Kindly note that lymphoblastic lymphoma and Burkitt lymphoma are oncological emergencies, and an early provisional report must be given to the pediatric oncologist. Turnaround time for a lymphoma histopathology report may be 3–4 working days, and 7–8 days when IHC has been performed.

Hematopathologist must be aware of other common causes of abnormal lymphoid proliferations including nonspecific lymphadenitis, EBV infection, tuberculosis, HIV, dermatopathic lymphadenitis, toxoplasmosis, Kikuchi Fujimoto disease, Rosai Dorfman disease, etc.

Pathologists must remember:

1. Common tumors occur at common sites, and the clinical history is extremely important, including site and the age of the patient. Radiological investigations are mandatory as

part of staging and can also give a clue in reaching decisions.
2. Request for a re-biopsy in case of inadequate/crushed or poorly processed tissue.
3. Mimics of lymphomas are many, from benign lesions to other malignant lesions.
4. Second opinion may be sought in difficult cases.
5. To err is human, and the pathologist must admit any mistake if it happens.
6. There are gray areas in pathology. Communication is important between the pathologist and the treating physician/oncologist.

There are many limitations in histopathological diagnosis, including tiny biopsy, crushed sample, necrotic tumor, gray zone lymphomas, etc. There are also problems in reporting core biopsy, like differentiating HL versus mediastinal DLBCL, thymic hyperplasia, and T-LL, BLL, and DLBCL, HL versus DLBCL versus reactive node/viral infections. It may be difficult to opine on small crushed biopsies. Second opinion may be sought, and a re-biopsy should be asked for without wasting time.

Checklist for reporting lymphoma
– Classification according to current WHO classification.
– T- or B-cell phenotype (CD20 and CD3 positive or negative).
– Incorporate IHC in the final report. Mention about the reaction of IHC with the tumor cells (cells of interest) and also the reactive cells in the background. All stains done should be reported.
– Incorporating results of other ancillary techniques.

16.12 Disposal and Storage of Tissues

Each laboratory should follow the local/national laws for waste management/disposal for the remaining specimen, used reagents, garbage, infectious waste, etc. Retention period for tissues may be at least 2 months from the date of dis-

patch of the final report. These specimens are retrieved, formalin is discarded and the tissue is wrapped in appropriate containers, which may be given to authorized agencies for disposal/incineration. Chemicals like 10% buffered formalin, xylene, and alcohols are hazardous and should be discarded as per guidelines and waste disposal policy of the laboratory.

No diagnostic material should be discarded until all investigations are complete. NABL recommends that paraffin blocks are stored for a minimum of 20 years. Stained slides should be stored for a minimum of 10 years, and preferably longer, especially in case of pediatric patients and in small biopsy specimens where material permitting diagnosis may no longer be contained within the paraffin blocks.

16.13 Fine Needle Aspirate Examination (FNAC)

Cytology is an easy, simple, and economical technique, which is extremely popular among cytopathologists. Experienced cytologists offer an extremely high degree of reliability. FNA material may be used for FCM and molecular tests. Lymphoma diagnosis is best done on a biopsy, and FNAC is not recommended to diagnose lymphomas. In context of lymphomas, FNAC may be useful in the following circumstances:

1. In a known case of lymphoma, for documentation of relapse.
2. In emergency situations, such as in a patient having a mediastinal mass and superior vena cava syndrome, FNAC may be performed before instituting therapy. The sample may be sent for morphology and for FCM. Biopsy should still be advised for proper typing of the lymphoma.
3. FCI is performed for diagnosis and subtyping of HLN; however, subtypes (like HL) may be missed by this technique.
4. FCM may be used to establish a primary diagnosis of hematolymphoid neoplasm when there is no other readily available tissue. In difficult cases, where the biopsy interpretation

is inconclusive, FCM might provide invaluable additional information as elaborate markers are available for FCM. On the contrary, diagnosis and subtyping of myeloid neoplasm and chronic lymphoproliferative disorders (CLPDs) is best done by FCM.

5. FNAC may be performed in suspected cases of tuberculosis.

16.13.1 WHO 2017 Classification of HLN

The WHO 2017 Classification of hematolymphoid neoplasms is expected to be on the stands later this year. Newer defined entities in B-cell lymphomas include small/indolent clonal lymphoid populations, pediatric-type follicular lymphoma, large cell and borderline (gray zone) categories, DLBCL versus BL and "double hit" lymphomas, THRLBCL versus NLPHL, and also a few new genetically defined entities [2]. New entities in T-cell neoplasms include indolent T/NK-cell proliferations, EATL I/II subtypes, which have been further clarified, and few new genetically defined entities. Indolent clonal populations like intrafollicular neoplasia/follicular lymphoma in situ include similar entities like "FL-like B-cells of undetermined significance" and "in situ follicular neoplasia." Other indolent clonal proliferations include mantle cell lymphoma "in situ," indolent NK/T-cell proliferations of the GI tract, CD8+ indolent cutaneous LPD, and seroma-associated ALK-negative ALCL. Pediatric FL are more common than "pediatric-type FL." Pediatric FL are nodal, localized, purely follicular, have high Ki67, are BCL2-negative, and do not reveal any rearrangement of BCL2/BCL6. Not all FL in children are "pediatric type" and such cases may also occur in adults. Follicular lymphoma grade 3B+/−DLBCL with MUM1 expression should be separated from other FL as it behaves more like DLBCL. Similarly, grade 3B FL/DLBCL with IG/IRF4 translocation is a distinct entity within most of DLBCL and few FL, seen in younger patients, at Waldeyer's ring, requires treatment and has a good prognosis.

Diffuse large B-cell lymphoma remains the most intriguing category. In distinguishing GCB from non-GCB types, we may use any of the published IHC algorithms accepted (should be mentioned in the report). Morphologic subtypes may be optional; however, anatomic location is important (CNS, skin, etc.) and should be mentioned in the final report. "Double-hit" B-cell lymphomas are defined as MYC+ with BCL2 and/or BCL6 rearrangements; they have morphology like DLBCL or BL-like (BCL-U). They may be recognized either as a separate category, subdivided by morphology, or as separate categories within DLBCL and BCL-U. IHC for MYC and bcl2 may be performed; however, its co-expression is not clinically actionable at present. We may perform MYC FISH in all new cases of DLBCL, but it is expensive and not available at all places. So FISH may be done in all GC subtype, in double expressor lymphomas (MYC and BCL2 expression) or else high-grade morphology cases of DLBCL. Treatment wise, most of these are still treated with R-CHOP; hence, it is debatable how much is the adequate IHC panel. DHL (2–8% of all DLBCLs) are though treated more aggressively by protocols like dose adjusted R-EPOCH. In the entity EBV+ DLBCL of the elderly, elderly has been removed, and it has been relabeled as EBV + DLBCL NOS. EBV+ mucocutaneous ulcer is a close differential diagnosis (of HL in mucocutaneous sites) and has an indolent behavior (history of immunosuppression). Gray zone between THRLBCL versus NLPHL is still debatable. It is not clear whether diffuse areas/progression in NLPHL may be considered equivalent to THRLBCL. It is important to comment on variant patterns in NLPHL at diagnosis. Few hematolymphoid neoplasms have been defined based on new genetic information like BRAF mutations in HCL, MYD88 mutations in LPL, NOTCH1/2mutations in CLL, MCL, and SMZL, ID3 mutations in BL, BCL-U IG/IRF4 translocations in DLBCL/FL, and DUSP22 translocations/p63 mutations in ALK-negative ALCL.

Next-generation sequencing will be an important tool in the coming years. There are studies to show the contribution of NGS with a consensus gene panel to personalized therapy in DLBCL, highlighting subtypes' molecular heterogeneity and identifying somatic mutations with therapeutic and prognostic impact [27].

16.14 SOPs and Policies for Tissue Processing

1. Sample accession
2. Grossing procedure: as per standard grossing manuals
3. Fixation
4. Decalcification
5. Tissue processing
6. Embedding
7. Routine staining (hematoxylin and eosin)
8. Mounting procedure
9. Submission of slides
10. Reporting of results (text, comment, impression, signature)
11. Procedure for telephonic reporting
12. Procedure for handling pending reports
13. Slide and block filing
14. Discarding of slides and blocks
15. Medical records
16. Special stains (AFB, GMS, PAS, Congo red, reticulin, Perls', Giemsa, etc.)
17. IHC
18. Karyotyping and FISH studies
19. Molecular studies
20. Internal quality control
21. Proficiency testing program (external quality assurance program)

References

1. Swerdlow SH, Campo E, Harris NL, Jaffe ES, Pileri SA, Stein H, Jurgen T. WHO classification of tumors of hematopoeitic and lymphoid tissues 2017, vol. 2. Revised 4th ed. Lyon: IARC; 2017.
2. Swerdlow SH, Campo E, Pileri SA, Harris NL, Stein H, Siebert R, Advani R, Ghielmini M, Salles GA, Zelenetz AD, Jaffe ES. The 2016 revision of the World Health Organization classification of lymphoid neoplasms. Blood. 2016;127(20):2375–90.
3. Arber DA, Orazi A, Hasserjian R, Thiele J, Borowitz MJ, Le Beau MM, Bloomfield CD, Cazzola M, Vardiman JW. The 2016 revision to the World Health Organization classification of myeloid neoplasms and acute leukemia. Blood. 2016;127(20):2391–405.
4. Willemze R, Jaffe ES, Burg G, Cerroni L, Berti E, Swerdlow SH, Ralfkiaer E, Chimenti S, Diaz-Perez JL, Duncan LM, Grange F, Harris NL, Kempf W, Kerl H, Kurrer M, Knobler R, Pimpinelli N, Sander C, Santucci M, Sterry W, Vermeer MH, Wechsler J, Whittaker S, Meijer CJ. WHO-EORTC classification for cutaneouslymphomas. Blood. 2005;105(10):3768–85.
5. Burg G, Kempf W, Cozzio A, Feit J, Willemze R, S Jaffe E, Dummer R, Berti E, Cerroni L, Chimenti S, Diaz-Perez JL, Grange F, Harris NL, Kazakov DV, Kerl H, Kurrer M, Knobler R, Meijer CJ, Pimpinelli N, Ralfkiaer E, Russell-Jones R, Sander C, Santucci M, Sterry W, Swerdlow SH, Vermeer MH, Wechsler J, Whittaker S. WHO/EORTC classification of cutaneous lymphomas 2005: histological and molecular aspects. J Cutan Pathol. 2005;32(10):647–74.
6. Carbone PP, Kaplan HS, Musshoff K, Smithers DW, Tubiana M. Report of the committee on Hodgkin's disease staging classification. Cancer Res. 1971;31:1860–1.
7. Cheson BD, Fisher RI, Barrington SF, Cavalli F, Schwartz LH, Zucca E, Lister TA. Recommendations for initial evaluation, staging, and response assessment of Hodgkin and non-Hodgkin lymphoma: the Lugano classification. J Clin Oncol. 2014;20;32(27):3059–68.
8. Deshpande V, Zen Y, Chan JK, Yi EE, Sato Y, Yoshino T, Klöppel G, Heathcote JG, Khosroshahi A, Ferry JA, Aalberse RC, Bloch DB, Brugge WR, Bateman AC, Carruthers MN, Chari ST, Cheuk W, Cornell LD, Fernandez-Del Castillo C, Forcione DG, Hamilos DL, Kamisawa T, Kasashima S, Kawa S, Kawano M, Lauwers GY, Masaki Y, Nakanuma Y, Notohara K, Okazaki K, Ryu JK, Saeki T, Sahani DV, Smyrk TC, Stone JR, Takahira M, Webster GJ, Yamamoto M, Zamboni G, Umehara H, Stone JH. Consensus statement on the pathology of IgG4-related disease. Mod Pathol. 2012;25(9):1181–92.
9. Staudt LM. Molecular diagnosis of the hematologic cancers. N Engl J Med. 2003;348(18):1777–85. Review. Erratum in: N Engl J Med. 2003 Jun 19;348(25):2588.
10. Hans CP, Weisenburger DD, Greiner TC, Gascoyne RD, Delabie J, Ott G, Müller-Hermelink HK, Campo E, Braziel RM, Jaffe ES, Pan Z, Farinha P, Smith LM, Falini B, Banham AH, Rosenwald A, Staudt LM, Connors JM, Armitage JO, Chan WC. Confirmation of the molecular classification of diffuse large B-cell lymphoma by immunohistochemistry using a tissue microarray. Blood. 2004;103(1):275–82.
11. Naresh KN, Srinivas V, Soman CS. Distribution of various subtypes of non-Hodgkin's lymphoma in India: a study of 2773 lymphomas using R.E.A.L. and WHO classifications. Ann Oncol. 2000;11(Suppl 1):63–7.
12. Srinivas V, Soman CS, Naresh KN. Study of the distribution of 289 non-Hodgkin lymphomas using the WHO classification among children and adolescents in India. Med Pediatr Oncol. 2002;39(1):40–3.

13. Craig FE, Foon KA. Flow cytometric immuno-phenotyping for hematologic neoplasms. Blood. 2008;111(8):3941–67.

14. Jennings CD, Foon KA. Recent advances in flow cytometry: application to the diagnosis of hematologic malignancy. Blood. 1997;90(8): 2863–92.

15. Gujral S, Polampalli SN, Badrinath Y, Kumar A, Subramanian PG, Nair R, Gupta S, Sengar M, Nair C. Immunophenotyping of mature B-cell non Hodgkin lymphoma involving bone marrow and peripheral blood: critical analysis and insights gained at a tertiary care cancer hospital. Leuk Lymphoma. 2009;50(8):1290–300.

16. Gujral S, Subramanian PG, Patkar N, Badrinath Y, Kumar A, Tembhare P, Vazifdar A, Khodaiji S, Madkaikar M, Ghosh K, Yargop M, Dasgupta A. Report of proceedings of the national meeting on "Guidelines for Immunophenotyping of Hematolymphoid Neoplasms by Flow Cytometry". Indian J Pathol Microbiol. 2008;51(2):161–6.

17. Gujral S, Badrinath Y, Kumar A, Subramanian PG, Raje G, Jain H, Pais A, Amre Kadam PS, Banavali SD, Arora B, Kumar P, Hari Menon VG, Kurkure PA, Parikh PM, Mahadik S, Chogule AB, Shinde SC, Nair CN. Immunophenotypic profile of acute leukemia: critical analysis and insights gained at a tertiary care center in India. Cytom B Clin Cytom. 2009;76(3):199–205.

18. Gujral S, Polampalli S, Badrinath Y, Kumar A, Subramanian PG, Nair R, Sengar M, Nair C. Immunophenotyping of mature T/NK cell neoplasm presenting as leukemia. Indian J Cancer. 2010;47(2):189–93.

19. Foucar K, Reichard K, Czuchlewski D. Bone marrow pathology. Chicago: ASCP; 2010.

20. Bain BJ. Bone marrow trephine biopsy. J Clin Pathol. 2001;54(10):737–42.

21. Naresh KN, Lampert I, Hasserjian R, Lykidis D, Elderfield K, Horncastle D, Smith N, Murray-Brown W, Stamp GW. Optimal processing of bone marrow trephine biopsy: the Hammersmith protocol. J Clin Pathol. 2006;59(9):903–11.

22. Hyun BH, Gulati GL, Ashton JK. Bone marrow examination: techniques and interpretation. Hematol Oncol Clin North Am. 1988;2(4):513–23.

23. Thiele J, Kvasnicka HM, Facchetti F, Franco V, van der Walt J, Orazi A. European consensus on grading bone marrow fibrosis and assessment of cellularity. Haematologica. 2005;90(8):1128–32.

24. Campo E, Chott A, Kinney MC, Leoncini L, Meijer CJ, Papadimitriou CS, Piris MA, Stein H, Swerdlow SH. Update on extranodal lymphomas. Conclusions of the workshop held by the EAHP and the SH in Thessaloniki, Greece. Histopathology. 2006;48(5):481–504.

25. Li JY, Guitart J, Pulitzer MP, Subtil A, Sundram U, Kim Y, Deonizio J, Myskowski PL, Moskowitz A, Horwitz S, Querfeld C. Multicenter case series of indolent small/medium-sized CD8+ lymphoid proliferations with predilection for the ear and face. Am J Dermatopathol. 2014;36(5):402–8.

26. Wang L, Gao T, Wang G. Primary cutaneous CD8+ cytotoxic T-cell lymphoma involving the epidermis and subcutis in a young child. J Cutan Pathol. 2015;42(4):271–5.

27. Dubois S, Viailly PJ, Mareschal S, Bohers E, Bertrand P, Ruminy P, Maingonnat C, Jais JP, Peyrouze P, Figeac M, Molina TJ, Desmots F, Fest T, Haioun C, Lamy T, Copie-Bergman C, Brière J, Petrella T, Canioni D, Fabiani B, Coiffier B, Delarue R, Peyrade F, Bosly A, André M, Ketterer N, Salles G, Tilly H, Leroy K, Jardin F. Next-generation sequencing in diffuse large B-cell lymphoma highlights molecular divergence and therapeutic opportunities: a LYSA study. Clin Cancer Res. 2016;22(12):2919–28.

Part III

Hemostasis

Inherited Platelet Defects and Mutations in Hematopoietic Transcription Factor RUNX1

17

Natthapol Songdej and A. Koneti Rao

17.1 Introduction

Patients with inherited platelet related bleeding disorders are frequently encountered in the clinical practice of hematology. In most such patients with inherited thrombocytopenias and platelet dysfunction, the genetic mechanisms are unknown. Studies over the last two decades have established that some of these patients have mutations in hematopoietic transcription factors (TFs) that regulate the expression of genes involved in platelet and megakaryocyte biology—starting with hematopoietic stem cell (HSC) differentiation and megakaryocyte (MK) lineage commitment to MK maturation and eventual platelet release (Fig. 17.1) [1]. TFs are proteins that bind to specific DNA sequences and regulate expression of genes. They function in a combinatorial manner as activators and repressors [2, 3]. Each TF regulates multiple genes and thus can induce multiple effects by influencing diverse mechanisms and pathways. Several

hematopoietic TFs have been implicated in platelet disorders including the runt related transcription factor 1 (RUNX1), Fli-1 proto-oncogene, ETS transcription factor (FLI1), GATA-binding protein 1 (GATA1), growth factor independent 1B transcriptional repressor (GFI1B), ETS variant 6 (ETV6), ecotropic viral integration site 1 (EVI1), and homeobox A11 (HOXA11). These regulate processes involved in hematopoiesis, MK lineage commitment and maturation, and platelet biogenesis [4, 5]. In addition to alterations in platelet number and function, some mutations are associated with a predisposition to leukemias. Of the TF mutations implicated in platelet disorders to date, the best characterized are the abnormalities associated with mutations in *RUNX1* and they are reviewed here. Others have been reviewed elsewhere [6].

17.2 RUNX1

RUNX1 belongs to RUNX family of three TFs coded by the genes, *RUNX1, RUNX2,* and *RUNX3* [7, 8]; all three proteins share the conserved runt-homology domain. RUNX1, also known as core-binding factor subunit alpha-2 (CBFA2), is encoded by the *RUNX1* gene on chromosome 21q22.3. It has a 128 amino acid conserved runt homology domain near the N-terminus that associates with its co-factor, core-binding factor subunit beta (CBFB) and binds to sequence-specific DNA to regulate gene expression [9]. RUNX1 is transcribed from two alternate promoters, a distal

N. Songdej
Department of Medicine and Pediatrics, Penn State College of Medicine, Hershey, PA, USA

A. K. Rao (✉)
Sol Sherry Thrombosis Research Center, Lewis Katz School of Medicine at Temple University, Philadelphia, PA, USA

Department of Medicine, Lewis Katz School of Medicine at Temple University, Philadelphia, PA, USA
e-mail: koneti.rao@temple.edu

© Springer Nature Singapore Pte Ltd. 2019
R. Saxena, H. P. Pati (eds.), *Hematopathology*, https://doi.org/10.1007/978-981-13-7713-6_17

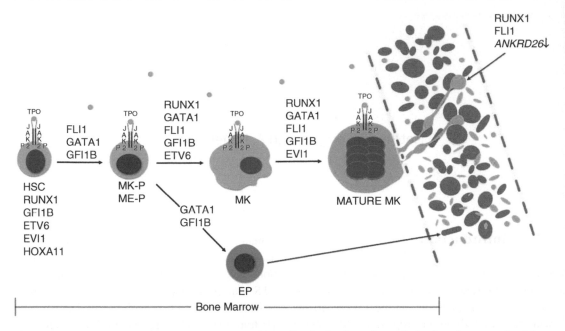

Fig. 17.1 Hematopoietic transcription factors (TFs) involved in normal platelet genesis. RUNX1, GFI1B, ETV6, EVI1, and HOXA11 are expressed in hematopoietic stem cells (HSCs). As denoted above by black arrows, various hematopoietic TFs, in combination with thrombopoietin (TPO) stimulation, function to promote HSC differentiation, megakaryocyte (MK) lineage commitment and maturation, proplatelet formation, and platelet release. Proplatelet formation and platelet release are also driven by RUNX1 and FLI1 silencing of *ANKRD26*. *MK-P* megakaryocyte progenitor, *ME-P* megakaryocyte-erythroid progenitor, *EP* erythroid progenitor, *P* phosphorylated, *TPO* thrombopoietin (green dots). Reproduced with permission from Songdej, N and Rao. AK, *Blood*. 2017;129 (21):2873–2881

P1 and a proximal P2 promoter, and leads to the formation of at least three isoforms and multiple splice variants [8, 10, 11]. The three isoforms have the runt domain, differ in their amino acid sequence, are expressed in a distinct temporal and tissue-specific form and have different functions. RUNX1 is indispensable for definitive hematopoiesis. *RUNX1* knockout mice lack primary hematopoiesis during embryogenesis and die in utero because of bleeding [12].

17.3 RUNX1 Haplodeficiency and Human Disease

RUNX1 mutations are associated with familial thrombocytopenia, impaired platelet function, and a predisposition to acute leukemia. In 1985, Dowton et al. [13] described kindred of 22 members with a bleeding tendency, autosomal dominant thrombocytopenia, and impaired platelet aggregation responses; 6 family members devel-

oped hematologic malignancies, including leukemia in 4 patients. Several investigators reported other families [13–15] and this entity came to be referred as Familial Platelet Disorder with Predisposition to Acute Myeloid Leukemia (FPD/AML; MIM 601399). Linkage analysis of FPD/AML patients mapped a potential locus to the long arm of chromosome 21q22 [15, 16]. In 1999, studies of Song et al. [17] identified heterozygous mutations in *RUNX1* in affected members of six families to establish the causal link, subsequently shown in several other families [18, 19].

Recent studies in patient with bleeding disorders using state-of-the-art approaches, such as next generation sequencing (NGS), indicate that TF mutations may be the genetic basis of platelet defects more frequently than generally considered [20–22]. In one study [20], *RUNX1* or *FLI1* mutations were found in 6 of 13 index patients with clinical bleeding and impaired platelet aggregation and dense granule secretion; this was also observed in other studies [22, 23]. Germline alterations in hematopoietic TFs therefore need to be considered in the pathogenesis of inherited platelet defects.

Patients with *RUNX1* mutations typically have a mild to moderate bleeding tendency due to the platelet dysfunction and thrombocytopenia, with normal-sized platelets; some patients may not have thrombocytopenia or bleeding symptoms [20, 24, 25]. It is likely that *RUNX1* mutations are under-recognized in patients with platelet defects.

Most of the reported mutations in *RUNX1* have been within the conserved runt domain with decreased RUNX1 binding to the target DNA [19, 26, 27], though a mutation in the transactivation domain near the C-terminus has also been reported [19]. The mutations usually result in haplodeficiency, but in some patients there is markedly decreased RUNX1 activity due to a dominant negative effect [19, 28]. Murine heterozygous *RUNX1* mutations do not recapitulate the human disease [29].

17.4   RUNX1 and Impaired Megakaryopoiesis

Conditional *RUNX1* knockouts in mouse models show impaired MK maturation, with abnormal micro-megakaryocytes and decreased MK polyploidization [30]. In patients with *RUNX1* mutations, MKs demonstrate defects in differentiation and polyploidization [17, 31]. This has been associated with dysregulated non-muscle myosin IIA (MYH9) and IIB (MYH10) expression, with impaired *MYH10* silencing and reduced *MYL9* and *MYH9* expression [31]. Reconstitution of *MYH10* silencing promotes MK polyploidization and progression from mitosis to endomitosis [31, 32]. Persistent platelet MYH10 protein expression has been proposed as a marker for defects in *RUNX1* and *FLI1* [33].

17.5   RUNX1 Mutations and Platelet Dysfunction

The platelet dysfunction associated with RUNX1 haplodeficiency is complex and recent studies have provided major insights, driven by identification

and understanding of some of the genes regulated by RUNX1 in platelets. Numerous platelet function abnormalities are documented in patients with *RUNX1* mutations and include decreased platelet aggregation and secretion upon activation with different agonists, deficiencies of dense granules (DG) or α-granules (or both) and decreased phosphorylation of myosin light chain and pleckstrin, activation of αIIbβ3, production of 12-hydroxyeicosatetraenoic acid (12-HETE, a product of 12-lipoxygenase) and protein kinase C-θ (which phosphorylates pleckstrin and other proteins) (Fig. 17.2) [19, 31, 34–36]. Recently, it has been reported that RUNX1 regulates *TREML1* (TREM-like transcript-1) and the integrin subunit α2 (*ITGA2*) of the platelet receptor α2β1 [37]; both are involved in platelet collagen interactions.

One of the hallmarks of the platelet defect in patients with *RUNX1* mutations is decreased platelet granules or their contents (storage pool deficiency, SPD), involving both the protein-bearing α-granules and DG. Some patients previously described with the storage pool deficiency have more recently been identified to have mutations in *RUNX1* or another TF [19, 20, 22, 23, 38]. In 1969, Weiss et al. described a family with an autosomal dominant inherited platelet disorder due to decreased DG contents [39]. This family was subsequently found to also have partial α-granule deficiency [40] and in 2002 reported to have a heterozygous Y260X mutation in *RUNX1* [19]. Similarly, an underlying TF mutation has been found in other patients previously reported as SPD [22, 23, 38, 41]. Further, it has become clear that the same platelet phenotype may result from mutations in more than one TF or underlying mechanism. For example, α-granule deficiencies have been shown to be associated with mutations in *RUNX1* [19, 22, 42], *GATA1* [41], and *GFI1B* [23, 38] in addition to *NBEAL2* [35].

The protein pallidin is involved in DG biogenesis, and platelets from the pallid mouse and patients with the human Hermansky–Pudlak syndrome 9 (both deficient in pallidin) have decreased DG [43, 44]. Platelet expression of *PLDN* is decreased in *RUNX1* haplodeficiency, and *PLDN* is a direct transcriptional target of RUNX1 [45]. This provides a potential mechanism for the DG

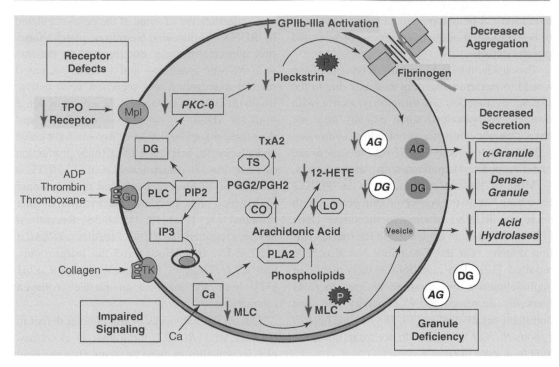

Fig. 17.2 Schematic representation of abnormalities in platelet responses to activation associated with *RUNX1* mutations. Platelet receptor activation results in the formation of intracellular mediators that regulate the end-responses, such as aggregation and secretion from α-granules (AG) and dense granules (DG) and from vesicles bearing acid hydrolases. Receptor activation leads to hydrolysis of phosphatidylinositol bisphosphate (PIP₂) by phospholipase C to form diacylglycerol (DAG), which activates protein kinase C (PKC), and inositoltrisphosphate (IP₃), which mediates the rise in cytoplasmic Ca²⁺ levels. PKC phosphorylates numerous proteins including pleckstrin. The increase in Ca²⁺ levels leads to other responses, such as activation of myosin light chain kinase (MYLK) to phosphorylate myosin light chain (MLC) and activation of phospholipase A₂ (PLA₂), which mediates the release of free arachidonic acid from phospholipids. Arachidonic acid is converted by cyclooxygenase (CO) and thromboxane synthase (TS) to thromboxane A₂. Numerous defects in platelet function have been described

in platelets with *RUNX1* haplodeficiency. These are shown with downward arrows (blue). Included below in this legend in parenthesis are some of the relevant genes that are RUNX1 targets and downregulated in *RUNX1* haplodeficiency. The abnormalities include reduction in the surface receptors for thrombopoietin (*MPL*); defects in signaling mechanisms, including impaired pleckstrin and myosin light chain phosphorylation, decreased protein kinase C-theta (*PRCKQ*) and myosin light chain (*MYL9*); decreased 12-lipoxygenase activity (*ALOX12*) and 12-HETE production; impaired activation of GPIIb-IIIa and aggregation on platelet activation; dense granule (*PLDN*) and alpha granule (*PF4*) deficiency; impaired secretion of α- and dense granule contents and from vesicles containing acid hydrolases. Other genes shown to be downregulated and not shown in the figure include *PCTP, NFE2,* and *NOTCH4*. Reproduced with permission from Songdej, N and Rao, AK, *Blood.* 2017;129 (21):2873–2881

deficiency in patients with *RUNX1* mutations. α-granules contain numerous proteins—some synthesized by MK (e.g., PF4, von Willebrand factor, p-selectin) and others not synthesized by MK but incorporated by endocytosis (albumin, IgG, fibrinogen, factor V). Platelet α-granule contents are decreased in patients with *RUNX1* haplodeficiency [6]. The mechanisms leading to

α-granule deficiency in these patients are poorly understood and it is likely that multiple mechanisms are involved, including the synthesis of the granule proteins, their trafficking between various endosomal compartments, endocytosis from outside, and specific targeting to the granules. There is evolving evidence to implicate several abnormalities. Platelet levels of the α-granule protein platelet factor 4 are decreased and *PF4* is regulated by RUNX1 [42]. There is evidence of decreased expression of *RAB1B,* a small GTPase linked to vesicle trafficking from the endoplasmic reticulum to the Golgi, with a potential effect in the handling of α-granule proteins, such as von Willebrand factor [46]. Consistent with this platelet VWF levels were decreased in patients with *RUNX1* mutations [46]. In these studies, *RUNX1* downregulation in megakaryocytic cells induced Golgi dispersion. Another small GTPase *RAB31* implicated in endosomal trafficking is a direct target of RUNX1 and its expression is decreased in platelets in these patients [47]. Lastly, platelet albumin and IgG, two α-granule proteins not synthesized by MKs, were also reduced in one patient, suggesting a defect in platelet uptake and trafficking into granules [34].

As described earlier, patients with *RUNX1* mutations have defects in platelet activation mechanisms that regulate agonist-stimulated responses and secretion from granules, including from the acid hydrolase containing vesicles, unrelated to a deficiency of granule contents [20, 48–50]. Thus, the platelet dysfunction is a result of dysregulation of multiple RUNX1-regulated genes and the defective secretion reflects abnormalities in granule biogenesis and in the secretory mechanisms (Fig. 17.2).

RUNX1 regulates expression of numerous genes and pathways in MK/platelet genes [37, 51, 52]. Platelet and MK transcript profiling of patients with heterozygous *RUNX1* mutation showed downregulation of multiple MK/platelet genes involved in diverse aspects of platelet production and function [37, 52]. Several genes are direct transcriptional targets of RUNX1, including 12-lipoxygenase (*ALOX12*) [36], platelet factor 4 (*PF4*) [42], platelet myosin light chain (*MYL9*) [53], protein kinase C-θ (*PRKCQ*) [54], pallidin (*PLDN*) [45], *RAB1B* [46], *TREML1* [37], ITGA2 [37], and the thrombopoietin receptor (*MPL*) [55]. Another gene downregulated and a target of RUNX1 is *PCTP* [56], which encodes for a protein implicated in platelet responses to PAR4 agonist activation [57]. Transcription factor NF-E2 (*NFE2*) is also a transcriptional target of RUNX1 [58]. NF-E2 has been implicated in

platelet granule development and αIIbβ3 signaling [58]. *NOTCH4* is a key RUNX1 target in MK differentiation and is negatively regulated by RUNX1 [59]. These alterations impact different aspects of MKs and platelets. Using induced pluripotent stem cells (IPSCs) from skin fibroblasts of two patients with RUNX1 Y260X mutation, Connelly et al. [60] demonstrated impaired MK production and abnormalities, including presence of vacuoles and reduction in α-granules and DG. Targeted in vitro mutation correction rescued the defects in MK production and phenotype in these and other studies using IPSCs [59, 61, 62]. These findings validated the causative role of *RUNX1* mutations and advance the potential for gene therapy.

RUNX1 has recently been shown to regulate *A4GALT,* which encodes alpha-1, 4-galactosyltransferase, an enzyme involved in the synthesis of P1 blood group antigens [63]. These studies implicate RUNX1 in the expression of glycosphingolipids and blood group antigens on red cells. The impact of this in patients with *RUNX1* haplodeficiency remains unclear.

17.6   RUNX1 and Cardiovascular Disease

Recent studies implicate RUNX1 regulation of MK/platelet genes in cardiovascular disease (CVD), extending the role of RUNX1 from bleeding disorders to atherothrombotic disease [64]. Aspirin is widely used in the treatment of CVD. Voora et al. [65] administered 325 mg/day of aspirin to 50 healthy volunteers and performed simultaneous peripheral blood gene expression profiling before and after aspirin exposure, and identified an aspirin response signature (ARS) as a set of 62 tightly co-expressed genes in peripheral blood RNA that was correlative of aspirin effects on platelet aggregation responses. They validated the ARS in an independent cohort of 53 healthy volunteers and 132 patients with cardiovascular disease [65]. A majority (60%, 37/62) of ARS genes in this study was noted to overlap with genes downregulated in inherited *RUNX1* haplodeficiency and 48% (28/62) of ARS genes contained putative RUNX1 binding sites. RUNX1 expression in hematopoietic cells is regulated by two alternative promoters, a distal promoter P1 and a proximal promoter P2. Most interestingly, in CVD patients, *RUNX1* P1 expression in blood was negatively associated with future death or MI. In megakaryocytic cells, in vitro exposure to aspirin and its metabolite (salicylic acid, a weak COX1 inhibitor) upregulated *RUNX1* P1 isoform. In human subjects, *RUNX1* P1 expression in blood and RUNX1-regulated platelet proteins, including MYL9, were aspirin-responsive and associated with platelet function. These studies advance the concept that RUNX1 is an aspirin-sensitive transcription factor.

The potential role of RUNX1 regulation of platelet genes in CVD is further advanced by the studies showing that *PCTP* (phosphatidylcholine transfer protein) is regulated by RUNX1 [56]. Edelstein et al. [57] have reported an association between the increased thrombin receptor PAR4 agonist-induced platelet aggregation among healthy black subjects and increased expression of platelet PCTP. PCTP has a wide tissue distribution [66] and is abundantly expressed in human platelets [57]. Studies of Mao et al. [56] show that platelet PCTP protein and mRNA are decreased in patients with *RUNX1* mutations and that *PCTP* is a direct RUNX1 target. Studies in CVD patients showed that *RUNX1* expression in blood correlated with *PCTP* gene expression and associated with future death/myocardial infarction. There were differential effects of *RUNX1* isoforms on PCTP expression with a negative correlation in blood between RUNX1 expressed from the P1 promoter and *PCTP* expression. These studies suggest that regulation of *PCTP* by RUNX1 may play a role in the pathogenesis of platelet-mediated CV events.

17.7 RUNX1 and Hematologic Malignancies

The bleeding symptoms in patients with germline mutations are mild to moderate in most patients. The most serious consequence of germline *RUNX1* mutation is the predisposition to acute myeloid leukemia and myelodysplastic syndrome (MDS), with the life time risk approaching 44% [10, 24, 67, 68]. It is important to note that mutations in *RUNX1* occur at a high frequency in patients with sporadic leukemias and MDS, and this may represent a different biology relative to germline inherited mutations [10, 67]. Interestingly, *RUNX1* mutations appear to be distinctly uncommon among individuals with the age-related clonal hematopoiesis of indeterminate potential (CHIP) [69–71]. The malignant transformation in patients with germline *RUNX1* mutations is heralded by the development of additional somatic mutations in other genes, such as *ASXL1, CBL, CDC25C, FLT3, PHF6, SRSF2*, and *WT1* [10, 67, 72–74]. In some patients, there were loss-of-function mutations in the second *RUNX1* allele [75]. RUNX1 activity level appears to be important in predisposition to leukemic transformation [28]. In one study of individuals with germline *RUNX1* mutations and without evidence of leukemia, 6 of 9 patients had clonal hematopoiesis [74]. Sporadic germline deletions involving chromosome 21q22 that include the *RUNX1* gene may result in syndromic features (dysmorphic facies, mental retardation, and organ abnormalities) and predisposition to hematologic malignancies [24]. In patients with *RUNX1* mutations who develop MDS or leukemia, use of an undiagnosed *RUNX1* haplodeficient sibling donor has been associated with recurrence of leukemia [25]. It has been suggested that patients undergo surveillance for MDS and leukemia with clinical examination and blood counts every 6–12 months [76].

17.8 Conclusions

RUNX1 mutations are emerging as an important genetic mechanism for inherited platelet disorders and may be more common than previously appreciated. Recognizing *RUNX1* and other TF mutations in patients with thrombocytopenia and/or platelet dysfunction is important—to prevent unnecessary therapies, such as based on an erroneous diagnosis of immune thrombocytopenic purpura, and because these patients have an increased risk of hematologic malignancy. Studies in patients with *RUNX1* and TF mutations are likely to provide important insights into the genetic and molecular mechanisms governing MK/platelet biology and into leukemogenesis.FundingThis study was supported by research funding from NIH (NHLBI) R01HL109568 and RO1HL137376.

Authorship: NS and AKR co-wrote the paper.

Conflict-of-interest Declaration: The authors declare no competing financial interests.

References

1. Eto K, Kunishima S. Linkage between the mechanisms of thrombocytopenia and thrombopoiesis. Blood. 2016;127(10):1234–41.
2. Tijssen MR, Cvejic A, Joshi A, Hannah RL, Ferreira R, Forrai A, et al. Genome-wide analysis of simultaneous GATA1/2, RUNX1, FLI1, and SCL binding in megakaryocytes identifies hematopoietic regulators. Dev Cell. 2011;20(5):597–609.
3. Dore LC, Crispino JD. Transcription factor networks in erythroid cell and megakaryocyte development. Blood. 2011;118(2):231–9.
4. Rabbolini DJ, Ward CM, Stevenson WS. Thrombocytopenia caused by inherited haematopoietic transcription factor mutation: clinical phenotypes and diagnostic considerations. EMJ Hematology. 2016;4(1):100–9.
5. Tijssen MR, Ghevaert C. Transcription factors in late megakaryopoiesis and related platelet disorders. J Thromb Haemost. 2013;11(4):593–604.
6. Songdej N, Rao AK. Hematopoietic transcription factor mutations: important players in inherited platelet defects. Blood. 2017;129(21):2873–81.
7. de Bruijn MF, Speck NA. Core-binding factors in hematopoiesis and immune function. Oncogene. 2004;23(24):4238–48.
8. Levanon D, Groner Y. Structure and regulated expression of mammalian RUNX genes. Oncogene. 2004;23(24):4211–9.
9. Coffman JA. Runx transcription factors and the developmental balance between cell proliferation and differentiation. Cell Biol Int. 2003;27(4):315–24.
10. Sood R, Kamikubo Y, Liu P. Role of RUNX1 in hematological malignancies. Blood. 2017;129(15):2070–82.
11. Cantor AB. Choosing wisely: RUNX1 alternate promoter use. Blood. 2017;130(3):236–7.
12. Wang Q, Stacy T, Binder M, Marin-Padilla M, Sharpe AH, Speck NA. Disruption of the Cbfa2 gene causes necrosis and hemorrhaging in the central nervous system and blocks definitive hematopoiesis. Proc Natl Acad Sci U S A. 1996;93(8):3444–9.
13. Dowton SB, Beardsley D, Jamison D, Blattner S, Li FP. Studies of a familial platelet disorder. Blood. 1985;65(3):557–63.
14. Gerrard JM, Israels ED, Bishop AJ, Schroeder ML, Beattie LL, McNicol A, et al. Inherited platelet-storage pool deficiency associated with a high incidence of acute myeloid leukaemia. Br J Haematol. 1991;79(2):246–55.
15. Ho CY, Otterud B, Legare RD, Varvil T, Saxena R, DeHart DB, et al. Linkage of a familial platelet disorder with a propensity to develop myeloid malignancies to human chromosome 21q22.1-22.2. Blood. 1996;87(12):5218–24.
16. Arepally G, Rebbeck TR, Song W, Gilliland G, Maris JM, Poncz M. Evidence for genetic homogeneity in a familial platelet disorder with predisposition to acute myelogenous leukemia (FPD/AML) [letter]. Blood. 1998;92(7):2600–2.
17. Song WJ, Sullivan MG, Legare RD, Hutchings S, Tan X, Kufrin D, et al. Haploinsufficiency of CBFA2 causes familial thrombocytopenia with propensity to develop acute myelogenous leukaemia. Nat Genet. 1999;23(2):166–75.
18. Preudhomme C, Warot-Loze D, Roumier C, Grardel-Duflos N, Garand R, Lai JL, et al. High incidence of biallelic point mutations in the Runt domain of the AML1/PEBP2 alpha B gene in Mo acute myeloid leukemia and in myeloid malignancies with acquired trisomy 21. Blood. 2000;96(8):2862–9.
19. Michaud J, Wu F, Osato M, Cottles GM, Yanagida M, Asou N, et al. In vitro analyses of known and novel RUNX1/AML1 mutations in dominant familial platelet disorder with predisposition to acute myelogenous leukemia: implications for mechanisms of pathogenesis. Blood. 2002;99(4):1364–72.
20. Stockley J, Morgan NV, Bem D, Lowe GC, Lordkipanidze M, Dawood B, et al. Enrichment of FLI1 and RUNX1 mutations in families with excessive bleeding and platelet dense granule secretion defects. Blood. 2013;122(25):4090–3.
21. Lentaigne C, Freson K, Laffan MA, Turro E, Ouwehand WH, Consortium B-B, et al. Inherited platelet disorders: toward DNA-based diagnosis. Blood. 2016;127(23):2814–23.
22. Simeoni I, Stephens JC, Hu F, Deevi SV, Megy K, Bariana TK, et al. A high-throughput sequencing test for diagnosing inherited bleeding, thrombotic, and platelet disorders. Blood. 2016;127(23):2791–803.
23. Stevenson WS, Morel-Kopp MC, Chen Q, Liang HP, Bromhead CJ, Wright S, et al. GFI1B mutation causes a bleeding disorder with abnormal platelet function. J Thromb Haemost. 2013;11(11):2039–47.
24. Liew E, Owen C. Familial myelodysplastic syndromes: a review of the literature. Haematologica. 2011;96(10):1536–42.
25. Owen CJ, Toze CL, Koochin A, Forrest DL, Smith CA, Stevens JM, et al. Five new pedigrees with inherited RUNX1 mutations causing familial platelet disorder with propensity to myeloid malignancy (FPD/AML). Blood. 2008;112(12):4639–45.
26. Morgan NV, Daly ME. Gene of the issue: RUNX1 mutations and inherited bleeding. Platelets. 2017;28(2):208–10.

27. Brown AL, Churpek JE, Malcovati L, Dohner H, Godley LA. Recognition of familial myeloid neoplasia in adults. Semin Hematol. 2017;54(2):60–8.

28. Antony-Debre I, Manchev VT, Balayn N, Bluteau D, Tomowiak C, Legrand C, et al. Level of RUNX1 activity is critical for leukemic predisposition but not for thrombocytopenia. Blood. 2015;125(6):930–40.

29. Sun W, Downing JR. Haploinsufficiency of AML1 results in a decrease in the number of LTR-HSCs while simultaneously inducing an increase in more mature progenitors. Blood. 2004;104(12):3565–72.

30. Ichikawa M, Asai T, Saito T, Seo S, Yamazaki I, Yamagata T, et al. AML-1 is required for megakaryocytic maturation and lymphocytic differentiation, but not for maintenance of hematopoietic stem cells in adult hematopoiesis. Nat Med. 2004;10(3):299–304.

31. Bluteau D, Glembotsky AC, Raimbault A, Balayn N, Gilles L, Rameau P, et al. Dysmegakaryopoiesis of FPD/AML pedigrees with constitutional RUNX1 mutations is linked to myosin II deregulated expression. Blood. 2012;120(13):2708–18.

32. Lordier L, Bluteau D, Jalil A, Legrand C, Pan J, Rameau P, et al. RUNX1-induced silencing of non-muscle myosin heavy chain IIB contributes to megakaryocyte polyploidization. Nat Commun. 2012;3:717.

33. Antony-Debre I, Bluteau D, Itzykson R, Baccini V, Renneville A, Boehlen F, et al. MYH10 protein expression in platelets as a biomarker of RUNX1 and FLI1 alterations. Blood. 2012;120(13):2719–22.

34. Sun L, Mao G, Rao AK. Association of CBFA2 mutation with decreased platelet PKC-θ and impaired receptor-mediated activation of GPIIb-IIIa and pleckstrin phosphorylation: proteins regulated by CBFA2 play a role in GPIIb-IIIa activation. Blood. 2004;103(3):948–54.

35. Rao AK. Inherited platelet function disorders: overview and disorders of granules, secretion, and signal transduction. Hematol Oncol Clin North Am. 2013;27(3):585–611.

36. Kaur G, Jalagadugula G, Mao G, Rao AK. RUNX1/core binding factor A2 regulates platelet 12-lipoxygenase gene (ALOX12): studies in human RUNX1 haplodeficiency. Blood. 2010;115(15):3128–35.

37. Glembotsky A, Sliwa D, Bluteau D, Balayn N, Marin Oyarzun CP, Raimbault A, et al. Downregulation of TREM-like transcript (TLT)-1 and collagen receptor 2 subunit, two novel RUNX1-targets, contribute to platelet dysfunction in familial platelet disorder with predisposition to acute myelogenous leukemia. Haematologica. 2019;104(6):1244–55. https://doi.org/10.3324/haematol.2018.188904.

38. Monteferrario D, Bolar NA, Marneth AE, Hebeda KM, Bergevoet SM, Veenstra H, et al. A dominant-negative GFI1B mutation in the gray platelet syndrome. N Engl J Med. 2014;370(3):245–53.

39. Weiss HJ, Chervenick PA, Zalusky R, Factor A. A familial defect in platelet function associated with impaired release of adenosine diphosphate. N Engl J Med. 1969;281:1264–70.

40. Weiss HJ, Witte LD, Kaplan KL, Lages BA, Chernoff A, Nossel HL, et al. Heterogeneity in storage pool deficiency: studies on granule-bound substances in 18 patients including variants deficient in alpha-granules, platelet factor 4, beta-thromboglobulin, and platelet-derived growth factor. Blood. 1979;54(6):1296–319.

41. Tubman VN, Levine JE, Campagna DR, Monahan-Earley R, Dvorak AM, Neufeld EJ, et al. X-linked gray platelet syndrome due to a GATA1 Arg216Gln mutation. Blood. 2007;109(8):3297–9.

42. Aneja K, Jalagadugula G, Mao G, Singh A, Rao AK. Mechanism of platelet factor 4 (PF4) deficiency with RUNX1 haplodeficiency: RUNX1 is a transcriptional regulator of *PF4*. J Thromb Haemost. 2011;9(2):383–91.

43. Huang L, Kuo YM, Gitschier J. The pallid gene encodes a novel, syntaxin 13-interacting protein involved in platelet storage pool deficiency. Nat Genet. 1999;23(3):329–32.

44. Cullinane AR, Curry JA, Carmona-Rivera C, Summers CG, Ciccone C, Cardillo ND, et al. A BLOC-1 mutation screen reveals that PLDN is mutated in Hermansky-Pudlak syndrome type 9. Am J Hum Genet. 2011;88(6):778–87.

45. Mao GF, Goldfinger LE, Fan DC, Lambert MP, Jalagadugula G, Freishtat R, et al. Dysregulation of PLDN (Pallidin) is a mechanism for platelet dense granule deficiency in RUNX1 haplodeficiency. J Thromb Haemost. 2017;15:792–801.

46. Jalagadugula G, Goldfinger LE, Mao G, Lambert MP, Rao AK. Defective RAB1B-related megakaryocytic ER-to-Golgi transport in RUNX1 haplodeficiency: impact on von Willebrand factor. Blood Adv. 2018;2(7):797–806.

47. Jalagadugula G, Mao G, Goldfinger L, Wurtzel J, Lambert M, Rao A. RAB31-mediated endosomal trafficking is defective in RUNX1 haplodeficiency. Blood. 2018;132:519.

48. Rao AK. Spotlight on FLI1, RUNX1, and platelet dysfunction. Blood. 2013;122(25):4004–6.

49. Gabbeta J, Yang X, Sun L, McLane M, Niewiarowski S, Rao AK. Abnormal inside-out signal transduction-dependent activation of GPIIb-IIIa in a patient with impaired pleckstrin phosphorylation. Blood. 1996;87:1368–76.

50. Rao AK, Poncz MP. Defective acid hydrolase secretion in RUNX1haplodeficiency: evidence for a global platelet secretory defect. Haemophilia. 2017;23:784–92.

51. Michaud J, Simpson KM, Escher R, Buchet-Poyau K, Beissbarth T, Carmichael C, et al. Integrative analysis of RUNX1 downstream pathways and target genes. BMC Genomics. 2008;9:363.

52. Sun L, Gorospe JR, Hoffman EP, Rao AK. Decreased platelet expression of myosin regulatory light chain polypeptide (MYL9) and other genes with platelet dysfunction and CBFA2/RUNX1 mutation: insights from platelet expression profiling. J Thromb Haemost. 2007;5(1):146–54.

53. Jalagadugula G, Mao G, Kaur G, Goldfinger LE, Dhanasekaran DN, Rao AK. Regulation of platelet myosin light chain (*MYL9*) by RUNX1: implications for thrombocytopenia and platelet dysfunction in *RUNX1* haplodeficiency. Blood. 2010;116(26):6037–45.

54. Jalagadugula G, Mao G, Kaur G, Dhanasekaran DN, Rao AK. Platelet PKC-θ deficiency with human RUNX1 mutation: *PRKCQ* is a transcriptional target of RUNX1. Arterioscler Thromb Vasc Biol. 2011;31(4):921–7.

55. Heller PG, Glembotsky AC, Gandhi MJ, Cummings CL, Pirola CJ, Marta RF, et al. Low Mpl receptor expression in a pedigree with familial platelet disorder with predisposition to acute myelogenous leukemia and a novel AML1 mutation. Blood. 2005;105(12):4664–70.

56. Mao G, Songdej N, Voora D, Goldfinger LE, Del Carpio-Cano FE, Myers RA, et al. Transcription factor RUNX1 regulates platelet PCTP (phosphatidylcholine transfer protein): implications for cardiovascular events. Circulation. 2017;136(10):927–39.

57. Edelstein LC, Simon LM, Montoya RT, Holinstat M, Chen ES, Bergeron A, et al. Racial differences in human platelet PAR4 reactivity reflect expression of PCTP and miR-376c. Nat Med. 2013;19(12):1609–16.

58. Glembotsky AC, Bluteau D, Espasandin YR, Goette NP, Marta RF, Marin Oyarzun CP, et al. Mechanisms underlying platelet function defect in a pedigree with familial platelet disorder with a predisposition to acute myelogenous leukemia: potential role for candidate RUNX1 targets. J Thromb Haemost. 2014;12(5):761–72.

59. Li Y, Jin C, Bai H, Gao Y, Sun S, Chen L, et al. Human NOTCH4 is a key target of RUNX1 in megakaryocytic differentiation. Blood. 2018;131(2):191–201.

60. Connelly JP, Kwon EM, Gao Y, Trivedi NS, Elkahloun AG, Horwitz MS, et al. Targeted correction of RUNX1 mutation in FPD patient-specific induced pluripotent stem cells rescues megakaryopoietic defects. Blood. 2014;124(12):1926–30.

61. Sakurai M, Kunimoto H, Watanabe N, Fukuchi Y, Yuasa S, Yamazaki S, et al. Impaired hematopoietic differentiation of RUNX1-mutated induced pluripotent stem cells derived from FPD/AML patients. Leukemia. 2014;28(12):2344–54.

62. Iizuka H, Kagoya Y, Kataoka K, Yoshimi A, Miyauchi M, Taoka K, et al. Targeted gene correction of RUNX1 in induced pluripotent stem cells derived from familial platelet disorder with propensity to myeloid malignancy restores normal megakaryopoiesis. Exp Hematol. 2015;43(10):849–57.

63. Westman JS, Stenfelt L, Vidovic K, Moller M, Hellberg A, Kjellstrom S, et al. Allele-selective RUNX1 binding regulates P1 blood group status by transcriptional control of A4GALT. Blood. 2018;131(14):1611–6.

64. Voora D, Rao AK, Jalagadugula GS, Myers R, Harris E, Ortel TL, et al. Systems pharmacogenomics finds RUNX1 is an aspirin-responsive transcription factor linked to cardiovascular disease and colon cancer. EBioMedicine. 2016;11:157–64.

65. Voora D, Cyr D, Lucas J, Chi JT, Dungan J, McCaffrey TA, et al. Aspirin exposure reveals novel genes associated with platelet function and cardiovascular events. J Am Coll Cardiol. 2013;62(14):1267–76.

66. Kang HW, Wei J, Cohen DE. PC-TP/StARD2: of membranes and metabolism. Trends Endocrinol Metab. 2010;21(7):449–56.

67. Bellissimo DC, Speck NA. RUNX1 mutations in inherited and sporadic leukemia. Front Cell Dev Biol. 2017;5:111.

68. Godley LA. Inherited predisposition to acute myeloid leukemia. Semin Hematol. 2014;51(4):306–21.

69. Genovese G, Kahler AK, Handsaker RE, Lindberg J, Rose SA, Bakhoum SF, et al. Clonal hematopoiesis and blood-cancer risk inferred from blood DNA sequence. N Engl J Med. 2014;371(26):2477–87.

70. Jaiswal S, Fontanillas P, Flannick J, Manning A, Grauman PV, Mar BG, et al. Age-related clonal hematopoiesis associated with adverse outcomes. N Engl J Med. 2014;371(26):2488–98.

71. Xie M, Lu C, Wang J, McLellan MD, Johnson KJ, Wendl MC, et al. Age-related mutations associated with clonal hematopoietic expansion and malignancies. Nat Med. 2014;20(12):1472–8.

72. Yoshimi A, Toya T, Kawazu M, Ueno T, Tsukamoto A, Iizuka H, et al. Recurrent CDC25C mutations drive malignant transformation in FPD/AML. Nat Commun. 2014;5:4770.

73. Sakurai M, Kasahara H, Yoshida K, Yoshimi A, Kunimoto H, Watanabe N, et al. Genetic basis of myeloid transformation in familial platelet disorder/acute myeloid leukemia patients with haploinsufficient RUNX1 allele. Blood Cancer J. 2016;6:e392.

74. Churpek JE, Pyrtel K, Kanchi KL, Shao J, Koboldt D, Miller CA, et al. Genomic analysis of germ line and somatic variants in familial myelodysplasia/acute myeloid leukemia. Blood. 2015;126(22):2484–90.

75. Antony-Debre I, Duployez N, Bucci M, Geffroy S, Micol JB, Renneville A, et al. Somatic mutations associated with leukemic progression of familial platelet disorder with predisposition to acute myeloid leukemia. Leukemia. 2016;30(4):999–1002.

76. The University of Chicago Hematopoietic Malignancies Cancer Risk Team, Drazer MW, Feurstein S, West AH, Jones MF, Churpek JE, et al. How I diagnose and manage individuals at risk for inherited myeloid malignancies. Blood. 2016;128(14):1800–13.

Update in the Investigation of von Willebrand Disease

Vishrut K. Srinivasan and Jasmina Ahluwalia

18.1 Introduction

Von Willebrand disease (VWD) is considered to be the commonest inherited bleeding disorder in the world. It is more commonly diagnosed in females, despite the autosomal inheritance pattern, due to increased reporting of bleeding as a result of female-specific haemostatic challenges. VWD has a prevalence of 0.6–1.3% based on population studies or approximately 1 case per 10,000 persons on the basis of referrals to specialized centres [1]. The prevalence is, however, dependent on the cut-off levels defining von Willebrand factor (VWF) used for the diagnosis (ranging from 30 to 50% at different centres), since current classifications do not specify cut-off values for VWF levels [2].

VWF is synthesized by endothelial cells and megakaryocytes as a multimeric glycoprotein with the multimers varying in size from 500 to 20,000 kDa. The *VWF* gene is located on chromosome 12 (12p13.2), having 52 exons and spanning about 178 kb. The product of *VWF* gene is composed of 2813 amino acids. This protein has three subunits: a pre-peptide (signal peptide) with 22 amino acids, a pro-peptide having 741 amino acids and a 2050 amino acid-containing mature VWF subunit [3]. VWF

protein is secreted into the plasma and the subendothelial space. The secreted VWF is proteolysed into an array of multimers by the enzyme ADAMTS-13 (a disintegrin and metalloproteinase with a thrombospondin type 1 motif, member 13). The main physiological function of VWF is to facilitate adhesion of platelet with subendothelium, interaction between platelets and platelet aggregation, promoting further clotting. VWF binds to glycoprotein-Ib (GPIb) and glycoprotein-IIb/IIIa (GPIIb-IIIa) receptors on platelets, allowing long VWF molecules to bind the platelets to sites of vascular injury and to each other during clot formation. High molecular weight (HMW) VWF multimers are the most effective at binding to the platelet Gp receptors as well as collagen molecules in the subendothelium. Both low and high molecular weight VWF multimers bind to factor VIII (FVIII) and stabilize it in the circulation. This prevents degradation of FVIII by activated protein C (APC) in plasma [4].

VWD results from a quantitative or qualitative defect in VWF leading to defective platelet adhesion and aggregation. VWD is subdivided into three main types, phenotypically—VWD type 1, 2 and 3. VWD type 1 is the most common, accounting for 70–80% of all cases. It is characterized by a partial quantitative defect of VWF and has an autosomal dominant inheritance pattern. Mechanisms causing VWD type 1 include reduced VWF synthesis caused by promoter polymorphisms, decreased VWF secretion with

V. K. Srinivasan · J. Ahluwalia (✉)
Department of Hematology, Postgraduate Institute of Medical Education and Research, Chandigarh, India

intracellular retention/degradation and increased clearance of VWF from plasma (VWD type 1C/VWD Vicenza type). VWD type 3 is the most severe form; however, it is rare accounting for less than 5% cases. It is an autosomal recessive disorder with nearly total absence of VWF in plasma and platelets. VWD type 2, accounting for 15–20% cases, is caused by altered functional activity of VWF normal or reduced VWF antigen levels. VWD type 2 is further divided into four subtypes: VWD type 2A, 2B, 2M and 2N.

VWD type 2A and 2B are characterized by the absence or loss of HMW VWF multimers in plasma; however, in VWD type 2B, VWF protein has an increased affinity for platelet receptor, GpIbα. VWD type 2M is associated with qualitatively abnormal VWF protein that has decreased platelet-dependent function and a normal multimer distribution pattern. There is decreased VWF-mediated platelet adhesion without loss of HMW VWF multimers in type 2M. VWD type 2B and 2M are autosomal dominant disorders, whereas VWD type 2A can have either autosomal dominant or recessive inheritance. In VWD type 2N, a defect in the N-terminal region of the VWF where the FVIII binding domain is present, leads to decreased VWF and FVIII binding. VWD type 2N is an autosomal recessive disorder [5].

In rare cases, VWD is acquired, rather than inherited, termed as acquired von Willebrand syndrome (AVWS) and is generally associated with an underlying disorder. AVWS is associated with a qualitative, structural or functional defect caused by immune and non-immune mechanisms resulting in rapid degradation or clearance of VWF [6].

The clinical manifestations of VWD vary among patients, and the severity is dependent on the residual VWF functional activity and, to some extent, on the secondary deficiency of FVIII, the age and sex. The clinical expression of VWD type 1 is usually mild, with VWD type 2 and 3 being characterized by increasing disease severity. In the paediatric population, the most common symptoms include epistaxis and bruising. In adults, the most common symptoms are menorrhagia, bleeding from minor wounds, and hema-

tomas. Bleeding after surgery or dental extractions is reported in up to 80% patients [1]. Gastrointestinal bleeding can also occur and is more common in patients with absent high molecular weight VWF molecules in plasma [7].

18.2 Diagnosis of VWD

18.2.1 Clinical Assessment and Bleeding Scores

Prior to proceeding with the laboratory tests, an appropriate personal bleeding history and/or family history should be considered for a diagnosis of VWD. The risk of over-treating patients with doubtful or mild bleeding can be avoided by eliciting a definitive bleeding history [8]. Bleeding questionnaires or Bleeding Assessment Tools (BATs) are being increasingly used to reduce both intra- and inter-observer variability. A bleeding score taking into account both the frequency and the severity of the bleeding symptoms is useful to define what constitutes a significant bleeding history. The standardization of these tools and bleeding scores for the diagnosis of VWD has seen significant development in the past decade.

The notable scoring system studied for assessment of bleeding in VWD are Vicenza bleeding questionnaire, "European Molecular and Clinical Markers for the Diagnosis and Management of Type 1 von Willebrand disease" (MCMDM-1VWD) Bleeding Questionnaire, Condensed MCMDM-1VWD Bleeding Questionnaire, ISTH Bleeding Assessment Tool (ISTH-BAT) and Self-BAT [9]. In the setting of VWD, the ISTH-BAT is a popular tool due to its development and endorsement by ISTH. A score of ≥4 for males and ≥6 for females (≥3 for children) is considered abnormal in ISTH-BAT and Self-BAT scoring systems. In Vicenza Bleeding Questionnaire, a score of ≥3 for males and ≥5 for females is abnormal, while the Condensed MCMDM-1VWD Bleeding Questionnaire classifies a score of ≥4 (for both sexes) as abnormal.

The application of these questionnaires helps in prioritizing laboratory testing. In individuals already diagnosed with VWD, bleeding scores can also help assess the disease severity. However, the diagnostic use of these tools is especially problematic in the case of young children, who have not yet undergone surgery or dental intervention. An additional limitation of the bleeding assessment tools is that they use cumulative scoring, which means that once a patient has had a severe bleeding episode, the bleeding score will remain high even if bleeding does not recur [1].

18.2.2 Laboratory Diagnosis of VWD

Currently, there is no single test that can provide information regarding platelet-endothelial-FVIII interaction with an acceptable degree of sensitivity and specificity. The large size of the VWF gene makes confirmation by molecular genetic testing, a challenge for most small and mid-level laboratories. Hence, a number of assays are required and have been devised to establish the diagnosis of VWD with reasonable degree of confidence.

Due to phenotypic heterogeneity, the diagnosis of VWD, especially of type 1, may be difficult. The diagnosis is also influenced by the modifying effect of different environmental and physiological variables and difficulties in standardizing diagnostic tests. The basic panel consisting of Prothrombin Time (PT), Activated Partial Thromboplastin Time (APTT), Thrombin Time (TT), Platelet Count and fibrinogen assay is recommended when screening for any bleeding disorder. However, these tests may yield normal results in a large majority of patients with VWD type 1. Some authorities recommend upfront screening with VWF antigen, ristocetin cofactor activity assay, and FVIII levels. Other common haemostatic defects in an undiagnosed case with bleeding should be excluded before proceeding with testing for VWD [10].

In patients with most VWD subtypes, the platelet count is normal. However, a mild to moderate degree of thrombocytopenia can be found in VWD type 2B. PT is normal, whereas APTT may be prolonged, depending on the FVIII levels in plasma. A defect in primary haemostasis can be identified by an increased closure time on PFA-100. This test has utility in screening for the more severe types of bleeding as in Bernard–Soulier syndrome, severe VWD and Glanzmann thrombasthenia [11]. However, the sensitivity of PFA-100 is low and may fail in identifying the various forms of VWD.

The basic diagnostic tests ("first level" tests) for VWD include measurements of VWF antigen (VWF:Ag) levels; measurement of VWF activity (VWF-dependent platelet adhesion), historically measured with the use of VWF-ristocetin cofactor activity (VWF:RCo) assay; and coagulant activity of factor VIII (FVIII:C). Additional subtyping assays are required when these "first level" tests are indicative of VWD type 2.

18.2.3 VWF Antigen Levels

The VWF:Ag levels in plasma are currently measured by enzyme-linked immunosorbent assay (ELISA) or automated latex immunoassay (LIA). Other methods including flow cytometry have also been described for the measurement of VWF:Ag, but are not routinely used. LIA has the advantage of being an automated assay providing reproducible quick results within hours. The current LIA assays are less reliable when measuring VWF levels at the lower end (less than 10 IU/dL) or towards the higher ends of more than 125 IU/dL [12]. Therefore, these assays may not be able to differentiate between severe form of VWD type 1 and 3. The lower limit of detection (LLOD) is usually 5 IU/dL with many VWF:Ag ELISA kits. However, the VWF:Ag ELISA yields less reproducible results compared to the LIA. Additionally, slow turn-around time and the need for batch testing are limitations of ELISA-based assay. Chemiluminescence assays (CLIA) may be able to provide a lower limit of detection and improve the discrimination between VWD type 1 and 3. This technology is currently available on some automated platforms.

ABO blood group type plays an important role in influencing plasma VWF levels. VWF antigen levels in individuals with blood group O are 25–35% lower than individuals with other blood groups [13]. VWF antigen levels are also influenced by various physiological and pathological factors. VWF:Ag levels increase with age, during pregnancy and in inflammation. Exercise and stress increase VWF:Ag levels and may lead to a false-negative test result (masking VWD diagnosis). A diagnosis of mild VWD cannot be excluded by a single normal value of VWF:Ag, especially if the patient was stressed when the test sample was collected. Repeat testing is recommended in order to avoid missing a VWD diagnosis. There are difficulties and differences in defining what cut-off values would be conclusive in defining VWD. Generally, VWF:Ag levels less than 30 IU/dL are considered diagnostic. VWF:Ag levels can yield a conclusive diagnosis only in cases of VWD type 3. However, values below the reference range may not always be indicative of VWD. VWF:Ag levels of 30–50 IU/dL are usually termed as "low VWF" and should be interpreted taking into account the bleeding phenotype [2].

Using two standard deviations as the cut-off for normal range for any given laboratory, it can be expected that VWF:Ag levels will be low in around 2.5% of normal individuals using any local reference range for that particular laboratory. By current standards, they may be classified as having "low VWF" without bleeding. Therefore, care needs to be taken to avoid over-diagnosis of VWD which can lead to unnecessary costly medications and unjustified labelling of patients. It is likely that the "low VWF" or borderline low VWF levels have a role as a risk factor for bleeding rather than being a case of VWD [14].

18.2.4 VWF-Platelet Binding Activity

Different assays can be used to determine the VWF-platelet binding activity. VWF-ristocetin cofactor activity (VWF:RCo) assay has remained the gold standard for measuring VWF activity for many years. Ristocetin is an antibiotic that is added to patient's platelet-poor plasma to agglutinate formalin-fixed platelets derived from an external source. Ristocetin produces a conformational change in VWF that allows VWF to bind to GPIb receptor on platelets. This assay serves a surrogate for VWF-platelet binding activity, and low values in VWF:RCo assay indicate a defect in VWF-platelet binding. Despite being a non-physiological assay, VWF:RCo has a good correlation with the VWF activity and distribution of VWF multimers.

However, the major drawback of the classical VWF:RCo assay is the low sensitivity and precision. This is more evident when the assay protocols are based on the assessment of agglutination by visual method or platelet aggregometry. The inter-laboratory coefficient of variation (CV) is usually high (30–40%), especially with samples having low VWF content. The limit of detection (LOD) may be 10–20 U/dL. Identification and discrimination between types of VWD with low activities using VWF:RCo assay can be challenging. This necessitates repeated measurements for correct diagnosis, when using VWF:RCo due to a high CV of this assay [15, 16]. The A1 domain in VWF has the binding site for ristocetin, and certain mutations in A1 domain can affect ristocetin-mediated VWF activation, and therefore, the results of the VWF:RCo assay, which may lead to a false-positive VWD diagnosis.

In recent years, several new versions/modifications of the classical VWF:RCo assay have been developed in order to overcome the above limitations. Ristocetin-mediated GPIb binding (VWF:GPIbR) assay has an improved CV and LOD [17]. In the VWF:GPIbR assay, a recombinant GPIb fragment replaces the formalin-fixed platelets. This fragment is usually bound to latex, magnetic particles or a monoclonal antibody. The variations in the ristocetin binding site also affect this assay. Additionally, substitution of reagents is not possible due to variation of GPIb sources and monoclonal antibodies in the different assays.

The drawback caused by the use of ristocetin can be circumvented by utilizing recombinant GPIb fragments possessing gain-of-function mutations (VWF:GPIbM assay). The mutant GPIb fragments are able to bind to VWF spontaneously without the need for ristocetin. By using these mutant GPIb peptides, ELISA-based assays and particle-based automated assays (Innovance™ VWF:Ac assay) have been developed [18]. In another assay, the exogenous platelets are swapped for a monoclonal antibody against an epitope in the A1 domain (GPIb binding site) of VWF (indicated as VWF:Ab, "monoclonal antibody capture"). The results of VWF:Ab assay correlated well with the VWF:RCo assay [19]. VWF:RCo assays based on flow cytometry and latex particle-enhanced immunoturbidimetry have also been described.

18.2.5 VWF Activity/Antigen Ratio

Quantitative and qualitative defects among VWD types can be distinguished by the ratio between VWF activity (platelet binding) and VWF:Ag. A proportionate reduction in VWF:Ag and VWF:RCo fits the diagnosis of VWD type 1. Qualitative VWF defects (with the exception of VWD type 2N) are associated with decreased VWF-platelet binding resulting in a disproportionate decrease in VWF:RCo as compared with VWF:Ag (ratio of VWF:RCo/VWF:Ag ≤ 0.6). Usually, a value below 0.6 indicates a diagnosis of VWD type 2A, 2B or 2M. In VWD type 2N, this ratio is normal as there is no defect in platelet binding [20, 21]. When the values of either VWF:RCo or VWF:Ag are very low, the ratio loses its reliability in distinguishing between qualitative and quantitative defects.

18.2.6 Factor VIII Activity (FVIII:C)

FVIII levels are measured typically by a one-stage clotting assay that evaluates the FVIII coagulant activity (FVIII:C). Decreased FVIII:C in VWD can be due to defective VWF-FVIII binding or decreased VWF levels. In VWD type 3, FVIII:C is markedly reduced due to the absence of VWF as FVIII is not protected by VWF from clearance in the circulation. VWD type 3 patients with very low FVIII:C values (less than 5 IU/dL) may also experience joint and muscle hematomas similar to those in haemophilia patients. Other than VWD type 2N, a FVIII/VWF:Ag ratio ≥ 1.0 may be encountered in type 1 and 2, since factor VIII levels may be variable [22]. In VWD type 2N, the

only detectable defect may be decreased FVIII:C levels with FVIII/VWF:Ag ratio < 0.7. Therefore, the diagnosis of VWD type 2N may be missed when laboratories rely only on VWF:Ag and VWF:RCo levels as VWD diagnostic tests [23].

18.2.7 Tests for Subclassifying VWD

When the results of all "first-level" tests are normal, VWD is ruled out; however, the tests should be repeated if values are at the low end of the normal range or if VWD is strongly suspected clinically. If the above-mentioned "first-level" tests reveal definitive abnormalities, a diagnosis of VWD can be made; however, the confirmatory diagnosis of specific VWD types often requires additional tests. The assays mentioned below ("second level" tests) are helpful for subtyping VWD and when initial testing leads to equivocal results and for the correct categorization of the VWD.

18.2.8 VWF Collagen Binding

After vascular injury, the A3 domain of ultra-large VWF (ULVWF) multimers bind collagen types I and III and the A1 domain bind to collagen types IV and VI. This VWF-collagen interaction is not assessed by most of the VWD screening tests. In VWD type 1 and 3, reduced collagen binding may result from a reduction in VWF levels. Whereas in VWD type 2 variants, decreased collagen binding is due to lack of HMW VWF multimers (in types 2A and 2B) or specific defects in collagen binding itself (in type 2M). The VWF collagen binding assay (VWF:CB) measures the ability of VWF to bind collagen. This assay is increasingly used in some parts of the world to identify mutations in the A3 domain of VWF.

The VWF:CB assay is generally performed by ELISA method utilizing various collagen types. The ELISA-based assays use collagen type I and/or III, with varying assay sensitivity. A recently developed automated VWF:CB chemiluminescence-based assay (AcuStar VWF:CB) has shown good assay reproducibility, sensitivity for low VWF levels, and is able to more consistently distinguish VWD type 1 vs. 2 [24, 25]. VWF:CB assay is especially sensitive to VWD subtypes in which the larger VWF multimers are missing. Therefore, VWF:CB assay can serve as a surrogate for VWF multimer analysis with VWF:CB/Ag ratio of 0.6–0.7, differentiating type 2A from type 2M.

The different sources of collagen and reference plasmas used lead to issues in optimizing and standardization of VWF:CB assay [26]. Also, assays using only collagen type I and III will miss patients with binding defects to collagen type IV and VI. Abnormal collagen VI and IV binding has been seen in control subjects who have not bled. So, with the current evidence, abnormal binding to collagen may add to the risk for bleeding rather than actually adding to the diagnosis for VWD [27, 28].

Currently, the VWF collagen binding (VWF:CB) assay is not generally included among the "first level" tests for VWD and is yet to be approved for diagnostic purposes in certain countries. However, there is a case for including VWF:CB in standard diagnostic VWD testing. Patients with exclusive collagen defects can be missed with the omission of VWF:CB assay. Cases of VWD type 2M are more likely to be diagnosed by using both VWF:RCo and VWF:CB assays for testing VWF activity. Laboratories using only one of the two assays are more likely to miss these cases. Additional information regarding VWF activity can be obtained by including VWF:CB in the commonly used testing panel consisting of VWF:Ag, VWF:RCo and FVIII:C assays. VWF:CB assay also serves to provide a "check" to VWF:RCo assay in diagnosis of VWD type 2 [29]. VWF:CB assay may also be used as a surrogate for VWF multimer analysis, which is technically challenging. This can be helpful in the diagnosis of patients with decreased HMW VWF multimers [30].

18.2.9 Analysis of VWF Multimers

A specific lack of HMW VWF multimers (in types 2A, 2B) or an intrinsic defect in VWF binding

affinity to GPIb receptor (in type 2M) can lead to defective VWF-mediated platelet adhesion. Definitive differentiation between these VWD type 2 variants requires VWF multimer analysis [31].

VWF multimer analysis involves agarose gel electrophoresis of plasma. This is followed by either transfer of the electrophoretic product to a membrane or fixation of the gel. The VWF protein is then measured by immunodetection and quantification in the gel or membrane. Low-resolution gels with agarose concentrations of less than 1.0% are very porous, and VWF multimers of all sizes can be run in the gel. These gels can establish the presence and the irregularity of the largest multimers. VWD type 2 is characterized by the absence of larger VWF multimers when compared with VWD type 1 and 3. More subtle changes of the inner electrophoretic structure of smaller multimers in low resolution can be used to differentiate between VWD type 2 variants. High-resolution gels, having agarose concentration more than 2.0%, are less porous and resolve the inner VWF multimeric structure. This enables visualization of non-reduced VWF. Each smaller multimer is usually made up of at least three bands (triplet structure) [32, 33].

VWF multimer analysis is technically complex and labour intensive. Currently, it is restricted to highly specialized laboratories that have the prerequisite expertise and resources to perform the test. However, the multimeric analysis has a high error rate, plagued by varying interpretations of multimer profiles and false VWD subtype classification. Subtle variations in multimer distribution associated with VWD subtypes can be missed [15]. The multimer analysis can also be hampered by artefacts produced due to improper specimen handling, which may lead to a wrong diagnosis of VWD type 2 [34].

18.2.10 Ristocetin-Induced Platelet Aggregation (RIPA)

The mutant VWF molecules in VWD type 2B patients are able to spontaneously bind to platelet GPIb as a result of conformational change in the GPIb binding site on the VWF protein. Lesser ristocetin concentrations in vitro, are sufficient to induce VWF-GPIb binding in such cases. RIPA assay using low concentrations of ristocetin (typically ≤0.6 mg/mL) can be used to separate cases of VWD type 2B from VWD types 2A and 2M [20]. On the other hand, patients with a mutant platelet GPIb receptor that has high affinity for VWF will also demonstrate similar abnormalities in this assay. Cases with such gain of function GPIb receptor mutations are categorized as platelet-type VWD (PT-VWD) [35]. RIPA assay is cumbersome to perform, and the resources to conduct this assay are not available in all laboratories. Additionally, the assay generally requires relatively larger quantities of blood for the preparation of platelet-rich plasma (PRP) from patients and controls which is most often not feasible in paediatric population. The drawbacks of RIPA by light transmission aggregometry (LTA) can be circumvented by using flow cytometry-based aggregometry. This enables detection of platelet aggregates in small blood volumes and lower platelet numbers. Also, flow cytometry is available in many haematology laboratories and allows for diagnosis of platelet-type VWD in laboratories not specifically involved in platelet function studies [36].

As VWD type 2B and PT-VWD require differential clinical management but yield very similar results with standard VWF tests including RIPA, further testing is required for their differentiation. Crossover mixing studies using plasma and platelets in the low-dose RIPA assay (mixing studies) can be used to determine if the enhanced response is plasma-based (in VWD type 2B) or platelet-based (in PT-VWD). It is difficult to distinguish between these two entities only on the basis of this test. Therefore, mutation testing of exon 28 of *VWF* and platelet glycoprotein-Ib (*GPIB*) genes is suggested for confirmatory diagnosis [37].

18.2.11 VWF-FVIII Binding Assay (VWF:FVIIIB)

An ELISA-based assay is employed to capture VWF on antibody-coated plate with subsequent removal of endogenous FVIII and addition of recombinant FVIII to detect VWF binding capacity to FVIII [38]. In VWD type 2N, a mutation in the FVIII binding site of VWF results in reduced FVIII coagulant activity. VWD type 2N is characterized with defects in the capacity of VWF to bind to FVIII, resulting in reduced VWF:FVIIIB. This assay helps in distinguishing mild haemophilia from VWD type 2N as the former has normal VWF:FVIIIB. The VWD type 2N patients with heterozygous mutations have a VWF:FVIIIB/VWF:Ag ratio of around 0.5. The more severe 2N VWD cases having homozygous or complex variant mutations show VWF:FVIIIB/VWF:Ag ratio of less than 0.3. In VWD type 3, VWF-FVIII binding cannot be measured due to very low levels of VWF. In the other VWD subtypes, the VWF:FVIII binding is within the normal range [39].

An algorithmic approach may be employed using these parameters for a diagnosis and subcategorisation. One such approach is depicted in Fig. 18.1

18.2.12 VWF Propeptide and VWFpp/VWF:Ag Ratio

VWF propeptide (VWFpp) and VWF proteins are non-covalently linked and stored in the Weibel–Palade bodies (WBP) of endothelial cells or α-granules of megakaryocytes/platelets. These are released in a regulated manner and in plasma, and after propeptide is cleaved, it circulates independently of the mature VWF. VWF propeptide circulates as a homodimer in plasma, with a half-life of 2–3 h. Mature VWF multimers in circulation have a half-life of 8–12 h [40].

VWFpp in a sample can be measured by performing an ELISA-based assay. Reduced levels of VWFpp indicate decreased VWF synthesis or defective secretion of VWF from the endothelial cells. This can be found in VWD type 1 patients with a null mutation or endoplasmic reticulum VWF retention. The propeptide assay can also distinguish between severe VWD type 1 with extremely low mature VWF (VWF:Ag) levels and VWD type 3 with a complete absence of both the propeptide and VWF:Ag [41].

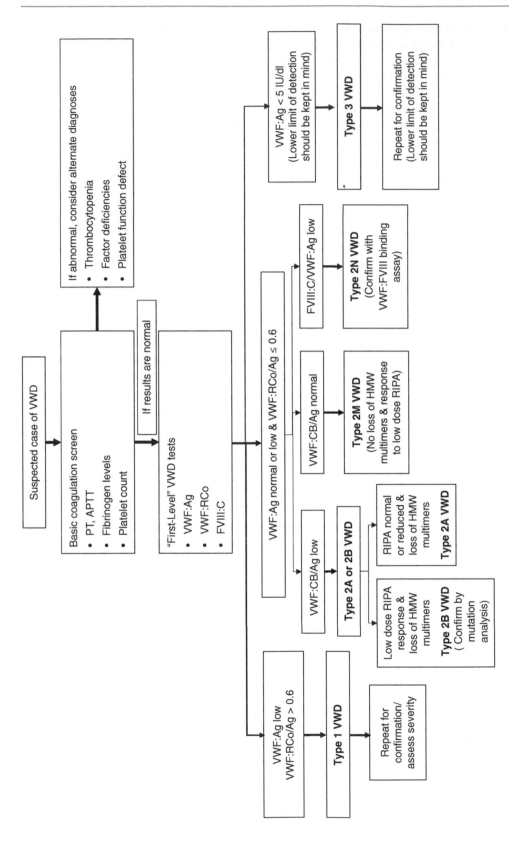

Fig. 18.1 Diagnostic algorithm for VWD classification

The clearance rate of mature VWF can be assessed by VWFpp/VWF:Ag ratio, assuming a constant clearance rate for VWFpp. Patients with VWD type 1 having reduced VWF survival (Vicenza or VWD type 1C) can be identified by this ratio. These patients have an increased VWF clearance and as a result, have an increased ratio of VWFpp/VWF:Ag [42]. Diagnosis of a clearance defect has treatment implications. The treatment of choice in VWD type 1 patients is desmopressin, but this drug may not be effective in patients having a major defect in VWF clearance. The increased VWF clearance from circulation also presents problem for long-term management (e.g. bleeding during surgical procedures). Therefore, VWF-containing products are recommended for such situations [43].

18.2.13   Platelet VWF Levels

Recent studies have shown significant differences between plasma and platelet VWF. Platelets are richer in ultra-large VWF multimers which are more haemostatically active, and more resistant to proteolysis by ADAMTS13 than plasma VWF. Plasma VWF levels are influenced by ABO blood group type; however, this has no determined effect on platelet VWF levels. The phenotypic heterogeneity of VWD also affects the platelet VWF levels and, hence, can be used as an additional tool in characterizing different types of VWD by revealing when VWD synthesis is defective.

Platelet VWF:Ag can be measured by ELISA-based assay utilizing washed platelets obtained from platelet-rich plasma (PRP). Laboratory-specific standard curves can be obtained by performing the assay with samples from a minimum of 20 normal subjects. The normal range for platelet VWF is usually 70–140 U/dL. Platelet VWF content can be useful in distinguishing between qualitative and quantitative defects, especially in VWD type 1 patients, in whom plasma VWF levels are not informative. Platelet VWF levels are also helpful in grading severity of defective VWF synthesis, identifying VWD type 1C (with Vicenza mutation) and VWD type

2N cases with quantitative mutations. It also predicts patient response to desmopressin, and the bleeding risk of VWD patients, especially for those with a quantitative defect [44].

18.2.14   VWD Testing in Resource Constrained Settings

A basic coagulation laboratory should include the following tests for testing patients suspected to have VWD based on clinical features: platelet count, BT, PT, APTT, correction studies, qualitative test for FXIII, along with FVIII levels and ristocetin-induced platelet aggregation (RIPA, manual). With this approach, most cases of severe VWD can be diagnosed and other bleeding defects can be screened. The milder cases can be missed and not subclassified. A more comprehensive testing can be taken up by laboratories in tertiary or specialized centres. The testing panel can be expanded to include VWF:Ag assays, VWF activity assays (VWF:RCo, VWF:CBA and immunoassays). Genetic testing can be performed at referral laboratories (1–2 per country) along with FVIII binding assay and multimer analysis for confirmation of VWD diagnosis [45].

18.2.15   Mutation Analysis

In a majority of VWD cases, mutation testing is not required, as the above-mentioned battery of tests can be used for a proper diagnosis and classification. Mutation analysis should only be performed when the first- and second-level assays are not clearly diagnostic and when required for patient counselling and management. The *VWF* gene located on chromosome 12 shares considerable homology with the *VWF* pseudogene. The latter is located on chromosome 22, and parts of *VWF* gene (particularly, exons 23–34) have 97% similarity with the *VWF* pseudogene. This should be kept in mind while planning for *VWF* gene sequencing.

Approximately 65% cases of VWD type 1 have candidate VWF mutations with 70% being missense mutation involving VWF trafficking, storage and secretion. VWF mutations are found in 85–90% cases with deletions, nonsense, splice site and missense mutations. VWD type 2A cases have missense mutations involving A2, CTCK domains and D1/D2/D'D3 assemblies. VWD type 2B and 2M result from missense mutation in A1 domains and A1 or A3 domains, respectively. VWD type 2N has missense mutation affecting D'D3 assembly [40].

Mutation analysis for confirmation of VWD can be done by direct Sanger sequencing of genomic DNA or mRNA, multiplex ligation-dependent probe amplification (MLPA) and next-generation sequencing (NGS). In VWD type 2 variants, the majority of mutations are clustered to exon 28. Hence, direct sequencing of target exons is better suited for such cases. In contrast, for VWD type 1 and 3, the mutations are random and scattered in location. In such cases, sequencing should include the whole VWF coding region, intronic flanking regions, the 5' and 3' untranslated regions (UTRs) and the proximal promoter of *VWF* gene [46].

Large gene deletions and duplications can be found in rare cases. Heterozygous deletions are not detected by PCR-based sequencing techniques. However, the MLPA technique can identify both heterozygous and homozygous gene deletions and/or duplications [46]. NGS techniques are faster and are becoming increasingly cheaper, enabling better and wider analysis of VWF mutations at a reasonable cost. NGS especially allows for study of the entire VWF coding region in a relatively short period of time, and hence NGS-based approach is particularly indicated for investigating mutations in VWD type 1 and 3 variants.

The large size of *VWF* gene and increased occurrence of non-pathological genetic variations hinder the genetic diagnosis of VWD. A detectable mutation in the VWF coding sequence may not be detected in all patients, especially those with VWD type 1. Conventional PCR-based sequencing may not be able to detect large gene deletions, resulting in low VWF levels. However, new developments, such as next-generation sequencing, can enable better characterization of the mutational landscape of VWD.

18.2.16 Acquired von Willebrand Syndrome (AVWS)

AVWS is characterized by a non-inherited structural or functional VWF defect associated with an increased risk of bleeding. It is usually associated with an underlying disorder. AVWS is associated with lymphoproliferative disorders (48%), cardiovascular (21%), myeloproliferative (15%), other neoplastic (5%) and autoimmune disorders (2%) [47]. Three main mechanisms are implicated in the AVWS pathogenesis. These include increased shear stress-induced loss, adsorption of VWF onto cellular surfaces and specific or non-specific VWF autoantibodies that form circulating VWF immune complexes leading to its increased clearance. A diagnosis of AVWS should be considered mainly in patients with bleeding having laboratory findings suggestive of VWF abnormalities and in patients known to have an underlying disorder associated with AVWS, expected to undergo procedures with high risk of bleeding [6].

The testing panel for diagnosis of AVWS is the same as that for inherited VWD. AVWS is associated with a reduced VWF:RCo/VWF:Ag or VWF:CB/VWF:Ag ratio (less than 0.6), even if the absolute levels of individual parameters are within normal limits. Multimer analysis shows loss or decrease in HMW multimers with disturbed triplet structure, even when activity/antigen ratios are normal. An increased VWF propeptide/VWF:Ag ratio can also be found in AVWS reflecting accelerated clearance of VWF from plasma [47]. In-house ELISA-based assays have been used to detect inhibitory (neutralizing) and non-neutralizing VWF-binding autoantibodies [48]. However, no standardized assays are available to detect these autoantibodies.

18.3 Conclusion

Even though von Willebrand disease is the commonest inherited bleeding disorder, not many laboratories are equipped to diagnose this condition. The phenotypic heterogeneity and influence of VWF levels by several physiological and pathological variables also add to the diagnostic difficulty. The recent decade has provided new pathophysiological insights into VWD. Newer diagnostic modalities and algorithms have been put forth to improve detection and help with better subtyping of VWD. Diagnosis will be further improved by the introduction of more reproducible and rapid assays of VWF function. The use of NGS will facilitate better and faster identification of mutations in VWF. For now, basic coagulation laboratories should at the least have expertise in performing and interpreting the "first level" VWD screening tests. This will enable better detection of VWD cases and provide a clear picture regarding the prevalence. Reference laboratories should be equipped to perform most of the "second level" tests for confirmatory diagnosis. Prospective studies are needed to address the issue of patients with "low VWF" levels and to assess the benefit of haemostatic treatment in them.

References

1. Leebeek FW, Eikenboom JC. von Willebrand's disease. N Engl J Med. 2016;375:2067–80.
2. Sadler JE, Budde U, Eikenboom JC, et al. Update on the pathophysiology and classification of von Willebrand disease: a report of the subcommittee on von Willebrand factor. J Thromb Haemost. 2006;4:2103–14.
3. Mancuso DJ, Tuley EA, Westfield LA, et al. Human von Willebrand factor gene and pseudogene: structural analysis and differentiation by polymerase chain reaction. Biochemistry. 1991;30:253–69.
4. Adcock DM, Bethel M, Valcour A. Diagnosing von Willebrand disease: a large reference laboratory's perspective. Semin Thromb Hemost. 2006;32:472–9.
5. Federici AB. Current and emerging approaches for assessing von Willebrand disease in 2016. Int J Lab Hematol. 2016;38(Suppl 1):41–9.
6. Federici AB, Budde U, Castaman G, et al. Current diagnostic and therapeutic approaches to patients with acquired von Willebrand syndrome: a 2013 update. Semin Thromb Hemost. 2013;39:191–201.
7. Castaman G, Federici AB, Tosetto A, et al. Different bleeding risk in type 2A and 2M von Willebrand disease: a 2-year prospective study in 107 patients. J Thromb Haemost. 2012;10:632–8.
8. Castaman G, Goodeve A, Eikenboom J, et al. Principles of care for the diagnosis and treatment of von Willebrand disease. Haematologica. 2013;98:667–74.
9. Bowman ML, James PD. Bleeding scores for the diagnosis of von Willebrand disease. Semin Thromb Hemost. 2017;43:530–9.
10. Castaman G, Linari S. Diagnosis and treatment of von Willebrand disease and rare bleeding disorders. J Clin Med. 2017;6. pii: E45.
11. Hayward CP, Harrison P, Cattaneo M, et al. Platelet function analyzer (PFA)-100 closure time in the evaluation of platelet disorders and platelet function. J Thromb Haemost. 2006;4:312–9.
12. Castaman G, Tosetto A, Cappelletti A, et al. Validation of a rapid test (VWF-LIA) for the quantitative determination of von Willebrand factor antigen in type 1 von Willebrand disease diagnosis within the European multicenter study MCMDM-1VWD. Thromb Res. 2010;126:227–31.
13. Gallinaro L, Cattini MG, Sztukowska M, et al. A shorter von Willebrand factor survival in O blood group subjects explains how ABO determinants influence plasma von Willebrand factor. Blood. 2008;111:3540–5.
14. Sadler JE. Von Willebrand disease type 1: a diagnosis in search of a disease. Blood. 2003;101:2089–93.
15. Meijer P, Haverkate F. An external quality assessment program for von Willebrand factor laboratory analysis: an overview from the European concerted action on thrombosis and disabilities foundation. Semin Thromb Hemost. 2006;32:485–91.
16. Kitchen S, Jennings I, Woods TA, et al. Laboratory tests for measurement of von Willebrand factor show poor agreement among different centers: results from the United Kingdom National External Quality Assessment Scheme for blood coagulation. Semin Thromb Hemost. 2006;32:492–8.
17. Bodo I, Eikenboom J, Montgomery R, et al. Platelet-dependent von Willebrand factor activity. Nomenclature and methodology: communication from the SSC of the ISTH. J Thromb Haemost. 2015;13:1345–50.
18. Flood VH, Gill JC, Morateck PA, et al. Gain-of-function GPIb ELISA assay for VWF activity in the Zimmerman program for the molecular and clinical biology of VWD. Blood. 2011;117:e67–74.
19. Favaloro EJ, Henniker A, Facey D, et al. Discrimination of von Willebrand's disease (VWD) subtypes: direct comparison of von Willebrand factor:collagen binding assay (VWF:CBA) with monoclonal antibody (MAB) based VWF-capture systems. Thromb Haemost. 2000;84:541–7.
20. Nichols WL, Hultin MB, James AH, et al. von Willebrand disease (VWD): evidence-based diagnosis and management guidelines, the National Heart, Lung, and Blood Institute (NHLBI) expert panel report (USA). Haemophilia. 2008;14:171–232.
21. Geisen U, Zieger B, Nakamura L, et al. Comparison of Von Willebrand factor (VWF) activity VWF:Ac with VWF ristocetin cofactor activity VWF:RCo. Thromb Res. 2014;134:246–50.

22. Federici AB. Diagnosis of inherited von Willebrand disease: a clinical perspective. Semin Thromb Hemost. 2006;32:555–65.

23. Mazurier C, Meyer D. Factor VIII binding assay of von Willebrand factor and the diagnosis of type 2N von Willebrand disease—results of an international survey. On behalf of the subcommittee on von Willebrand factor of the scientific and standardization committee of the ISTH. Thromb Haemost. 1996;76:270–4.

24. Favaloro EJ, Mohammed S. Evaluation of a von Willebrand factor three test panel and chemiluminescent-based assay system for identification of, and therapy monitoring in, von Willebrand disease. Thromb Res. 2016;141:202–11.

25. Jousselme E, Jourdy Y, Rugeri L, et al. Comparison of an automated chemiluminescent assay to a manual ELISA assay for determination of von Willebrand factor collagen binding activity on VWD plasma patients previously diagnosed through molecular analysis of VWF. Int J Lab Hematol. 2018;40:77–83.

26. Favaloro EJ. Evaluation of commercial von Willebrand factor collagen binding assays to assist the discrimination of types 1 and 2 von Willebrand disease. Thromb Haemost. 2010;104:1009–21.

27. Flood VH, Schlauderaff AC, Haberichter SL, et al. Crucial role for the VWF A1 domain in binding to type IV collagen. Blood. 2015;125:2297–304.

28. Flood VH, Gill JC, Christopherson PA, et al. Critical von Willebrand factor A1 domain residues influence type VI collagen binding. J Thromb Haemost. 2012;10:1417–24.

29. Favaloro EJ. Utility of the von Willebrand factor collagen binding assay in the diagnosis of von Willebrand disease. Am J Hematol. 2017;92:114–8.

30. Flood VH, Gill JC, Friedman KD, et al. Collagen binding provides a sensitive screen for variant von Willebrand disease. Clin Chem. 2013;59:684–91.

31. Budde U, Pieconka A, Will K, et al. Laboratory testing for von Willebrand disease: contribution of multimer analysis to diagnosis and classification. Semin Thromb Hemost. 2006;32:514–21.

32. Ott HW, Griesmacher A, Schnapka-Koepf M, et al. Analysis of von Willebrand factor multimers by simultaneous high- and low-resolution vertical SDS-agarose gel electrophoresis and Cy5-labeled antibody high-sensitivity fluorescence detection. Am J Clin Pathol. 2010;133:322–30.

33. Budde U, Schneppenheim R, Eikenboom J, et al. Detailed von Willebrand factor multimer analysis in patients with von Willebrand disease in the European study, molecular and clinical markers for the diagnosis and management of type 1 von Willebrand disease (MCMDM-1VWD). J Thromb Haemost. 2008;6:762–71.

34. Favaloro EJ, Facey D, Grispo L. Laboratory assessment of von Willebrand factor. Use of different assays can influence the diagnosis of von Willebrand's disease, dependent on differing sensitivity to sample preparation and differential recognition of high molecular weight VWF forms. Am J Clin Pathol. 1995;104:264–71.

35. Frontroth JP, Hepner M, Sciuccati G, et al. Prospective study of low-dose ristocetin-induced platelet aggregation to identify type 2B von Willebrand disease (VWD) and platelet-type VWD in children. Thromb Haemost. 2010;104:1158–65.

36. De Cuyper IM, Meinders M, van de Vijver E, et al. A novel flow cytometry-based platelet aggregation assay. Blood. 2013;121:e70–80.

37. Favaloro EJ. Phenotypic identification of platelet-type von Willebrand disease and its discrimination from type 2B von Willebrand disease: a question of 2B or not 2B? A story of nonidentical twins? Or two sides of a multidenominational or multifaceted primary-hemostasis coin? Semin Thromb Hemost. 2008;34:113–27.

38. Veyradier A, Caron C, Ternisien C, et al. Validation of the first commercial ELISA for type 2N von Willebrand's disease diagnosis. Haemophilia. 2011;17:944–51.

39. Caron C, Mazurier C, Goudemand J. Large experience with a factor VIII binding assay of plasma von Willebrand factor using commercial reagents. Br J Haematol. 2002;117:716–8.

40. Lillicrap D. von Willebrand disease: advances in pathogenetic understanding, diagnosis, and therapy. Blood. 2013;122:3735–40.

41. Sanders YV, Groeneveld D, Meijer K, et al. von Willebrand factor propeptide and the phenotypic classification of von Willebrand disease. Blood. 2015;125:3006–13.

42. Haberichter SL, Balistreri M, Christopherson P, et al. Assay of the von Willebrand factor (VWF) propeptide to identify patients with type 1 von Willebrand disease with decreased VWF survival. Blood. 2006;108:3344–51.

43. Castaman G, Lethagen S, Federici AB, et al. Response to desmopressin is influenced by the genotype and phenotype in type 1 von Willebrand disease (VWD): results from the European study MCMDM-1VWD. Blood. 2008;111:3531–9.

44. Casonato A, Cattini MG, Daidone V, et al. Diagnostic value of measuring platelet Von Willebrand factor in Von Willebrand disease. PLoS One. 2016;11:e0161310.

45. Nair SC, Viswabandya A, Srivastava A. Diagnosis and management of von Willebrand disease: a developing country perspective. Semin Thromb Hemost. 2011;37:587–94.

46. Baronciani L, Goodeve A, Peyvandi F. Molecular diagnosis of von Willebrand disease. Haemophilia. 2017;23:188–97.

47. Tiede A, Rand JH, Budde U, et al. How I treat the acquired von Willebrand syndrome. Blood. 2011;117:6777–85.

48. Siaka C, Rugeri L, Caron C, et al. A new ELISA assay for diagnosis of acquired von Willebrand syndrome. Haemophilia. 2003;9:303–8.

Hepatic Coagulopathy: Intricacies and Challenges

19

Rakhee Kar

19.1 Introduction

Liver is an elegant factory which synthesizes several plasma proteins, transport proteins, and most of the clotting factors to name just a few of its immense synthetic function. Virtually every arm of the complex hemostatic pathway gets deranged in liver disease. Hence, it is quite natural to find abnormal tests of hemostasis in patients with chronic liver disease (CLD). A bleeding as well as a clotting tendency does exist simultaneously in liver disease. These are due to a set of complex and multifactorial process leading to a state of rebalanced hemostasis in stable cirrhosis patients [1].

Variceal hemorrhage, which is one of the most severe forms of bleeding in liver cirrhosis, is mainly a consequence of local vascular abnormalities and increased splanchnic blood pressure; the contribution of a hemostatic impairment here is debatable [2]. So, the concept of a causal relationship between deranged hemostasis and bleeding is questionable. It is also debatable whether screening patients with hemostasis tests and treating those with abnormal values prior to liver biopsy or other potentially hemorrhagic procedures are required. Recent findings of the literature question the usefulness of conventional

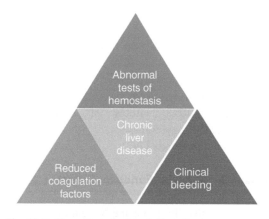

Fig. 19.1 Hemostasis in chronic liver disease

tests in assessing the hemorrhagic risk, as well as the appropriateness of therapeutic strategies aimed at correcting abnormal hemostasis tests [3]. Hence CLD is an intriguing situation characterized by reduced levels of clotting factors, deranged tests of hemostasis, and a bleeding tendency (Fig. 19.1) but not strictly a causal relationship between them.

19.2 Hemostatic Defects in Liver Disease

19.2.1 Defect in Primary Hemostasis

Patients who have liver disease can present with significant alterations in the primary hemostatic system. Thrombocytopenia and defects in platelet function are common and traditionally have

R. Kar (✉)
Department of Pathology, Jawaharlal Institute of Postgraduate Medical Education and Research, Puducherry, India

© Springer Nature Singapore Pte Ltd. 2019
R. Saxena, H. P. Pati (eds.), *Hematopathology*, https://doi.org/10.1007/978-981-13-7713-6_19

been thought to contribute to the impaired hemostasis in both acute and chronic liver disease [4, 5]. The causes of reduced platelet numbers and function are as follows [3–5].

19.2.1.1 Thrombocytopenia

Multiple factors can lead to thrombocytopenia:

- Increased splenic or hepatic sequestration
- Decreased production of thrombopoietin (TPO) by liver
- Bone marrow suppression by chronic hepatitis C infection
- Antiviral treatment with interferon-based therapy
- Increased platelet destruction
- Autoimmune mechanism
- Alcoholic cirrhosis
    - Folic acid deficiency
    - Direct toxic effects of ethanol on megakaryocytopoiesis
- Chronic low-grade DIC

19.2.1.2 Platelet Function Defect

- Thrombocytopathy
    - Defective thromboxane A_2 synthesis
    - Storage pool deficiency
    - Abnormalities of the platelet glycoprotein Ib
- Extrinsic factors
    - Abnormal high-density lipoproteins
    - Reduced hematocrit
    - Increased levels of endothelium-derived nitric oxide and prostacyclin, two potent platelet inhibitors

Recent observations suggest that patients with CLD have elevated levels of vWF and decreased levels of ADAMTS13 that may partially compensate for thrombocytopenia and/or reduced functional capacity (Fig. 19.2).

19.2.2 Defect in Secondary Hemostasis

A complex interplay between pro- and anticoagulant pathways occurs in liver disease. A delicate

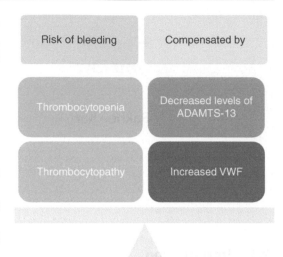

Fig. 19.2 Defect in primary hemostasis

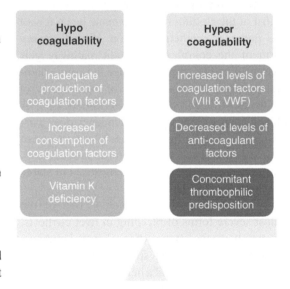

Fig. 19.3 Defect in secondary hemostasis

balance between these opposing pathways is able to sustain normal hemostasis whereas its disruption leads to either hypo or hypercoagulability (Fig. 19.3).

19.2.2.1 Hypocoagulability

Inadequate Production of Coagulation Factors

Liver is the primary source for the production of many of the coagulation factors. Hence, the levels of these factors may be significantly reduced in patients who have liver failure [6]. Although liver is the principal site of synthesis for factor VIII, other tissues have also been shown to produce factor VIII messenger RNA, and protein synthesis in these tissues may be stimulated by liver disease [7].

Increased Consumption of Coagulation Factors

There is evidence that cirrhotic patients may have enhanced consumption of coagulation factors [8]; however, clinically evident DIC in a cirrhotic patient is relatively uncommon and typically is seen in a critically ill patient before death following a severe associated illness such as variceal bleeding, sepsis, or both [6].

Vitamin K Deficiency

Patients who have impaired bile production from end-stage liver disease, especially cholestatic liver disease, may be at increased risk for vitamin K deficiency, although clinically relevant vitamin K deficiency is rare [6].

19.2.2.2 Hypercoagulability

Increased Levels of Coagulation Factors

FVIII and von Willebrand Factor (vWF) are synthesized by both the liver and endothelial cells. Both are also acute phase reactants. Normal or elevated FVIII and vWF levels are typically seen in patients with liver disease because of (1) continued endothelial cell FVIII production despite decreased hepatic FVIII production, (2) increased synthesis because of acute disease or inflammation, and (3) decreased clearance of FVIII due to decreased synthesis of low-density lipoprotein receptor-related protein which binds to FVIII in a dose-dependent manner, and the complex is cleared from the circulation by endocytosis [9].

Decreased Levels of Anticoagulant Factors

Decreased levels of protein C and S, antithrombin III, heparin cofactor II, and α2-macroglobulin are found in patients with liver disease. Moreover, protein C and S molecules lacking γ carboxylation may be produced [10].

Concomitant Thrombophilic Predisposition

Patients with liver disease may occasionally be exposed to acquired or genetic risk factors leading to thrombosis. Portal vein thrombosis is not an infrequent event especially in cirrhotics who are carriers of prothrombotic gain of function mutations like factor V Leiden or prothrombin G20210A [3, 11].

19.2.3 Defect in Fibrinolytic Pathway

The balance of fibrinolysis is important to prevent unwanted plasmin generation, and the perturbation of this balance may cause either hyper- or hypofibrinolysis. The literature and textbooks state that cirrhosis is characterized by hyperfibrinolysis. This complex defect is documented either by measuring the individual plasma-based components of fibrinolysis or rarely through global tests. The measurement of the individual components cannot give a clear picture of the balance of fibrinolysis because of the complex interplay between activators and anti-activators that regulates the plasminogen–plasmin conversion [12]. Recent attention has focused on thrombin-activatable fibrinolysis inhibitor (TAFI), and researchers have speculated that its deficiency which is seen in cirrhosis may explain the hyperfibrinolytic state. Investigations [13, 14] on this topic however show conflicting results, possibly because of the different designs of the global assays used in these studies. Nevertheless, it is estimated that between 5 and 10% of patients with decompensated cirrhosis will have clinical evidence of hyperfibrinolysis. The presence of hyperfibrinolysis indicates that though a clot is formed, it gets prematurely dissolved. Hyperfibrinolysis should be suspected in patients with mucosal bleeding, oozing from puncture sites, or late bleeding after a procedure [1].

19.2.4 Superimposed Coagulopathic Conditions in Cirrhosis

Several superimposed coagulopathic conditions can occur in patients who have CLD. The pivotal role of **infection** in variceal bleeding is well established. It leads to abnormalities in coagulation. One of the pathways through which this occurs is shown to depend on endogenous heparinoids. **Renal failure** may contribute to hemostatic imbalance in CLD through "uremic bleeding." Multifactorial platelet defects play a central role in the cause of uremic bleeding. **Endothelial dysfunction** plays an important role in the development of portal hypertension in patients who have cirrhosis [15].

19.3 Tests of Hemostasis in Liver Disease

19.3.1 Conventional Tests

1. **Bleeding Time**: The bleeding time is prolonged in up to 40% of patients who have liver disease [16]. However, it is not firmly established whether this prolongation is of clinical relevance. A former study showed that a prolonged bleeding time (more than 12 min) was associated with a fivefold increased risk of hemoglobin reduction after liver biopsy, but the association with other clinical manifestations of bleeding was not evaluated [17]. Desmopressin, an analog of vasopressin, shortens the bleeding time in these patients, probably by enhancing endothelial-derived vWF levels [18]. Randomized trials [19, 20], however, did not show that desmopressin had any efficacy in controlling variceal bleeding or in reducing blood loss in patients undergoing partial liver resections or liver transplantation. Lisman and associates using a test system carried out under flow conditions to replicate in vivo conditions showed that the high levels of von Willebrand factor found in cirrhosis support normal platelet adhesion in these patients, thus compensating for the defects of platelet numbers and function [21]. So, it appears that bleeding time is a poor reflector of the defect in primary hemostasis in liver disease and hence a poor predictor of the risk of bleeding in cirrhotics.

2. **Platelet Counts**: Thrombocytopenia has been used as a marker of advanced liver fibrosis and portal hypertension, but its clinical significance needs to be known. Thrombocytopenia is mostly mild to moderate in patients who have stable liver disease. Mild reduction in platelet counts is in general not associated with severe bleeding. However, thrombocytopenia can impact routine care of patients with CLD, by causing postponement or interference with diagnostic and therapeutic procedures like liver biopsy, antiviral therapy, and elective surgery due to concern over possible complications. Data on the safety of laparoscopic and transjugular liver biopsies suggests that few complications occur with a platelet count above 50,000/μL [22–24]. Moreover, a platelet level that is over about 50,000/μL is associated with improved thrombin production [1].

3. **Prothrombin Time and Activated Partial Thromboplastin Time**: PT is responsive to congenital or acquired deficiencies of factors VII, X, V, and II and fibrinogen (extrinsic and common pathway). The type of thromboplastin is the main factor governing the responsiveness of the test to the coagulation defect. The aPTT is responsive to congenital or acquired deficiencies of all coagulation factors except factors VII and XIII (intrinsic and common pathway). The type, concentration, and combination of activators and phospholipids determine the responsiveness of the test [12]. PT and aPTT are sometimes used to investigate patients who have cirrhosis although these tests are known to be poor predictors of bleeding in such patients [25, 26]. This apparent paradox can be explained by the fact that the PT and aPTT which reflect the competence of parts of the coagulation cascade are inadequate to reflect the balance of coagulation as occurs in vivo, especially in cirrhosis, where levels of naturally occurring anticoagulants are reduced in parallel with the procoagulants [12]. Normally, protein C in vivo is activated by thrombin along with its endothelial receptor thrombomodulin [27]. Antithrombin activation is brought about by

glycosaminoglycans such as heparan sulfate and others, which are located on endothelial cells [27]. Neither the plasma nor the reagents needed to perform PT and aPTT contain thrombomodulin or glycosaminoglycans. As a result, PT and aPTT are responsive only to the thrombin generated as a function of procoagulants but are less responsive to the inhibition of thrombin mediated by the anticoagulants. PT and aPTT are suitable tests to investigate congenital deficiency of procoagulant factors, but they are unfit to investigate congenital deficiencies of anticoagulants or acquired deficiencies of both the pro- and the anticoagulant factors as occurs in liver cirrhosis. Hence these tests are poor predictors of bleeding in cirrhotics.

4. **International Normalized Ratio (INR)**: Several studies have demonstrated a wide variation in prothrombin time based on the type of thromboplastin reagent and measuring device [6]. INR is subject to the same variations and does not adequately normalize differences between clinical laboratories. Studies [28, 29] using different thromboplastins found significant variation in the mean INR in patients who had liver impairment but no difference in patients receiving warfarin. Similar findings were also observed by us [30]. Hepatologists and transplant surgeons may be surprised by this finding. The INR was devised primarily to standardize the anticoagulation effects of warfarin and was not designed to provide a reproducibly precise assessment of severity of illness in patients who have end-stage liver disease. The reasons for the wide variation in INR in patients who had liver impairment compared with patients receiving anticoagulation therapy are not known. One explanation may be the different mechanisms of prolonged prothrombin time caused by warfarin and liver disease. Warfarin causes prolonged prothrombin time through the inhibition of vitamin K-dependent gamma-carboxylation of coagulation factors II, VII, IX, and X. In liver disease, the elevated prothrombin time is caused in large part by decreased production of coagulation factors,

including the vitamin K-dependent factors II, VII, IX, and X [6]. The differences in INR from laboratory to laboratory may be relevant for patients listed for liver transplantation based on Model for End-stage Liver Disease (MELD) score, which has INR as the most heavily weighted determinant [31].

19.3.2 Functional Hemostasis and Other Tests

5. **Platelet functional analyzer (PFA-100)**: The PFA-100 has been advocated as a simple substitute for the bleeding time, but it has not yet been evaluated widely for its clinical usefulness in predicting the risk of bleeding in patients with liver cirrhosis.

6. **Thrombin generation test**: The thrombin generation test is a global test in which platelet-free plasma is incubated with small amounts of tissue factor as coagulation trigger and phospholipids that act as platelet substitutes [32]. The test is performed in the presence or absence of soluble thrombomodulin as protein C activator. The amount of thrombin generated over time is monitored by means of a synthetic fluorogenic substrate. The area under the thrombin generation curve is called "endogenous thrombin potential (ETP)." ETP is expressed as fluorogenic units (FU min) or thrombin concentration (nM min) and represents the balance between the action of pro- and anticoagulant factors in plasma [3]. In fact, the balance of pro- and anticoagulants in stable cirrhosis was found to be normal when assessed by thrombin generation measured in the presence of thrombomodulin [33], and this balance was seen even though the PT and aPTT were prolonged [33]. Platelets contribute to the generation of thrombin [34]; therefore, the occurrence of thrombocytopenia and/or thrombocytopathy often found in cirrhosis could affect the generation of thrombin in this condition. A recent study showed that thrombin generation, when measured in platelet-rich plasma from stable cirrhotics in the presence of thrombomodulin,

was indistinguishable from that of control subjects under the same experimental conditions, provided that the platelet levels were higher than $60 \times 10^9/L$ [35]. The conclusion drawn from these studies is that coagulation in patients who have stable cirrhosis is normal if the platelet levels are sufficiently high to sustain the normal thrombin generation elicited by plasma.

7. **Thromboelastography**: Thromboelastography is a technique that can provide continuous observation and tracing of all the hemostatic functions that lead to clot formation and dissolution. It can be considered as the prototype of a global test for hemostasis because it takes into account primary hemostasis, coagulation, and fibrinolysis. To be consistent with in vivo conditions, however, it should incorporate thrombomodulin to secure optimal protein C activation. Further work is needed to explore its clinical utility.

19.4 Therapeutic Decision-Making

So, from this ongoing discussion, it appears that there is a state of a precarious rebalanced hemostasis in patients with CLD. While a bleeding and clotting tendency both coexist, bleeding events are more common among hospitalized patients and those with decompensated cirrhosis [1]. Patients in whom platelet count is above 50,000/mL are usually not at risk for acute bleeding or bleeding during small invasive procedures. The platelet count increment following platelet transfusion may be markedly less in a patient with liver failure compared to patients with intact liver function due to sequestration of the transfused platelets in the enlarged spleen [10]. Drugs that stimulate TPO and increase platelet levels, such as the oral platelet growth factor eltrombopag, are currently in development for the prevention and/or treatment of thrombocytopenia. The ability to increase platelet levels could significantly reduce the need for platelet transfusions and facilitate the use of interferon-based antiviral therapy and other medically indicated treatments in patients with liver disease [4]. Splenic artery embolization and splenectomy are often, but not always, effective in increasing platelet counts in patients with portal hypertension. Possible complications of these procedures include splenic abscesses and portal vein thrombosis. Transjugular intrahepatic portosystemic shunt (TIPS) placement can decrease sinusoidal portal pressure, but it is unclear if portal decompression can reduce the degree of thrombocytopenia in cirrhotic patients [36, 37]. Vasopressin (DDAVP) can correct prolonged bleeding time in patients with liver failure, but has failed to prove efficacy in acute variceal bleeding in cirrhotic patients [19].

All guidelines for plasma transfusion include the multiple clotting factor deficiencies of liver disease when hemostasis is needed for bleeding or invasive procedures. Vitamin K deficiency should be corrected first, if present and if time permits. Most of the criteria justify plasma transfusion when PT or partial thromboplastin time (PTT) values are more than 1.5 times normal [38]. Disadvantages of FFP are the large volumes required for correction of a severe coagulopathy and the brief duration of action because of the short biological half-life of some clotting factors, particularly factor VII [10]. Observational studies in common invasive procedures such as liver biopsy, paracentesis, and central venous cannulation indicate that modest elevations in PT and PTT are not detrimental for bleeding risk [38]. A fibrinogen level over 120 mg/dL is preferred because fibrinogen is the main target of thrombin and a final step in clot formation [1].

Studies assessing the use of rFVIIa have shown that it can reduce the PT in liver disease but that its benefit for bleeding is less clear to date. Some benefits have been reported in the early control of variceal bleeding and in ability to place intracranial pressure transducers [39, 40]. As an alternative to plasma, rFVIIa can help correct clotting tests, but further randomized trials are needed to better define its efficacy in reducing bleeding [38].

Antifibrinolytic agents such as e-aminocaproic acid, tranexamic acid, and aprotinin may be administered if a hyperfibrinolytic state is shown. However, since a hyperfibrinolytic state in patients with chronic liver failure is still somewhat controversial, and because of the risk for thromboembolic complications, the general therapeutic value of antifibrinolytics in these patients remains uncertain [10].

Acute kidney injury (AKI) frequently occurs in patients who have cirrhosis experiencing an acute decompensation in liver function. Hepatorenal syndrome (HRS) is a leading cause of AKI in these patients, but other causes may coexist. Renal replacement therapies are frequent adjuncts in the care of patients who have cirrhosis with acute decompensation or who require bridge therapy to liver transplantation [41].

19.5 Conclusion

The pathophysiology and assessment of coagulopathy in liver disease have undergone revision. The abnormality of coagulation in stable cirrhosis is more of a state of rebalanced hemostasis where a potential bleeding and thrombotic risk coexists. This understanding helps explain the apparent paradox of the prolonged global coagulation tests and their poor prediction of bleeding risk. However, randomized clinical trials addressing the value of old and newer tests and treatment vs. placebo in mild to moderate hemostatic defects are needed. The best approach rests on clinical judgment based on prior bleeding and on the awareness that any prophylactic procedure may expose the patient to unnecessary risks [3].

Take Home Message
- The typical cirrhotic patient has multiple and frequently opposing factors that influence hemostasis and clot formation.
- Alterations in the primary hemostatic system tilting the balance in favor of a bleeding diathesis include abnormal platelet numbers and function. This is compensated by elevated levels of vWF and decreased ADAMTS13 activity.
- A complex interplay between pro- and anticoagulant pathways occurs in liver disease.

- Decreased production of procoagulant factors, increased consumption of coagulation factors, and vitamin K deficiency favor the balance toward a hypocoagulable state while increased levels of factor VIII and vWF, decreased levels of anticoagulants, and a concomitant thrombophilic predisposition tilt the balance toward a hypercoagulable state.
- Thrombin-activatable fibrinolysis inhibitor (TAFI) deficiency has been speculated to explain the hyperfibrinolytic state often described in cirrhosis.
- Several superimposed coagulopathic conditions like infection, renal failure, and endothelial dysfunction can occur in patients who have liver cirrhosis.
- The PT and aPTT are poor predictors of bleeding as they are inadequate to reflect the balance of coagulation as occurs in vivo.
- Significant variation in the mean INR is seen in patients with liver impairment compared to patients receiving warfarin.
- Alternative tests mimicking more closely what occurs in vivo like platelet functional analyzer (PFA-100), thrombin generation test, and thromboelastography should be developed and investigated in appropriate clinical trials to determine their value in the management of bleeding in cirrhosis.
- Several measures to correct the defective hemostatic test results have been adopted earlier. However, randomized clinical trials addressing the value of old and newer tests and treatment vs. placebo in mild to moderate hemostatic defect are needed. So long, therapeutic approach should be individualized based on clinical judgment and prior bleeding history.

References

1. Caldwell SH. Management of coagulopathy in liver disease. Gastroenterol Hepatol (N Y). 2014;10(5):330–2.
2. Sharara AI, Rockey DC. Gastroesophageal variceal hemorrhage. N Engl J Med. 2001;345(9):669–81.
3. Tripodi A, Mannucci PM. Abnormalities of hemostasis in chronic liver disease: reappraisal of their clinical significance and need for clinical and laboratory research. J Hepatol. 2007;46:727–33.

4. Afdhal N, McHutchison J, Brown R, Jacobson I, Manns M, Poordad F, Weksler B, Esteban R. Thrombocytopenia associated with chronic liver disease. J Hepatol. 2008;48(6):1000–7.

5. Hugenholtz GG, Porte RJ, Lisman T. The platelet and platelet function testing in liver disease. Clin Liver Dis. 2009;13(1):11–20.

6. Trotter JF. Coagulation abnormalities in patients who have liver disease. Clin Liver Dis. 2006;10:665–78.

7. Hollestelle MJ, Thinnes T, Crain K, Stiko A, Kruijt JK, van Berkel TJ, et al. Tissue distribution of factor VIII gene expression in vivo—a closer look. Thromb Haemost. 2001;86:855–61.

8. Ben-Ari Z, Osman E, Hutton RA, et al. Disseminated intravascular coagulation in liver cirrhosis: fact or fiction? Am J Gastroenterol. 1999;94:2977–82.

9. Ng VL. Liver disease, coagulation testing, and hemostasis. Clin Lab Med. 2009;29:265–82.

10. Lisman T, Leebeek FWG, de Groot PG. Haemostatic abnormalities in patients with liver disease. J Hepatol. 2002;37:280–7.

11. Amitrano L, Brancaccio V, Guardascione MA, Margaglione M, Iannaccone L, D'Andrea G, et al. Inherited coagulation disorders in cirrhotic patients with portal vein thrombosis. Hepatology. 2000;31:345–8.

12. Tripodi A. Tests of coagulation in liver disease. Clin Liver Dis. 2009;13:55–61.

13. Lisman T, Leebeek FW, Mosnier LO, et al. Thrombin-activatable fibrinolysis inhibitor deficiency in cirrhosis is not associated with increased plasma fibrinolysis. Gastroenterology. 2001;121:131–9.

14. Colucci M, Binetti BM, Branca MG, et al. Deficiency of thrombin activatable fibrinolysis inhibitor in cirrhosis is associated with increased plasma fibrinolysis. Hepatology. 2003;38:230–7.

15. Smalberg JH, Leebeek FWG. Superimposed coagulopathic conditions in cirrhosis: infection and endogenous heparinoids, renal failure, and endothelial dysfunction. Clin Liver Dis. 2009;13:33–42.

16. Violi F, Leo R, Vezza E, et al. Bleeding time in patients with cirrhosis: relation with degree of liver failure and clotting abnormalities. C.A.L.C. Group. Coagulation Abnormalities in Cirrhosis Study Group. J Hepatol. 1994;20(4):531–6.

17. Boberg KM, Brosstad F, Egeland T, Egge T, Schrumpf E. Is a prolonged bleeding time associated with an increased risk of hemorrhage after liver biopsy? Thromb Haemost. 1999;81:378–81.

18. Cattaneo M, Tenconi PM, Alberca I, et al. Subcutaneous desmopressin (DDAVP) shortens the prolonged bleeding time in patients with liver cirrhosis. Thromb Haemost. 1990;64(3):358–60.

19. de Franchis R, Arcidiacono PG, Carpinelli L, et al. Randomized controlled trial of desmopressin plus terlipressin vs. terlipressin alone for the treatment of acute variceal hemorrhage in cirrhotic patients: a multicenter, double-blind study. New Italian Endoscopic Club. Hepatology. 1993;18(5):1102–7.

20. Wong AY, Irwin MG, Hui TW, et al. Desmopressin does not decrease blood loss and transfusion requirements in patients undergoing hepatectomy. Can J Anaesth. 2003;50(1):14–20.

21. Lisman T, Bongers TN, Adelmeijer J, Janssen HL, de Maat MP, de Groot PG, et al. Elevated levels of von Willebrand factor in cirrhosis support platelet adhesion despite reduced functional capacity. Hepatology. 2006;44:53–61.

22. McVay PA, Toy PT. Lack of increased bleeding after liver biopsy in patients with mild hemostatic abnormalities. Am J Clin Pathol. 1990;94:747–53.

23. Cobb WS, Heniford BT, Burns JM, Carbonell AM, Matthews BD, Kercher KW. Cirrhosis is not a contraindication to laparoscopic surgery. Surg Endosc. 2005;19:418–23.

24. Inabnet WB, Deziel DJ. Laparoscopic liver biopsy in patients with coagulopathy, portal hypertension, and ascites. Am Surg. 1995;61:603–6.

25. Ewe K. Bleeding after liver biopsy does not correlate with indices of peripheral coagulation. Dig Dis Sci. 1981;26:388–93.

26. Segal JB, Dzik WH. Paucity of studies to support that abnormal coagulation test results predict bleeding in the setting of invasive procedures: an evidence-based review. Transfusion. 2005;45:1413–25.

27. Huntington JA. Mechanisms of glycosaminoglycan activation of the serpins in hemostasis. J Thromb Haemost. 2003;1:1535–49.

28. Kovacs MH, Wong A, MacKinnon K, et al. Assessment of the validity of the INR system for patients with liver impairment. Thromb Haemost. 1994;71:727–30.

29. Denson KWE, Reed SV, Haddon ME, et al. Comparative studies of rabbit and human recombinant tissue factor reagents. Thromb Res. 1999;94:255–61.

30. Kar R, Kar SS, Sarin SK. Hepatic coagulopathy-intricacies and challenges; a cross-sectional descriptive study of 110 patients from a superspecialty institute in North India with review of literature. Blood Coagul Fibrinolysis. 2013;24(2):175–80.

31. Wiesner R, Edwards E, Freeman R, et al. Model for end-stage liver disease (MELD) and allocation of donor liver. Gastroenterology. 2003;124:91–6.

32. Hemker HC, Giesen P, Al Dieri R, et al. Calibrated automated thrombin generation measurement in clotting plasma. Pathophysiol Haemost Thromb. 2003;33:4–15.

33. Tripodi A, Salerno F, Chantarangkul V, et al. Evidence of normal thrombin generation in cirrhosis despite abnormal conventional coagulation tests. Hepatology. 2005;41:553–8.

34. Bevers EM, Comfurius P, Zwaal RF. Platelet procoagulant activity: physiological significance and mechanisms of exposure. Blood Rev. 1991;5:146–54.

35. Tripodi A, Primignani M, Chantarangkul V, et al. Thrombin generation in patients with cirrhosis: the role of platelets. Hepatology. 2006;44:440–5.

36. Wong F. The use of TIPS in chronic liver disease. Ann Hepatol. 2006;5:5–15.

37. Jabbour N, Zajko A, Orons P, Irish W, Fung JJ, Selby RR. Does transjugular intrahepatic portosystemic shunt (TIPS) resolve thrombocytopenia associated with cirrhosis? Dig Dis Sci. 1998;43:2459–62.
38. Ramsey G. Treating coagulopathy in liver disease with plasma transfusions or recombinant factor VIIa: an evidence-based review. Best Pract Res Clin Haematol. 2006;19(1):113–26.
39. Bosch J, Thabut D, Bendtsen F, et al. Recombinant factor VIIa for upper gastrointestinal bleeding in patients with cirrhosis: a randomized, double-blind trial. Gastroenterology. 2004;127:1123–30.
40. Shami VM, Caldwell SH, Hespenheide EE, et al. Recombinant activated factor VII for coagulopathy in fulminant hepatic failure compared with conventional therapy. Liver Transpl. 2003;9: 138–43.
41. Argo CK, Balogun RA. Blood products, volume control, and renal support in the coagulopathy of liver disease. Clin Liver Dis. 2009;13:73–85.

Antiphospholipid Syndrome

20

Abhishek Purohit and Mayank Kumar

20.1 Introduction

Antiphospholipid syndrome (APS) is a prothrombotic condition with immune pathogenesis that is characterized by thrombosis in the venous or arterial vasculature and/or pregnancy morbidity, which occurs in the presence of persistent laboratory evidence of antiphospholipid antibodies (aPLs). aPLs are autoantibodies that target phospholipid-bound proteins, especially β2-glycoprotein I (β2-GPI). The presence of these antibodies is the defining feature of this syndrome; however, the mechanism by which aPLs cause a hypercoagulable state is not fully understood [1].

Since this condition was first described by GR Hughes almost three decades ago, after whom it is also referred to as "Hughes syndrome," there have been significant advances in the understanding of the pathogenesis of this disease, its clinical manifestations and associations, and improved diagnostic accuracy. The various advances have led to optimization of therapy [2]. Information regarding this disease is being updated to fill in the gaps that are existing in its understanding.

The aim of this review is to summarize the current knowledge on this enigmatic disease, incorporating the most recent advances.

A. Purohit (✉) · M. Kumar
Department of Pathology, All India Institute of Medical Sciences, Jodhpur, Rajasthan, India
e-mail: purohita@aiimsjodhpur.edu.in

20.2 History

The history of APS can be traced back to the mid-twentieth century when screening programs for syphilis, an infection of high incidence at that time, were conducted.

Treponema pallidum, the causative organism for syphilis, was identified in the beginning of the twentieth century by light microscopy. The first serological test for diagnosis, based on complement fixation technique, was described by Wasserman et al. Cardiolipin, now known to be a component of the inner mitochondrial membrane, was extracted from beef heart, and this allowed assay standardization which led to the development of Venereal Disease Research Laboratory (VDRL) microflocculation assay. This assay was then used for population screening. The widespread use of this test for screening purpose demonstrated significant occurrence of false-positive reactions, positive tests in individuals who were not thought to have been exposed to syphilis. These false-positive reactions were attributed to malaria, leprosy, infectious mononucleosis, disseminated lupus erythematosus, rheumatoid arthritis, and collagen diseases by various authors [2].

In 1950s, it was recognized that some patients with systemic lupus erythematosus (SLE) had a circulating anticoagulant and that these patients also tested false-positive for syphilis. Also, it was discovered over time that many of the patients with SLE also had high levels of anticardiolipin

R. Saxena, H. P. Pati (eds.), *Hematopathology*, https://doi.org/10.1007/978-981-13-7713-6_20

(aCL). The term "antiphospholipid antibody syndrome" was first coined in the 1980s and soon abbreviated to "antiphospholipid syndrome."

By 1990s, it had become clear that β2-GPI, a member of the complement control family, was a key target for antibody binding, rather than phospholipid itself [2].

20.3 Nomenclature

APS can be classified as [3]:

1. Primary APS
2. Secondary APS
3. Seronegative APS
4. Catastrophic APS
5. Suggested categories—probable APS, micro-angiopathic APS

Primary APS is the occurrence of the disease without association with other autoimmune disease. Secondary APS occurs in the setting of a preexisting autoimmune disease. The commonly associated autoimmune diseases are SLE and rheumatoid arthritis. Seronegative APS is the condition where the individuals have highly suggestive clinical features of the disease but are persistently negative for aPLs. Catastrophic APS, described in detail later, is an accelerated form of APS where the patients present with coagulopathy and ischemic necrosis of the extremities along with presence of aPLs.

20.4 Laboratory Diagnosis

20.4.1 Recognizing APS

The clinical presentation of APS is not specific, with a variety of presenting features being associated with the disease. However, the defining feature of this syndrome is the persistent presence of aPLs.

The patient may present with both venous and arterial thrombosis. Deep vein thrombosis of the lower extremity is the most common clinical presentation. However, the most common arterial manifestation is stroke [4].

Pregnancy-related complications are seen, the most common being recurrent pregnancy loss. Other features seen in patients with APS include thrombocytopenia, hemolytic anemia, valvular heart disease, livedo reticularis, and neurologic findings which range from mild cognitive deficits to white matter lesions. The presence of one or more of these features should alert the treating physician to consider the diagnosis of APS.

20.4.2 Diagnosing APS

The diagnosis of APS is based on the Sydney Consensus Statement of 2006 which was an update to the Sapporo criteria proposed in 1999.

The clinical criteria include arterial, venous, or small vessel thrombosis that is objectively confirmed or pregnancy complications. These pregnancy complications, in order to be included in the criteria, should be attributed to placental insufficiency and include pregnancy loss or premature birth.

The laboratory criteria state that a positive laboratory test for aPLs be found on two or more occasions, at least 12 weeks apart. Laboratory tests for lupus anticoagulant (LA), anticardiolipin (aCL) antibody (IgG or IgM), or anti-β2-GPI antibody (IgG or IgM) are performed, as per guidelines.

The summary of the Sydney Consensus Statement for the diagnosis of APS is as follows [1]:

Clinical criteria
1. Vascular thrombosis
     One or more episodes of arterial, venous, or small vessel thrombosis in any tissue, which have been confirmed by objective validated criteria. For histologic confirmation, thrombosis should be present without significant vessel wall inflammation.
2. Pregnancy morbidity
     (a) One or more unexplained deaths of a morphologically normal fetus at or beyond the tenth week of gestation, with normal

fetal morphology documented by ultrasound or direct examination of the fetus, or

(b) One or more premature births of a morphologically normal neonate before the 34th week of gestation because of eclampsia or preeclampsia diagnosed by standard definitions, or recognized features of placental insufficiency, or

(c) Three or more unexplained consecutive spontaneous abortions before the tenth week of gestation, with maternal or hormonal abnormalities, and maternal and paternal chromosomal causes excluded.

Laboratory criteria

1. LA present in plasma, on two or more occasions, detected according to the guidelines of the International Society of Thrombosis and Hemostasis. The two tests should be performed at least 12 weeks apart.

2. aCL of IgG and/or IgM isotype in serum or plasma, present in medium or high titer (>40 GPL or MPL, or >99th percentile), on two or more occasions, measured by a standardized ELISA. The two tests should be performed at least 12 weeks apart.

3. Anti-β2-GPI of IgG and/or IgM isotype in serum or plasma with a titer >99th percentile, on two or more occasions, measured by a standardized ELISA. The two tests should be performed at least 12 weeks apart.

It is recommended to classify APS patients into one of the following categories [5]:

- I: More than one laboratory criteria present (any combination)
- IIa: LA present alone
- IIb: aCL present alone
- IIc: anti-β2-GPI present alone

False-positive LA results can sometimes occur. These are usually seen when the testing is performed while patients are receiving anticoagulants or in the presence of a factor deficiency.

Transient aPLs can be induced by certain infections and medications, but these usually disappear on drug discontinuation or on repeat testing. This emphasizes the importance of repeated aPL measurements for the diagnosis.

These three laboratory tests are currently the key diagnostic tests used in the assessment of APS.

At present, patients who have aPLs that are currently not recognized in the diagnostic criteria or who have clinical manifestations other than thrombosis or pregnancy morbidity are not recognized as having APS. However, the diagnostic criteria continue to evolve. In current clinical practice, testing for non-criteria aPLs is not recommended. This is because prospective studies are needed to be carried out in order to assess whether these antibodies provide any additional information. Also, there is a lack of standardization of the assays for these antibodies [1].

The International Society on Thrombosis and Haemostasis (ISTH) criteria for diagnosis of LAs are as follows [6]:

1. Positive screening test (phospholipid-dependent coagulation assay)
   - Two or more screening tests are recommended:
     – Dilute Russell's viper venom time (DRVVT)
     – Sensitive aPTT (low phospholipids with silica as activator)

2. Evidence of inhibition in mixing studies (factor deficiency has to be excluded)
   - 1:1 mixing of patient plasma with normal plasma does not correct the prolonged clotting time
   - If thrombin time is prolonged, LA cannot be conclusively identified

3. Evidence that inhibition is phospholipid-dependent
   - Confirmatory test(s) in which increased phospholipid reduces or corrects the prolonged clotting time
   - Examples: DRVVT confirm, platelet neutralization test, hexagonal phase phospholipid

4. Exclusion of coagulation inhibitors
   - Heparin
   - Direct thrombin or factor Xa inhibitors (DOAC)
   - Individual factor inhibitors

Key points in diagnosis of APS

1. In routine practice, patients may be suspected to have APS without necessarily meeting all the strict investigational criteria. This is because the consensus criteria for APS are meant to identify patients for research studies, who can be labeled as having "definite APS."
2. Laboratory testing for aPLs should usually be limited to patients who present with thrombosis and/or complications related to pregnancy.
3. It is better not to rely on a single negative test for LA assays. For diagnosis, at least two tests with different testing principles should be used.
4. In cases having prolonged aPTT, multiple coagulation factor deficiencies, and no clinical evidence for a bleeding tendency, the deficiencies may represent laboratory artifacts induced by the LA effect.
5. In cases of bleeding in APS patients with a normal platelet count, the differential diagnosis should include prothrombin deficiency, an inhibitor against a specific coagulation factor, AVWS, an acquired thrombocytopathy, or acquired inhibitor to factor XIII.
6. Infections should always be ruled out, as they are potential cause for positive aCL immunoassays.
7. The possibility of seronegative APS should be considered in patients who are negative for standard aPL assay results with clinical appearance of APS [7].

Assessment of thrombotic risk

- It is difficult to identify individuals who are at risk for thrombosis and to predict the risk of occurrence of first episode of thrombosis in asymptomatic aPL carriers [8, 9].
  - Anti-β2-GPI has been proposed to be the strongest risk factor for arterial and venous thrombosis.
  - LA positivity is a stronger risk factor compared to aCL.
  - Also, positivity for two or more aPLs is more strongly associated with the occurrence of thrombosis.
  - Obstetrical complications are usually seen in the presence of IgG anti-β2-GPI-domain I antibodies.

20.5 Pathogenesis

Formation of aPLs is necessary, though not sufficient, for the development of APS. There are secondary factors that lead to thrombosis, in the presence of predisposing aPLs. These include, among others, infections, inflammation, intake of procoagulant factors, endothelial injury, recent surgery, and immobility due to any cause [5]. Also, a critical variable for the development of clinical features of APS is the patient's genetic constitution. Mutations in prothrombin gene, factor V Leiden, and activated protein C resistance are associated with an increased risk of venous thromboembolism [10].

20.5.1 Anti-β2-GPI

β2-GPI, a natural inhibitor of coagulation, is a member of the complement control family. It functions as a cofactor in the binding of aPL to cardiolipin. Structurally, it consists of 326 amino acids which are arranged in five (designated I to V) highly homologous protein domains.

The pathogenicity of antibodies against β2-GPI can be demonstrated from the fact that infusion of these from APS patients to mice with injured blood vessels leads to thrombus formation [11]. It has also been seen that purified anti-β2-GPI IgG autoantibodies potentiate thrombus size in a dose-dependent manner. β2-GPI exists in two different conformations—a circular "inactivated" form in plasma and an open "activated" form. The circular form is maintained by interaction between the first and fifth domains. Unfolding of the molecule occurs in the presence of anionic phospholipids. This leads to exposure of the antigenic determinants, which plays a pivotal role in the formation of autoantibodies. One

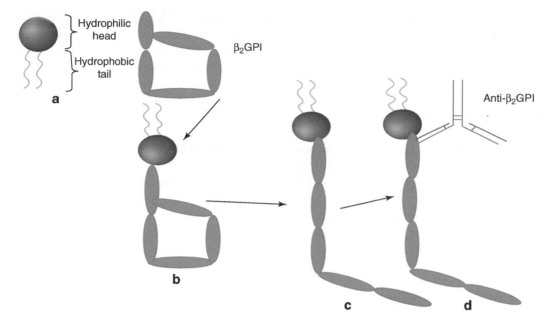

Fig. 20.1 Schematic representation of folded (circular) and unfolded conformation of β2-GPI and subsequent binding to anti-β2-GPI antibodies. In the presence of anionic phospholipids, the circular conformation of the protein unfolds, exposing antigenic determinants that are normally shielded from the circulation (**a–c**) which facilitate the binding to antibodies (**d**)

such important epitope is located within domain I (DI) (Fig. 20.1).

After attachment to the endothelial surface, unfolding of β2-GPI can be brought about by reduction in surface thiols by thioredoxin, and in response to oxidative stress. In normal circumstances, this plays a protective role against oxidative cell injury. However, antibody binding fixes β2-GPI in an open configuration, and these complexes bind and activate various receptors on different cell types, which may be a trigger for the initiation of intracellular signaling and inflammatory responses [12, 13].

20.5.2 Non-criteria Antibodies

There are several antibodies whose role in the pathogenesis of APS is under evaluation. These antibodies are collectively referred to as non-criteria antibodies. It is essential to carry out prospective studies with uniform methodology in order to study their definitive role in the pathogenesis. The antibodies in this group include anti-vimentin/cardiolipin complex, antiphospha-tidylserine/prothrombin, anti-protein C/S, anti-phosphatidic acid, and a variety of autoantibodies with other specificities, such as factor X, factor XII, annexin A2, and annexin A5 [2].

20.5.3 Other Pathways

Supposedly, excess generation of C3a and C5a during complement activation plays a role in thrombotic manifestations in APS.

It is postulated that mTOR complex (mTORC) pathway activation plays a role in the manifestation of microthrombosis, peripheral ischemia, skin ulcers, aPL nephropathy, and diffuse alveolar hemorrhage. Ig antibodies from patients with APS stimulate the target of rapamycin (mTOR) through the phosphatidylinositol 3-kinase (PI3K)–AKT pathway, which leads to cell proliferation [14].

Acquired activated protein C resistance, due to interference with anticoagulant activity of activated protein C, may lead to thrombosis. Upregulation of TF pathway, which may occur due to downregulation of TF pathway inhibitor

(TFPI), is postulated as another mechanism by which risk of thrombosis may increase. Autoantibodies against TFPI have been demonstrated in patients with APS [15].

20.5.4 Microparticles

These are fragments of cell surface membranes that are released from apoptotic, activated, and damaged cells. It is seen that plasma concentration of microparticles that are derived from endothelial cells is increased among patients with APS [16]. These may play a role in the pathogenesis and lead to thrombotic manifestations.

20.5.5 Pregnancy Complications

Presence of aPLs is an important cause for recurrent pregnancy loss and late placenta-mediated obstetric complications. Pathophysiology of obstetric APS differs from that of thrombotic APS. Here, the thrombosis may be neither a specific nor a universal feature.

The various mechanisms for aPL-medicated fetal loss or obstetric complications include inflammation, complement activation, intraplacental thrombosis, inhibition of syncytium-trophoblast differentiation, interference with annexin V function, and defective placentation or placental apoptosis.

In normal individuals, anticoagulant annexin V aggregates on trophoblast membranes and blocks binding of factor Xa and prothrombin. There is disrupted and reduced annexin V binding in women with APS. This is postulated to play an important role in the occurrence of obstetric complications.

20.6   Epidemiology and Clinical Associations

The prevalence of various autoantibodies in patients with SLE has been well demonstrated—about 40% have aPLs, 12–30% have aCLs, and 15–34% have LA. In about 50–70% of the patients with SLE who demonstrate laboratory evidence for aPLs, the condition progress to APS. Also, aPLs are present in about 20% of patients who have had stroke at a young age, and 10–15% of women with recurrent pregnancy loss are diagnosed with APS [17, 18].

20.6.1 Thrombotic Events

Thromboses are the hallmark of APS, with venous thromboses being more common than arterial thromboses. Individuals with positive tests for LA activity or with medium or high levels of aCL are at an increased risk of thrombosis and/or thromboembolism. Further, the risk of recurrent thrombosis and/or thromboembolism is enhanced in those patients who show positivity to three aPLs (LA, aCL, and anti-β2-GPI antibodies) upon repeated testing.

The most common sites of venous thrombosis are the deep veins of the lower extremities. Other sites include the pulmonary, hepatic, pelvic, renal, axillary, portal, ocular, subclavian veins and cerebral sinuses, and also the inferior vena cava. There may also be episodes of superficial vein thrombosis.

The most common site of arterial thrombosis is in the cerebral vasculature. This usually manifests in the form of transient ischemic attack or a stroke. Occlusions in the retinal, renal, coronary, and mesenteric arteries may also occur [19].

20.6.2 Pregnancy Complications

Pregnancy complications are the hallmark of APS. These complications include fetal death, and premature birth due to placental insufficiency or severe preeclampsia [18].

20.6.3 Neurological Involvement

Central nervous system abnormalities are a common feature of APS. These are attributed to vascular thrombosis and direct injury to neuronal tissue by aPLs.

The most common neurologic manifestations of APS are transient ischemic attack and stroke. Cognitive deficits and/or white matter lesions have been associated. These may range from subtle findings to transient global amnesia and permanent, profound loss in cognitive functioning [20].

20.6.4 Hematologic Abnormalities

Thrombocytopenia is frequently observed in APS patients. The occurrence of thrombocytopenia is higher in SLE-associated APS than in primary APS. With a platelet count in the range of 100,000–140,000/μL, the degree of thrombocytopenia is usually moderate. It is rarely associated with any hemorrhagic events. It should be kept in mind that the presence of thrombocytopenia does not preclude the occurrence of thrombotic complications of APS.

Other hematologic abnormalities have been reported in patients with APS. These include autoimmune hemolytic anemia, bone marrow necrosis, and thrombotic microangiopathic syndromes like thrombotic thrombocytopenic purpura (TTP) and hemolytic uremic syndrome (HUS) [21]. Bone marrow necrosis is usually seen in cases which have widespread thrombosis.

20.6.5 Cardiac Involvement

APS most commonly involves the heart valves, leading to valvular thickening and valve nodules. The occurrence of these is known as Libman–Sacks endocarditis, with the mitral valve being most frequently involved, followed by the aortic valve. Patients with LA or IgG aCL have a higher risk of valvular involvement.

Patients with APS also have an increased risk for developing coronary artery disease. Myocardial infarction may occur and can be attributed to thrombosis in the microvasculature, coronary thromboembolism, or accelerated atherosclerosis leading to a plaque rupture [22].

20.6.6 Cutaneous Manifestations

The cutaneous abnormalities associated with APS are splinter hemorrhages, cutaneous necrosis and infarction, livedo reticularis, digital gangrene with skin ulcerations, superficial vein thrombosis, lesions resembling vasculitis, and livedoid vasculopathy.

Livedo reticularis, the most common cutaneous manifestation of APS, is associated with arterial lesions and multiple thromboses [23].

The rarer clinical associations include

- Renal disease—Glomerular capillaries, and other renal vessels, may be affected. The disease may be silent in the initial stages and may progress to acute or chronic renal failure with proteinuria.
- Gastrointestinal (GI) involvement—Ischemia involving the GI tract may result in abdominal pain, gastrointestinal bleeding, or may sometimes present as an acute abdomen. Splenic or pancreatic infarction can also occur. However, the liver is rarely involved.
- Ocular involvement—Retinal venous and arterial occlusion, amaurosis fugax, and anterior ischemic optic neuropathy can occur in patients with aPLs.
- Adrenal disease—Bilateral adrenal vein thrombosis, resulting in hemorrhagic infarction, may lead to loss of adrenal function. This may present as abdominal, lumbar, pelvic, or thoracic pain.

To summarize, the most common associations of APS include deep vein thrombosis, thrombocytopenia, pulmonary embolism, livedo reticularis, fetal loss, transient ischemic attacks, stroke, and superficial thrombophlebitis [4].

20.7 Catastrophic APS (CAPS)

The term "CAPS" is used for an accelerated form of APS in which the patients having aPLs present with coagulopathy and ischemic necrosis of the extremities.

The diagnostic and classification criteria for CAPS are as follows:

Criteria

1. Evidence of involvement of three or more organs, systems, and/or tissues
2. Development of manifestations simultaneously or within 1 week
3. Confirmation of small vessel occlusion in at least one organ or tissue, by histopathology
4. Laboratory confirmation of the presence of aPLs

Classification criteria

1. Definite CAPS
   - All four criteria present
2. Probable CAPS
   - All four criteria but with involvement of only two organs, systems, and/or tissues
   - All four criteria but with the absence of repeat detection of aPLs at least 12 weeks apart, due to the early death of a patient who had never been tested for aPLs before the CAPS event
   - Criteria 1, 2, and 4
   - Criteria 1, 3, and 4 and the development of a third event after more than 1 week but before 1 month, despite anticoagulation

CAPS develops in less than 1% of patients with APS. However, among these almost 50% do not have a prior diagnosis of APS [24].

In most of the cases of CAPS, a precipitating factor can be identified. The most common precipitating factors are infection and surgery.

The thrombotic manifestations of CAPS differ in their anatomical distribution. They manifest as small vessel occlusion and most commonly present with abdominal pain and intra-abdominal thrombosis. Systemic inflammatory response syndrome, which is triggered in response to the tissue necrosis from underlying small vessel occlusion, is an important feature of CAPS.

20.8   Treatment

Long-term anticoagulation with a vitamin K antagonist is the mainstay of therapy for thrombotic APS. However, this will not be able to prevent recurrent thrombosis in a significant proportion of patients.

20.8.1 Venous Thrombosis

Unfractionated heparin or low molecular weight heparin transitioned to warfarin is commonly used. A target international normalized ratio (INR) of 2.0–3.0 is recommended in such cases.

The duration of anticoagulation must be determined based upon the risk–benefit ratio of the individual patients, taking into account the risk of recurrent thrombosis, the likelihood of bleeding, and compliance [1]. Usually, the treatment has to be continued indefinitely.

If thrombosis develops in the setting of a reversible risk factor, and in patients who subsequently test negative for aPLs, short-term anticoagulation may be considered. This may also be advocated in children with APS, who have a lower risk of recurrent thrombosis compared with adults [25].

20.8.2 Arterial Thrombosis

Antiplatelet and anticoagulant therapy has to be usually continued indefinitely, for patients with APS and non-stroke arterial events. In patients with high-risk aPL profile and other cardiovascular risk factors, secondary prophylaxis can be considered, in case the potential benefits outweigh the risk of bleeding.

20.8.3 Non-anticoagulant Treatment of Thrombotic APS

New therapeutic approaches have been identified that may be useful in patients with recurrent thrombosis and underlying SLE. These include use of novel antiplatelet agents, inhibition of intracellular signaling pathways, and immunomodulatory therapies using B-cell-directed therapy, hydroxychloroquine, and statins.

20.8.4 CAPS

The treatment of CAPS is based on addressing thrombosis as well as inflammatory response. Complement-directed therapies, defibrotide, and plasma exchange have proved to be useful for treatment [26].

20.8.5 Approach to Asymptomatic Cases with Positive aPLs
(Fig. 20.2) [26]

Individuals who have not had prior episodes of thrombosis or pregnancy morbidity but demonstrate laboratory evidence of positive aPLs should be advised repeat testing for aPLs after a gap of at least 12 weeks. In such cases, if the repeat test is negative, no further evaluation is necessary. However, if the repeat test is positive, the individual should be labeled as having "persistent asymptomatic aPLs."

These individuals should be evaluated for the presence of other risk factors for thrombosis and associated autoimmune diseases to determine the need for initiation of primary prophylaxis. It is not advisable to administer primary prophylaxis in individuals without any other risk factors. Hydroxychloroquine and aspirin may be used in patients with SLE, and short-term anticoagulation may be considered during high-risk situations. However, prophylaxis with daily aspirin is recommended in individuals with cardiovascular risk factors.

20.9 Management During Pregnancy

The approach to antithrombotic treatment of pregnant women with APS varies depending on whether they have APS based on a prior thrombosis or an APS-associated pregnancy morbidity.

If only laboratory criteria for APS are present but no clinical criteria are seen, then low-dose aspirin will be sufficient for antepartum management.

In cases with APS based on laboratory criteria for aPLs and APS defining pregnancy morbidity of ≥1 fetal losses at ≥10 weeks of gestation or ≥3 unexplained consecutive spontaneous pregnancy losses <10 weeks of gestation with no history of arterial or venous thrombosis, prophylactic-dose low molecular weight heparin (LMWH) and low-dose aspirin should be administered in the antepartum period.

Women with APS by laboratory criteria for aPLs and a prior history of arterial or venous thrombosis are at high risk of recurrence. These cases are generally on an indefinite period of anticoagulation with warfarin, which

Fig. 20.2 Approach to the asymptomatic cases with aPLs

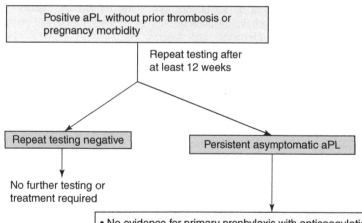

should be resumed postpartum. Heparin and warfarin are not contraindicated in breastfeeding mothers [27].

20.10 Conclusion

APS, a prothrombotic disorder, commonly manifests with venous and arterial thromboembolism and recurrent pregnancy loss. Variations in clinical associations and heterogeneity in antibodies that are essential for the diagnosis lead to the challenges in diagnosis and treatment of this entity. Further studies are necessary to refine our understanding of this entity, characterize thrombotic risk, and evaluate various modalities for therapy.

References

1. Lim W. Antiphospholipid Syndrome. Hematology. 2013;2013:675–80.
2. Arachchillage DRJ, Greaves M. The chequered history of the antiphospholipid syndrome. Br J Haematol. 2014;165:609–17.
3. Deka R, Saxena R. Antiphospholipid syndrome – revisited. In: Purohit A, Bohra GK, editors. Haematology pearls 2017. Jodhpur: Haematology Update 2017; 2017. p. 207–19.
4. Cervera R, Piette JC, Font J, Khamashta MA, Shoenfeld Y, et al. Antiphospholipid syndrome: clinical and immunologic manifestations and patterns of disease expression in a cohort of 1,000 patients. Arthritis Rheum. 2002;46:1019–27.
5. Miyakis S, Lockshin MD, Atsumi T, Branch DW, Brey RL, et al. International consensus statement on an update of the classification criteria for definite antiphospholipid syndrome (APS). J Thromb Haemost. 2006;4:295–306.
6. Pengo V, Banzato A, Denas G, Jose SP, Bison E, et al. Correct laboratory approach to APS diagnosis and monitoring. Autoimmun Rev. 2013;12:832–4.
7. Rand JH, Wolgast LR. Dos and don'ts in diagnosing antiphospholipid syndrome. Hematology. 2012;2012:455–9.
8. Bucciarelli S, Espinosa G, Cervera R. The CAPS Registry: morbidity and mortality of the catastrophic antiphospholipid syndrome. Lupus. 2009;18:905–12.
9. Urbanus RT, de Groot PG. Antiphospholipid antibodies: we are not quite there yet. Blood Rev. 2011;25:97–106.
10. Brouwer JL, Bijl M, Veeger NJ, Kluin-Nelemans HC, van der Meer J. The contribution of inherited and acquired thrombophilic defects, alone or combined with antiphospholipid antibodies, to venous and arterial thromboembolism in patients with systemic lupus erythematosus. Blood. 2004;104:143–8.
11. Arad A, Proulle V, Furie RA, Furie BC, Furie B. β2-glycoprotein-1 autoantibodies from patients with antiphospholipid syndrome are sufficient to potentiate arterial thrombus formation in a mouse model. Blood. 2011;117:3453–9.
12. de Laat B, Derksen RH, van Lummel M, Pennings MT, de Groot PG. Pathogenic anti-beta2-glycoprotein I antibodies recognize domain I of beta2-glycoprotein I only after a conformational change. Blood. 2006;107:1916–24.
13. de Groot PG, Meijers JC. β(2)-Glycoprotein I: evolution, structure and function. J Thromb Haemost. 2011;9:1275–84.
14. Canaud G, Bienaimé F, Tabarin F, Bataillon G, Seilhean D. Inhibition of the mTORC pathway in the antiphospholipid syndrome. N Engl J Med. 2014;371:303–12.
15. Liestøl S, Sandset PM, Mowinckel MC, Wisløff F. Activated protein C resistance determined with a thrombin generation-based test is associated with thrombotic events in patients with lupus anticoagulants. J Thromb Haemost. 2007;5:2204–11.
16. Dignat-George F, Camoin-Jau L, Sabatier F, Arnoux D, Anfosso F, et al. Endothelial microparticles: a potential contribution to the thrombotic complications of the antiphospholipid syndrome. Thromb Haemost. 2004;91:667–73.
17. Mok CC, Tang S, To C, Petri M. Incidence and risk factors of thromboembolism in systemic lupus erythematosus: a comparison of three ethnic groups. Arthritis Rheum. 2005;52:2774–82.
18. Yetman DL, Kutteh WH. Antiphospholipid antibody panels and recurrent pregnancy loss: prevalence of anticardiolipin antibodies compared with other antiphospholipid antibodies. Fertil Steril. 1996;66:540–6.
19. Pengo V, Ruffatti A, Legnani C, Gresele P, Barcellona D, et al. Clinical course of high-risk patients diagnosed with antiphospholipid syndrome. J Thromb Haemost. 2010;8:237–42.
20. Muscal E, Brey RL. Neurologic manifestations of the antiphospholipid syndrome: integrating molecular and clinical lessons. Curr Rheumatol Rep. 2008;10:67.
21. Uthman I, Godeau B, Taher A, Khamashta M. The hematologic manifestations of the antiphospholipid syndrome. Blood Rev. 2008;22:187–94.
22. Denas G, Jose SP, Bracco A, Zoppellaro G, Pengo V. Antiphospholipid syndrome and the heart: a case series and literature review. Autoimmun Rev. 2015;14:214–22.
23. Francès C, Niang S, Laffitte E, Pelletier F, Costedoat N, et al. Dermatologic manifestations of the antiphospholipid syndrome: two hundred consecutive cases. Arthritis Rheum. 2005;52:1785–93.
24. Cervera R, Bucciarelli S, Plasin MA, Gómez-Puerta JA, Plaza J, et al. Catastrophic antiphospholipid syn-

drome (CAPS): descriptive analysis of a series of 280 patients from the "CAPS Registry". J Autoimmun. 2009;32:240–5.

25. Hunt BJ. Pediatric antiphospholipid antibodies and antiphospholipid syndrome. Semin Thromb Hemost. 2008;34:274–81.

26. Chaturvedi S, McCrae KR. The antiphospholipid syndrome: still an enigma. Hematology. 2015;2015:53–60.

27. Lockwood CJ, Lockshin MD. Management of antiphospholipid syndrome in pregnant and postpartum women. In: Berghella V, Pisetsky DS, editors. UpToDate. Waltham: UpToDate; 2017.

Seema Tyagi, Debdas Bose, and Prasad Dange

21.1 Introduction

The term thrombophilia (or hypercoagulability) denotes the presence of risk factors for the development of venous or/and arterial thrombosis. It could be inherited or acquired defect of haemostatic system [1].

In USA, the incidence is 1.92/1000 person-years, and it constitutes 1% of all hospital admissions. The global disease burden is 0.75–2.69/1000 individuals in population. Incidence of venous thrombo-embolism (VTE) is difficult to estimate, and studies regarding Indian data are few. In a study from a teaching hospital in south India, the incidence is 17.4 cases per 10,000 person admitted in hospital. However, it is less in general population. Malignancy and surgery were the prominent predisposing factors [2]. However, being a tertiary care institute, the incidence and distribution of cases may not be representative of the general population.

Thrombophilia, inherited or acquired, is among the various factors that predispose to VTE. This chapter mainly deals with inherited thrombophilia testing along with antiphospholipid syndrome which is an important acquired thrombophilic condition.

21.2 Pathophysiology

Thrombus formation involves activation of platelets followed by the activation of coagulation cascade. The inhibitory pathway involving antithrombin and protein C regulates the coagulation cascade (Fig. 21.1). Simultaneously, fibrinolytic system (plasminogen and tissue plasminogen activator) with anti-fibrinolytic (plasminogen activator inhibitor) system helps to control excess thrombus formation and in recanalization.

Venous thrombi consist of fibrin, red cells, platelets, and leucocytes [3]. In 1854, German pathologist Rudolph Virchow postulated his famous Virchow triad comprising abnormal blood flow, endothelial injury and hypercoagulability. Abnormal blood flow occurs typically in the setting of hypertension, venous stasis hyperviscosity, etc. Endothelial injury, as a cause of thrombosis, occurs in a variety of settings like atherosclerosis, hyperhomocysteinemia, infections, toxins, etc. These factors, either independently or often in combination, precipitate thrombosis (Fig. 21.2).

The haemostatic system consists of endothelium, platelets, coagulation factors, natural anticoagulants, fibrinolytic and antifibrinolytic proteins. Normal haemostasis is achieved by maintaining a delicate balance between the procoagulant and anticoagulant factors (Fig. 21.3). Overactivity of the procoagulant factors or defect in the fibrinolytic system tilts the balance in

S. Tyagi (✉) · D. Bose · P. Dange
Department of Hematology, AIIMS, New Delhi, India

© Springer Nature Singapore Pte Ltd. 2019
R. Saxena, H. P. Pati (eds.), *Hematopathology*, https://doi.org/10.1007/978-981-13-7713-6_21

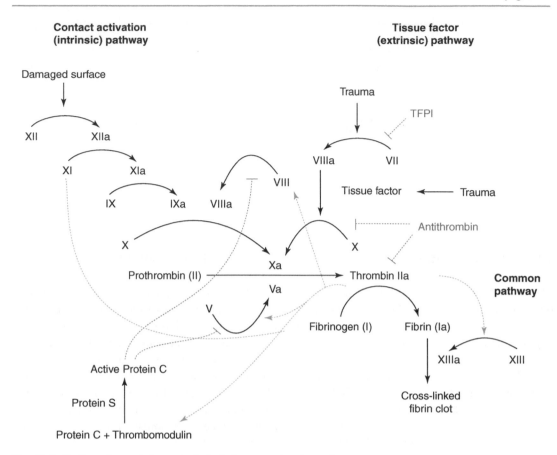

Fig. 21.1 Outline of coagulation cascade including natural anticoagulants

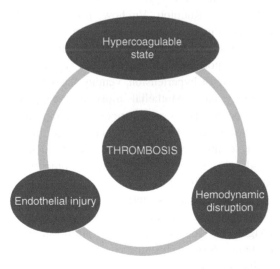

Fig. 21.2 The three components of the Virchow's triad

favour of thrombosis. These defects may be inherited or acquired, secondary to variety of illnesses.

Thrombophilia (or hypercoagulability) is an inherited or acquired defect in haemostatic system that predisposes to venous or/and arterial thrombosis. Given below is a list of some common causes of thrombophilia that disturbs the delicate balance of the haemostatic system. It is important to remember that many of the conditions can be thrombogenic by more than one mechanism. For example in cancer patients, stasis (due to immobility), endothelial injury (due to infections, chemo-radiotherapy, etc.) and hypercoagulability (secretion of procoagulant molecules by tumour cells) all contribute to VTE.

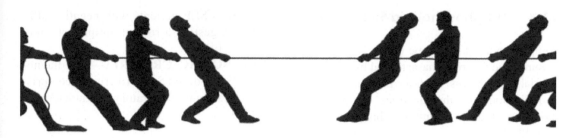

Pro coagulant like platelets, coagulation factors, anti-fibrinolytics

Anti coagulant like protein C, AT, fibrinolytics

Fig. 21.3 Normal hemostasis is achieved by a delicate balance of the two tendencies. Imbalance leads to thrombophilia

Inherited Thrombophilia
1. Protein C, protein S deficiency
2. Antithrombin (formerly called as antithrombin III) deficiency
3. Activated protein C resistance and factor V Leiden mutation
4. Prothrombin G20210A mutation
5. Hyperhomocysteinaemia (may also be acquired)
6. Others like elevated factor VIII level, plasminogen deficiency, tissue plasminogen activator deficiency, tissue factor pathway inhibitor, etc.

Acquired Thrombophilia
1. Antiphospholipid syndrome (APS)
2. Myeloproliferative neoplasm
3. Paroxysmal nocturnal haemoglobinuria (PNH)
4. Immobilisation, fracture, prolonged surgery
5. Oestrogen therapy (including contraceptive pills), pregnancy
6. Nephrotic syndrome
7. Cancer

Certain authors classify the inherited thrombophilia into weak and strong thrombophilia based on the risk of thrombosis. Weak thrombophilia has minimal risk for venous thrombo-embolism (VTE) events while strong thrombophilia poses signifi-

cant risk for VTE. Strong thrombophilia includes homozygous factor V Leiden, protein C and S deficiency, AT deficiency and APS [4]. However, since VTE is multifactorial disease, there are considerable overlaps in this risk classification and hence this classification, though sometimes a useful guide for management is not universally followed.

Clinical presentation—Inherited thrombophilias are predominantly associated with venous thrombo-embolism events. Factor V Leiden has slightly increased risk for arterial thrombosis However, no consistent association has been found [5]. Antiphospholipid syndrome (APS), on the other hand, is an important acquired predisposing condition for both venous and arterial thrombosis.

Pregnancy-related complications are another important presentation of APS as well as the inherited thrombophilias. These include recurrent pregnancy loss, pregnancy-induced hypertension, etc. However, studies have failed to find significant association between inherited thrombophilia and pregnancy outcomes [6].

Clinical indicators for thrombophilia include young age at presentation (usually <40 years), strong family history, unusual site of thrombosis, VTE either unprovoked or after weak provoking situations [7].

21.3   Antiphospholipid Syndrome

Antiphospholipid syndrome (APS) is a systemic autoimmune disorder characterised by venous or arterial thrombosis and/or pregnancy-related complications in the presence of persistent laboratory evidence of antiphospholipid antibodies (aPL) [8].

Pathophysiology—APS is caused by the presence of circulating anticoagulant antibodies. Though associated with thrombosis, in vitro testing shows prolonged aPTT, hence the name. These antibodies bind to the phospholipid complex causing a pro-thrombotic state. Recent studies have shown that these antibodies act through multiple mechanisms and result in inflammation, vasculopathy, and thrombosis [9]. Many different antibodies are implicated, some of them include anti-cardiolipin (aCL), anti-beta-2 glycoprotein-1 (anti-B2GP1), anti-prothrombin and anti-annexin V antibody. aCL and anti-B2GP1 are the most significant ones.

Clinical presentation—APS may be primary or may be associated with a connective tissue disease like SLE, Sjogren's syndrome, etc. [10]. In either case, major manifestations of APS can be conveniently described as follows [9, 11]:

Thrombotic—Venous (e.g. DVT, pulmonary embolism), arterial (stroke, transient ischaemic attack, etc.) or microcirculation thrombosis. One particular microvessel thrombotic complication is termed catastrophic APS characterised by widespread small vessel thrombosis, sometimes mimicking DIC [10].

Obstetric—These include recurrent pregnancy loss, prematurity and pre-eclampsia.

Non-thrombotic—These are less recognised manifestations and include thrombocytopenia, haemolytic anaemia, renal impairment, thrombotic microangiopathy, cardiac valve thickening, cognitive impairment and livedo reticularis. These complications may represent the complications of underlying connective tissue disease. However, these are usually more common in the aPL-positive SLE patients as compared to SLE patients with negative aPL, thereby suggesting a role of antiphospholipid antibodies [9].

DIAGNOSTIC CRITERIA—For diagnosis of APS, modified Sapporo criteria comprising clinical and laboratory parameters is used [12].

21.4   Clinical

21.4.1 Vascular Thrombosis

Unequivocally diagnosed (by imaging or histopathology) one or more episodes of thrombosis (arterial, venous or small vessel). In tissue section, thrombosis should not be accompanied by inflammation in the vessel wall. However, superficial vein thrombosis is excluded from the criteria.

Pregnancy Morbidity

(a) One or more unexplained pregnancy loss beyond 10th week in an otherwise morphologically normal foetus OR

(b) One or more premature births (before 34 weeks) attributable to either eclampsia/pre-eclampsia or accompanied by placental insufficiency OR

(c) Three or more unexplained consecutive pregnancy loss before 10 weeks

Laboratory

1. Positive for lupus anticoagulant (LA) on two occasions at least 12 weeks apart

2. Anti-cardiolipin antibody, IgG and/or IgM isotype present in medium to high titre (i.e. >40 GPL or MPL, or more than the 99th percentile), on two occasions tested at least 12 weeks apart

3. Anti-beta-2 glycoprotein-I (anti-B2GP1) antibody, IgG and/or IgM isotype, in titre more than the 99th percentile, present on two or more occasions, at least 12 weeks apart.

For APS diagnosis, at least one of the clinical criteria and one of the laboratory criteria must be met.

ASSOCIATIONS—Many different conditions may give rise to circulating aPL. These conditions include:

1. Primary APS
2. Autoimmune diseases like SLE, RA and others. In one study [8], aPL profile has been detected in approximately 30% of patients with SLE. However, mere presence of aPL on screening should not be diagnosed as APS unless the clinical criteria are also fulfilled.
3. Transient antibodies due to drugs (like phenytoin, quinine, amoxicillin, propranolol, etc.).
4. Infections including bactrial, viral as well as parasitic.
5. Malignancy including haematopoietc as well as solid organ malignancy
6. Asymptomatic individuals.

Due to numerous associations, laboratory testing for APS should be undertaken only under appropriate clinical settings. Generalised testing performed on asymptomatic individuals is highly discouraged to avoid false-positive results. Also, in view of conditions with transient antibodies, a positive result must be repeated at least 12 weeks after the initial testing.

The appropriateness to search for LA can be graded according to clinical characteristics into low, moderate and high.

Low: venous (VTE) or arterial thromboembolism in elderly patients.

Moderate: accidentally found prolonged aPTT in asymptomatic subjects, recurrent spontaneous early pregnancy loss, provoked VTE in young patients.

High: unprovoked VTE and (unexplained) arterial thrombosis in young patients (<50 years of age), thrombosis at unusual sites, late pregnancy loss, any thrombosis or pregnancy morbidity in patients with autoimmune diseases [12].

21.5 Laboratory Testing

Laboratory testing includes LA testing as well as aCL and anti-B2GP1 antibody. These tests are complementary since all are not positive in a given patient. Hence, LA testing as well as antibody detection is necessary to avoid false-negative laboratory testing.

aCL and anti-B2GP1 antibody titre are measured by ELISA. The cutoff values may differ according to the kit used. IgG and IgM antibodies are usually measured. There is no compelling evidence to include IgA isotype of these antibodies in the routine diagnostic workup for APS. However, the Systemic Lupus International Collaborating Clinics (SLICC) revised classification criteria for SLE include IgA isotype of aCL and anti-B2GP1 as part of the definition of aPL positivity as IgA isotype is more common in SLE patients. Antibodies such as antiprothrombin antibodies and others are not used routinely because of lack of standardisation and uncertainty about their clinical significance [13].

LA testing, on the other hand, is a two-step procedure.

1. Screening test—Demonstration of a prolonged phospholipid-dependent screening test like aPTT or dilute Russel viper venom test (dRVVT). It may also involve mixing patient plasma with normal plasma. Kaolin clotting time testing is based on the mixing principle.
2. Confirmatory test—Addition of excess phospholipid shortens or corrects the prolonged coagulation test (demonstration of phospholipid dependence).
3. Recent guidelines do not prefer mixing studies as mixing may dilute the LA in cases with low titre leading to false-negative results [14].

Two tests should be used for LA screening to enhance sensitivity. dRVVT is the choice for the first test. Second test is usually lupus-sensitive aPTT. Any one positive result should be considered as positive for LA. Positive screening should be confirmed by confirmatory assay. Kaolin clotting time, dilute PT and ecarin venom-based assays are not recommended [15].

A brief description of the commonly employed tests is given below:

(a) PTT-LA—Routinely used aPTT is not sensitive for LA. PTT-LA is a modified aPTT with low content of phospholipid (cephalin) derived from rabbit brain and silica as the activator. Low phospholipid makes it more sensitive for LA. Factor deficiency and anticoagulants may give false-positive results.

(b) dRVVT—As it involves direct activation of factor X, effect of deficiency of some of the factors is eliminated. Also, dilution of both the venom and phospholipid makes it very sensitive and the screening test of choice. Result is often expressed as a ratio between dRVVT of the test and normal pooled plasma (ratio = test/pooled plasma).

(c) Confirmatory assay—Addition of excess phospholipid (derived from platelets) to aPTT- or dRVVT-based assays leads to saturation of the LA, thereby correcting the prolonged clotting time. Coagulation factor defects or a very high titre of LA will lead to negative test result. Mixing study is useful in such instances [14].

Summary
1. APS is an acquired thrombophilia for which both clinical and laboratory criteria must be satisfied.
2. Lab testing for APS includes LA testing along with aCL and anti-B2GP1 testing.
3. These tests may be transiently positive in many other circumstances as well. Hence, a repeat testing after 12 weeks is necessary
4. Not every positive aPL test result is clinically significant. The interpretation of 'clinically significant aPL positivity' should take into account the type, isotype, titre, persistency and the number of positive aPL tests.

21.6 Factor V Leiden and Activated Protein C Resistance

Factor V Leiden (FVL) results from a single point mutation in the factor V gene leading to replacement of arginine with glutamine at amino acid 506 (FVA506G) resulting in alteration of the cleavage site for aPC in factor V and factor Va. Normally, aPC cleavage of the procoagulant factor Va causes factor Va degradation and cleavage of factor V increases factor V function which acts as a cofactor in degradation of factor Va and VIIIa. FVL (mutated form) is insensitive to both of these cleavages because it lacks the Arg506 cleavage site. Because activated FVL are not cleaved, they are available for continued thrombin generation [16].

The FVL mutation accounts for more than 95% cases of hereditary aPC resistance, with the remainder of aPC resistance cases being due to other inherited mutations and acquired factors. Other causes of aPC resistance include Factor V Cambridge (replacement of Arg306 with threonine), Factor V Nara (replacement of Trp1920 with arginine), Factor V Liverpool (replacement of Ile359 with threonine), Factor V Bonn (replacement of Ala512 with valine) and Factor V Hong Kong (replacement of Arg306 with glycine).

FVL is an autosomal dominant condition with 99% heterozygotes and 1% homozygotes, and rarely with pseudo-homozygosity due to a mutation on the other allele causing factor V deficiency in heterozygotes [17].

21.7 Clinical Manifestations

Factor V Leiden mutation is associated with venous thrombo-embolism and also implicated in arterial thrombosis and some cases of unexplained recurrent late pregnancy loss. Homozygous individuals are at a higher risk for VTE as compared to the heterozygous individuals [18].

Diagnostic tests—Diagnostic testing includes the functional assays and the genetic testing for the mutation.

Functional assays—It is based on the inhibition of factor V (in the test plasma) by the exogenously added aPC leading to prolongation of aPTT. The result is expressed as a ratio of aPTT to aPTT without added aPC. A modified method involves dilution with factor V-deficient plasma to normalise and controls the levels of other coagulation factor except factor V [19].

Presence of LA and anticoagulant therapy can cause false-positive results.

Mutation testing—The FVL mutation can be detected directly by analysing genomic DNA from peripheral blood cells by polymerase chain reaction (PCR). The principle used is restriction fragment length polymorphism (RFLP). The amplified factor V gene product is treated with restriction enzymes. Mutation results in loss of the cleavage site for the enzyme, resulting in different amplification products as compared to the normal individuals [20]. The amplification products are analysed by agarose gel electrophoresis.

Genetic testing is unaffected by anticoagulants and other drugs. However, it does not detect other acquired or hereditary causes of aPC resistance like variant genotypes. It can be done in following situation:

1. For individuals with a family history of FVL who require testing, genetic testing is preferable because it provides definitive evidence of the mutation.
2. For individuals with lupus anticoagulant or those who are on anticoagulants which might interfere with the results (e.g. direct thrombin inhibitor, direct factor Xa inhibitor), genetic testing will circumvent these potential sources of test interference.
3. For individuals who have a positive functional assay for aPC resistance, to confirm the diagnosis and to determine if the patient is homozygous or heterozygous for the FVL mutation.

21.8 Antithrombin Deficiency

Antithrombin (AT), with heparin as its co-factor, regulates coagulation by inactivating thrombin and other procoagulant enzymes, including factors Xa, IXa, XIa and XIIa (Fig. 21.1).

AT deficiency is manifested primarily by recurrent VTE. Heparin resistance is another possible manifestation of AT deficiency.

AT deficiency may be in the form of reduced levels (type 1) or in the form of structural defect (type 2). Most AT-deficient patients are heterozygotes; homozygous AT deficiency is believed to be fatal in utero [21–23].

Numerous acquired conditions may cause AT deficiency including pre-eclampsia, surgery, massive venous thrombosis, heparin therapy, renal and hepatic diseases, etc. These conditions must be ruled out before testing for AT [21].

21.9 Laboratory Diagnosis

The types of tests available for AT assay are described below. The chromogenic assays are the most preferred ones [20].

1. Chromogenic method—Test plasma is incubated with excess thrombin and added heparin. The AT will neutralise the thrombin. In next step, the residual thrombin is quantitated by its amidolytic action on a chromogenic substrate added. Thus, the amount of residual thrombin measured is inversely proportional to the plasma AT level. Newer assays use enzymatic activity of factor X instead of thrombin.
2. Immunogenic assay—For example Laurell rocket immunoelectrophoresis, microlatex-particle immunoassay, radial immunodiffusion or enzyme-linked immunosorbent assay (ELISA) methods.
3. Clotting based assay—It is based on the ability of AT to neutralise exogenously added thrombin leading to prolongation of the clotting time.

21.10 Hyperhomocysteinaemia

INTRODUCTION—Homocysteine is an intermediate metabolite in the methionine pathway. The transsulphuration of homocysteine to cysteine is by cystathionine-beta-synthase with the help of pyridoxal phosphate (vitamin B6) as a cofactor. Remethylation of homocysteine produces methionine by methionine synthase or by betaine-homocysteine methyltransferase. Vitamin B12 (cobalamin) is the precursor of methylcobalamin, which is the cofactor for methionine synthase.

Many conditions like genetic defects in enzyme, vitamin/folate deficiency, drugs (like nicotinic acid, fibrates), cigarette smoking and chronic kidney disease may cause hyperhomocysteinaemia.

The most common form of genetic hyperhomocysteinaemia is due to substitution of cytosine to thymine at nucleotide 677 producing a thermolabile variant of methylene tetrahydrofolate reductase enzyme (MTHFR) with reduced enzymatic activity. Homozygosity causes mildly elevated plasma homocysteine levels in the general population, often occurring in association with low serum folate levels [24, 25].

Pathophysiology—High homocysteine levels appear to be clearly associated with an increased risk of cardiovascular and cerebrovascular disease. Patients with the MTHFR TT genotype have a higher chance of having coronary heart disease compared with controls. Risk for recurrent VTE and obstetric complications is also increased There are multiple mechanisms by which homocysteine may induce vascular injury like endothelial cell desquamation, low-density lipoprotein (LDL) oxidation, increased thrombin generation, monocyte adhesion to endothelium and factor V activation. Platelet aggregation is also enhanced, probably secondary to endothelial damage [26–28].

LABORATORY   DIAGNOSIS—Total plasma homocysteine concentration is measured by ELISA. Rapid separation of the plasma is required because homocysteine quickly leaks out of red blood cells.

Approximately 75–85% is protein-bound and 15–25% found in free forms. Normal homocysteine concentrations range between 5 and 15 μmol/ L. Hyperhomocysteinaemia has been classified as moderate (15–30 μmol/L), intermediate (30–100 μmol/L) and severe (>100 μmol/L) [29].

Oral methionine challenge may be helpful in diagnosis in some cases, particularly with cystathionine-beta-synthase deficiency [30].

21.10.1 Protein C

Protein C (PC) is a vitamin K-dependent anticoagulant protein synthesised in the liver. After activation by thrombin, activated Protein C (aPc) inactivates coagulation factors Va and VIIIa with the help of cofactor Protein S (Fig. 21.1). It is transmitted as an autosomal dominant disorder, most individuals being heterozygous for the defect causing deficiency in the form of reduced protein C level (type 1) or of reduced protein C function (type 2) [31].

PC levels in healthy adults are normally distributed, with 95% of the values ranging from 70% to 140% of normal. Among randomly selected healthy adults, the prevalence of deficiency is about 0.2–0.5% while it is found in 2–5% of VTE patients [32].

Clinical Presentation—Due to varied mutations, the deficient patients may have varied presentation ranging from asymptomatic adults at one end to purpurafulminans in the severely deficient babies. In between are the individuals with increased risk for venous thrombo-embolism or for warfarin-induced skin necrosis. Neonatal purpurafulminans occurs in severely deficient neonates and is characterised by widespread arterial and venous thrombosis mimicking DIC. It is a potentially fatal condition unless promptly treated. Warfarin-induced skin necrosis occurs in deficient individuals who started on warfarin without any bridging parenteral anticoagulation [33].

Laboratory testing—The laboratory testing may be done by ELISA or a chromogenic assay.

Chromogenic method: PC is converted into its active form by venom of a copperhead snake *Agkistrodon contortrix* (Protac). Activated PC cleaves a specific chromogenic substrate and releases p-nitro-alanine which is measured in a spectrometer at 405 nm.

Immunological assay: may also be carried out with an ELISA-based kit which will distinguish between type 1 and type 2 deficiencies.

Clotting-based protein C assay: PC clotting assays use a modified APTT.

Diagnostic pitfalls—Circulating levels of protein C may be reduced in liver diseases such as right heart failure with hepatic congestion, severe liver disease or disseminated intravascular coagulation, and in acute inflammation/infections, trauma/surgery or acute respiratory distress syndrome, uraemia, cancer and vitamin K deficiency/warfarin therapy.

Causes of increased protein C—nephrotic syndrome, hyperlipidemia and normal ageing.

- Type II—Type II deficiency (normal total and free protein S; reduced protein S function) is rare (qualitative defect).
- Type III—Selectively reduced free protein S and protein S function; normal total protein S.

For patients who have had a VTE or those with a strong family history of VTE, plasma levels of total or free protein S antigen less than 60–65 international units/dL are considered to be in the deficient range. For individuals who are asymptomatic or who have a first VTE in the absence of a strong family history, lower levels of free protein S (e.g. <33 units/dL) are more predictive for an increased risk of VTE.

Clinical presentation—Since it is a co-factor for protein C, the deficiency of protein S has similar clinical presentation to protein C deficiency.

21.10.2 Protein S

Pathophysiology—Protein S is named for Seattle, Washington, where it was originally discovered. Protein S is synthesised by hepatocytes, endothelial cells and megakaryocytes. Protein S is the co-factor for protein C that inactivates factor V and VIII (Fig. 21.1).

Protein S circulates in two states: free and bound to the complement component C4b-binding protein. The free form comprises 30–40% of total protein S and is the active form.

Total protein S levels change with age, but free protein S levels remain constant. In healthy neonates, free protein S predominates and functional protein S levels are only slightly reduced compared with those in adults [34–36]. It is an autosomal dominant condition due to mutations in the PROS1 gene on chromosome 3. Inherited protein S deficiency can be subdivided according to whether the abnormality affects total protein S level, free protein S level, and/or protein S function [37]:

- Type I—Type I deficiency (reduced total protein S, free protein S and protein S function) is the classic type of inherited protein S deficiency.

21.11 Laboratory Testing

Protein S level may be determined by ELISA or by using the functional assay.

ELISA—Using specific monoclonal antibodies, free as well as total protein S can be measured using ELISA. However, measurement of free protein S is preferred since it is the functional form. Earlier assays used polyethylene glycol precipitation to remove protein S bound to C4b-binding protein [38].

Functional assay—Dilute normal and test plasmas with commercially available PS-deficient plasma. Then a reagent containing factor Xa, APC and phospholipid is mixed. After a 5 min incubation, calcium chloride is added and clot formation is noted. Under these conditions, the prolongation of the clotting time is directly proportional to the concentration of PS in the patient plasma (e.g. Staclot). The use of factor Xa as the activator minimises the potential interference by high levels of factor VIII. It may also be based on the PT, in which case the effect of factor VIII is bypassed. Because the assays are subject to interference by other plasma factors, it is recommended that the test plasma be assayed at two different dilutions to ensure parallelism with the standard curve.

Potential pitfalls—Low levels of PS may be an acquired phenomenon during pregnancy, oral anticoagulation, nephrotic syndrome, use of oral contraceptives, systemic lupus erythematosus, human immunodeficiency virus (HIV) infection and liver disease. Catastrophically low levels have been reported in children after varicella infection owing to auto-antibody production.

In addition, the functional assays are prone to confounding by other factors: factor V Leiden (FVL), LAC and levels of other coagulation factors.

21.12 Prothrombin G20210A Mutation

Prothrombin G20210A mutation is seen more commonly in the Caucasian population. It is infrequent in the Asians [39].

Prothrombin G20210A mutation—The G20210A mutation results from a substitution of adenine (A) for guanine (G) at position 20,210 in a non-coding region of the prothrombin gene, causing base pair change in the terminal nucleotide of the 3′ untranslated region of the gene responsible for polyadenylation of messenger RNA. The mutation is considered a gain-of-function mutation because it increases prothrombin biosynthesis and also increases its stability [35].

Most individuals with the mutation are heterozygous. Transmission is considered to be autosomal dominant. Heterozygotes for the G20210A mutation have approximately 30% higher plasma prothrombin levels than controls. Homozygotes have even higher levels. However, prothrombin levels cannot be used to make the diagnosis, because there is overlap with the normal range and the coefficient of variation in coagulation assays is relatively large.

Other prothrombin gene variants include prothrombin Yukuhashi and C20209T [40].

DIAGNOSIS—Polymerase chain reaction on peripheral blood is the most straightforward and cost-effective genetic test for the G20210A mutation. The presence of the mutation is detected using restriction enzyme digestion with electro-phoresis or an enzyme-based immunoassay. Some laboratories use multiplex PCR to identify the prothrombin G20210A mutation and the factor V Leiden mutation in the same reaction [41, 42].

21.13 Special Circumstances

Isolated distal DVT—Almost every case of DVT starts in calf veins and then extend proximally. However, for cases with thrombosis confined to calf veins, the risk of extension into proximal veins and pulmonary embolism is low. Only about 15–25% of symptomatic distal DVT will extend to proximal vein [43].

Only the cases with severe symptoms or with high risk for extension into proximal veins should be treated. Other patients are serially monitored with Doppler ultrasound examination for extension into proximal veins. The risk factors for extension include positive D-dimer, extensive involvement of calf veins, no reversible provoking factor, active cancer, past history of VTE and inpatient status [44]. If treatment is indicated, treatment approach for distal DVT is same as that for proximal vein DVT.

Superficial vein thrombosis—Lower limb followed by upper limb are the commonest sites for SVT. The risk factors for superficial vein thrombosis are very similar to those for DVT and include conditions like trauma, immobility, surgery, pregnancy as well as thrombophilia [45]. In fact, systematic review by Leon et al has found that though variable, in a significant number of cases, the SVT may co-exist or propagate to a DVT and may even give rise to PE. However, it is not known whether the PE arises from the SVT or from its extension into deep vein [46]. However, secondary causes like varicose veins, malignancy (e.g. Trousseau syndrome), autoimmune disease need to be excluded.

A case of SVT needs ultrasound evaluation to rule out co-existing DVT. There is no agreed upon therapy for SVT. However, it is now agreed that at least the high-risk patients like those involving at least 5 cm of the vein, presence of thrombus near sapheno-femoral junction, etc.

need anticoagulation. NSAIDs may be used in other patients who are not anticoagulated [46]. Prospective studies addressing issues like duration of anticoagulation, thrombophilia testing in isolated SVT are lacking.

Thrombosis at unusual sites—Abdominal vein thrombosis, cerebral vein and cortical vein thrombosis are some unusual sites for thrombosis and are often a suggestive feature for underlying thrombophilia. Infections, myeloproliferative neoplasms, PNH, cirrhosis (for abdominal vein thrombosis), oestrogen therapy/OC pills (for cerebral vein thrombosis), however, are important secondary causes that must be ruled out. On the contrary, other unusual sites like upper extremity vein, retinal vein thrombosis are not strongly associated with thrombophilia. PE however may occur with upper limb venous thrombosis [47].

Management of these conditions is by anticoagulation. However, for incidentally detected abdominal vein thrombosis, anticoagulation is not recommended [44]. Also, duration for anticoagulation is controversial, especially when no secondary cause like PNH or MPN is found. Thus, thrombophilia testing is often advocated. If positive, such patients may be prescribed indefinite anticoagulation.

21.14 Management of Thrombosis

Management of venous thrombosis can be discussed under the following headings:

1. Initial phase and long-term anticoagulation
2. Risk assessment for recurrence
3. Extended anticoagulation
4. Anticoagulant agents
5. Indication for thrombophilia testing

Initial and long-term anticoagulation therapy—Anticoagulation with oral anticoagulant (vitamin K antagonist, VKA) is the mainstay of treatment for all DVT patients irrespective of the underlying provoking factor. Since VKA has a slow onset of action, fast-acting parenteral anticoagulation with heparins is simultaneously administered for initial 5–7 days till the INR value reaches between 2 and 3 for 2 consecutive days. Anticoagulant therapy should be initiated even in patients with moderate to high suspicion of VTE for whom the investigation reports are pending. Low molecular weight heparins (LMWH), unless contraindicated, are now chosen over unfractionated heparin (UFH) for the parenteral therapy because of the safety profile. If used, UFH may be given subcutaneously or intravenously. The dosage for UFH is monitored by using heparin-sensitive aPTT corresponding to 0.3—0.7 U/mL. LMWH usually do not need laboratory monitoring, and once daily dosing is sufficient.

The initial treatment can be carried out on outpatient basis if the patient is otherwise healthy and has easy access to hospital emergency services. Certain guidelines like PESI score, Hestia criteria are useful while deciding for outpatient therapy [48]. Other treatment options like thrombolytic therapy, catheter-directed or operative thrombectomy, IVC filters are used in a certain special circumstances only and are not included in the routine management of VTE.

Initial anticoagulation should be completed within 5–7 days. Once the INR is stabilised in the therapeutic range, the parenteral anticoagulant is discontinued. Long-term anticoagulation with oral anticoagulant is continued for 3 months.

Thrombophilia status usually has no effect on initial and long-term phase with possible exception of protein C/S and AT deficiency. In protein C/S deficiency, due to the possibility of warfarin-induced skin necrosis, warfarin is either avoided in favour of newer anticoagulant (DOAC) or administered with a lower starting dose and a longer overlap with parenteral anticoagulation. AT deficiency may cause heparin resistance rarely and AT replacement or use of direct thrombin inhibitor might be considered. However, in cases with first episode of VTE, thrombophilia status is often unknown.

Risk assessment for recurrence—Once the long-term anticoagulation is complete at 3 months, patient risk assessment for recurrence is the most crucial step in deciding the further anticoagulation. Patients with high risk of recurrence usually need extended (often indefinite) anticoagulation. For example, recurrence following transient strong provoking factors is only 1% after 1 year and 3% at 5 years after stopping therapy [49]. Extended anticoagulation is not warranted in these cases. On the other hand, risk following unprovoked DVT 10% at 1 year and 30% at 5 year [50]. Thus, unprovoked DVT patients need extended anticoagulation. Hence, active search should be made for provoking factors before labelling a DVT episode as 'unprovoked'. Overall, male sex, unprovoked DVT, pulmonary embolism, past history of DVT are predictors of higher risk for recurrence.

Various scoring systems have been proposed for risk assessment. They consider various parameters for risk assessment and help decide the duration for anticoagulation. DASH score includes four parameters—D-dimer at 1 month after stopping anticoagulation, age, sex, hormone use during VTE [51]. Vienna model is another such score that includes sex, location of VTE along with D-dimer measured at 3–15 months after stopping anticoagulation [52]. However, APS and AT deficiency patients were excluded while formulating DASH score, and all the thrombophilia patients were excluded for Vienna predicting model, making them suboptimal for decision-making in patients with thrombophilia. Though none of the scoring models include thrombophilia as a parameter, it is still considered by many while deciding the duration for anticoagulation.

Apart from risk of recurrence, risk of bleeding due to anticoagulant and patient choice are other important factors under consideration. Risk factors for bleeding include old age, liver or renal dysfunction, wide fluctuations in INR during therapy, other co-morbidities like diabetes, malignancy, simultaneous anti-platelet agents, alcohol abuse, etc. [53]. Patient's informed choice whether to continue or discontinue the therapy despite the risk of recurrence is another important factor.

Thus, the risk of recurrence needs to be balanced with the risk of bleeding and patient's choice while deciding the duration of anticoagulation (Fig. 21.4). Thrombophilia status is at best a moderate indicator for risk of recurrence [4]. However, it does enable the patient and the treating physician to decide further anticoagulation when the other factors are indeterminate. For example, positive thrombophilia status in a DVT patient following minor provoking factors like oral contraceptive (OC), minor surgery, and short-duration immobilisation may tilt the balance in favour of extended anticoagulation. Thrombophilia testing and its impact in various scenarios are described in detail in subsequent sections.

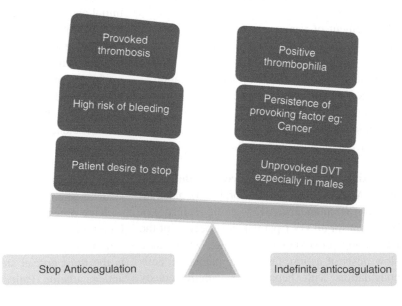

Fig. 21.4 The decision regarding the duration of anticoagulation includes multiple factors. Scoring models that help the decision are described in the text

Extended anticoagulation—Once decided, vitamin K antagonist is usually the most commonly used agent for extended anticoagulation. Cost, ease of availability, easy monitoring, and vast experience with them make VKA the obvious choice. However, newer oral anticoagulants with a better safety profile, though expensive, are now available.

Newer anticoagulants—Apart from heparin, LMWH and VKA, many newer therapeutic options, termed as Direct Oral Anticoagulants (DOAC), are now available. All of them have been approved for the treatment of DVT/PE, for extended anticoagulation in DVT/PE, for VTE prophylaxis in non-valvular atrial fibrillation and in patients undergoing surgery, especially hip/knee replacement. They have not yet been approved for cancer-related or pregnancy-related VTE [12]. All of them have predictable dose-responses, limited drug interactions and food interactions. They have emerged as very good alternatives for VKA for patients with significant drug interactions [54]. Also, they do not need routine monitoring in all patients due to predictable dose-response. However, cost factor and lack of easy monitoring assays for high-risk patients impede their routine use in all patients.

Dabigatran—It is an orally acting direct thrombin inhibitor. It has been approved for stroke prevention in atrial fibrillation patients.

Oral factor Xa inhibitors—These include rivaroxaban, apixaban and edoxaban. They too have renal clearance, and hence, dose modification in renal failure is necessary.

Indications for thrombophilia testing— Several studies have been conducted to scrutinise the practise of thrombophilia testing. It is a popular saying 'do not perform a test whose result you do not want to know'. In short, any investigation should be performed only if it will alter the management of the patient. The perceived role of thrombophilia testing is to guide the long-term management of the patient and family counselling of the asymptomatic family members. High cost for testing and anxiety of a positive result are other factors to be considered before testing for thrombophilia.

Various authorities [55, 56] have published recently updated guidelines. Despite minor differences, the important principles of these guidelines in context to various scenarios can be summarised:

1. Provoked VTE—The risk of recurrence after provoked VTE is similar between thrombophilia-positive and -negative patients. A positive thrombophilia workup does not form an indication for extended duration anticoagulation. Hence, it is not advised to test after provoked VTE [4].
2. Unprovoked DVT—Unprovoked DVT itself is a risk factor for recurrence and warrants extended duration anticoagulation irrespective of thrombophilia status. Thus, thrombophilia testing should be done only in those patients of unprovoked DVT who are desirous of stopping the anticoagulant.
3. Primary prevention in relatives of VTE patients—There is an increased risk of VTE in first-degree relatives, even in thrombophilia-negative patients, and the relatives may be counselled to use prophylaxis during high-risk situation like surgery, prolonged immobilisation, etc. Hence, routine testing for thrombophilia of the asymptomatic family members of VTE patients is not recommended.
4. Arterial thrombosis—Inherited thrombophilia, except APS and factor V Leiden, have no or minimal risk for arterial thrombosis and hence should not be tested for cases of stroke, myocardial infarction or peripheral arterial thrombosis.
5. Oestrogen use/pregnancy—Thrombophilia positivity synergistically increases the risk for VTE in women using OC pills or those who are pregnant. Negative testing may falsely reassure the patients. It is not cost-effective to screen all women for thrombophilia who are contemplating OC pill use. Hence, it is not usually recommended to test for inherited thrombophilia in this group of patients unless it will alter the decision to use OC pills [57].

To summarise, testing for thrombophilia is an extensive and costly process and testing is helpful in following scenarios:

(a) Unprovoked VTE patients who are contemplating discontinuation of anticoagulation.

(b) VTE provoked by minor risk factors like minor surgery or short duration air travel, etc. It may help in better risk assessment and a 'strong' thrombophilia might be a basis for long-term anticoagulation.

(c) Obstetric complications like recurrent pregnancy loss. Guidelines vary for this scenario, but at least APS testing is usually recommended if not other thrombophilia testing [6].

(d) Arterial thrombosis in the young. Focus should be more on APS and factor V Leiden.

(e) Unusual site (e.g. abdominal) thrombosis. However, in these cases, investigations should be more focussed on acquired causes like PNH and myeloproliferative neoplasm.

(f) Patient choice—Some patients may want to find the reason for the unprovoked VTE episode. Detailed counselling regarding the tests must be done before commencing testing.

21.15 Precautions While Testing

Various pre-analytical and analytical factors affect the thrombophilia testing. Certain precautions are recommended to be followed to ensure reliable results.

1. History of anticoagulation—Clot-based assays like LA and APC-R will be affected by anticoagulant therapy. Also, both protein C and protein S are vitamin K-dependent proteins. Hence, their levels will be low in patients on warfarin. Heparin, on the other hand, affects only AT level testing in addition to clot-based assays [5]. On the other hand, certain assay like aCL antibody, beta2 microglobulin and the genetic assays will not be affected by anticoagulant therapy. Hence, a detailed history of anticoagulant therapy is mandatory before performing the assays. A gap of at least 2 weeks after stopping warfarin is necessary before considering for the above-mentioned tests. For direct oral anticoagulants, the recommended gap is at least five half-lives (minimum 3 days) [7].

2. <<Interval after acute thrombosis—Many thrombophilia tests like protein C, protein S, LA, AT may yield erroneous results if tested at the time of presentation because of acute thrombosis, inflammation, pregnancy. Hence, it is advisable to test these after the acute thrombotic event is treated adequately [7].

3. Other confounding factors—Other factors like liver disease, pregnancy, oestrogen therapy may cause alteration in test results.

Salient Points

1. Thrombophilia-inherited or acquired is one of the factors that increases the risk for venous and arterial thrombosis

2. Provoking factor for the thrombosis should be carefully sought.

3. Duration of anticoagulation depends on the balance between risk of recurrence and risk for bleeding

4. Thrombophilia status affects the long term management and testing should be done in cases where the management decision is altered

5. Factors like anticoagulant therapy, acute inflammation and others may affect the test results

6. Patient counselling regarding the implications of positive as well as negative thrombophilia testing is necessary

7. Thrombophilia includes various entities that are tested using a battery of investigations using genetic, antigenic (ELISA) and functional assays

References

1. Pendleton RC, Rodgers GM. Chapter 55: Thrombosis and anti-thrombotic therapy. In: Wintrobe's clinical hematology. 13th ed. Philadelphia: Wolters Kluwer Lippincott Williams & Wilkins Health; 2014. p. 1218–1257.

2. Lee AD, Stephen E, Agarwal S, Premkumar P. Venous thrombo-embolism in India. Eur J Vasc Endovasc Surg. 2009;37:482–5.

3. Agarwal S, Lee AD, Raju RS, Stephen E. Venous thrombo-embolism: a problem in Indian/Asian polulation? Indian J Urol. 2009;25(1):11–6.

4. Moll S. Thrombophilia: clinical–practical aspects. J Thromb Thrombolysis. 2015;39:367–78.

5. Middeldorp S. Inherited thrombophilia: a double edged sword. Hematology Am Soc Hematol Educ Program. 2016;(1):1–9.

6. American College of Obstetricians and Gynecologists Women's Health Care Physicians. ACOG practice bulletin no.138: inherited thrombophilia in pregnancy. Obstet Gynecol. 2013;122(3):706–17.

7. Connors JM. Thrombophilia testing and venous thrombosis. N Engl J Med. 2017;377(12):1177–87.

8. APLA Pengo V, Tripodi A, Reber G, et al. Update of the guidelines for lupus anticoagulant detection. Subcommittee on Lupus Anticoagulant/Antiphospholipid Antibody of the Scientific and Standardisation Committee of the International Society on Thrombosis and Haemostasis. J Thromb Haemost. 2009;7:1737.

9. Garcia D, Erkan D. Diagnosis and management of the antiphospholipid syndrome. N Engl J Med. 2018;378(21):2010–21.

10. Harris EN, Pierangeli SS. Primary, secondary, and catastrophic antiphospholipid syndrome: what's in a name? Semin Thromb Hemost. 2008;34(3):219–26.

11. Rodriguez-Garcia JL, Bertolaccini ML, Cuadrado MJ, Sanna G, Ateka-Barrutia O, Khamashta MA. Clinical manifestations of antiphospholipid syndrome (APS) with and without antiphospholipid antibodies (the so-called 'seronegative APS'). Ann Rheum Dis. 2012;71(2):242–4.

12. Miyakis S, Lockshin MD, Atsumi T, et al. International consensus statement on an update of the classification criteria for definite antiphospholipid syndrome (APS). J Thromb Haemost. 2006;4:295.

13. Ruiz-Irastorza G, Crowther M, Branch W, Khamashta MA. Antiphospholipid syndrome. Lancet. 2010;376:1498.

14. CLSI. Laboratory testing for the lupus anticoagulant; approved guideline. CLSI document H60-A. Wayne: Clinical and Laboratory Standards Institute; 2014.

15. Moore GW. Recent guidelines and recommendations for laboratory detection of lupus anticoagulants. Semin Thromb Hemost. 2014;40(2):163–71.

16. Castoldi E, Brugge JM, Nicolaes GA, et al. Impaired APC cofactor activity of factor V plays a major role in the APC resistance associated with the factor V Leiden (R506Q) and R2 (H1299R) mutations. Blood. 2004;103:4173.

17. Guasch JF, Lensen RP, Bertina RM. Molecular characterization of a type I quantitative factor V deficiency in a thrombosis patient that is "pseudo homozygous" for activated protein C resistance. Thromb Haemost. 1997;77:252.

18. Alhenc-Gelas M, Nicaud V, Gandrille S, et al. The factor V gene A4070G mutation and the risk of venous thrombosis. Thromb Haemost. 1999;81:193.

19. Trossaërt M, Conard J, Horellou MH, et al. The modified APC resistance test in the presence of factor V deficient plasma can be used in patients without oral anticoagulant. Thromb Haemost. 1996;75:521.

20. Bertina RM, Koeleman BP, Koster T, et al. Mutation in blood coagulation factor V associated with resistance to activated protein C. Nature. 1994;369:64.

21. AT Kumar R, Chan AK, Dawson JE, et al. Clinical presentation and molecular basis of congenital antithrombin deficiency in children: a cohort study. Br J Haematol. 2014;166:130.

22. https://www1.imperial.ac.uk/departmentofmedicine/divisions/experimentalmedicine/haematology/coag/antithrombin/

23. Mammen EF. Antithrombin: its physiological importance and role in DIC. Semin Thromb Hemost. 1998;24:19.

24. Gaustadnes M, Rüdiger N, Rasmussen K, Ingerslev J. Intermediate and severe hyperhomocysteinemia with thrombosis: a study of genetic determinants. Thromb Haemost. 2000;83(4):554–8.

25. D'Angelo A, Coppola A, Madonna P, et al. The role of vitamin B12 in fasting hyperhomocysteinemia and its interaction with the homozygous C677T mutation of the methylenetetrahydrofolatereductase (MTHFR) gene. A case-control study of patients with early-onset thrombotic events. Thromb Haemost. 2000;83:563.

26. Klerk M, Verhoef P, Clarke R, et al. MTHFR 677C-->T polymorphism and risk of coronary heart disease: a meta-analysis. JAMA. 2002;288:2023.

27. Kohara K, Fujisawa M, Ando F, et al. MTHFR gene polymorphism as a risk factor for silent brain infarcts and white matter lesions in the Japanese general population: the NILS-LSA Study. Stroke. 2003;34:1130.

28. Nappo F, De Rosa N, Marfella R, et al. Impairment of endothelial functions by acute hyperhomocysteinemia and reversal by antioxidant vitamins. JAMA. 1999;281:2113.

29. Kang SS, Wong PW, Malinow MR. Hyperhomocyst(e)inemia as a risk factor for occlusive vascular disease. Annu Rev Nutr. 1992;12:279.

30. Gallagher PM, Meleady R, Shields DC, et al. Homocysteine and risk of premature coronary heart disease. Evidence of a common gene mutation. Circulation. 1996;94:2154.

31. Reitsma PH. Protein C deficiency: from gene defects to disease. Thromb Haemost. 1997;78:344.

32. Mateo J, Oliver A, Borrell M, et al. Laboratory evaluation and clinical characteristics of 2,132 consecutive unselected patients with venous thromboembolism—results of the Spanish Multicentric Study on Thrombophilia (EMET-Study). Thromb Haemost. 1997;77:444.

33. Sallah S, Abdallah JM, Gagnon GA. Recurrent warfarin-induced skin necrosis in kindreds with protein S deficiency. Haemostasis. 1998;28:25.

34. Koenen RR, Tans G, van Oerle R, et al. The APC-independent anticoagulant activity of protein S in plasma is decreased by elevated prothrombin levels due to the prothrombin G20210A mutation. Blood. 2003;102:1686.

35. Takeyama M, Nogami K, Saenko EL, et al. Protein S down-regulates factor Xase activity independent of activated protein C: specific binding of factor VIII(a)

to protein S inhibits interactions with factor IXa. Br J Haematol. 2008;143:409.

36. Dahlbäck B. C4b-binding protein: a forgotten factor in thrombosis and hemostasis. Semin Thromb Hemost. 2011;37:355.

37. Gandrille S, Borgel D, Sala N, et al. Protein S deficiency: a database of mutations—summary of the first update. Thromb Haemost. 2000;84:918.

38. Comp PC, Doray D, Patton D, Esmon CT. An abnormal plasma distribution of protein S occurs in functional protein S deficiency. Blood. 1986;67:504.

39. Rosendaal FR, Doggen CJ, Zivelin A, et al. Geographic distribution of the 20210 G to A prothrombin variant. Thromb Haemost. 1998;79:706.

40. Mannucci PM, Franchini M. Classic thrombophilic gene variants. Thromb Haemost. 2015;114:885–9.

41. Cooper PC, Rezende SM. An overview of methods for detection of factor V Leiden and the prothrombin G20210A mutations. Int J Lab Hematol. 2007;29:153.

42. Gomez E, van der Poel SC, Jansen JH, et al. Rapid simultaneous screening of factor V Leiden and G20210A prothrombin variant by multiplex polymerase chain reaction on whole blood. Blood. 1998;91:2208.

43. Kearon C. Natural history of venous thromboembolism. Circulation. 2003;107(23 Suppl 1):I22–30.

44. Kearon C, Akl EA, Comerota AJ, Prandoni P, Bounameaux H, Goldhaber SZ, et al. Antithrombotic therapy for VTE disease: antithrombotic therapy and prevention of thrombosis, 9th ed: American college of chest physicians evidence-based clinical practice guidelines. Chest. 2012;141(2 Suppl):e419S–94S.

45. Kitchens CS. How I treat superficial venous thrombosis. Blood. 2011;117(1):39–44.

46. Leon L, Giannoukas AD, Dodd D, Chan P, Labropoulos N. Clinical significance of superficial vein thrombosis. Eur J Vasc Endovasc Surg. 2005;29(1):10–7.

47. Baglin T, Keeling D. Chapter 47, Management of venous thromboembolism. In: Postgraduate haematology. 7th ed. West Sussex: Wiley Blackwell; 2016. p. 830–7.

48. Streiff MB, Agnelli G, Connors JM, Crowther M, Eichinger S, Lopes R, et al. Guidance for the treatment of deep vein thrombosis and pulmonary embolism. J Thromb Thrombolysis. 2016;41:32–67.

49. Iorio A, Kearon C, Filippucci E, Marcucci M, Macura A, Pengo V, et al. Risk of recurrence after a first episode of symptomatic venous thromboembolismprovoked by a transient risk factor: a systematic review. Arch Intern Med. 2010;170(19):1710–6.

50. Boutitie F, Pinede L, Schulman S, Agnelli G, Raskob G, Julian J, et al. Influence of preceding length of anticoagulant treatment and initial presentation of venous thromboembolism on risk of recurrence after stopping treatment: analysis of individual participants' data from seven trials. BMJ. 2011;343:d3036.

51. Tosetto A, Iorio A, Marcucci M, Baglin T, Cushman M, Eichinger S, et al. Predicting disease recurrence in patients with previous unprovoked venous thromboembolism: a proposed prediction score (DASH). J Thromb Haemost. 2012;10(6):1019–25.

52. Eichenger S, Heinze G, Jandeck LM, Kyrle PA. Risk assessment of recurrence in patients with unprovoked deep vein thrombosisor pulmonary embolism: the Vienna prediction model. Circulation. 2010;121(14):1630–6.

53. Kearon C, Akl EA. Duration of anticoagulant therapy for deep vein thrombosis and pulmonary embolism. Blood. 2014;123(12):1794–801.

54. Milling TJ Jr, Frontera J. Exploring indications for the use of direct oral anticoagulants and the associated risks of major bleeding. Am J Manag Care. 2017;23(4 Suppl):S67–80.

55. Hicks LK, Bering H, Carson KR, Kleinerman J, Kukreti V, Ma A, et al. The ASH Choosing Wisely campaign: five hematologic tests and treatments to question. Blood. 2013;122:3879–83.

56. National Clinical Guideline centre (UK). Venous thromboembolic diseases: the management of venous thromboembolic diseases and the role of thrombophilia testing [Internet]. London: Royal College of Physicians (UK); 2012.

57. Stevens SM, Woller SC, Bauer KA, Kasthuri R, Cushman M, Streiff M, et al. Guidance for the evaluation and treatment of hereditary and acquired thrombophilia. J Thromb Thrombolysis. 2016;41(1):154–64.

Laboratory Monitoring of Anticoagulant therapy

22

Aastha Gupta, D. S. Udayakumar,
and Renu Saxena

22.1 Introduction

Worldwide, millions of patients are put on short-term and long-term anticoagulant therapy for several thrombotic indications. The critical balance of the inherent risk of bleeding and the anticoagulant effect of these drugs needs to be maintained. There is an increasing use of new oral anticoagulants apart from the conventional agents such as heparin and vitamin K antagonists, and it is imperative to know the appropriate assay(s) that are used for each drug monitoring. Hence, both clinical and laboratory personnel should be aware of assays to monitor different anticoagulant therapy and various physiological as well as laboratory variables affecting these results.

The conventional agents include heparins (unfractionated heparin, low molecular weight heparin) and vitamin K antagonists (VKAs). Dabigatran (Pradaxa), rivaroxaban (Xarelto), apixaban (Eliquis), and edoxaban (Savaysa and Lixiana) are direct acting oral anticoagulants (DOACs) that have been approved for the prevention of stroke or systemic embolic events (SEE) in patients with non-valvular atrial fibrillation (NVAF) and for the treatment of VTE [1, 2]. DOACs act by inhibiting either factor Xa (rivaroxaban, apixaban, and edoxaban) or thrombin (dabigatran). In comparison with warfarin, the advantages of DOACs include the much faster onset of action, simpler dosing, reduced monitoring requirements, reduced food and drug interactions, and a decreased risk of bleeding [2].

We will discuss the laboratory monitoring of each group of anticoagulants.

22.2 Heparins

22.2.1 Structure and Anticoagulant Activity

Unfractionated heparin (UFH) and low molecular weight heparin (LMWH) are negatively charged compounds which contain the mixture of glycosaminoglycans. Fondaparinux is a synthetic compound which is similar to the active site of heparin. The mechanism underlying the anticoagulant effect of these drugs is the potentiation of antithrombin (AT) activity. Heparins greatly enhance the AT-mediated inhibition of factor II, X, IX, XI, and XII, thus inhibiting the clot formation.

For this anticoagulant property, a specific pentasaccharide sequence is required for binding to antithrombin and potentiating its effect. This pentasaccharide sequence is present in all heparins. UFH and low molecular weight heparins (LMWH and fondaparinux) vary considerably in their molecular size. This variation in size is mainly due to the long side chain of alternating

A. Gupta · D. S. Udayakumar · R. Saxena (✉)
Department of Hematology, All India Institute of
Medical Sciences, New Delhi, India

© Springer Nature Singapore Pte Ltd. 2019
R. Saxena, H. P. Pati (eds.), *Hematopathology*, https://doi.org/10.1007/978-981-13-7713-6_22

uronic acid and glucosamine. The molecular weight of UFH ranges from 5000 to 35,000 Da while that of LMWH ranges from 3000 to 5000 Da [3].

This variation in size will determine both the anticoagulant property and pharmacokinetics (Fig. 22.1). Heparins with molecular weight more than 5000 Da (UFH) will have an increased tendency to bind thrombin and bring it close to the antithrombin, thus potentiating its inhibition. UFH accounts for anti-Xa activity to anti-IIa activity ratio of 1:1. Whereas for all LMWHs (molecular weight less than 5000 Da), the anti-Xa activity exceeds anti-IIa activity with a ratio ranging from 1.6: 1 to 4.2:1 [4].

22.2.2 Pharmacokinetics

Larger molecules (UFH) have unpredictable pharmacokinetic as they bind to several acute phase proteins and are rapidly cleared by a saturable cellular mechanism. UFH in therapeutic doses produces variable drug levels leading to wavering degree of anticoagulation. Thus, it requires close monitoring to prevent any bleeding or subtherapeutic effect. Smaller molecules, i.e., LMWH and fondaparinux, bind very less with the plasma proteins and are cleared by a predictable non-saturable renal route. Hence, LMWH and fondaparinux do not require monitoring except for some special situations. The dose–response relationship of

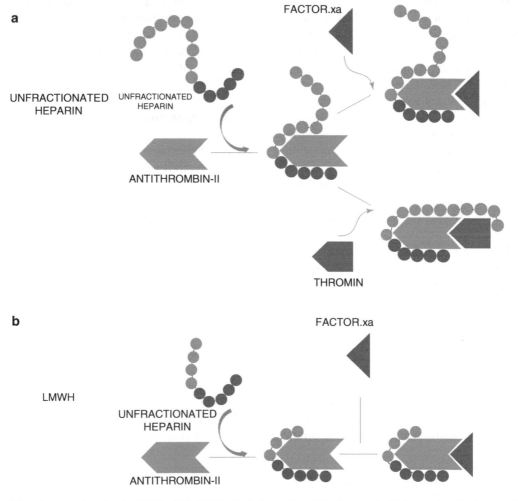

Fig. 22.1 Large molecular size UFH which inhibits both factor II and X with equal affinity (**a**). Small size LMWH inhibiting factor X but unable to bind factor II (**b**)

LMWH is quite predictable and can be given on the basis of "units per kg." Treatment should be monitored when the pharmacokinetics is expected to be altered as in renal failure, pregnancy, and extremes of weight.

22.2.2.1 UFH Monitoring

Before starting UFH, certain baseline information must be looked for which include thorough history suggestive of any bleeding disorder including the family history, history of any recent surgery or trauma, complete blood count (CBC) to note baseline hemoglobin and platelet count, baseline coagulation tests including PT and APTT to look for any coagulopathy or any inhibitors like lupus anticoagulants which could later interfere with heparin monitoring, and liver function tests to know the baseline transaminase levels. Renal function tests are not required for heparin dosing but it is always good to know the baseline levels.

Therapeutic UFH is given by a starting bolus dose followed by continuous intravenous infusion or as a continuous infusion without a bolus. This will depend on the rapidity with which anticoagulant effect is needed or if there is an underlying risk of bleeding. At this dose, UFH requires monitoring which should be a combination of clinical assessment and laboratory testing. For laboratory monitoring, blood samples should be taken every 4–6 h after starting heparin till a therapeutic range is achieved on two occasions, and then it must be repeated at least once a day. The sample should be drawn 6 h after every dose change.

22.2.3 Methods

Tests that can be used to monitor UFH are whole blood clotting time, APTT, TT, protamine neutralization test, and anti-Xa assay. They have little or no effect on PT.

Whole blood clotting time and protamine neutralization tests are time-consuming tests and not used in routine laboratories.

APTT and anti-Xa assay are routinely used for heparin monitoring. There is no strong evidence to suggest the superiority of one over the other

Table 22.1 Advantages and disadvantages of APTT- and anti-Xa assay-based heparin monitoring

Test	Advantages	Disadvantages
APTT	• Easily available • Simple • Cost-effective	• Many variables affect baseline APTT • It is not sensitive to doses less than 0.2 IU/mL • Not all APTT reagents are heparin sensitive • Not sensitive to LMWH
Anti-Xa assay	• Expensive • Not easily available	• Sensitive to all concentrations of heparin and LMWH

[5]. Each of these tests comes with its own advantages and disadvantages (Table 22.1). The choice also depends on the cost of the test and familiarity with the result. An important disadvantage common to both tests is the unavailability of standards to normalize APTT or anti-Xa values.

22.2.4 APTT-Based Heparin Monitoring

APTT has been the most commonly used test for heparin monitoring. It is a cost-effective and most familiar method. However, it has a few shortcomings which need to be considered beforehand. First of all, different APTT reagents have different sensitivity to different heparins. To determine this, normal platelet-poor pooled plasma is spiked with different concentrations of a particular brand of heparin. APTT is plotted against heparin concentrations on a linear-linear graph. A combination which gives a linear relation of APTT and heparin concentration in therapeutic range is selected. Heparin ratio denotes a ratio of APTT of plasma with added heparin to that without heparin (APTT of heparinized plasma/APTT of plasma without heparin).

Traditionally, APTT ranging from 1.5 to 2.5 times the mean of reference range covers the therapeutic range for most of the sensitive reagents. However, studies have shown this to be an underestimation of the amount of heparin required [6]. Hence, it is important to design a heparin response curve. There are two methods to determine a heparin response curve.

1. In vitro heparin response curve [6]:
   (a) Platelet-poor pooled normal plasma is prepared from normal healthy individuals which is spiked with known concentrations of heparin of a particular brand and lot.
   (b) APTT is performed using the sensitive reagent for each plasma which has been spiked with different heparin concentrations.
   (c) These APTT values are plotted on a linear-linear graph on Y-axis against the known heparin concentrations on the X-axis.
   (d) The APTT range which corresponds to the heparin therapeutic range (0.2–0.4 U/ mL) will be the APTT therapeutic range.
2. Ex vivo heparin response curve [6]:
   In this method, patient sample fully anticoagulated with UFH is collected, and APTT is performed for each patient. Heparin activity on these samples is established by using the anti-Xa assay. A graph is then plotted with APTT and heparin concentrations, and the APTT range which corresponds to the therapeutic range is selected.

The advantage of an in vitro test is that it is easier to perform when compared to ex vivo test. However, the disadvantage is that it does not truly represent the heparin activity in patients who must be having an underlying inflammation and acute phase changes.

The second disadvantage of APTT-based monitoring is that it is affected by several pre-analytical variables like factor deficiency, liver diseases, DIC, the presence of fibrin degradation products, lupus anticoagulants, or raised factor VIII concentration during acute phase response.

Situations with prolonged baseline APTT should be investigated prior to starting anticoagulant therapy. If this is not possible, then reliable monitoring by APTT is questionable and should be determined on a case-by-case basis. If the APTT prolongation is due to lupus anticoagulant, then it is advisable to use a reagent not sensitive to lupus which should be calibrated.

22.2.5 Anti-Xa Assay for Heparin

Principle: Anti-Xa activity of antithrombin is enhanced by heparin. Residual factor Xa level is measured to establish the heparin activity. An advantage of anti-Xa is less susceptible to pre-analytical variables [7].

Method: Clotting-based or chromogenic-based measurement of residual factor Xa is done. A standard curve is made using normal pooled plasma (source of antithrombin) added with heparin of different concentrations. $CaCl_2$ and a known amount of factor Xa are added. After incubation, factor X-deficient plasma along with platelet substitute is added, and the clotting time is observed. Patient plasma is tested undiluted and plotted on the standard curve to get the heparin concentration.

22.2.5.1 LMWH and Fondaparinux Monitoring

As discussed earlier, these heparins will require monitoring only in special situations.

These agents prolong APTT in an unpredictable manner which will depend on the sensitivity of the reagents and on the drug dose being administered to the patient. Hence, APTT is not used to monitor these drugs.

LMWH and fondaparinux are monitored by anti-Xa assay described above. The appropriate standard curve must be made for each. Unlike UFH, different standard curves are not needed for different LMWHs. The blood sample should be drawn 4 and 3 h after the subcutaneous injection of LMWH and fondaparinux, respectively [8].

22.3 Guideline for the Management of Bleeding in a Patient on UFH

1. Stop UFH infusion.
2. General hemostatic measures are often sufficient to stop or prevent bleeding.
3. Protamine sulfate (1 mg per 80–100 units UFH) will fully reverse UFH but should be given slower than 5 mg/min to minimize the risk of adverse reactions.

4. The maximum recommended dose of 50 mg protamine is sufficient to reverse UHF in most settings [9].

22.4 Vitamin K Antagonists

Despite a plethora of newer anticoagulants now available, warfarin still remains the most widely used oral anticoagulant in the world. In 1940, Karl Link and his student Harold Campbell in Wisconsin identified the anticoagulant in sweet clover as 3,3'-methylene-bis (4-hydroxycoumarin) which was oxidized to its active agent called dicoumarol [7]. Further work by Link led to the synthesis of warfarin in 1948, which was approved for human use in 1954. The name warfarin is derived from WARF (Wisconsin Alumni Research Foundation) and -arin from coumarin.

22.4.1 Mechanism of Action

Warfarin acts as a water-soluble vitamin K antagonist which interferes with the synthesis of the vitamin K-dependent clotting factors including prothrombin (factor II) and factors VII, IX, and X. It also inhibits the synthesis of anticoagulant proteins C and S.

Vitamin K-dependent factors are functionally active after the addition of a carboxyl group to generate γ-carboxy glutamic acid which is catalyzed by a vitamin K-dependent enzyme known as gamma-glutamyl carboxylase. This facilitates the calcium-dependent binding of these factors to the negatively charged phospholipid surfaces. Vitamin K hydroquinone is a cofactor for gamma-carboxylase, and during this process, vitamin K hydroquinone is oxidized to vitamin K epoxide. The oxidized form of vitamin K is then converted back to the reduced hydroquinone form by vitamin K epoxide reductase which is required for a constant supply of the cofactor for gamma carboxylation [10].

Warfarin inhibits the C1 subunit of the vitamin K epoxide reductase (VKORC1) enzyme complex, thus blocking the conversion of vitamin K to its active reduced form, thereby inter-

fering with the process of gamma-carboxylation (Fig. 22.2). This, in turn, results in the production of partially carboxylated clotting factors which have reduced or absent biological activity [8].

The onset of action of warfarin is delayed until the newly synthesized clotting factors with reduced activity gradually replace their fully active counterparts. During this time, warfarin treatment requires supplementation with concomitant administration of rapidly acting parenteral anticoagulants to cover for the delayed onset of warfarin anticoagulation.

22.4.2 Pharmacokinetics

Warfarin is a racemic mixture of R- and S-isomers, latter being 2–5 times more active than the former. It is rapidly and almost completely absorbed from the gastrointestinal tract with peak levels attained approximately 90 min after administration. More than 97% of circulating warfarin is bound to albumin. However, only the unbound fraction of warfarin is biologically active [11].

Warfarin is accumulated in the liver where it is extensively metabolized by the cytochrome P450 system. The R and S enantiomers follow different metabolic pathways. The more potent S isomer is metabolized by CYP2C9 which has two common variants, CYP2C9*2 and CYP2C9*3. Minimally active metabolites are excreted in urine and a small amount in bile. The effective half-life of racemic warfarin is 36–42 h.

22.4.3 Monitoring of Warfarin

The anticoagulant effect of warfarin is influenced by a large number of factors affecting both pharmacodynamics and pharmacokinetics. Fluctuations in dietary vitamin K intake, diarrhea, and malnutrition may have a significant effect on the anticoagulant response of warfarin. A wide variety of drugs can alter absorption, clearance, or metabolism of warfarin. Various disease states like hepatic and renal dysfunction, heart failure, and thyroid disorders may alter the

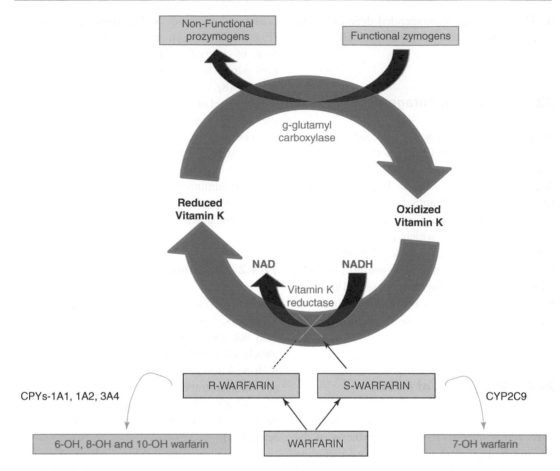

Fig. 22.2 Mechanism of action of warfarin

bioavailability of warfarin. In addition to this, various polymorphisms in the target enzyme VKORC1 may lead to altered in vivo response to warfarin. Furthermore, genomic variants of CYP2C9 (*2 and *3 alleles) with reduced metabolic activity may potentiate the anticoagulant effects of warfarin, thus necessitating a decrease in dosage. However, to date, the guidelines do not recommend the use of routine pharmacogenomic testing to guide warfarin therapy.

All these factors lead to a marked variation in the individual response to warfarin therapy and thus warrant vigilant monitoring and tailored treatment based on a comprehensive patient review.

Warfarin therapy is most often monitored using the Prothrombin Time (PT), a test which reflects the reductions in the levels of prothrombin, factor VII, and factor X. Thromboplastins vary in their sensitivity to reductions in the levels of the vitamin K-dependent clotting factors [12]. The international normalized ratio (INR) was developed to circumvent these problems associated with the PT test. To calculate the INR, the patient's prothrombin time is divided by the geometric mean normal prothrombin time (GMNPT), and this ratio is then multiplied by the international sensitivity index (ISI).

$$INR = [PT \text{ of patient}/GMNPT]^{ISI}$$

ISI is a measure of the sensitivity of test thromboplastin when compared to the reference thromboplastin. Highly sensitive thromboplastins have an ISI of 1.0. Most current thromboplastins have ISI values that range from 1.0 to 1.4. Therapeutic INR for most indications is targeted between 2 and 3 [8].

22.5   Point of Care Testing (POC)

Efforts are being made to develop POC testing devices which can help patients to monitor their anticoagulant therapy at home only. However, proper training should be given to these patients regarding the working and quality control of these devices. They should be well informed to visit a hospital if they notice a major variation in INR and regarding warfarin dose changes. An INR of more than 4.0 must be confirmed by a standard laboratory [13].

22.6   Guideline for the Management of Bleeding in a Patient on Warfarin [9, 14]

The approach to a patient with warfarin-associated coagulopathy depends on the degree of INR elevation, the presence of clinically significant bleeding (Table 22.2).

Table 22.2 Management of warfarin-associated bleeding [14]

INR	Bleeding	Recommended action
3–6 (Target INR 2.5) 4–6 (Target INR 3.5)	Absent	Reduce warfarin dose or stop Restart warfarin when INR <5
>6–8	Absent/minor bleeding	Stop warfarin and restart when INR <5
>8	Absent/minor bleeding	Stop warfarin and restart when INR <5 If other risk factors for bleeding present, give oral/IV vitamin K (0.5–2.5 mg)
Major bleeding	Intracranial, gastrointestinal	Stop warfarin Give PCC 25–50 U/kg or FFP 15 mL/kg if PCC not available Give 5 mg of vitamin K (oral/IV)

22.7   Direct Acting Oral Anticoagulants (DOAC)

The DOACs include direct thrombin inhibitor (dabigatran) and factor Xa inhibitors (rivaroxaban, apixaban, and edoxaban). DOACs have favorable pharmacokinetic and pharmacodynamic properties and have been shown to have an equal or superior efficacy with an improved safety profile compared with warfarin (Table 22.3) [2, 15]. DOACs have shorter half-lives and require stricter adherence. Other shortcomings with DOACs are the lack of standardized laboratory monitoring and lack of reversal agents. Monitoring of DOACs can be done by qualitative and quantitative tests.

DOACs do not require routine laboratory monitoring for dose adjustments. But there are many situations when assessment of a DOAC effect is desirable such as emergency situations (i.e., trauma), urgent surgery, major bleeding, attempted suicide, acute thrombosis, renal failure, liver failure, and potential drug–drug interactions [1]. Many authors have suggested that young and healthy patients do not require regular monitoring, whereas patients who are 75 years of age and older would require monitoring [16]. There are no evidence-based recommendations for drug concentration measurements, coagulation tests, assay standardization/calibration, or target therapeutic ranges for DOACs [1, 17].

Qualitative assessment of DOACs can be done by routinely available coagulation assays such as activated partial thromboplastin time, prothrombin time, and thrombin time. The quantitative assessment of DOACs can be done by plasma drug concentrations, ecarin clotting time, dilute thrombin time, and anti-factor Xa concentrations. Serum creatinine, liver function tests, and complete blood counts are also important in monitoring patients on DOACs. Routine assessment of adherence, bleeding risks, and drug interactions should be done in every clinical visit. The frequency of monitoring depends on

Table 22.3 Properties of DOACs [1, 15]

	Dabigatran	Rivaroxaban	Apixaban	Edoxaban
FDA-approved indication	Reduction of stroke and SEE risk for patients with NVAF Treatment of DVT and PE following 5–10 days of parenteral anticoagulant Reduction of recurrence risk for DVT and PE	Reduction of stroke and SEE risk for patients with NVAF Treatment of DVT and PE and reduction of recurrence risk for DVT and PE Prophylaxis of DVT in patients undergoing knee or hip replacement surgery		Reduction of stroke and SEE risk for patients with NVAF Treatment of DVT and PE following 5–10 days of parenteral anticoagulant
Time to Cmax (h)	1–2	2–4	3–4	1–2
Half-life (h)	12–17	5–13	12	10–14
Renal elimination	80% of the absorbed dose	66% of the oral dose	27% of the absorbed dose	50% of the absorbed dose
Transporters	P-gp	P-gp/BCRP	P-gp/BCRP	P-gp
CYP450 metabolism	No	Yes	Yes	Minimal
Bioavailability (%)	3–7	≥80	50	62
Potential drug interactions	Potent P-gp inhibitors and P-gp/CYP3A4 dual inducer rifampin	Potent dual CYP3A4and P-gp inhibitors or inducers		Potent P-gp inhibitors and P-gp/CYP3A4 dual inducer rifampin

NVAF non-valvular atrial fibrillation, *BCRP* breast cancer resistance protein, *max* maximum observed plasma concentration, *CYP3A4* cytochrome P450 3A4 enzyme, *DVT* deep-vein thrombosis, *P-gp* P-glycoprotein, *PE* pulmonary embolism, *SEE* systemic embolic event, *VTE* venous thromboembolism

patient-specific characteristics such as age, renal impairment, hepatic impairment, and concomitant drug therapy [1, 15].

22.8 Laboratory Monitoring

So far there are no studies that have suggested if drug concentration measurement or dose adjustment based on coagulation parameters affects clinical outcomes during chronic therapy.

APTT, PT, and TT are widely available tests with rapid turnaround times. But they have poor sensitivity and specificity and lack optimal dose–response relationships for monitoring DOACs. Other tests like plasma drug concentrations, ecarin clotting time (ECT), dilute thrombin time (dTT), and anti-FXa concentration test require specialized laboratories and are not widely available. ECT, dTT, and anti-FXa concentrations have potential utility as quantitative tests to measure DOAC intensity [15].

Other quantitative measures of DOACs such as dilute PT, HepTest, and prothrombinase-induced clotting time (PiCT) are not widely available [15].

22.9 Direct Thrombin Inhibitors

22.9.1 Activated Partial Thromboplastin Time (aPTT)

Many studies have evaluated the aPTT and dabigatran etexilate levels simultaneously. The aPTT is somewhat more sensitive to dabigatran compared with PT. aPTT is often prolonged in these patients. However, the degree of prolongation correlates poorly with drug concentrations. Although an aPTT range of 46–54 s has been shown to correspond to a therapeutic dabigatran concentration of 90–180 ng/mL, it is insensitive at supratherapeutic concentrations of dabigatran and hence may underestimate high concentrations. The sensitivity of different aPTT assays varies with reagents used, and hence, checking the sensitivity of aPTT to dabigatran at each institution is recommended. A normal aPTT does not exclude clinically relevant dabigatran activity [1, 15, 17].

22.9.2 Chromogenic Anti-FXa Assay

In this assay, factor Xa is added to plasma containing a factor Xa substrate that is tagged with a chromophore. When FXa cleaves the chromophore, a color change occurs that is proportional to the concentration of FXa present in the assay. The assay must be calibrated for a specific anticoagulant. While the chromogenic anti-FXa assay is commonly available, a calibrated assay for the individual DOACs is not widely available. Dabigatran has no effect on the anti-FXa assay [1, 15].

22.9.3 Thrombin Time

TT is overly sensitive, and at even subtherapeutic concentrations, dabigatran prolongs TT. TT is not suited for quantitative assessment. A normal TT excludes even low concentrations of dabigatran [1, 15].

22.9.4 Dilute Thrombin Time (dTT)

Various assays are available, including Hemoclot thrombin inhibitor assay, Technoview, and Hemosil.

Dabigatran prolongs the dTT in a linear dose relationship in therapeutic concentrations and hence is suitable for quantitative assessment of dabigatran. A normal dTT indicates no clinically relevant anticoagulation [1, 15, 17].

22.9.5 Ecarin Clotting Time (ECT)

The ECT directly measures thrombin generation. Coagulation is initiated with ecarin, which cleaves prothrombin to an active intermediate meizothrombin which is inhibited by dabigatran.

ECT has a concentration-dependent, linear response in dabigatran-treated patients. It is a useful test for quantitative assessment of anticoagulant activity from dabigatran. An ECT near baseline indicates no clinically relevant dabigatran effect [1, 15, 17].

22.9.6 Prothrombin Time/ International Normalized Ratio

The INR system is not recommended for assessing DOACs because the International Sensitivity Index (ISI) was developed specifically for vitamin K antagonists. Although dabigatran prolongs PT, it has poor sensitivity. Hence, PT/INR is not suitable for quantitative assessment. Supratherapeutic concentrations of dabigatran have more pronounced effects on PT [1, 15, 17].

22.9.7 Prothrombinase-Induced Clotting Time (PiCT)

The assay is composed of FXa, phospholipids, and an enzyme that activates FV on the addition of plasma to the assay. Although a concentration-dependent relationship has been demonstrated with PiCT and dabigatran, it lacks sensitivity [1, 15].

22.10 FXa Inhibitors

22.10.1 Activated Partial Thromboplastin Time (aPTT)

FXa inhibitors prolong aPTT to a variable degree but show poor correlation with drug concentrations. At therapeutic doses, all three FXa inhibitors cause a small prolongation of aPTT with a high degree of variability. aPTT assay sensitivity varies with reagents used and has wider interlaboratory variability.

The aPTT should not be used for qualitative or quantitative assessment of FXa inhibitors [1, 15].

22.10.2 Chromogenic Anti-FXa Assay

The calibrated anti-FXa assays for the anticoagulant effects of rivaroxaban, edoxaban, and apixaban is precise, sensitive, and accurate. These assays have the best correlation with plasma drug concentrations. It is now the preferred method for quantitative assessment of anticoagulant activity when calibrated to rivaroxaban, apixaban, and edoxaban [1, 15, 17].

22.10.3 Dilute Thrombin Time (dTT)

No effect is expected on dTT from FXa inhibitors.

22.10.4 Ecarin Clotting Time (ECT)

FXa inhibitors have no effect on ECT.

22.10.5 Prothrombin Time/ International Normalized Ratio

The effect on PT varies with the drug used. In general, all FXa inhibitors can result in normal/prolonged PT at therapeutic concentrations. At therapeutic doses, rivaroxaban has a relatively weak effect on PT and has a more pronounced effect on PT at supratherapeutic concentrations [15].

The effects of apixaban and edoxaban on PT have a high degree of variability at therapeutic concentrations. The PT/INR is not recommended for use with FXa inhibitors.

22.10.6 Prothrombinase-Induced Clotting Time (PiCT)

Although concentration-dependent relationship and a sensitive response have been shown with PiCT and rivaroxaban, paradoxically low doses of rivaroxaban have been shown to shorten PiCT. Apixaban and edoxaban have not been studied with PiCT [15].

22.10.7 Thrombin Time (TT)

FXa inhibitors have been shown to have no effect on TT.

22.10.8 Plasma Drug Concentrations

Plasma concentrations can be measured for all four DOACs (dabigatran, apixaban, edoxaban, and rivaroxaban). The liquid chromatography-tandem mass spectrometry is the most accurate way of measuring plasma concentrations [18].

22.11 Clinical Monitoring

Surrogate qualitative testing methods such as renal function, liver function, and hemoglobin/hematocrit are also used in the monitoring of DOACs. It is recommended to monitor renal and liver function at baseline and every 6–12 months or more frequently depending on age and other comorbidities in a particular individual [1, 15] (Fig. 22.3) (Table 22.4).

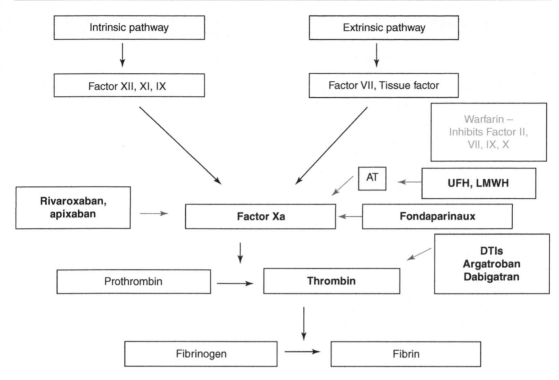

Fig. 22.3 Coagulation cascade with targets of anticoagulants

Table 22.4 Summary of Laboratory Coagulation Monitoring assays for DOACs [1, 15, 17]

Assay	Direct thrombin inhibitors (dabigatran)		Factor Xa inhibitors (apixaban, edoxaban, rivaroxaban)	
	Sensitivity	Utility	Sensitivity	Utility
APTT	Low	Qualitative assessment, availability support use	Low	Not useful
Chromogenic anti-factor Xa assay	N/A	N/A	High	Quantitative assessment if calibrated to specific anticoagulant
Dilute thrombin time (dTT)	Sensitive	Quantitative assessment	N/A	N/A
Ecarin clotting time (ECT)	Sensitive	Quantitative assessment	N/A	N/A
Prothrombin time (PT)	Low	Therapeutic doses—no utility. Qualitative in supratherapeutic doses	N/A	Qualitative assessment if calibrated reagents
Plasma drug concentration	Sensitive	Quantitative assessment	Sensitive	Quantitative assessment
Thrombin time	Sensitive	Qualitative assessment only	N/A	N/A

N/A not applicable

22.12 Conclusion

Even in the era of newer anticoagulants, the majority of patients are managed by conventional anticoagulants like heparin and warfarin. This is not only because of the familiarity with the drugs but also because the laboratory tests to monitor these agents are more established and well standardized. Clinical studies have demonstrated that DOACs are at least as effective as warfarin for the prevention of NVAF-related stroke, the treatment of acute VTE, and the prevention of recurrent VTE and are associated with similar or decreased risks of bleeding. Bleeding is a concern for all anticoagulants, and the lack of specific laboratory measurements and reversal agents poses additional challenges to its management in patients using DOACs. Overall, DOACs represent effective, safe, and likely cost-effective alternatives to warfarin.

References

1. Peacock W, Rafique Z, Singer A. Direct-acting oral anticoagulants: practical considerations for emergency medicine physicians. Emer Med Int. 2016;2016:1–13.
2. Ruff C, Giugliano R, Braunwald E, Hoffman E, Deenadayalu N, Ezekowitz M, et al. Comparison of the efficacy and safety of new oral anticoagulants with warfarin in patients with atrial fibrillation: a meta-analysis of randomized trials. Lancet. 2014;383(9921):955–62.
3. Smythe MA, Priziola J, Dobesh PP, Wirth D, Cuker A, Wittkowsky AK. Guidance for the practical management of the heparin anticoagulants in the treatment of venous thromboembolism. J Thromb Thrombolysis. 2016;41:165–86.
4. Baglin T, Barrowcliffe TW, Cohen A, et al. Guidelines on the use and monitoring of heparin. Br J Haematol. 2006;133(1):19–34.
5. Zehnder J, Prince E, Jin J. Controversies in heparin monitoring. Am J Hematol. 2012;87(Suppl 1):S137–40.
6. Bates SM, Weitz JI, Johnston M, Hirsh J, Ginsberg JS. Use of a fixed activated partial thromboplastin time ratio to establish a therapeutic range. Arch Int Med. 2001;161:385–91.
7. Vandiver JW, Vondracek TG. AntifactorXa levels versus activated partial thromboplastin time for monitoring unfractionated heparin. Pharmacotherapy. 2012;32:546–58.
8. Funk DM. Coagulation assays and anticoagulant monitoring. Hematology. 2012;2012:460–5.
9. Makris M, Van Veen J, Tait C, Mumford A, Laffan M. Guideline on the management of bleeding in patients on antithrombotic agents. Br J Haematol. 2012;160(1):35–46.
10. Hirsh J, Dalen JE, Anderson DR, et al. Oral anticoagulants: mechanism of action, clinical effectiveness, and optimal therapeutic range. Chest. 2001;119(Suppl):8–21.
11. Breckenridge A, Orme M, Wesseling H, et al. Pharmacokinetics and pharmacodynamics of the enantiomers of warfarin in man. Clin Pharmacol Ther. 1974;15:424–30.
12. Favaloro EJ, Adcock DM. Standardization of the INR: how good is your laboratory's INR and can it be improved? Semin Thromb Hemost. 2008;34(7):593–603.
13. Dorfman DM, Goonan EM, Boutilier MK, Jarolim P, Tanasijevic M, Goldhaber S. Point-of-care (POC) versus central laboratory instrumentation for monitoring oral anticoagulation. Vasc Med. 2005;10(1):23–7.
14. Lewis S, Bain B, Bates I, Dacie J, Dacie J. Dacie and Lewis practical haematology. Philadelphia: Churchill Livingstone; 2006.
15. Conway S, Hwang A, Ponte C, Gums J. Laboratory and clinical monitoring of direct-acting oral anticoagulants: what clinicians need to know. Pharmacotherapy. 2017;37(2):236–48.
16. Ten Cate H. New oral anticoagulants: discussion on monitoring and adherence should start now! Thromb J. 2013;11(1):8.
17. Ramos-Esquivel A. Monitoring anticoagulant therapy with new oral agents. World J Methodol. 2015;5(4):212.
18. Gous T, Couchman L, Patel J, Paradzai C, Arya R, Flanagan R. Measurement of the direct oral anticoagulants apixaban, dabigatran, edoxaban, and rivaroxaban in human plasma using turbulent flow liquid chromatography with high-resolution mass spectrometry. Ther Drug Monit. 2014;36(5):597–605.

Inhibitors in Coagulation

23

Prashant Sharma

23.1 Introduction

Inhibitors in coagulation are acquired antibodies that act by either neutralizing or inhibiting the activity of specific clotting factors or, alternatively, enhancing their degradation and clearance [1]. Clinically, these occur in two pathogenetically distinct scenarios. The **first** is when these antibodies occur idiopathically, or in association with other disorders like malignancies, pregnancy, drug exposures, or systemic autoimmune disorders. Such autoantibodies ("auto" since they are directed against the affected individual's own antigens) usually result in a bleeding diathesis as their most common clinical manifestation. Antiphospholipid antibodies (APLA) are a special subset of this group, since their unique properties cause thromboses more often than abnormal bleeding [2].

The **second** major group of inhibitors develop in patients who have inherited deficiencies of various coagulation factors like hemophilia A and B. They usually develop when these patients are exposed to exogenous factors as replacement therapy. These are alloantibodies (the modern preferred term is isoantibodies), i.e., they are targeted against an antigen of another individual of the same species. They bind to and neutralize the

specific deficient factor and often worsen the bleeding phenotype in these patients, posing challenges in clinical management [3].

As opposed to the above two "pathological" conditions, a third group of inhibitors in coagulation are the natural anticoagulants—proteins C and S, and antithrombin, whose deficiencies either cause or modify several disorders that result in a prothrombotic state. Pharmacological inhibition of clotting pathway factors may also be achieved by various agents like heparin and the newer oral anticoagulants [4]. This chapter, however, focuses on the first two groups of "acquired" inhibitors, dealing sequentially with their pathogenesis, clinical features, laboratory diagnosis, and management. Only a last brief section is devoted to exclusion of heparin contamination in blood samples, a common artifact in the hemostasis laboratory.

23.2 Section 1: Autoantibodies to Coagulation Factors: Acquired Hemophilia and Related Disorders

Acquired inhibitory antibodies directed against various clotting factors cause rare, but usually severe, bleeding disorders with increased morbidity and mortality in previously healthy individuals, mostly adults. The most common of these antibodies bind to and interfere with coagulation factor VIII activity, leading to acquired

P. Sharma (✉)
Hematology Department, Postgraduate Institute of Medical Education and Research, Level 5, Research Block A, Sector 12, Chandigarh, India
e-mail: sharma.prashant@pgimer.edu.in

© Springer Nature Singapore Pte Ltd. 2019
R. Saxena, H. P. Pati (eds.), *Hematopathology*, https://doi.org/10.1007/978-981-13-7713-6_23

hemophilia Λ [2, 4]. The section below mostly deals with acquired hemophilia A with laboratory tests common to all entities summarized in Table 23.1 and acquired inhibitors to other factors summarized in Table 23.2.

23.2.1 Epidemiology

Acquired hemophilic disorders are much rarer than the inherited form of the disease with a 2007 UK-based survey estimating them to affect approximately two per million of the general population [5]. Acquired hemophilia occurs worldwide in all ethnic groups. The condition carries a high risk of under- or delayed recognition and may be mistaken for another acquired bleeding disorder like disseminated intravascular coagulation (DIC). Patients are usually middle-aged to elderly (median age 64 years) with a wide range of 8–93 years. It is rare in children [2, 5].

23.2.2 Pathogenesis

Acquired hemophilia has a varied etiology. About 50% patients have no associated disease. The remaining are associated with autoimmune diseases like rheumatoid arthritis, SLE, polymyalgia (17–18%), post-partum states (7–21%), solid malignancies (lungs, GIT, breast), lymphomas and monoclonal gammopathies, dermatological disorders (pemphigus, psoriasis), pharmacological agents (phenytoin, penicillin, methyldopa, fludarabine, etc.), infections (mycoplasma, hepatitis B or C), respiratory disorders (obstructive airway diseases like bronchial asthma), and post-influenza vaccination [5, 6].

The circulating immunoglobulins that are acquired are predominantly IgG, mostly IgG4. They do not show complement-binding activity. They are polyclonal and most often bind to the FVIII molecule's A2 domain (that binds factor IX and activated protein C) or C2 domain

Table 23.1 Major tests for laboratory-based detection of inhibitors of coagulation [2–6, 9, 10]

- **Prothrombin time (PT):** Prolonged in cases with inhibitors of factors VII, II, V, X and fibrinogen. The international normalized ratio (INR) allows comparability by reagent standardization across various laboratories.
- **Activated partial thromboplastin time (aPTT):** Prolonged in patients with inhibitors of factors VIII, IX, II, X, XI, XII and fibrinogen. Causes of an isolated prolonged aPTT include the following, which must be considered before initiating mixing studies:
  - Normal: ~5% of healthy individuals exceed reference range upper limit
  - Preanalytical error: lavender or green-cap tube, lipemia, hemolysis, clotted sample
  - Drugs: Dabigatran, unfractionated heparin
  - Congenital deficiency with bleeding: VIII, IX, or XI (hemophilias A, B, or C, respectively) or vWD
  - Congenital deficiency without bleeding: FXII, prekallikrein, or HMWK
  - FVIII or FIX inhibitor (acquired hemophilia)
  - Lupus anticoagulant (LA)
- **Mixing studies on PT or/and aPTT:** Performed by mixing patient plasma and normal plasma in a 1:1 ratio. Correction occurs in cases with factor deficiencies. Inhibitors prevent complete correction. Factor VIII inhibitors are usually time-dependent.
- Calculation of the index of circulating anticoagulant (**ICA**, also known as **Rosner index**) is recommended. ICA = $(b - c)/a \times 100$ (a, b, and c denote clotting times of patient plasma, 1:1 mix, and normal pooled plasma, respectively). Typically, values <11 suggest correction while values ≥15 suggest inhibitors.
- The **Chang formula** of %correction = $(a - b)/(a - c) \times 100$ (same key as above) where ≥75% value suggests that correction has also been used.
- **Specific coagulation factor assays:** Reduced factor activity is usual on functional assays. Non-parallelism of serial dilutions is indicative of an inhibitor
- **Bethesda assay:** Functional assay yields factor VIII inhibitor titer. Assesses the ability of a patient's plasma to neutralize factor VIII in normal plasma. Can be modified for other coagulation factors as well.
- **Immunological assays for specific factor inhibitors:** Enzyme-linked immunosorbent assays (ELISA) and microtitration plate-based immunoassays have been tested. Some factors (e.g., von Willebrand factor) give frequent false-positive results, necessitating caution.

Table 23.2 Acquired inhibitors to coagulation factors—a summary of salient features and management strategies [1–6, 9]

Factor/antibody target	Features	Frontline treatment strategies	Alternative treatment strategies
VIII	Mainly present with mucocutaneous bleeding; most antibodies (often IgG4) bind to the C2 or A2 domains	rFVIIa or FEIBA	FVIII with immunoadsorption, desmopressin, IVIg, IST
I (fibrinogen) or fibrin polymerization	Antibodies may be of IgG, IgA, IgM subtypes. Inhibit polymerization or release of fibrinopeptides. High-titer asymptomatic antibodies may arise due to cryptic or neoantigen exposure during high turnover of fibrinogen in pregnancy	Fibrinogen concentrate	Cryoprecipitate/fibrinogen concentrate with immunoadsorption, rFVIIa
II (prothrombin) or thrombin	Seen most often in APLA syndrome, cause bleeding due to increased clearance, lab results are consistent with factor deficiency rather than inhibitors. Thrombin antibodies may form following exposure to exogenous thrombin or surgery	FEIBA or PCC; FFP or even plasma exchange for severe active bleeding	FEIBA or PCC with immunoadsorption, rFVIIa, IST
V	Associated with bleeding; antibodies usually directed against C2 domain (phosphatidylserine binding on activated platelets + endothelial cells). Triggers may include exposure to fibrin glue or bovine thrombin	Platelets with FFP	FEIBA, rFVIIa, immunoadsorption + FFP, IST
VII	Rare. Isolated prolonged PT is seen. Mixing studies require prolonged incubation	FEIBA	rFVIIa, FVII, FFP, immunoadsorption + rFVIIa, FVII
IX	IgG4 antibodies; may arise post-partum	rFVIIa or FEIBA	Alternative bypassing agent, FFP, FIX concentrate + immunoadsorption, IST
X	Present with sudden onset bleeding, long PT and aPTT with transient, severe factor X deficiency. Often have recent acute respiratory infection	FEIBA or PCC	Immunoadsorption + FEIBA/PCC, rFIIa
XI	Often associated with SLE. Usually have mild or no clinical bleeding	rFVIIa or FEIBA	Alternative bypassing agent, IST
XII	Anti-XII antibodies common in SLE, associated with poor obstetric outcome and arterial thromboses. Impair fibrinolysis	Manage as for SLE and secondary APS	Manage as for SLE and secondary APS
XIII	Present with delayed bleeding post-surgery/invasive procedures. High mortality. Normal PT and aPTT. Clot solubility with 5 M urea, 2% acetic acid or 1% monochloroacetic acid is required	FXIII concentrate	Immunoadsorption + FXIII/cryoprecipitate, rFVIIa, IST
von Willebrand factor	Over 300 cases of acquired vWS described, common associations are SLE, gammopathies, myelo- and lymphoproliferative disorders and solid tumors. Antibodies inhibit RiCof and collagen binding, cause loss of HMW multimers	Treatments of inciting medical condition	Desmopressin, vWF concentrates, IVIg, plasmapheresis or rFVIIa, IST

APS antiphospholipid antibody syndrome, *aPTT* activated partial thromboplastin time, *FEIBA* factor VIII inhibitor bypassing agents, *FFP* fresh frozen plasma, *HMW* high molecular weight, *IST* immunosuppressive therapy including corticosteroids. cyclophosphamide, rituximab, etc. (see text); *PCC* prothrombin complex concentrates, *PT* prothrombin time, *rFVIIa* recombinant facto VIIa, *SLE* systemic lupus erythematosus (phospholipid/membrane-binding). The inciting cause for the production of autoantibodies remains unexplained in most cases, but similar to other immune phenomena, studies have implicated autoreactive T-cell clones that may arise from environmental influences aided by polymorphisms in HLA class II locus genes as well as in the cytotoxic T-cell-associated protein 4 or CTLA-4 gene. HLA DRB1*16 and DRB1*0502 are overrepresented while DRB1*15 and DQB1*0602 are reduced in acquired hemophilia A patients vis-à-vis healthy controls [7].

Interestingly, naturally occurring anti-FVIII IgG antibodies have been found in healthy individuals. These antibodies inhibit FVIII procoagulant activity *in vitro*, but *in vivo* they are neutralized by anti-idiotypic antibodies. Innate FVIII-reactive CD4+ T cells also occur among healthy persons. These are kept under control by T-regulatory cells. This apparent paradox only illustrates that autoimmune disorders arise from an imbalance between immunogenic versus tolerogenic signals that trigger host immune systems [7].

Antibody-factor neutralization kinetics. Interactions between the inactivating antibody and its target factor in acquired hemophilia show type II kinetics, i.e., a nonlinear inactivation pattern wherein the antibody-factor complex retains some residual catalytic activity. Practically, this means that patients may retain measurable baseline factor levels even if high-titer inhibitory antibodies are present. This phenomenon explains the non-correlation between measurable factor levels and bleeding severity in these cases [8].

23.2.3 Clinical features

Inhibitory autoantibodies against coagulation factors display a wide spectrum of clinical manifestations that range from life-threatening conditions to those with minimal or no bleeding. The latter include a few cases where antibodies are incidentally detected during the investigation of a suspected autoimmune condition or routine coagulation tests for another indication.

Bleeding in symptomatic acquired hemophilia is unlike that of the inherited form. Hemarthroses are typical in severe inherited hemophilia but are unusual in acquired disease. Principal manifestations of acquired hemophilia comprise skin and soft tissue bleeds. Reasons underlying this different bleeding pattern remain unknown; specifically, platelet dysfunction or abnormal fibrin polymerization has not been demonstrated. Soft tissue bleeding can lead to a limb-compromising compartment syndrome. Less common presentations include hematuria, gastrointestinal tract bleeding, and peripartum bleeding. The condition is potentially fatal. Mortality ranges from 8% to 22%. Risk of death is highest within the first few weeks after the onset of symptoms [1, 2, 4–6].

Clinical diagnosis before confirmatory lab testing is often difficult in these patients, since the associated medical conditions like autoimmune disorders, malignancies, and pregnancy are all by themselves also associated with multifactorial bleeding risks. Awareness of this entity is essential, and the sudden unexplained appearance of multiple hematomas or expansive ecchymoses in an elderly person without a known bleeding disorder should always raise the clinical possibility of an acquired coagulation factor inhibitor [2, 9].

23.2.4 Laboratory diagnosis

Typical initial laboratory results in acquired hemophilia A include prolonged activated partial thromboplastin time (aPTT) with reduced factor VIII coagulant activity (Fig. 23.1). Prothrombin and thrombin times are normal and, if prolonged, suggest inhibitors to other clotting factors. The thrombocyte count and platelet function are normal [4].

Mixing studies form the backbone of diagnostic assessment and are usually sufficient to clinch the diagnosis of a time-dependent (factor VIII) or immediate-acting inhibitor (factor IX and lupus anticoagulants). This distinction between factor VIII inhibitors versus the more common antiphospholipid antibodies or lupus anticoagulant is also important clinically. In the

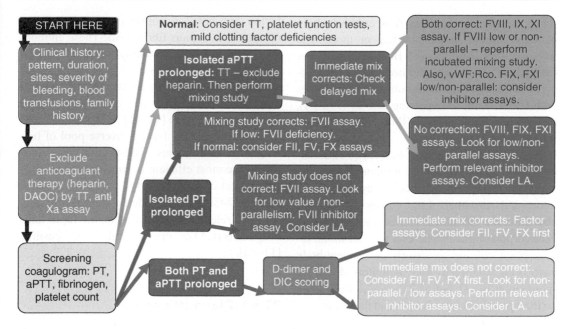

Fig. 23.1 A suggested scheme for laboratory investigation of patients suspected to have acquired inhibitors of coagulation. *aPTT* activated partial thromboplastin time, *DAOC* direct-acting oral anticoagulant, *DIC* disseminated intravascular coagulation, *LA* lupus anticoagulant, *PT* prothrombin time, *TT* thrombin time, *VWF:RCo* von Willebrand factor:ristocetin cofactor activity

latter, no correction of the baseline prolonged aPTT is seen immediately post-mixing of patient plasma with normal control plasma (Table 23.1). On the other hand, delayed-acting FVIII inhibitors are characterized by a loss of the initial correction once the mix sample is incubated for 2 h [2, 4, 9].

The definition of *correction* of clotting times in the 1:1 mix has varied in literature, from a value in the reference range of normal plasma to a more practical definition of corrected if the time becomes ≤10% longer than the control plasma. Certain formulae like the index of circulating anticoagulant (ICA, also referred to as Rosner index) are recommended for more objective interpretation of mixing studies (Table 23.1). A modified formula, called the Chang formula has been used especially with 4:1 mixes of patient:control plasmas [2, 4, 9, 10].

While interpreting laboratory tests, one must remember that markedly increased PT or aPTT due to a moderate/severe factor deficiency may not correct to within the reference range in mixing studies. On the other hand, a low-titer inhibitor can get diluted during mixing by the normal plasma to yield partial PT/aPTT correction. Also, it is possible for lupus anticoagulant and factor deficiency to coexist. Patients on oral direct thrombin inhibitors may secondarily acquire antibodies that may prolong the aPTT disproportionate to the PT. Bleeding patients with normal-range aPTT, or patients with prolonged aPTT but normal factor assay results, should ideally undergo two-stage or chromogenic assays for FVIII-coagulant activity [4, 9].

23.2.5 Principles of Management

Initial management of acquired hemophilia is based on the bleeding severity and inhibitor titer. It focuses on two major steps. The first is to control the active bleeding and the second is to avoid any interventions that may precipitate bleeding (e.g., antiplatelet medications, intramuscular injections, invasive procedures, or surgeries). Strategies for the former include administration of desmopressin (DDAVP), factor VIII concentrates (once acquired hemophilia A is established) in patients without severe bleeding or those who have low-titer inhibitors (<5 Bethesda units). For patients with high-titer inhibitors or severe bleeding, activated prothrombin complex concentrates with FVIII inhibitor bypassing activity (FEIBA), recombinant human factor VIIa and porcine factor VIII are suitable [1, 3, 9].

Subsequent management focuses on eliminating the inhibitor using immunosuppressive approaches like glucocorticoids, cyclophosphamide, and rituximab. Less commonly, intravenous immune globulin (IVIG), cyclosporine, and extracorporeal plasmapheresis with an immunoadsorption column to absorb the autoantibody have been attempted. Rare inhibitors disappear spontaneously (31 out of 215 in one study with no therapy except transfusions and factor concentrates) [1, 3, 9].

Monitoring of response to treatment is mainly clinical by observing the cessation of bleeding along with basic laboratory parameters. Decrease in inhibitor titer is very slow, and monitoring may be done monthly once immunosuppressive therapy is initiated. One in five patients relapse after complete resolution, but even among them 70% second complete remissions are seen. Relapse rates of pregnancy-associated inhibitors are lower. Low-titer inhibitors tend to remit in months, but antibodies with titers ≥5 Bethesda units may persist for years [2–4].

23.3 Section 2: Autoantibodies to Coagulation Factors: Inhibitory Antibodies in the Antiphospholipid Antibody Syndrome

The antiphospholipid antibody syndrome (APS) is a well-recognized systemic autoimmune syndromic disorder with protean manifestations. It is diagnosed by the presence in the patient of at least one clinical event (arterial or venous thrombosis or obstetric morbidity) and at least one persistent antiphospholipid antibody (APLA) that is directed against and influences a phospholipid associated/cofactor component including serum proteases, protein C, annexin V, FXII, tissue factor, anti-beta2-glycoprotein (GP)-I, toll-like receptors, or impairs fibrinolysis. These antibodies in addition to exacerbating the risk of arterial and venous thromboses and gestational losses also alter vascular elements, increasing susceptibility to atherosclerosis and cardiovascular and neurological damage [11–13].

Patients typically have a diverse pool of heterogeneous antibodies. The high-affinity antibodies are most efficient in causing activation of endothelial cells, monocytes, and platelets. The anti-beta2-GP-I is considered pathogenetically the most relevant antibody, while the lupus anticoagulants (LA) are diagnostically most sensitive [11–13].

23.3.1 Diagnostic criteria

The revised Sapporo or Sydney criteria (reproduced below) stipulate that APS is present in patients meeting at least one clinical and one laboratory criteria out of the following [14]:

Clinical criteria (at least one)
1. **Vascular thrombosis**—One or more episodes of venous, arterial, or small vessel thrombosis in any tissue or organ, with unequivocal imaging or histologic evidence of thrombosis. Superficial venous thrombosis does not satisfy the criteria for thrombosis for APS.
2. **Pregnancy morbidity**—One or more unexplained demise of a morphologically normal fetus at ≥10 weeks gestation, or one or more premature births of a morphologically normal neonate before 34 weeks gestation because of eclampsia, preeclampsia, or placental insufficiency, or three or more consecutive spontaneous pregnancy losses at <10 weeks gestation, unexplained by chromosomal abnormalities or by maternal anatomic or hormonal causes.

Laboratory criteria. Presence of at least one of the following antiphospholipid antibodies (aPL) on at least two occasions that are at least 12 weeks or more apart:

1. Immunoglobulin G (IgG) and/or IgM anticardiolipin antibodies (aCL) of a high or

moderate titer (>40 GPL or MPL units, respectively, or a titer >99th percentile for the testing laboratory), measured by a standardized enzyme-linked immunosorbent assay (ELISA).

2. IgG and/or IgM anti-beta2-GP I > 40 GPL or MPL units, respectively, or a titer >99th percentile for the testing laboratory, measured by a standardized ELISA according to recommended procedures.

3. LA activity detected by a three-step procedure.
   - **Step 1.** Demonstration of a prolonged phospholipid-dependent screening clotting assay. Common screening tests include dilute Russell viper venom time (dRVVT) and activated partial thromboplastin time (aPTT) optimized for this purpose (lupus-sensitive aPTT).
   - **Step 2.** Mixing patient plasma with normal plasma fails to correct the prolonged screening test(s). This eliminates the possibility that prolongation of the screening test is due to a coagulation factor deficiency. If the coagulation test remains prolonged after the addition of normal plasma, an inhibitor is present.
   - **Step 3.** Addition of excess phospholipid either shortens or completely corrects the prolonged coagulation test (evidence of phospholipid-dependence).

The revised Sapporo criteria [14] also indicate that the presence or absence of further substantial risk factors for thrombosis should be recognized among patients. While the ELISA immunoassays for anti-beta-2GP-1 are more straightforward to interpret, tests for LA typically are prone to more inter-laboratory variation. The LA/APLA Subcommittee of the Scientific and Standardization Committee (SSC) under the International Society on Thrombosis and Haemostasis (ISTH) issued guidance in 2009 on technical aspects of these tests [15], and this is summarized briefly below.

The ISTH SSC recommends collection of sample before initiation of anticoagulants. Patients already on anticoagulants need deferral until a suitable period after cessation of therapy. Testing is best done on fresh venous blood in a 9:1 ratio with 3.2% (0.109 M) trisodium citrate from which platelet-poor plasma (<10,000 platelets/microliter) is obtained by double centrifugation. If test is to be postponed, rapid freezing and storage at −70 °C or lower is recommended. At the time of testing, the sample should be thawed at 37 °C for at least 5 min by total immersion in a warm water bath and mixed well [15].

Screen, mix, and confirm steps are advised with at least two tests with *different* underlying principles being mandatory. The ISTH recommends a dRVVT as the first test followed by a sensitive aPTT with low phospholipids and silica as activator as the second. For mixing tests, a 1:1 proportion of patient to normal pooled plasma (NPP) is advised without a preincubation step with testing being done within 30 min. In-house NPP is preferred but commercial NPP can also be used if adequate. Screening test cutoff value should be at the 99th percentile of a normal population so as to maximize sensitivity or can be determined by the Rosner index (please see Table 23.1) [15].

Confirmatory testing is performed by increasing phospholipid content of the screening test. Ideally, bilayer or hexogonal (II) phase phospholipids should be used. The cutoff value is determined by % correction [(screen minus confirm) divided by screen value] × 100 or LA ratio (screen/confirm). Results are expressed as ratio of patient-to-NPP for screening, mixing, and confirmatory tests, and the final report should explain the results released beyond just numerical values [15].

Non-criteria Antiphospholipid Antibodies. These include candidates with less clear links to pathogenesis and in whom less-standardized assays are typically available including anti-annexin A2, -annexin A5, -ethanolamine, -glycerol, -inositol, -phosphatidic acid, -phosphatidylcholine, -protein S, -prothrombin, and -serine antibodies. They are not included in the Sydney criteria, but may be considered in an individual case where the diagnosis remains unclear using conventional testing.

23.3.2 Recent Advances in Diagnostic Testing

Although laboratory assays for aCL, anti-β2-GP-1 antibodies, and LA correlate with clinical manifestations of APS, none of them is uniformly specific for patients with this disorder. Many alternative diagnostic approaches are under evaluation to improve the accuracy of diagnostic testing for antiphospholipid antibodies [10–14, 16]. Chief among them are:

1. **Domain I-specific anti-β2-GP-I antibodies.** Autoantibodies that are specific for β2-GP-I domain I are linked more closely with thrombosis vis-à-vis other anti-β2-GP-I antibodies.
2. **High-risk antiphospholipid antibody profiles.** Triple positivity (LA, anti-β2-GP-I, and aCL antibodies) comprises a high-risk profile for APLA syndrome manifestations. Hence, current recommendations are that tests for APLA in patients suspected to have the syndrome should include all three assays.
3. **Endogenous thrombin potential.** This test identifies patients at risk for thrombotic complications especially in conjunction with factor VII and soluble P-selectin levels.
4. **Annexin A5 resistance testing.** Annexin A5 displays high-affinity binding with anionic phospholipids. In doing so, it forms a protective cover over membrane surfaces that restricts availability of anionic phospholipids for critical coagulation reactions. This physiological barrier can be disrupted by APLA, leading to exposure of negatively charged thrombogenic surfaces. Coagulation-based assays to test this resistance are available. These distinguish APS patients from otherwise healthy individuals with APLA-type antibodies and from persons with venous thromboembolism but no evidence of APS. Annexin A5 resistance also correlates with domain 1-specific anti-β2-GP-I antibodies, further corroborating a dual testing strategy to detect high-risk APS.

23.4 Section 3: Factor VIII and Factor IX Inhibitors in Inherited Hemophilia Patients

Development of an inhibitor is a relatively common and dreaded complication of hemophilia treatment. It occurs in ~25–30% patients with severe hemophilia A and 3–5% patients with severe hemophilia B. It often occurs subsequent to commencement of factor replacement in young children, early in the course of treatment, and is much less frequent in patients with moderate or mild disease. The inhibitory antibodies are directed against the specific deficient factor and are usually of IgG subclass. Inhibitor development is typically reported in terms of the number of exposure days (i.e., days elapsed on which the patient received replacement factor). For hemophilia A, the severity of factor VIII deficiency and the type of replacement product used are major predisposing factors [17–19].

Although the development of an inhibitor does not *per se* lead to a marked increase in frequency of bleeding, their presence can convert an individual with moderate or mild factor deficiency to a more severe phenotype. Bleeding episodes are much more difficult to suppress. An overall increase in the rate of bleeds over time leads to more rapid development of musculoskeletal and locomotor complications like acute and chronic synovitis. Although inhibitors occur more commonly in hemophilia A as compared to hemophilia B, the inhibitors in factor IX deficiency may have peculiar associations including nephrotic syndrome and anaphylaxis [17, 19, 20].

Hemophilia patients with inhibitors may be classified based on the degree of response in Bethesda units (BU) [2, 4, 9]:

1. **High responders**—Development of titers over 5 BU at any point of time indicates a high responder patient. There is an increase in antibody titers after successive exposures. The response begins within 2–3 days, peaks at 1–3 weeks, and can

persist for years in the absence of re-exposure. High responders require bypassing agents and are usually refractory to factor VIII preparations. Most hemophilia B patients developing inhibitors are high responders.

2. **Low responders**—Low responders have persistently low inhibitor titers (<5 BU) that stay stable even after factor infusion, and indeed may even disappear spontaneously. Patients may continue to respond to factor VIII replacement therapy with increased factor VIII dose.

23.4.1 Mechanism of Action

The inhibitory alloantibodies formed after factor VIII concentrate exposure target the factor VIII protein domains A2 and/or C2 as epitopes. Antibodies against A2 interfere with X to Xa conversion. Anti-C2 domain antibodies lead to loss of procoagulant activity due to interference with phospholipid binding and also lead to rapid clearance due to interference with vWF binding. C2 domain also contains the binding sites for thrombin and factor Xa, the former being responsible for factor VIII cleavage. Some antibodies can directly proteolyse factor VIII [21, 22].

Non-neutralizing antibodies also occur in these patients. In fact, congenital hemophilia patients with inhibitors often have multiple antibodies binding to distinct epitopes on the exogenous factor VIII. On the other hand, acquired hemophilia patients usually have a single antibody targeting a single factor VIII domain [2, 21, 22].

23.4.2 Predisposing factors

Both host and iatrogenic (replacement product-related) factors influence the chances of inhibitor formation.

Major risk markers for inhibitor development in patients with hemophilia a [21, 23–25]

Genetic risk markers
- Underlying *F8* gene mutation:
  - o Null mutations (including large deletions, stop-gain or nonsense mutations, and intron 22 inversion) confer highest risk
  - o Lower risk for missense, splice site, and indel mutations
  - o Higher risk for mutations in the 3′ half of the *F8* gene
- Afflicted family member with an inhibitor
- Ethnicity/race: Africans and Hispanics are at higher risk (may be partially explained by the fact that ~25% blacks with hemophilia A receive replacement products differing from their own factor VIII at one or two residues)
- Immune response traits: MHC class II system and cytokine (IL-10, TNF-α, CTLA-4) polymorphisms

Environmental risk factors
- Factor VIII replacement product: increased risk with recombinant products as compared to plasma-derived products (SIPPET trial) that contain vWF and other plasma proteins
- Intensity of first FVIII exposure: degree of tissue injury, surgical procedure, high frequency treatment
- Early prophylaxis: to prevent inhibitor formation

Based on the above, a risk score has been proposed for assessing risk of developing factor VIII inhibitors [26–28]:

- Family history of inhibitors—2 points
- High-risk gene mutation present—2 points
- Intensive treatment at first bleeding episode—3 points

Inhibitor incidence is 6%, 23%, and 57%, respectively, for risk scores of 0, 2, or 3 or more points. This otherwise robust score however requires mutation analysis and applies only to patients treated at least once, a potential disadvantage when used in patient being considered for first therapy [26].

23.4.3 Diagnosis and screening

The **Bethesda assay** both diagnoses and quantifies the inhibitor titer. For this, normal plasma is mixed with the patient's plasma in serial dilutions for 2 h at 37 °C. Residual factor VIII activity is then estimated using an aPTT-based clotting assay. The inhibitor titer in BU is the reciprocal of that dilution of the patient's plasma that results in 50%, i.e., half of residual factor VIII activity, since high-titer inhibitors require greater dilutions to show the residual factor VIII activity. A Nijmegen modification improves specificity and reliability of the Bethesda assay, especially with lower titer inhibitors, by enhancing the intrinsic buffering effect following serial dilution in the assay [2, 4].

Screening test for inhibitor development should be done at least annually. More frequent screening is required in severely deficient patients (once every 10 exposure days for the first 50 exposure days) and in patients with poor clinical responses or those with bleeding-increased severity or frequency. Lupus anticoagulants can confound the diagnosis of low-titer inhibitors [18–20].

23.4.4 Management principles

Therapy involves treatment of active bleeding followed by immune tolerance induction for long-term inhibitor elimination. The principles of the former are the same as those for acquired hemophilia. Immune tolerance induction, on the other hand, uses administration of repetitive doses of the deficient factor together with or even without accompanying immunosuppressive therapy for inhibitor eradication by resetting or toler-

izing the patient's immune system and thereby reduces antibody production. Younger patients with lower inhibitor titers (<10 BU) and a shorter time from onset of the inhibitor to therapy have superior outcomes. Hemophilia A cases also fare better than hemophilia B patients. The latter, in addition to lower success rates, also have a post-therapy risk of anaphylactoid reactions and development of nephrotic syndrome poorly responsive to corticosteroids. Rituximab may help in high-titer inhibitors that are unresponsive to immune tolerance therapy [3, 18, 20].

Recent years have seen the rapid development of novel alternative hemostatic preparations or agents for therapeutic use. These novel agents are based on technological maneuvering of coagulation pathway factors and its natural anticoagulants to obtain hemostasis. Approaches for their development include factor biomimics that resist natural anticoagulant systems and knock-down or disrupted effete natural anticoagulants that cannot degrade coagulation factors [29].

23.5 Section 4: Heparin as an *In Vitro* and *In Vivo* Inhibitor of Coagulation: Via Potentiation of Antithrombin

Heparin, although not an antibody, is a biological substance that is often included among the inhibitors of coagulation. Exclusion of heparin contamination is frequently required for samples received in the coagulation laboratory and may be carried out as follows [4]:

1. History, patient chart review.
2. Repeat on a fresh skin puncture specimen. If there is no other source of blood other than a heparinized line, then the line must be flushed thoroughly before sampling and the results scrutinized for possible artifacts.
3. Thrombin time (high NPV).
4. Reptilase time (the venom of the lancehead snake *Bothrops atrox* cleaves fibrinopeptide A but not fibrinopeptide B from fibrinogen to form fibrils of fibrin I. The enzyme is unaf-

fected by even a potentiated human inhibitor and generates a normal clotting time in the presence of heparin or, alternatively, dabigatran-like direct thrombin inhibitors. Abnormalities of fibrinogen prolong the reptilase time).

5. Heparinase treatment, for instance with Hepzyme (Baxter Diagnostics).
6. Mixing study with toluidine blue (toluidine blue neutralizes heparin but has no effect on hepatic or moderate level FDPs; hence, a prolonged TT even after mixing NPP + toluidine blue indicates fibrinogen deficiency or a very high-concentration FDP).

23.6 Conclusion

This chapter has attempted to cover the various pathological entities that are included under the umbrella term "inhibitors in coagulation." Together, this motley group of antibodies in inherited and acquired hemophilia as well as the APLA syndrome illustrates the multifaceted nature of human hemostatic pathways, and the various factors that control and modulate them.

References

1. Hurwitz A, Massone R, Lopez BL. Acquired bleeding disorders. Hematol Oncol Clin North Am. 2017;31(6):1123–45.
2. Giangrande P. Acquired hemophilia. Monograph published by the World Federation of Hemophilia (WFH) 2005, revised 2012. No. 38; Nov 2012. www.wfh.org/publication/files/pdf-1186.pdf. Accessed 31 Jul 2018.
3. Ljung RCR. How I manage patients with inherited haemophilia A and B and factor inhibitors. Br J Haematol. 2018;180(4):501–10.
4. Bain BJ, Bates I, Laffan MA, Lewis SM. Dacie and lewis' practical haematology. 12/e; 2017.
5. Collins P, Baudo F, Huth-Kühne A, Ingerslev J, Kessler CM, Castellano ME, Shima M, St-Louis J, Lévesque H. Consensus recommendations for the diagnosis and treatment of acquired hemophilia A. BMC Res Notes. 2010;3:161.
6. Kruse-Jarres R, Kempton CL, Baudo F, Collins PW, Knoebl P, Leissinger CA, Tiede A, Kessler CM. Acquired hemophilia A: updated review of evidence and treatment guidance. Am J Hematol. 2017;92(7):695–705.
7. Mahendra A, Padiolleau-Lefevre S, Kaveri SV, Lacroix-Desmazes S. Do proteolytic antibodies complete the panoply of the autoimmune response in acquired haemophilia A? Br J Haematol. 2012;156(1):3–12.
8. Ling M, Duncan EM, Rodgers SE, Somogyi AA, Crabb GA, Street AM, Lloyd JV. Classification of the kinetics of factor VIII inhibitors in haemophilia A: plasma dilution studies are more discriminatory than time-course studies. Br J Haematol. 2001;114(4):861–7.
9. Franchini M, Castaman G, Coppola A, Santoro C, Zanon E, Di Minno G, Morfini M, Santagostino E, Rocino A, AICE Working Group. Acquired inhibitors of clotting factors: AICE recommendations for diagnosis and management. Blood Transfus. 2015;13(3):498–513.
10. Depreter B, Devreese KM. Differences in lupus anticoagulant final conclusion through clotting time or Rosner index for mixing test interpretation. Clin Chem Lab Med. 2016;54(9):1511–6.
11. Keeling D, Mackie I, Moore GW, Greer IA, Greaves M, British Committee for Standards in Haematology. Guidelines on the investigation and management of antiphospholipid syndrome. Br J Haematol. 2012;157(1):47–58.
12. Danowski A, Rego J, Kakehasi AM, Funke A, Carvalho JF, Lima IV, Souza AW, Levy RA, Comissão de Vasculopatias da Sociedade Brasileira de Reumatologia. Guidelines for the treatment of antiphospholipid syndrome. Rev Bras Reumatol. 2013;53(2):184–92.
13. Groot N, de Graeff N, Avcin T, Bader-Meunier B, Dolezalova P, Feldman B, Kenet G, Koné-Paut I, Lahdenne P, Marks SD, McCann L, Pilkington CA, Ravelli A, van Royen-Kerkhof A, Uziel Y, Vastert SJ, Wulffraat NM, Ozen S, Brogan P, Kamphuis S, Beresford MW. European evidence-based recommendations for diagnosis and treatment of paediatric antiphospholipid syndrome: the SHARE initiative. Ann Rheum Dis. 2017;76(10):1637–41.
14. Miyakis S, Lockshin MD, Atsumi T, Branch DW, Brey RL, Cervera R, Derksen RH, DE Groot PG, Koike T, Meroni PL, Reber G, Shoenfeld Y, Tincani A, Vlachoyiannopoulos PG, Krilis SA. International consensus statement on an update of the classification criteria for definite antiphospholipid syndrome (APS). J Thromb Haemost. 2006;4(2):295.
15. Pengo V, Tripodi A, Reber G, Rand JH, Ortel TL, Galli M, De Groot PG, Subcommittee on Lupus Anticoagulant/Antiphospholipid Antibody of the Scientific and Standardisation Committee of the International Society on Thrombosis and Haemostasis. Update of the guidelines for lupus anticoagulant detection. Subcommittee on Lupus Anticoagulant/Antiphospholipid Antibody of the Scientific and Standardisation Committee of the International Society on Thrombosis and Haemostasis. J Thromb Haemost. 2009;7(10):1737–40.

16. Ortel TL. Antiphospholipid syndrome: laboratory testing and diagnostic strategies. Am J Hematol. 2012;87(Suppl 1):S75–81.

17. Miller CH. Laboratory testing for factor VIII and IX inhibitors in haemophilia: a review. Haemophilia. 2018;24(2):186–97.

18. Srivastava A, Brewer AK, Mauser-Bunschoten EP, Key NS, Kitchen S, Llinas A, Ludlam CA, Mahlangu JN, Mulder K, Poon MC, Street A, Treatment Guidelines Working Group on Behalf of The World Federation Of Hemophilia. Guidelines for the management of hemophilia. Haemophilia. 2013;19(1):e1–47.

19. Brown SA, Barnes C, Curtin J, Dunkley S, Ockelford P, Phillips J, Rowell J, Smith M, Tran H, Hematology Working Group. How we use recombinant activated Factor VII in patients with haemophilia A or B complicated by inhibitors. Working group of hematology experts from Australia and New Zealand, Melbourne, April 2011. Intern Med J. 2012;42(11):1243–50.

20. Gringeri A, Mannucci PM, Italian Association of Haemophilia Centres. Italian guidelines for the diagnosis and treatment of patients with haemophilia and inhibitors. Haemophilia. 2005;11(6):611–9.

21. Lai J, Hough C, Tarrant J, Lillicrap D. Biological considerations of plasma-derived and recombinant factor VIII immunogenicity. Blood. 2017;129(24):3147–54.

22. Clere AS, Diaz I, Lebreton A, Lavigne-Lissalde G, Schved JF, Biron-Andreani C. Are low-density lipoprotein receptor-related protein 1 or non-neutralizing antibodies predictors of FVIII in vivo recovery in haemophilia A patients? Haemophilia. 2014;20(6):e406–8.

23. Santagostino E, Young G, Carcao M, Mannucci PM, Halimeh S, Austin S. A contemporary look at FVIII inhibitor development: still a great influence on the evolution of hemophilia therapies. Expert Rev Hematol. 2018;11(2):87–97.

24. Rosendaal FR, Palla R, Garagiola I, Mannucci PM, Peyvandi F, SIPPET Study Group. Genetic risk stratification to reduce inhibitor development in the early treatment of hemophilia A: a SIPPET analysis. Blood. 2017;130(15):1757–9.

25. Lai JD, Lillicrap D. Factor VIII inhibitors: advances in basic and translational science. Int J Lab Hematol. 2017;39(Suppl 1):6–13.

26. ter Avest PC, Fischer K, Mancuso ME, Santagostino E, Yuste VJ, van den Berg HM, van der Bom JG, CANAL Study Group. Risk stratification for inhibitor development at first treatment for severe hemophilia A: a tool for clinical practice. J Thromb Haemost. 2008;6(12):2048–54.

27. Marcucci M, Mancuso ME, Santagostino E, Kenet G, Elalfy M, Holzhauer S, Bidlingmaier C, Escuriola Ettingshausen C, Iorio A, Nowak-Göttl U. Type and intensity of FVIII exposure on inhibitor development in PUPs with haemophilia A. A patient-level meta-analysis. Thromb Haemost. 2015;113(5):958–67.

28. Coppola A, Santoro C, Tagliaferri A, Franchini M, DI Minno G. Understanding inhibitor development in haemophilia A: towards clinical prediction and prevention strategies. Haemophilia. 2010;16(Suppl 1):13–9.

29. Ragni MV. Novel alternate hemostatic agents for patients with inhibitors: beyond bypass therapy. Hematology Am Soc Hematol Educ Program. 2017;2017(1):605–9.

Part IV

Miscellaneous

Role of Laboratory in Hematopoietic Stem Cell Transplantation

Dinesh Chandra and Ruchi Gupta

24.1 Introduction

Hematopoietic stem cell transplantation (HSCT) is considered as the standard of care for numerous hematological malignancies. A successful HSCT requires the support of a good clinical laboratory which performs various routine clinical tests as well as transplantation specific investigations. Transplant biology laboratory should be well equipped and have the infrastructure for performing investigations pertaining to tissue typing, CD34 enumeration by flow cytometry, assessment of graft viability/rejection, evaluation of minimal residual disease, and measurement of immunosuppressive drugs. The importance of the routine clinical laboratory tests like biochemical, hematological, serological, urinary, and microbiological examinations too cannot be undermined in a transplant setup. The clinical laboratory monitoring is important at each step and contributes to an early diagnosis, monitoring, and thereby enhancing prevention and treatment of the complications or adverse events. It is essential to provide information regarding engraftment, chimerism, diagnosing infections, veno-occlusive disease, therapy-related toxicities, graft versus host disease, and thrombotic microangiopathy which are the major causes of

mortality and morbidity in HSCT. In this chapter, the importance of a laboratory in different facets of HSCT will be discussed.

24.1.1 Pretransplant Workup

The role of the laboratory starts from the point of selection of a matched donor by HLA typing, which is followed by the screening of donor and patient samples for various infectious and biochemical parameters. A detailed evaluation of the donor is essential before allogeneic SCT (Allo SCT) to ensure that the harvest is disease free, particularly of any transmissible infections, and the donation is safe for the donor. The routine donor investigations performed before a HSCT are listed in Table 24.1. The recipient also undergoes a comprehensive pretransplant workup as listed below and other additional investigations to assess his comorbidities. Specialized pretransplant investigations are discussed in detail in the next section.

24.1.2 Human Leukocyte Antigen (HLA) Typing for Donor Selection

Every individual has a unique genome structure, and thus no two individuals can be genetically similar. Hence, the HSCT donor and recipient always differ in their genetic makeup. Among

D. Chandra (✉) · R. Gupta
Department of Hematology, Sanjay Gandhi Post Graduate Institute of Medical Sciences, Lucknow, Uttar Pradesh, India
e-mail: dineshc@sgpgi.ac.in

© Springer Nature Singapore Pte Ltd. 2019
R. Saxena, H. P. Pati (eds.), *Hematopathology*, https://doi.org/10.1007/978-981-13-7713-6_24

Table 24.1 Routine pretransplant investigations

Hematological parameters
CBC with peripheral smear examination
Coagulation profile including PT, APTT, Pl fibrinogen levels
Biochemical parameters
Liver function tests (serum protein, albumin, aminotransferase, bilirubin)
Renal function tests (creatinine and blood urea nitrogen)
Serum electrolytes
Serum glucose levels
Blood grouping
Infectious disease workup
Viruses—HIV, HTLV, HBV, HCV, CMV, EBV, VZV
Bacterial infections particularly tuberculosis
Parasitic infestations
Urine analysis
Imaging
Chest X-ray
Ultrasonography
Electrocardiogram
Pulmonary function test and endoscopy as indicated
Screening for carrier states of inherited disorders, if any

several others, the major and minor histocompatibility genes and killer cell immunoglobulin-like receptor (KIR) genes are of paramount importance in HSCT. These genetic variations result in the generation of numerous potentially immunogenic antigens in the recipient which in the course of HSCT may lead to graft versus host disease (GVHD), graft versus leukemia (GVL) effect, or graft rejection. Major histocompatibility complex (MHC) region of the genome encompasses the genes which encode for the transplant-related antigens [1].

The MHC region is located on the short arm of chromosome 6 and considered as one of the most complex regions (4 Mb) due to its enormous polymorphism [2]. The HLA region has approximately 200 genes of which six HLA genes—class I-A, B, C and class II-DR, DP, DQ—play a critical role in the recognition of self-antigens from non-self. The HLA proteins play a central role in triggering the immune response during infections, autoimmune disease, cancer, and drug reactions [3]. The HLA typing is widely used in solid organ as well as HSC

transplant and guides in identifying a suitable donor for the patient. The risk of GVHD and chances of transplant survival are better, where the HLA alleles of the donor and recipient are closely matched [4].

Various technologies are available to identify the HLA genes. With increasing knowledge of the human genetic database, the polymorphism of HLA system has been better understood. The HLA typing techniques have thus evolved from serological to advanced molecular methods. Serological approach was based on the complement-dependent cytotoxicity (CDC) and has been in use till date since its inception many years ago. For null allele identification, the serological methods are still applicable. However, in the molecular era and the advent of Polymerase Chain Reaction (PCR), the DNA-based techniques are preferred for typing as they are more accurate and reproducible. The DNA-based typing is preferred over the conventional serological typing as it has the advantage of (1) specificity—which is due to the primers and probes designed for a specific sequence of nucleotide, (2) flexibility—new primers can be synthesized to accommodate identification of the newly discovered alleles, and (3) robustness—in terms of the need for specific cell type and is unaffected by the patient health [5].

The different DNA-based methods include PCR-sequence-specific primers (SSP), real-time PCR, Sequencing-Based Typing (SBT), and PCR-sequence-specific oligonucleotide (SSO), and the latest addition to the list is the next-generation sequencing (NGS) [6]. The level of resolution of molecular methods is primarily due to the specificity of the probe used for the typing and varies according to the depth of information provided in defining the sequence of the nucleotide of an HLA gene [7].

(a) *Low Resolution*: Serologically defined antigen equivalent (HLA-A*02) is detected by low-resolution kits. SSP and SSO with limited number of probes can provide this basic sequence information about a particular gene. This is comparable to the serological typing.

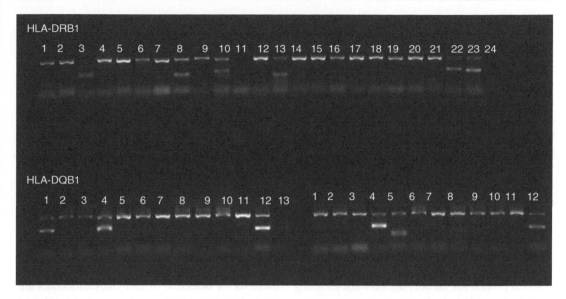

Fig. 24.1 Example of low-resolution HLA-DRB1 typing by SSP. The agarose gel shows the presence of internal control bands (arrow) and specific amplified products in lanes 3, 8, 10, 13, 22, and 23. A software-based analysis indicates the presence of HLA-DRB1*11 and HLA-DRB1*15 alleles. The specific amplification in lane 22 indicates the presence of DRB3* alleles, while the amplified product or band in lane 23 identifies the DRB5* alleles

(b) *Intermediate Resolution*: The HLA typing results are representative of two or more alleles. For example, the allele reported as A*02;01/02 can be either A*02:01 or A*02:02. This level of resolution may be obtained by SSO with more number of probes.

(c) *High Resolution*: This typing method allows precise identification of an HLA allele and is based on the nucleotide sequence information (HLA-B*01:02). It identifies only those set of alleles which encode the sequence of protein specific for the antigen-binding site. Sequence-based typing (SBT) is the most commonly employed technique for high-resolution HLA typing and identification of new alleles.

24.1.2.1 Sequence-Specific Primer (SSP)

HLA typing by sequence-specific primer (SSP) is one of the most widely practiced approach. A predefined set of primers is used to amplify the target gene sequence by PCR. Each primer is sequence specific, and when there is complete sequence complementarity to the sequence of the template, an amplification product is generated. The amplified products are detected by separation of the PCR products by gel electrophoresis [8]. A software-based data analysis is used for HLA allele assignment (Fig. 24.1).

24.1.2.2 Sequence-Specific Oligonucleotide Probes (SSOP)

Sequence-specific oligonucleotide probe hybridization (PCR-SSOP) is a very economical method for typing the HLA alleles. In this assay, specific primers are used for exon 2 and 3 in case of identification of class I, while primers are used for exon 2 to detect the class II alleles. These primers are designed for specific locus amplification. The amplified products are then hybridized to sequence-specific oligonucleotide probes, ~20 nucleotide in length, on a solid support media. As in the case of SSO by Luminex platform, microbeads are used as the support media. These microbeads are color coded and hybridized with labeled PCR products. Phycoerythrin dye is used to detect the PCR products which are biotinylated.

This is followed by rehydridization of the PCR products to the complementary DNA probes that are bound to the microbeads. The detection system consists of fluorescent intensity detection of the microbeads followed by interpretation using the software. Thus, the specific HLA alleles are detected using 50–100 probes for higher resolution, the limitation being its inability to detect polymorphism outside the amplified region [9]. DNA microarrays, reported as variant of the SSO method, have a limited use in clinical practice owing to their high cost [10].

24.1.2.3 Sequence-Based Typing (SBT)

The most powerful technique among the DNA-based approach for identifying new alleles along with high-resolution HLA typing is sequence-based typing (SBT). The first step consists of PCR amplification of specific locus. Sequencing is performed on amplified single-stranded DNA templates using specific DNA primers, a DNA polymerizing enzyme, deoxynucleotidephosphates (dNTPs), and fluorescently labeled dideoxynucleotidephosphates (ddNTPs). The fluorescently labeled dideoxynucleotidesterminate DNA strand elongation, after incorporating into the growing chain resulting in the formation of variable sized PCR products. With the help of modern sequencing machines which use capillary electrophoresis for size separation, these different DNA fragments are automatically separated. They have a fluorescence-detecting laser, built in the equipment, which detects the labeled ddNTPs as they pass through the capillary and generate data as peak traces on a chromatogram. Four-digit allele information is required for HSCT and thus necessitates the use of sequence-based typing. High-cost and long turnaround time along with resolution of ambiguous allele combinations constitute the limitations for SBT [11].

24.1.3 Anti-HLA Antibody Detection

Human leukocyte antigen (HLA)-identical siblings comprise about 30% of allogenic HSCT. In unrelated donors, with a 10/10 match, there is still a discrepancy in HLA compatibility between the donor and recipient. In solid organ transplant, it is a well-documented fact that anti-HLA immunization has delirious effects. The risk of primary graft failure varies as per the type of transplantation; in matched unrelated donor transplantation, it is about 3–4% while in cord blood transplantation and T-cell-depleted haploidentical stem cell transplantation, it is 15% [12]. Anti-HLA donor-specific antibody (DSA) screening is highly recommended in recipients with primary graft failure.

The CDC assay has been the gold standard for many years for the detection of anti-HLA antibodies. It is based on the expression level of HLA proteins on the donor lymphocytes and the amount, avidity, and subclasses of immunoglobulins. Other methods for detection of anti-HLA antibodies are solid phase assays (SPAs), fluorescent bead-based assay, as seen in Luminex platform, and found to have increased sensitivity and accuracy [13].

24.1.4 CD34+ Hematopoietic Stem Cell Enumeration

In addition to the phenotypic compatibility between the donor and patient, the number of CD34+ hematopoietic stem cells (HSC) in the graft plays a vital role in determining the success of HSCT [14]. The CD34+ hematopoietic progenitor cells (HPCs) occur only in low proportion in peripheral blood, i.e., typically between 0.1% and 2%; however, their percentage can be increased by using cytotoxic drugs and cytokines alone or in combination. This allows collection of these primitive cells by apheresis, from the peripheral blood itself, in sufficient quantities required for transplantation procedure. CD34 antigen is expressed on the cell membrane of HPCs and has been correlated with colony-forming units in cell cultures. Thus, multilineage hematopoiesis can be restored by infusing these CD34+ HPCs in non-myeloablated patients. Furthermore, the hematopoietic reconstitutive capacity of PBSC transplants can be assessed by enumerating cells per kilogram of the recipient's body weight using flow cytometry. A CD34+ cell dose of 3×10^6 cells/kg or more has been shown to improve all hematopoietic recoveries, decrease the incidence of fungal infections and transplant-related mortality, and improve overall survival [15].

Flow cytometry-based CD34 enumeration not only represents a rare event analysis but also has the advantage of being rapid and reliable along with the provision of continuous monitoring of CD34+ cell count in the peripheral blood and guiding for the appropriate timing of aphaeresis sessions [16].

Hematopoietic stem cells (HSCs) have the potential for self-renewal and differentiation into all lineages of blood cells. Transplantation studies with the injection of HSCs into myeloablated recipients allow for the analysis of the presence of donor cells and their capacity to proliferate and repopulate, thereby indicating HSC activity. Hematopoietic stem cells (HSCs) have the potential for self-renewal and differentiation into all lineages of blood cells. Transplantation studies with the injection of HSCs into myeloablated recipients allow for the analysis of the presence of donor cells and their capacity to proliferate and repopulate, thereby indicating HSC activity. To be clinically relevant, any flow cytometric assay must meet the following criteria:

1. It must correlate with a clinically meaningful outcome such as time to multilineage engraftment.
2. It must be applicable for the different stem cell product sources, via cord blood, peripheral blood, and bone marrow.
3. It must provide timely results (less than 2 h) and must be reproducible between institutions.
4. It should be sufficiently flexible to permit more sophisticated qualitative analysis of CD34+ cell subsets using a multi-parametric approach.
5. It should be able to determine the viability of the target (i.e., CD34+) population.
6. It should be a single-platform assay.

24.1.4.1 Dual-Platform Method of CD34 Enumeration

Earlier, dual-platform methods were used for CD34+ HPC enumeration. In dual-platform methods, the leukocyte count is obtained from an automated hematology analyzer, while percentage of CD34+ cells of the leukocytes is determined by flow cytometry. One of the initial attempts at enumerating CD34+ progenitors by flow cytometry was made by Siena et al.; the improvised version was later known as Milan/Mulhouse protocol [17]. It was a dual-platform method, based on the evaluation of CD34+ cells with a low light scatter (SSC). Debris, cell aggregates, platelets, red blood cells, and their nucleated precursors were excluded from the analysis after initial forward versus SSC live gating.

The International Society of Haematotherapy and Graft Engineering (ISHAGE) later in 1994 defined a set of guidelines for accurately determining the CD34+ cells. This protocol was based on four-parameter flow cytometry method (forward scatter, SSC, CD45PerCP, and CD34 PE staining). This approach allowed the discrimination of HPCs (which express relatively low levels of CD45 on their surface) from lymphocytes and monocytes, thus permitting the detection of "true" CD34+ cells, which have a dim CD45fluorescence and low side scatter (CD45^{dim}, SSC^{low}) [18].

Sequential Boolean gating is done to fulfill the characteristic of true stem cell, for example, CD34+ events, which are dim CD45+ (dimmer than mature lymphocytes), have a low side scatter (comparable to mature lymphocytes and lower than monocytes). Cells fulfilling these criteria are regarded as true CD34+ HPCs.

24.1.4.2 Single-Platform Method of CD34 Enumeration

The dual platform methods, however, have shown greater intra-assay and inter-assay variability. To overcome this, a single-platform method has now become the preferred enumeration method for CD34+ HPCs. A single-platform method allows direct quantification of CD34+ cell concentration from cell suspensions by incorporating a known number of fluorescent beads. All single-platform methods are based on the ISHAGE guidelines, allowing the enumeration of true CD34+ cells after exclusion of non-specific cells through sequential gating [19]. The addition of a viability dye for true CD34+ cells was recommended since dead cells could not be excluded on the basis of light scatter alone. The viability dye is a nucleic acid stain that does not cross intact cell membranes, and thus viable cells are detected on the basis of dye exclusion. Several single-platform stem cell enumeration (SCE) kits are available commercially, for example, SCE™ Kit (BD Biosciences), Stem-Kit (Beckman Coulter), and CD34Count Kit™ (Dako). These are largely based on the modified ISHAGE guidelines published by Sutherland et al. and have four main components: (1) tubes containing a lyophilized pellet of known number of fluorescently labeled beads, (2) pre-titrated antibody cocktail of CD34-phycoerythrin (PE) labeled and CD45—fluorescein isothiocyanate (FITC) labeled, (3) a nuclear stain, 7-AAD, for viability testing, and (4) a RBC lysing reagent.

Dual platform techniques have the limitation of lesser level of standardization between laboratories, thus single-platform techniques are preferred. Use of single-platform techniques reduces the intra-assay coefficient of variation as there is no need of another instrument like a hematology analyser for assessing the cell counts.

In our laboratory, we perform single-platform CD34+ HPC enumeration using BD SCE kit on a BD FACS Canto II platform. The kit contains a pre-mixed combination of anti-CD45 (FITC) antibody (clone 2D1)/anti-CD34-(PE) antibody (clone 8G12), BD Trucount ™ tubes containing the lyophilized pellet of fluorescently labeled beads, and a 10× non-fixating ammonium chloride-based reagent. Leukocyte counts for specimens are determined on an automated cell. Appropriate dilutions with phosphate-buffered saline (PBS) are made in specimens exceeding leukocyte count of 30×10^9/L. A lyse/no-wash protocol is used for staining of the surface antigens CD45/CD34. Briefly, 100 µL of the specimen is added to the BD Trucount tubes and incubated for 20 min with 20 µL of the pre-mixed antibody cocktail and 20 µL of 7-AAD, in dark at room temperature. After incubation, red blood cells are lysed for 10 min at 20–25 °C by adding 2.0 mL of freshly prepared 1× lysing reagent. Each specimen is stained in duplicate and analyzed by flow cytometry for evaluating the performance method (Fig. 24.2). The absolute CD34 count is derived as per the formula shown below:

$$CD34 + cells\,/\,\mu L = \frac{No.\,of\,CD34 + cells \times Bead\,count\,per\,test \times dilution\,factor}{No.\,of\,beads\,collected \times volume\,of\,sample}$$

24.1.5 Cryopreservation of Hematopoietic Stem Cells

Appropriate preservation of the apheresis product is essential to maintain viability and prevent microbial contamination. If the product is to be transfused within 24–48 h of collection, storage at 2–8 °C is acceptable for HSC viability. However, to increase the duration of storage, cryopreservation is mandatory. Ideally, the products should be cryopreserved as soon as possible after collection. Though there are no universally accepted cryopreservation guidelines, the majority of the cryopreservation protocols involve the following steps under aseptic conditions: volume reduction by centrifugation, re-suspension of the pellet in plasma, the addition of a cryopreservative, controlled rate freezing, and storage in

vapor-phase liquid nitrogen temperatures (≤−196 °C). Ten percent dimethylsulfoxide (DMSO) is the most widely used cryoprotectant [20]. Prior to the stem cell infusion, the product is rapidly thawed at a temperature of 37 °C.

24.2 Posttransplant Workup

24.2.1 Documentation of Engraftment After Transplant

Engraftment in hematopoietic stem cell transplant usually occurs 10–21 days after infusion of the stem cells. A number of factors can influence the engraftment kinetics, which includes the underlying disorder, pre-HSCT treatment protocols,

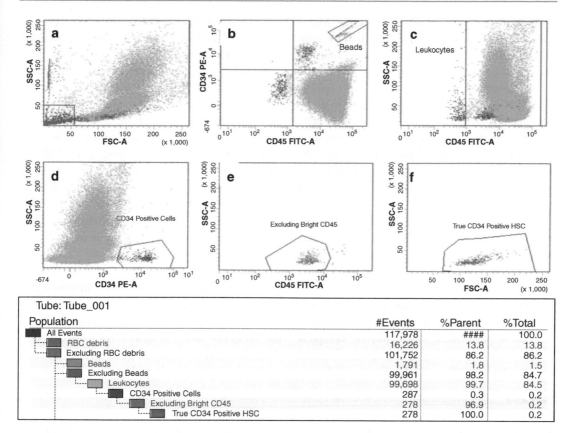

Tube: Tube_001			
Population	#Events	%Parent	%Total
All Events	117,978	####	100.0
RBC debris	16,226	13.8	13.8
Excluding RBC debris	101,752	86.2	86.2
Beads	1,791	1.8	1.5
Excluding Beads	99,961	98.2	84.7
Leukocytes	99,698	99.7	84.5
CD34 Positive Cells	287	0.3	0.2
Excluding Bright CD45	278	96.9	0.2
True CD34 Positive HSC	278	100.0	0.2

Fig. 24.2 Dot plots depicting the sequential gating in the single-platform method based on the modified ISHAGE guidelines for CD34 enumeration. **Plot a**: Represents all the acquired events and exclusion of RBC/debris in the first gate (invert gate). **Plot b**: The CD34 vs. CD45 plot shows the dual positive events or beads at the top right corner. These are gated to get the total number of beads acquired and also excluded from subsequent evaluation. **Plot c**: CD45 vs. SSC to gate the leukocytes. **Plot d**: Gating of the CD34+ events. **Plot e**: CD34+ events are re-plotted on CD45 vs. SSC plot to exclude the bright CD45+ (mature lymphoid) cells. **Plot f**: The dim CD45 and bright CD34+ events are plotted on FSC vs. SSC (to exclude the debris/platelets, etc.) and high SSC events (monocytes) and derive the true CD34+ HPCs. Absolute viable CD34+ HPCs count can be calculated by using the above formula

conditioning regimen, the quality of the graft, and post-HSCT complications like GVHD, medications, and infections.

The definition of engraftment may vary in different institutes, but minimally requires absolute neutrophil count of $\geq$500/mm^3 and platelet count of $\geq$20,000/m^3 for 3 consecutive days; a hematocrit of $\geq$25% for at least 20 days, in the absence of a transfusion support, is mandated. Documentation of engraftment is done by serial monitoring of complete blood counts [21].

Newer parameters in automated hematological analyzers have been used as indicators of engraftment, which bank upon the production and release of immature reticulocytes and platelets from the marrow. These cells have a higher RNA content, and thus, the immature reticulocyte fraction (IRF) and the immature platelet fraction (IPF) are derived in newer analyzers with the help of fluorescent nucleic acid-specific dyes. These parameters have shown good concordance in assessing marrow recovery [22].

24.2.2 Posttransplant Chimerism Analysis

The word "chimerism" is derived from a mythological creature consisting of the head of a lion, the body of a goat, and the tail of a serpent [23].

A chimera thus represents an individual whose cells are derived from genetically distinct individuals. Important indications for chimerism analysis in posttransplant patients are monitoring of engraftment process, detection of graft failure, the risk of relapse, GVHD, and response to therapies (such as DLI) [24]. Various terms have been used to describe the posttransplant chimerism:

Complete or full chimerism: When the patient shows only donor hematopoietic cells and no evidence of recipient cells at any time after transplant.

Mixed Chimerism: When the hematopoietic cells present in the patient are from the recipient as well as the donor. It is to be noted here that the recipient cells could be the normal hematopoietic cells or the leukemic cells.

Split Chimerism: The state of mixed chimerism is detected when lineage-specific chimerism analysis is performed. There may be complete chimerism (100% donor) in one or more cellular fractions, while other cellular fractions show a mixed chimerism or 100% recipient markers, for example, T cells are 100% host while the myeloid lineage cells are of 100% donor origin.

Chimerism testing is based on the differences in the genetic markers between donor and recipient. A variety of molecular techniques have been used for the detection of these differences in post-allogeneic HSCT: semi-quantitative fluorescent polymerase chain reaction (QF-PCR) of short tandem repeats, real-time quantitative PCR (qPCR) analysis of single-nucleotide polymorphisms (SNP), fluorescent in situ hybridization (FISH)/PCR for the sex chromosomes [25]. Different techniques have been used for post-transplant chimerism analysis, the details of which are listed in Table 24.2.

Chimerism analysis by sex chromosome-based amelogenin markers: Sex-mismatched HSCT is when there is difference in the gender of the recipient and the donor. In case of sex-mismatched HSCTs, amelogenin gene is used as a marker of choice as it enables the simultaneous

Table 24.2 Comparison of different methods for chimerism analysis [25]

Techniques	Sensitivity (%)	Advantages	Disadvantages	Informatively
Erythrocyte phenotyping	0.04–3	Easy to perform	Can be affected by transfusions; hence, not very sensitive/specific It may not be in rapidly proliferating disorders	Low
Cytogenetics	5–10	Particularly informative in cases of CML for detecting Ph +ve cells	Low sensitivity and high rate of false positivity	Low
FISH for X and Y chromosomes	0.1–0.5	Sensitive; applicable for screening a large number of cells and quantification	Limited for use in sex-mismatched transplants only	High
RFLP	5–10	Very informative and requires a small sample size. Can be used for lineage chimerism	Multiple restriction sites leads to low sensitivity and non-clear results	High
STR/VNTR	0.4–5	Widely used, highly informative. Independent of sex mismatch	There is low sensitivity due to competition of the primer for the major and minor cell population	High
Amelogenin	0.1–4	Very informative and reliable method in sex-mismatched transplants	False positivity rate is high owing to the use of the same set of primers for two different regions	High
Real-time qPCR	0.1–1	Rapid and powerful technique with high sensitivity and specificity. Provides exact quantification of mixed chimerism	Costly and efficient mainly with biallelic markers	High

RFLP restriction fragment length polymorphisms; *STR* short tandem repeat, *VNTR* variable tandem repeat; *FISH* fluorescence in situ hybridization, *qPCR* quantitative PCR

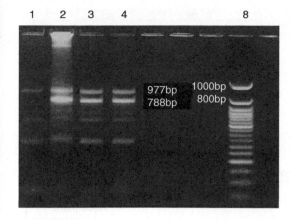

Fig. 24.3 Use of X, Y chromosome-based amelogenin marker. **Lane 1**: Recipient (female, a single amplicon of 977 bp), **Lane 2**: Donor (male, two amplicons of 977 and 788 bp, respectively), **Lane 3**: Day +30 posttransplant recipient sample, **Lane 4**: Day +90 posttransplant recipient sample. Lanes 3 and 4 show full chimerism. **Lane 8**: A 50 bp ladder

detection of cells of both genders by a single-step PCR. Thus, even a slight recurrence of recipient cells can be detected [26].

In our lab, we use the amelogenin marker in sex-mismatched cases, for analyzing the chimerism status of the recipient. Representative picture of agarose gel electrophoresis after PCR amplification in one of our cases is depicted in Fig. 24.3.

24.2.3 Chimerism Analysis by Short Tandem Repeat (STR)

The most widely deployed method for chimerism analysis is the fragment analysis of STRs. The PCR-amplified products are detected by capillary electrophoresis (CE) which has the advantage of being rapid, and the analysis of results is straightforward. In the CE-based sequencing equipment, the amplified DNA fragments migrate through the liquid polymer within a thin capillary with high voltage. The fluorescently labeled products are separated on the basis of their molecular weight. An optical detection device in the genetic analyzers detects the fluorescence, and software converts the fluorescence signal to digital data. As each dye emits light at a different wavelength,

following excitation by the laser, multiplex PCR experiments can be performed to simultaneously amplify the different loci. The differently sized PCR products can then be accurately sized or sorted into "bins" by the inclusion of a size marker [27].

The goal of the pretransplant analysis is to identify two or more informative STR alleles that differ between the donor and recipient and assist in monitoring chimerism after HSCT (Fig. 24.4).

24.2.3.1 Interpretation of STR Results

Posttransplant STR analysis is used to determine the percentage of residual recipient-specific allele(s) if present. The lack of recipient-specific alleles is compatible with complete engraftment. In the case of the presence of mixed chimerism, the calculations to assess donor chimerism are depicted in Fig. 24.5.

24.2.4 Detection of Minimal Residual Disease

The advent of newer techniques allows precise quantification of minimal residual disease (MRD) and also early detection of disease relapse. These techniques involve the study of novel leukemia-specific mRNA transcripts, few examples of which are listed in Table 24.3 [28, 29].

Different methods used to detect MRD for different diseases have been summarized in Table 24.3.

24.2.5 Monitoring of Posttransplant Infections

The risk of infection among the recipients of allogeneic HSCT is determined by various factors like the age of the patient, existing comorbid conditions, and adverse effects of treatment taken. The modality of the transplant, posttransplant immunological reconstitution as well as the severity of graft versus host disease play a major role in determining transplant outcome. It is also seen that the rate of mortality due to infection is significantly higher in cases who have infection post engraft-

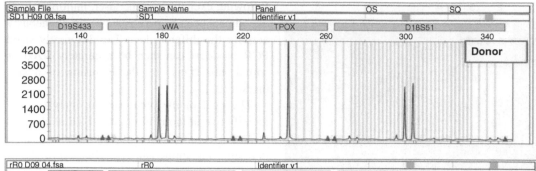

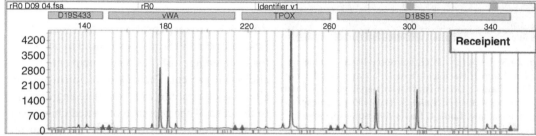

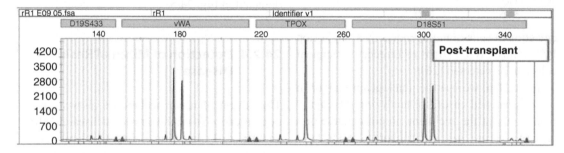

Fig. 24.4 STR-based chimerism analysis, in capillary gel electrophoresis. The figure shows electropherogram of fragment analysis of products obtained after multiplex amplification of three loci (listed in the gray bars) at day 70 post allogeneic stem cell transplantation. The top lane represents the amplified products from the donor (top), the pretransplant recipient (middle), and posttransplant recipient (bottom). In this case, informative marker was D18S51 alleles (different between the patient and recipient) while vWA and TPOX alleles were non-informative markers (similar alleles)

ment as compared to those having an infection in the short posttransplant neutropenia period [30].

The role of the clinical microbiology laboratory in support of stem cell transplant cannot be overemphasized as it accurately and on time identifies the various causative microorganisms viz. bacteria, fungus, and virus. Here, it is important to note that viral infections like Epstein–Barr virus (EBV), cytomegalovirus (CMV), and herpes virus 6 (HHV6) were found to be the underlying causative agents of morbidity as well as mortality after allogeneic HSCT [31].

During the period between engraftment and day 100 of BMT, infection by cytomegalovirus (CMV) has been found in a significant number of patients. In cases where the donor was seropositive for CMV infection, the rate of seroconversion was as high as 30% [32]. Thus, it is essential to diagnose the infection prematurely, in order to start presumptive treatment. Various tests available include detection of the virus in leukocytes and body fluids. The detection methods detect CMV-RNA, CMV-DNA, or CMV pp65 antigen depending on the method. Of these the most reliable result is that obtained by qualitative and quantitative monitoring of CMV-DNA as it aids in the monitoring of the treatment [33].

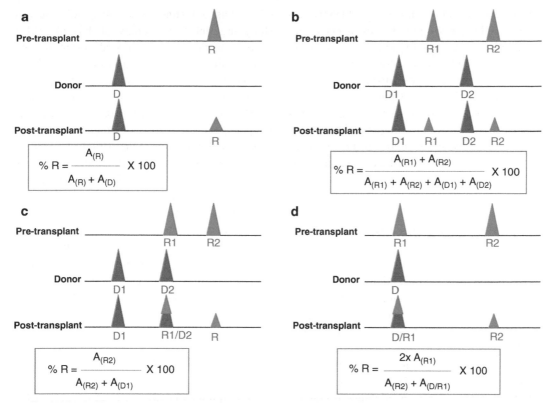

Fig. 24.5 Calculation of percent recipient cells: Four diagrammatic representative scenarios (**a–d**) for possible combinations of informative recipient (R) and donor (D) alleles are shown. For each scenario, the third line is a hypothetical posttransplant recipient sample showing a mixed chimeric pattern. The formula used to calculate the percent recipient cells is provided, where "A" represents the peak area of the appropriate peak. In case of heterozygous, the subscripts 1 and 2 indicate the two alleles

Table 24.3 Methods/markers used in the detection of MRD in different diseases

Disease	Identification markers	Technique
CML	BCR-ABL transcription	RT-PCR
AML	ETO/, CBFβ/ MYH11 fusion	RT-PCR
β-Thalassemia	β-Globin mutation and synthesis	PCR-based mutation analysis
B/T ALL	IgH TCR gene re-arrangment	PCR amplification of gene

Another pathogen known to significant morbidity as well as mortality is an invasive fungal infection (IFI) caused by Aspergillus [34]. The diagnosis needs to be made accurately as well as in a short time. The microbiological culture gives reliable results but is time-consuming and cannot be relied upon as the sole diagnostic method. Imaging techniques like high-resolution computed tomography aid in the detection of fungal infection even if it is deep-seated. Antigen detection technique detecting β-glucan and mannan helps in the early detection. Numerous molecular detection techniques are in the pipeline. Candida species is also known to be the causative agent. In addition to the microbiological culture, detection of the anti-mycelium antibody has been tried by some to make the diagnosis [35].

Detection of Galactomannan by enzyme-linked immunosorbent assay (ELISA) is found to be helpful in the early and prompt diagnosis of invasive Aspergillosis especially in high-risk patients with hematological malignancies. It is a sandwich type of ELISA. The test is interpreted as positive if the index value is more than 0.8 in a single sample or more than 0.5 in two consecutive samples. It has been found to have a sensitivity of 71% and specificity of 89% [36].

Detection of (1,3)-β-D-Glucan: It is present in the cell wall of numerous pathogenic and thus considered by some as a pan-fungal marker. It is detected by **the** ELISA technique and has a sensitivity of 82%. A limitation of this method is its false positivity in patients with bacterial infection [37, 38].

24.2.6 Monitoring and Workup for GVHD

All the patients who have undergone allogeneic HSCT should be evaluated for acute graft-versus-host disease (GVHD) as it can occur at any time after transplantation but more so in the initial few months posttransplantation. During the initial 100 days posttransplantation, the diagnosis can be made from clinical features alone which include diarrhea, skin rash, abdominal cramps, and elevated serum bilirubin levels [39].

Serial monitoring of biochemical parameters is the key to diagnose and detect acute GVHD at the earliest. The biochemical parameters indicative of liver involvement include increased levels of bilirubin, aspartate aminotransferase (AST), alanine aminotransferase (ALT), alkaline phosphatase, and reduced albumin. Hypoalbuminemia can be attributed to the GVHD-associated intestinal protein leak and a negative nitrogen balance while electrolyte abnormalities are due to decreased oral intake coupled with colossal diarrhea [40].

Further required investigations may include a biopsy for histopathological examination to rule out other differentials like drug reactions and infections. The biopsy is usually taken from the skin, liver, and/or gastrointestinal tract; it may be taken from all the sites or only the site with symptoms at the discretion of the treating physician. In the GI tract, the areas most commonly affected are caecum, ileum, and colon; however, the upper gastrointestinal tract involvement is not uncommon. The endoscopic findings include

edematous intestine with areas of mucosal sloughing and focal areas of bleeding [41]. Biopsy of the intestine reveals crypt abscess along with crypt-cell necrosis [42] while histopathological changes in the liver are dependent on the duration of insult on the liver due to GVHD. The changes can range from increased lymphocytes in the liver to irregular bile ducts, apoptosis of bile ducts along with dyskaryosis of hepatocytes. Inflammation of the endothelium is also not uncommon [43] while fibrosis of submucosa and serosa is evident in chronic GVHD [42]. Characteristic histopathological findings in skin biopsy include Langerhans cell depletion, dyskeratosis of keratinocytes, necrosis of basal cells, and exocytosis of lymphocytes. In chronic GVHD, there is a presence of dermal fibrosis along with inflammation of the sweat glands [44].

24.3 Conclusions

A well-equipped laboratory is an integral part of any transplant program, particularly HSCT. It not only is essential for the identification of the right donor but also aids in determining the adequacy of HSC in the harvest, their storage, viability assessment, engraftment, and subsequently delineating the chimeric status. Besides instrumentation, a certain degree of expertise and trained healthcare personnel are required for performing and interpreting the results of these specialized tests. Graft rejection, GVHD, and disease relapse are major potential complications of the transplant which can only be addressed and averted in the presence of an adequate clinical laboratory.

References

1. Kanda Y, Kanda J, Atsuta Y, et al. Changes in the clinical impact of high-risk human leukocyte antigen allele mismatch combinations on the outcome of unrelated bone marrow transplantation. Biol Blood Marrow Transplant. 2014;20:526–35.
2. Krausa P, Browning M. Detection of HLA gene polymorphism. In: Browning M, McMichael A, editors. HLA and MHC: genes, molecules and function. Oxford: BIOS Scientific; 1996. p. 113–37.

3. Piancatelli D. Human leukocyte antigen-A, -B, and -Cw polymorphism in a Berber population from North Morocco using sequence-based typing. Tissue Antigens. 2004;26:78–87.

4. Ferrer A, Fernandez ME, Nazabal M. Biotechnol Aplicada. 2005;22:91–101.

5. Erlich HA, Opelz G, Hansen J. Immunity. 2001;14:347–56.

6. Dunn PP. Novel approaches and technologies in molecular HLA typing. Methods Mol Biol. 2015;1310:213–0300.

7. Nunes E, Heslop H, Fernandez-Vina M, Taves C, Wagenknecht DR, Eisenbrey AB, et al. Definitions of histocompatibility typing terms. Blood. 2011;118:e180–3.

8. Olerup O, Zetterquist H. HLA-DRB1*01 subtyping by allele-specific PCR amplification: a sensitive, specific and rapid technique. Tissue Antigens. 1991;37:197–204.

9. Testi M, Andreani M. Luminex-based methods in high-resolution HLA typing. Methods Mol Biol. 2015;1310:231–45.

10. Zhang GL, Keskin DB, Lin HN, Lin HH, De Luca DS, Leppanen S, et al. Human leukocyte antigen typing using a knowledge base coupled with a high-throughput oligonucleotide probe array analysis. Front Immunol. 2014;5:597.

11. Erlich H. HLA DNA typing: past, present, and future. Tissue Antigens. 2012;80:1–11.

12. Hourmant M, Cesbron-Gautier A, Terasaki PI, Mizutani K, Moreau A, Meurette A, et al. Frequency and clinical implications of development of donor-specific and non-donor-specific HLA antibodies after kidney transplantation. J Am Soc Nephrol. 2005;16:2804–12.

13. Ottinger HD, Rebmann V, Pfeiffer KA, Beelen DW, Kremens B, Runde V, et al. Positive serum cross-match as predictor for graft failure in HLA mismatched allogeneic blood stem cell transplantation. Transplantation. 2002;73:1280–5.

14. Allan DS, Keeney M, Howson-Jan K, et al. Number of viable CD34(+) cells reinfused predicts engraftment in autologous hematopoietic stem cell transplantation. Bone Marrow Transplant. 2002;29:967–72.

15. Bittencourt H, Rocha V, Chevret S, Socié G, Espérou H, Devergie A, et al. Association of CD34 cell dose with hematopoietic recovery, infections, and other outcomes after HLA-identical sibling bone marrow transplantation. Blood. 2002;99:2726–33.

16. Sutherland RD, Michael Keeney M, Gratama JW. Enumeration of CD34+ hematopoietic stem and progenitor cells. Curr Protoc Cytom. 2003;25:6.4.1–6.4.23.

17. Siena S, Bregni M, Belli N. Flow cytometry for clinical estimation of circulating hematopoietic progenitors for autologous transplantation in cancer patients. Blood. 1991;77:400–9.

18. Sutherland DR, Anderson L, Keeney M. The ISHAGE guidelines for CD34+ cell determination by flow cytometry. J Hematother. 1996;5:213–36.

19. Sutherland DR, Nayyar R, Acton E, Giftakis A, Dean S, Mosiman VL. Comparison of two single-platform ISHAGEbased CD34 enumeration protocols on BD FACSCalibur and FACSCantoflow cytometers. Cytotherapy. 2009;11:595–605.

20. Aird W, Labopin M, Gorin NC, Antin JH. Long-term cryopreservation of human stem cells. Bone Marrow Transplant. 1992;9:487–90.

21. Gonçalves TL, Benvegnú DM, Bonfanti G. Specific factors influence the success of autologous and allogeneic hematopoietic stem cell transplantation. Oxidative Med Cell Longev. 2009;2:82–7.

22. Morkis IV, Farias MG, Rigoni LD, Scotti L, Gregianin LJ, Daudt LE, et al. Assessment of immature platelet fraction and immature reticulocyte fraction as predictors of engraftment after hematopoietic stem cell transplantation. Int J Lab Hematol. 2015;37:259–64.

23. Rose HJ. A handbook of Greek mythology. London: Routledge; 1989.

24. McCann SR, Lawler M. Mixed chimerism: detection and significance following BMT. Bone Marrow Transplant. 1993;11:91–4.

25. Khan F, Agarwal A, Agrawal S. Significance of chimerism in hematopoietic stem cell transplantation: new variations on an old theme. Bone Marrow Transplant. 2004;34:1–12.

26. Ghaffari SH, Chahardouli B, Gavamzadeh A, Alimoghaddam K. Evaluation of hematopoietic Chimerism following allogeneic peripheral blood stem cell transplantation with Amelogenin marker. Arch Iranian Med. 2008;11:35–41.

27. Lion T. Summary: reports on quantitative analysis of chimerism after allogeneic stem cell transplantation by PCR amplification of microsatellite markers and capillary electrophoresis with fluorescence detection. Leukemia. 2003;17:252–4.

28. Brunstein CG, Hirsch BA, Miller JS, et al. Non-leukemic autologous reconstitution after allogeneic bone marrow transplantation for Ph-positive chronic myelogenousleukemia: extended remission preceding eventual relapse. Bone Marrow Transplant. 2000;26:1173–7.

29. van der Velden VH, Hochhaus A, Cazzaniga G, et al. Detection of minimal residual disease in hematologic malignancies by real-time quantitative PCR: principles, approaches, and laboratory aspects. Leukemia. 2003;17:1013–34.

30. Maschmeyer G, Ljungman P. Infections in hematopoietic stem cell transplant recipients. In: Safdar A, editor. Principles and practice of cancer infectious diseases, current clinical oncology. Berlin: Springer Science+Business Media, LLC; 2011. https://doi.org/10.1007/978-1-60761-644-3_2.

31. Walter E, Bowden RA. Infection in the bone marrow transplant recipient. Infect Dis Clin N Am. 1995;9:823–47.

32. Nichols WG, Corey L, Gooley T, et al. High risk of death due to bacterial and fungal infection among cytomegalovirus (CMV)-seronegative recipients of stem cell transplants from seropositive donors: evi-

dence for indirect effects of primary CMV infection. J Infect Dis. 2002;185:273–82.

33. Tomblyn M, Chiller T, Einsele H, Gress R, Sepkowitz K, Storek J, John R, et al. Guidelines for preventing infectious complications among hematopoietic cell transplantation recipients: a global perspective. Biol Blood Marrow Transplant. 2009;15:1143–238.

34. Akan H, Antia VP, Kouba M, Sinkó J, Tănase AD, Vrhovac R, et al. Preventing invasive fungal disease in patients with haematological malignancies and the recipients of haematopoietic stem cell transplantation: practical aspects. J Antimicrob Chemother. 2013;68:5–16.

35. Richardson M, Ellis M. Clinical and laboratory diagnosis. Hosp Med. 2000;61:610–4.

36. Pfeiffer CD, Fine JP, Safdar N. Diagnosis of invasive aspergillosis using a galactomannan assay: a meta-analysis. Clin Infect Dis. 2006;42:1417–27.

37. Odabasi Z, Mattiuzzi G, Estey E, et al. Beta-d-glucan as a diagnostic adjunct for invasive fungal infections: validation, cutoff development, and performance in patients with acute myelogenous leukemia and myelodysplastic syndrome. Clin Infect Dis. 2004;39:199–205.

38. Pickering JW, Sant HW, Bowles CAP, Roberts WL, Woods GL. Evaluation of a (17→3)-b-d-glucan assay for diagnosis of invasive fungal infections. J Clin Microbiol. 2005;43:5957–62.

39. Glucksberg HR, storb R, Fefer A, Buckner cD, Neiman pE, clift RA, Lerner KG, Thomas ED. Clinical manifestations of graft-versus-host disease in human recipients of marrow from Hl-A-matched sibling donors. Transplantation. 1974;18:295–304.

40. Wakui M, Okamoto S, Ishida A, et al. Prospective evaluation for upper gastrointestinal tract acute graft-versus-host disease after hematopoietic stem cell transplantation. Bone Marrow Transplant. 1999;23:573.

41. Sale GE, Shulman HM, McDonald GB, Thomas ED. Gastrointestinal graft-versus-host disease in man. A clinicopathologic study of the rectal biopsy. Am J Surg Pathol. 1979;3:291–9.

42. Bone Marrow Transplantation. Cambridge, MA: Blackwell; 1994.

43. Shulman HM, Cardona DM, Greenson JK et al. NIH Consensus development project on criteria for clinical trials in chronic graft-versus-host disease: II. The 2014 Pathology Working Group Report. Biol Blood Marrow Transplant. 2015;21(4):589–603.

44. Esteban JM, Somlo G. Skin biopsy in allogeneic and autologous bone marrow transplant patients: a histologic and immunohistochemical study and review of the literature. Mod Pathol. 1995;8:59–64.

45. O'Shaughnessy EM, Shea YM, Witebsky FG. Laboratory diagnosis of invasive mycoses. Infect Dis Clin N Am. 2003;17:135–58.

Complement-Mediated Hematological Disorders

25

Neelam Varma and Shano Naseem

25.1 The Complement System

The complement system, which is part of the innate immune system, was first identified as a heat-labile component of serum that "complemented" antibodies in killing of bacteria. It is composed of over 30 proteins, which circulate as inactive precursors, and contributes 3 g/L to overall serum proteins. On activation of a complement system, a series of proteolysis-based activation cascade starts, which leads to the formation of membrane attack complex (MAC) and increased local immune response [1–3].

Complement kills microbes in following different ways

1. Opsonization—increases phagocytosis by opsonizing antigen. C3b and C4b have important opsonizing activity via binding to foreign organisms.
2. Chemoattractant/inflammation—by attracting macrophages and neutrophils to site of inflammation and increases their overall activity. Predominantly, C5a and, to a lesser extent, C3a and C4a act as inflammatory mediators.

3. Cytolysis—by rupturing cell membranes due to the formation of membrane attack complex (MAC). C5b–C9 form the MAC.
4. Agglutination—causes clustering and binding of pathogens.

25.1.1 Complement Activation

The complement system works as a cascade system, where one reaction triggers another and so on, and therefore grows exponentially.

Complement proteins are named by capital letter "C" and are inactive until they are split into products (e.g., C1), which are active and designated with a small letter "a" or "b" (e.g., C1a and C1b), with "b" being the active and larger part (except for C2). The smaller fragment (a) is released and acts as soluble mediator, whereas the larger active serine protease stays on the pathogen surface (b).

These complement proteins circulate as pro-enzymes (except for factor D) and become functionally active upon cleavage by a protease. However, the normal host cells are protected against complement attack, but foreign pathogens and altered host cells are susceptible to complement attack, which causes their phagocytosis and removal upon activation.

The complement pathway can be activated by either of the three distinct pathways. These require different molecules for initiation, but lead to finally activation of same effector molecules.

N. Varma (✉) · S. Naseem
Department of Hematology, PGIMER,
Chandigarh, India
e-mail: varma.neelam@pgimer.edu.in;
naseem.shano@pgimer.edu.in

© Springer Nature Singapore Pte Ltd. 2019
R. Saxena, H. P. Pati (eds.), *Hematopathology*, https://doi.org/10.1007/978-981-13-7713-6_25

1. Classical pathway (most specific—with antibody-dependent activation, binds C1)
2. Alternative (nonspecific, with auto-activation of C3)
3. Lectin pathway (some specificity—with mannose binding protein activation, binds C4)

All three pathways are mediated through C3 and C5 convertases that cleave molecules C3 and C5, respectively. This results in the production of two functional fragments each from C3 and C5: (1) inflammatory mediators—C3a and C5a; and (2) enzymatic cleavage components—C3b and C5b. These then lead to downstream inflammatory effects and amplification of the complement cascade, eventually forming cytolytic MAC, which is composed of C5b, C6, C7, C8, and polymeric C9 [4–6].

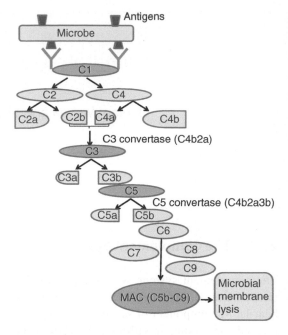

Fig. 25.1 Classical complement pathway

25.1.1.1 Classical Pathway

The classical pathway starts with binding of antibodies to cell surface and ends with lysis of cell. C1–C9 are proteins of this pathway.

Activation (Fig. 25.1)

– Only IgG and IgM antibodies can activate complement.
– C1 component contains three polypeptides (C1q, C1r, and C1s). The initiating molecule is C1q, which interacts with C1r and C1s to form activated C1.
– C1 attaches to Fc portion of antibody. C1 activates two other complement proteins, C2 and C4. C2 is cleaved into C2a and C2b, and C4 into C4a and C4b.
– **C3 convertase (C4b-C2a)**—C4b and C2a come together to form C4b2a which is the C3 convertase.
– Formation of C3 convertase represents the nodal point for all pathways of complement system activation. The C3 convertase causes activation of the common terminal complement cascade.

– C3 convertase activates C3 to C3a and C3b. C3b is an opsonin and it increases phagocytosis many fold.
  C3a increases the inflammatory response by binding to mast cells and subsequent release of histamine.
– **C5 convertase (C4b-C2a-C3b)**—When C3b binds to C2a and C4b, it forms C5 convertase (C4bC2aC3b), which activates C5 proteins by cleaving them into C5a and C5b.
  C5b begins to coat the surface of the target cell and is an opsonin, increasing phagocytosis.
  C5a binds to mast cells and increases inflammation.
– **Membrane attack complex (C5b-C6-C7-C8-C9)**—C5b on the surface of the target cell binds to C6, which activates C6. Subsequently C6 binds to C7, which binds to C8 and C8 binds to C9. Thus a circular complex of these proteins is formed called the MAC.
  The MAC causes cytolysis, by disrupting the inner integrity of cell membrane [6–8].

25.1.1.2 Alternate Pathway

The alternate pathway does not need antibodies to initiate and is therefore part of the nonspecific defense. It is slower than the classical pathway.

Activation

- Activation occurs by process known as tickover, which occurs by low level of constitutive activation of C3.
- C3 undergoes slow spontaneous hydrolysis to C3b and C3a. Subsequently, phagocytosis occurs by binding of C3b to foreign surface antigens. However, the mammalian cells are protected, as they contain sialic acid which inactivates C3b.
- C3b then binds to plasma protein factor B, on the surface of foreign cells. This causes factor D to cleave factor B to Ba and Bb.
- Factor Bb remains bound to C3b and factor D along with Ba separate away.
- **C3 convertase (C3b-Bb)**—Properdin (factor P), binds to the C3bBb and stabilizes it. The C3 convertase causes the production of more C3b, which results in the amplification of this pathway.
- **C5 convertase (C3b-Bb-C3b)**—When an additional C3b binds to the C3 convertase, C5 activation complex is formed, which cleaves C5 into C5a and C5b. C5b begins the production of the MAC.
  Membrane attack complex (C5b-C6-C7-C8-C9)—C5b is unstable and is stabilized by C6. C5b6 allows C6 and C7 to associate and penetrate a membrane. C5b67 recruits C8 which organizes C9 to form the MAC [9, 10].

25.1.1.3 Lectin Pathway

The lectin pathway is triggered by receptors, which identifies carbohydrates on microbial surfaces, as below:

- Mannose binding protein (MBP) or mannose binding lectin (MBL).

- The other three have a fibrinogen-like domain, including ficolins—M-ficolin (ficolin-1), L-ficolin (ficolin-2), and H-ficolin (ficolin-3).

Activation

- The lectin complement pathway is similar to the classical pathway, and instead of C1 complex, the MBL complex binds to the cell membrane of infectious agent, through MBL-associated serine proteases (MASP-1 and MASP-2).
- C3 convertase (C4b-2a) is formed when MASP cleaves C4 and C2.

Once the C3 convertase has formed at the pathogen surface, similar to classical pathway, it cleaves C3 to generate C3b and C3a. C3b acts as an opsonin and also binds to C3 convertase to form C5 convertase. C5 is cleaved by C5 convertase, to form C5a and C5b. C5b initiates assembly of a membrane attack complex, including C5b-C6-C7-C8-C9, that creates pores in the cell membrane of the pathogen and subsequent lysis [11–13].

25.1.2 Regulatory Proteins: For Complement Pathways

The complement activity is normally kept under control due to the requirement of a foreign pathogen to trigger activation and also due to the transient nature of the activation. However, uncontrolled activation can occur, which is prevented by regulatory proteins that keep control of the complement cascade. These regulatory proteins, present as both circulating in fluid phase and bound to the cell surface, are very important. They maintain the host defense against infection and immune homeostasis [4, 5, 8, 14–18].

Fluid phase regulators include

- **C1 inhibitor (C1 INH)**—binds to active C1r:C1s, leading to its dissociation from C1q, which limits cleaving of C4 and C2.
- C1 INH is also involved in the inhibition of several other proteases, including contact-

system proteases (plasma kallikrein, coagulation factor XIa, and coagulation factor XIIa), circulating complement proteases (MASP 1 and 2), and fibrinolytics (plasmin) [14].

- **C4 binding protein (C4BP)**—binds and degrades C4b to C4c and C4d. C4d limits amplification of classical and lectin pathways of complement activation, as it does not have protease activity [15].
- **Protein S**—binds to the C5bC6C7 complex to prevent insertion into the cell membrane and subsequent formation of a MAC [15].
- **Factor I**—cleaves C3b into iC3b and then C3dg and cleaves C4b into C4c and C4d, causing them both to become inactive. C4d remains covalently bound close to the site where the C4b was bound, and as C4d has a much longer half-life than C4b, it remains on the cell surface, while other molecules get cleared away.
- **Factor H**—along with Factor I inactivates C3b. This leads to inability of C3b to cleave C5 and factor B and the production of C3 and C5 convertases. This therefore affects the classical, lectin, and alternative pathway activation [16].
- **Anaphylatoxin inhibitor (AI)**

Cell-bound regulators include

- **CD55 (delay accelerating factor or DAF)**—promotes the dissociation of active C3 convertase. In lectin and classical pathway, it causes decay dissociation of C4b2a and formation of C3 convertases. In alternative pathway, it impacts the signal amplification by C3b, by inhibiting C3b formation [17].
- **CD59 [membrane inhibitor of reactive lysis (MIRL), MAC-inhibitory protein, or protection]**—inhibits C9 binding to the C5b678 complex, thereby impeding formation of MAC and preventing cytolysis [18].
- **Membrane cofactor protein (MCP, or CD46)**—serves as a cofactor for factor I-mediated proteolysis of plasma C3b.
- **Complement receptor 1 (CR1, or CD35)**—Similarly, CR1 also serves as a cofactor for factor I-mediated degradation of C3b.

- **CRIg (complement receptor of the immunoglobulin superfamily)**—recognizes C3b-opsonized surfaces and functions in immune clearance. In addition, extracellular domain of CRIg binds to C3b and interferes with substrate binding, limiting C3b-mediated amplification of activation of the alternative pathway.

These regulatory proteins function through different mechanisms:

- **By enzymatically attacking complement components, thereby inactivating them**—factor I inactivates C3b; anaphylatoxin inactivator inactivates anaphylatoxins (C3a, C4a, C5a).
- **By binding to and thus inhibiting complement components**—C1-INH inhibits C1; factor H acts with factor I in causing the inhibition of C3b; S protein binds to C5b67 and prevents MAC binding to cell membrane.
- **Regulatory proteins in cell membranes**—DAF (decay-accelerating factor)—it has the same function as factor H, the inactivation of C3b and C4b; membrane cofactor protein—it serves as a cofactor for inactivation of C4b and C3b.

Table 25.1 and Fig. 25.2 summarize the three complement pathways and their regulatory proteins.

25.2 Complement-Mediated Hematological Disorders

Dysregulation of the complement system is involved in a number of hematologic disorders and may be due to defects in pathways of activation, complement regulatory proteins, or deficiencies of complement proteins.

The main hematological diseases that are mediated by the complement system include

1. Paroxysmal nocturnal hemoglobinuria (PNH).
2. Atypical hemolytic uremic syndrome (aHUS).
3. Cold agglutinin disease (CAD).

Table 25.1 Complement pathways and their regulatory proteins

Pathway	Classic	Alternate	Lectin
Specificity	Most specific	Nonspecific	Some specificity
Activation	Antibody mediated	Spontaneous hydrolysis of C3	Mannose-binding lectin
Complement protein activated for initiation	C1	C3	C4
C3 convertase	C4bC2a	C3bBb	C4b2a
C5 convertase	C4b2a3b	C3bBbC3b	C4b2a3b
Membrane attack complex	C5bC6C7C8C9	C5bC6C7C8C9	C5bC6C7C8C9
Regulatory proteins	C1 inhibitor, C4BP, CR1, DAF, MIRL, anaphylatoxin inhibitor, MCP, Factor H, Factor I	CRIg, CR1, DAF, MIRL, anaphylatoxin inhibitor, MCP, Factor H, Factor I	C1 inhibitor, C4BP, CR1, DAF, MIRL, anaphylatoxin inhibitor, MCP, Factor H, Factor I
Hematological disease involved	PNH, cold agglutinin disease	aHUS	

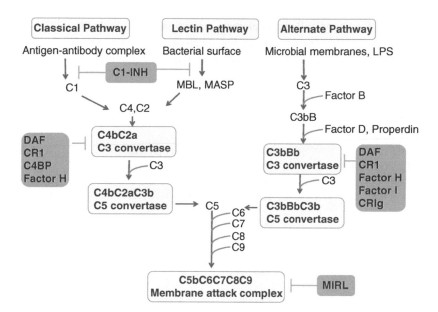

Fig. 25.2 Three complement pathways. The inhibitory proteins are shown in red boxes

25.2.1 Paroxysmal Nocturnal Hemoglobinuria

Paroxysmal nocturnal hemoglobinuria (PNH) is an acquired bone marrow disorder, characterized by triad of hemolytic anemia, bone marrow failure, and thrombosis.

It results due to uncontrolled complement activation, leading to complement-mediated intravascular hemolysis and also activation of monocytes, granulocytes, and platelets with the formation of prothrombotic microparticles, which together account for most of the clinical manifestations of PNH [19].

25.2.1.1 Epidemiology

PNH is a rare disorder with reported prevalence of clinical disease being approximately 16 cases per million population and an incidence rate of 1.3 cases per million population. However, it may be an underestimate as a subset of patients are likely to remain undiagnosed.

PNH is mostly a disease of adults, although reported in children also. The median age of onset is in the third decade. It affects males and females nearly equally despite being caused by mutation of a gene on the X-chromosome, because PNH results from acquired somatic mutation rather than a germline mutation [20, 21].

25.2.1.2 Pathophysiology

It arises due to acquired somatic mutation in the X-linked phosphatidylinositol glycan class A (*PIG-A*) gene in pluripotent hematopoietic stem cells. As not all stem cells of the bone marrow are affected, therefore, mosaic situation exists. The *PIG-A* gene product is responsible for the first step in the biosynthesis of glycosylphosphatidylinositol (GPI)-anchored proteins, and hence, the PNH stem cell and all of its progeny have GPI-anchored protein deficiency [22–25].

The deficiency of GPI-anchored complement inhibitory proteins, such as CD55 and CD59, accounts for uncontrolled complement activation and subsequently complement-mediated hemolysis that characterizes PNH. Till now, over 20 different antigens (e.g., CD16, CD24, CD52, CD55, CD59, CD58, CD66b/67, CD73, CD87, CD90, CD108, red cell acetylcholinesterase, neutrophil alkaline phosphatase, and homologous restriction factor) have been described that are missing from PNH cells. Table 25.2 mentions briefly the GPI-anchored proteins affected in PNH.

Platelets and granulocytes also have reduced GPI proteins, which result in infections and thrombosis seen in PNH patients.

CD55, CD59, and HRF all have roles in the protection of the cell against complement-mediated attack.

Therefore, after activation of complement pathway, red blood cells become susceptible to complement-mediated lysis due to the absence of complement inhibitory proteins. In addition, a proportion of granulocytes, platelets, and lymphocytes are also part of the PNH clone and

Table 25.2 GPI-linked proteins deficient in PNH

Protein/antigen	Function	Expression/distribution
CD55 (DAF)	Complement regulatory protein	All hematopoietic cells
CD59 (MIRL)	Complement regulatory protein	All hematopoietic cells
CD48	Adhesion molecule	Monocytes, lymphocytes
CD58 (LFA-3)	Adhesion molecule	Erythrocytes, neutrophils, lymphocytes
CD66/CD67	Adhesion molecule	Neutrophils
CD90/Thy-1		Stem cells
Acetylcholinesterase	Enzyme	Erythrocytes
Neutrophil alkaline phosphatase	Enzyme	Neutrophils
CD73 (5′-ectonucleotidase)	Enzyme	Lymphocytes
CD157/ADP-ribosyl cyclase	Enzyme	Monocyte, neutrophils
Comer antigen (DAF)	Blood group antigens	Erythrocytes
CD108/JMH antigen	Blood group antigens	Erythrocytes
Holley Gregory antigen	Blood group antigens	Erythrocytes
Yt antigens	Blood group antigens	
Dombrock residue	Blood group antigens	
CD14	Endotoxin receptor	Monocyte, neutrophils
CD16	Fc receptor IIIb	Neutrophils
CD87	Urokinase plasminogen activator receptor (u-PAR)	Monocyte, neutrophils
CD24	Receptor	Neutrophils, lymphocytes
CDw52 (CAMPATH-1)	Adhesion molecule	Monocytes, lymphocytes
CD109	Regulates signaling by TGF-beta	Lymphocytes, platelets
p50-80		Neutrophils
GP500	Platelet antigen	Platelets
GP175	Platelet antigen	Platelets

also lack GPI-linked proteins leading to their uncontrolled activation and further clinical symptoms, like thrombosis.

Therefore, bone marrow failure and thrombophilia are also seen in PNH patients. It also frequently arises in association with aplastic anemia and sometimes myelodysplastic syndrome (MDS) [26–28].

"According to the recommendations of the International PNH Interest Group, PNH is classified by the context under which it is diagnosed [29]:

1. De novo/Primary PNH: Evidence of PNH in the absence of another bone marrow disorder
2. Secondary PNH: PNH in the setting of another specified bone marrow disorder
3. Subclinical PNH: PNH clone on flow cytometry examination without signs of hemolysis."

Phenotypic mosaicism—characteristic feature of PNH, is based on sensitivity of the erythrocytes to complement-mediated lysis. This phenomenon of some red cells being sensitive to complement lysis and some being insensitive was studied quantitatively by Rosse and Dacie, and later, Rosse reported that in PNH patients, three populations of red cells can be demonstrated [30, 31].

1. Type III PNH red cells—are very sensitive cells, being 10–15 times more sensitive than normal cells.
2. Type II PNH red cells—are cells of medium sensitivity, being 3–5 times more sensitive than normal cells.
3. Type I PNH red cells—are cells of normal sensitivity.

Most PNH patients have a mixture of type I and type III cells, but mosaics of other two types are also seen.

In vivo the proportion of type III cells parallels the severity of the patient's hemolysis [27, 28].

In the presence of less than 20% PNH type III erythrocytes, visible hemoglobinuria is absent; when PNH type III erythrocytes are between 20% and 50%, paroxysms of gross hemoglobinuria occur; and when PNH type III erythrocytes are greater than 50%, constant hemoglobinuria is seen [28].

25.2.1.3 Clinical Presentation

PNH usually begins insidiously, with clinically apparent hemoglobinuria being the presenting symptom in only one quarter of patients. The illness ranges in severity from a mild, clinically benign process to a chronically debilitating, potentially lethal disease.

Most commonly, patients with classic PNH have symptoms of malaise, lethargy, asthenia, yellowish discoloration of the skin (jaundice), and darkly colored urine.

In addition, some patients present with features of bone marrow failure and thrombophilia.

Table 25.3 summarizes the frequency of clinical features reported at presentation in patients with PNH [32].

25.2.1.4 Laboratory Diagnosis of PNH

Initially, PNH diagnosis was based on tests that made use of the abnormal sensitivity of PNH red cells to lysis by complement. These include Ham test and the sucrose hemolysis test, both of which demonstrate the increased sensitivity of PNH red cells to complement. Although these tests are sensitive and specific, they are cumbersome to perform and are operator dependent.

Currently, traditional Ham and sucrose lysis tests have been replaced by quantitative and more sensitive flow cytometric immunophenotypic analysis of GPI-linked proteins.

Table 25.3 Presenting features in PNH from a study on 80 PNH patients [32]

Symptoms/signs	Frequency (%)
Anemia	35
Hemoglobinuria	26
Hemorrhagic signs and symptoms	18
Pancytopenia	13
Gastrointestinal symptoms	10
Hemolytic anemia	9
Iron deficiency anemia	6
Thrombosis	6
Infections	5
Neurologic signs and symptoms	4

Flow cytometric testing for PNH cells has certain advantages over the conventional lytic tests: it has higher sensitivity, performs a quantitative analysis, identifies the type of red cell abnormality (type I, II, or III), and also is the only method for the identification of PNH defect on platelets and granulocytes. The identification of size of PNH clone correlates with risk for thrombosis and identification of the PNH clone on granulocytes is also clinically relevant as granulocytes are unaffected by red cell transfusions [33, 34].

Analysis of somatic mutations of *PIG-A* gene can also be used for diagnosis. However, mutation analysis is less valuable for the diagnosis of PNH, as the development of PNH phenotype requires not only mutation of *PIG-A* gene but also a survival advantage of PNH clone. Therefore, currently, flow cytometry is used as a gold standard technique for PNH diagnosis and monitoring [35].

1. Acidified-Serum Lysis Test (Ham test)

In Ham test, at 37 °C, patient's red cells are exposed to the action of normal or patient's own serum, acidified to the optimum pH for lysis (pH 6.5–7.0).

A positive acidified-serum test, carried out with positive and negative controls, denotes the PNH abnormality. To increase sensitivity of the test, magnesium chloride is added. If there is lysis in inactivated serum (done by heating at 56 °C), the test should not be considered positive [27].

2. Sucrose Lysis Test

PNH-positive RBC undergo lysis in sucrose lysis test, as they absorb complement components from serum at low ionic concentrations. However, normal RBC do not undergo lysis, as they do not absorb complement components in the test conditions [27].

3. Gel Card Test

Sephacryl gel card technique is based on an antigen–antibody reaction. PNH cells lacking CD55 or CD59 do not agglutinate and pellet at the bottom of column, whereas normal RBC which express CD55 and CD59 agglutinate at top only [36].

4. Flow Cytometry Analysis

It is important to document deficiency of more than one GPI-anchored protein for PNH diagnosis, as in rare cases an inherited deficiency of one protein has been described [37, 38].

For GPI-anchored proteins on red cells— The patient's red cells are stained with a fluorochrome-labeled monoclonal antibody that is specific for one of several GPI-linked proteins—CD55, CD58, or CD59 which are deficient in PNH red cells.

For GPI-anchor or GPI-anchored proteins on neutrophils and monocytes—Similarly patients' neutrophils and monocytes are stained with fluorochrome-labeled monoclonal antibody that is specific for one of several GPI-linked proteins which are deficient on granulocytes— CD14, CD16, CD24, CD55, CD59, CD66a, and CD67.

Fluorescein-labeled pro-aerolysin (FLAER)—Analysis has been described recently for PNH testing. FLAER is a fluorochrome (Alexa fluor 488)-conjugated inactive variant of the bacterially (*Aeromonas hydrophila*) derived protein aerolysin, which binds specifically to GPI anchors. PNH granulocytes lack GPI-anchors and hence do not bind FLAER.

FLAER offers significant advantage as a reagent for PNH testing, compared to monoclonal antibodies against GPI-anchored protein normally studied, as its binding is less sensitive to the maturational stage of the cells, and also as it detects GPI-anchor, specific individual antibodies are not required. FLAER can also be used in multicolor combinations with monoclonal antibodies to GPI-linked and non-GPI antigens for the detection of PNH clones.

However, the main disadvantage is that the FLAER reagent does not bind to red cells, as red blood cells lack the enzyme that converts pro-aerolysin to aerolysin [39].

Table 25.4 summarizes the gating strategy and antibodies recommended for PNH testing by flow cytometry, and Fig. 25.3 shows flow cytometry plots of a case of PNH.

In Table 25.5 various laboratory tests for PNH diagnosis are outlined.

Table 25.4 Gating strategy and antibodies to be used for routine PNH testing [34]

Cells to be analyzed	Gating strategy	Antibodies
Red blood cells	– Log forward versus side scatter or – Glycophorin A versus side scatter	– CD59, CD55
Granulocytes	– CD45 versus side scatter or – CD15 versus side scatter	– FLAER, CD24, CD66b, CD16, CD157. Two antibodies preferred. CD55 and CD59 combination not recommended
Monocytes	– CD45 versus side scatter or – CD33 versus side scatter or – CD64 versus side scatter or – CD163 versus side scatter	– FLAER, CD14, CD48, CD55, CD157

25.2.1.5 Clinical Indications for PNH Testing [34]

PNH may present with varied signs and symptoms, and it being a rare disease, screening every patient with anemia or thrombosis is not suitable. However, some clinical presentations raise the suspicion of finding PNH clones, and these should be tested.

– Patients with unexplained intravascular hemolysis (e.g., with hemoglobinuria and increased plasma hemoglobin).
– Patients with Coombs-negative hemolytic anemia with no obvious infectious cause of the hemolysis.
– Thrombosis at unusual sites should warrant PNH testing. Although thrombosis as a complication is seen in 40% PNH patients, but as a presenting feature is seen in about 5% patients only and at unusual sites, such as intra-abdominal or cerebral thrombosis.
– Patients with coexistent thrombosis or intravascular hemolysis or cytopenias.
– Any young patient with cytopenia and a differential diagnosis of aplastic anemia.
– Based respectively on recent recommendation by the International PNH Interest Group and EXPLORE study, (1) all patients with aplastic anemia and (2) MDS should be screened yearly for PNH using high-sensitivity assays [29, 40].

25.2.1.6 Treatment

In 2007, eculizumab, which is a humanized monoclonal antibody, that binds complement C5, preventing its activation to C5b by the alternate complement pathway-C5 convertase and thereby inhibiting MAC formation, has been approved by both the US Food and Drug Administration and the European Union Commission for the treatment of hemolysis of PNH.

Treatment of classic PNH patients with eculizumab reduces transfusion requirements and improves anemia and quality of life [41–44].

Recent reports also show that eculizumab reduces the risk of thromboembolic complications [45, 46].

Prophylactic anticoagulation should be continued in patients on eculizumab with prior thromboembolic event; however, prophylactic anticoagulation is not recommended in patients who have no prior history of thromboembolic complications.

Eculizumab is well tolerated with minor adverse reactions. Although, meningococcal vaccination, followed by prophylactic antibiotics until 2 weeks after the vaccination, should be given to patients on eculizumab, as it may predispose them to fulminant *Neisseria meningitidis* infections.

The main limitation for treatment with eculizumab is its exorbitantly high cost—4,00,000 US dollars/year, and the therapy needs to be continued throughout life, as it only inhibits the formation of MAC, and the underlying stem cell abnormality continues as it is.

Therefore, in economically constrained countries, alternate treatment may be in the form of supportive therapy with folic acid, iron supplements, and blood transfusions. Prednisolone is

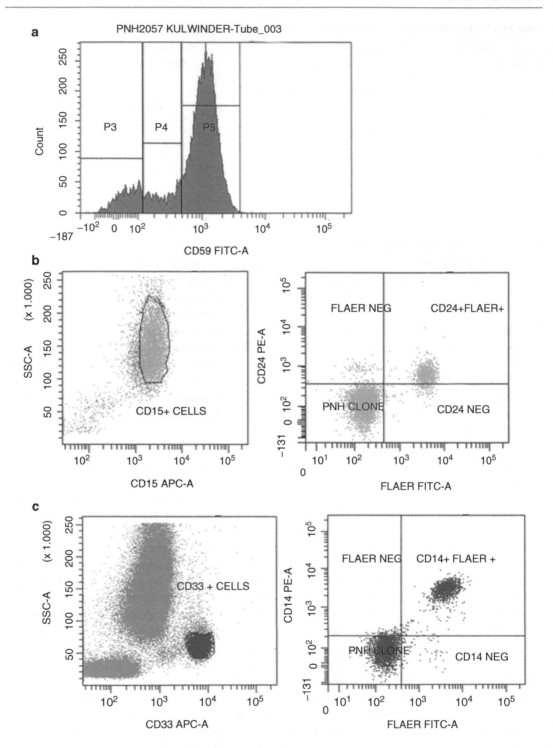

Fig. 25.3 Flow cytometry plots showing a case of PNH. (**a**) Red cells: P3 shows type III cells, P4—type II cells, P5—type I cells. (**b**) Neutrophils gated with CD15 anti-body, showing PNH clone, negative for both CD24 and FLAER. (**c**) Monocytes gated with CD33 antibody, show-ing PNH clone, negative for both CD14 and FLAER

Table 25.5 Laboratory tests for PNH diagnosis

Test	Remarks
Traditional tests	
– Ham test (acidified serum lysis test) – Sucrose lysis test	– Based on lysis of PNH red cells due to their increased sensitivity to activated complement pathway, because of deficiency of CD55 and CD59 on red cells – Are cheap, but labor intensive – Tests only for PNH red cells
Recent tests	
– Sephacryl Gel card test	– Uses the gel microtyping system – Is cheap and simple to perform, but has lower sensitivity and is not quantitative like flow cytometry analysis
– Flow cytometric analysis (RBC analysis, neutrophils and monocytes analysis, FLAER testing)	– Quantitative and highly sensitive – Identifies, the type of red cell abnormality- type I, II or III – Identifies PNH defect on granulocytes – As, granulocytes are unaffected by red cell transfusions, can be done in recently transfused patients
Genetic test	
– PIG-A gene mutation analysis	– Although specific for PNH defect, but is <u>not</u> recommended for routine diagnosis
Supportive laboratory tests	
– Increased lactate dehydrogenase levels – Low haptoglobulin – Increased unconjugated bilirubin – Increased plasma hemoglobin – Hemoglobinuria – Hemosidrinuria – Reticulocytosis	– are parameters of intravascular thrombosis – are supportive, but not diagnostic of PNH

also used during acute hemolytic exacerbations, but long-term administration of prednisolone even at low dosage is contraindicated. Patients with an episode of thrombosis should be put on regular anticoagulant.

The only curative treatment for PNH is hematopoietic stem cell transplantation. However, the decision of who should receive a transplantation has become all the more challenging, as reports have shown normal survival of PNH patients treated with eculizumab and successful control of recurrent life-threatening thrombosis and uncontrollable hemolysis with eculizumab [29, 45].

25.2.2 Atypical Hemolytic Uremic Syndrome (aHUS)

Hemolytic uremic syndrome presents classically as the clinical triad of nonimmune hemolytic anemia, thrombocytopenia, and renal impairment. It is classified as atypical HUS (aHUS), in the absence of Shiga-producing bacteria or streptococci.

aHUS is a thrombotic microangiopathy (TMA) that occurs due to defective complement regulation of the alternate pathway [47–49].

25.2.2.1 Pathogenesis

Mutations of the complement pathway are seen in approximately 50–60% of the familial and sporadic forms of aHUS.

Mutation of the factor H gene is the most common inherited abnormality in aHUS, causing dysregulation of alternative pathway activation. Hemolysis occurs due to less efficient binding of C3b and C3d on endothelial cells, resulting in increased vascular damage.

The other most common mutation seen in 10–15% of patients with aHUS is in CD46 (MCP). CD46 is a cofactor necessary for factor I, to cleave C3b and C4b on the cell surface.

In addition to factor H and CD46, other mutations have also been implicated in aHUS, including gain of function mutations of factor B and C3, loss of function mutations of factor I, thrombomodulin, and CFHR1/3 (complement factor H-related pseudogenes), all of which affect regulation of complement activation. Compound mutations are present in 10% or more of the patients [50].

aHUS patients have low C3 levels and high levels of activated complement components (C3b, C3c, C3d) and normal levels of C4, leading to selective activation of the alternative pathway [51].

When the complement system is triggered by infection or other factors, defective regulation of the alternative pathway leads to the generation of complement activation products. MAC (C5b-C9) causes direct injury of vascular endothelial cells, and C3a and C5a cause abnormal vascular permeability. This exposes the prothrombotic components in the subendothelium, leading to the activation of the coagulation system, microvascular thrombosis, thrombocytopenia, and ischemic organ injury. Microvascular thrombosis and vascular stenosis increase the shear stress, leading to fragmentation of red blood cells [49].

25.2.2.2 Clinical Presentation

aHUS is a systemic disease. The onset of aHUS crisis may occur spontaneously or after trigger of stress conditions such as infection, surgery, trauma, inflammation, pancreatitis, intravenous contrast agents, or pregnancy.

Gastrointestinal symptoms including diarrhea, abdominal pain, nausea, and vomiting are the most common acute presenting symptoms of aHUS.

aHUS can affect multiple organs, with renal failure, microangiopathic hemolysis, and thrombocytopenia being most common clinical features. Neurological symptoms such as headache, seizures, somnolence, or visual defects may occur. Cardiopulmonary symptoms such as chest pain and dyspnea may also occur. Advanced renal failure, hypertension, or complications of abnormal vascular permeability are more frequently seen in aHUS, than other TMA [thrombotic thrombocytopenic purpura (TTP)] [49].

25.2.2.3 Lab Diagnosis of aHUS

As there is no definitive test for the diagnosis of aHUS, its identification relies on exclusion of other TMA.

Although, decreased C3 levels may be seen in 30–50% patients and C4 levels in less than 10% patients, neither is specific for aHUS. Also, in patients with mutations of factor H/factor I, etc., the antigen levels of the affected proteins are decreased in around 30% cases. Mutation analysis will detect abnormalities in approximately 50% patients, also as compound mutations are common, all genes known to be involved in alternative complement regulation will have to be analyzed. The genetics of aHUS also involves single-nucleotide polymorphism, haplotypes, and combinations of common or uncommon variants of complement activators or regulators. Due to this complexity, genetic studies are not recommended for the diagnosis of aHUS.

aHUS should be suspected in patients presenting with microangiopathic hemolysis, renal function impairment, and thrombocytopenia, and the diagnosis is established after exclusion of TTP, typical HUS, etc., as detailed in Fig. 25.4.

ADAMTS13 (a disintegrin and metalloprotease with thrombospondin type 1 motif, member 13) assay should be done in patients presenting with thrombocytopenia, microangiopathic hemolytic anemia (MAHA), and neurologic deficits to exclude TTP. Shiga toxin assays are indicated for patients presenting with diarrhea to exclude typical HUS.

If ADAMTS13 activity is less than 10%, a diagnosis of TTP is considered; however, if ADAMTS13 activity is greater than 10% and Shiga toxin assay is negative, a diagnosis of aHUS must be considered.

In patients with suspected systemic infections, blood culture or viral studies should be done. Tissue biopsy/serological studies are required in patients with autoimmune diseases developing MAHA due to vasculitis.

In pregnant females with hemolysis and thrombocytopenia, HELLP (hemolysis and elevated liver enzymes and low platelets) syndrome should be excluded.

As few patients with aHUS may not have MAHA and overt renal failure, a high index of

Fig. 25.4 Approach to aHUS diagnosis and treatment

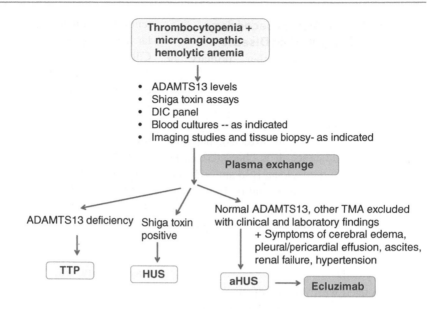

suspicion should be kept in the presence of hypertension, effusions (pleural or pericardial), edema (mesenteric, intestinal, airway, or brain), generalized anasarca, acute respiratory distress syndrome, exudative retinopathy, or posterior reversible encephalopathy syndrome (PRES) by imaging studies [49, 52–54].

25.2.2.4 Treatment

Plasma exchange is the initial therapy to be given till TTP is excluded.

Once diagnosis of aHUS is established, eculizumab is the treatment of choice and has been approved in 2011, by the United States Food and Drug Administration and European Medicines Agency for the treatment of aHUS.

Improvement in thrombocytopenia and mental status change occurs after one or two doses of eculizumab; however, recovery of renal function occurs slowly over many months.

Long-term therapy with eculizumab is usually considered for patients who have severe renal dysfunction or are predisposed to relapse/severe hypertension.

In patients, in whom eculizumab is discontinued, close monitoring with complete blood counts, renal functions, and hemolysis markers is required for the detection of impending relapse or organ injury [49, 52, 54].

25.2.3 Cold Agglutinin Disease (CAD)

CAD is a type of autoimmune hemolytic anemia (AIHA), having extravascular hemolysis, due to IgM autoantibodies fixing complement on the surface of red cells.

Overall, AIHA is characterized by autoantibodies that attach to and lead to the destruction of red blood cells resulting in hemolysis and anemia. AIHA is sub-characterized based on the temperature at which autoantibody acts.

- Warm-active antibodies—have greatest activity at 37 °C, are typically IgG, may or may not fix complement, and lead to red cell loss by splenic-mediated clearance of sensitized cells.
- Cold-active antibodies—have greatest activity at 4 °C are typically IgM, fix complement, and lead to immediate intravascular red cell destruction or hepatic-mediated clearance [27, 55].

Although, some activation of complement pathway may occur in few warm AIHA cases, but primarily it is not complement mediated, like cold AIHA/CAD. Therefore, here CAD which is complement mediated will be discussed.

25.2.3.1 Primary Versus Secondary Cold Agglutinin Disease

CAD is classified as either primary or secondary.

Primary or Idiopathic CAD

– Occurs in older adults, with peak age around 70 years. Both sexes are affected, but mild female preponderance. It is characterized by the presence of monoclonal IgM antibody and may be an indication of future B-cell neoplasms. However, mostly patients have a relatively benign, waxing, and waning hemolytic anemia.

Secondary CAD

– Is associated with various infectious and neoplastic disorders, including B-cell neoplasms, squamous cell carcinoma of the lung, metastatic adrenal adenocarcinoma, metastatic adenocarcinoma of the colon, and basal cell carcinoma, occurs after *Mycoplasma pneumoniae* infection or infectious mononucleosis, and is more commonly seen in younger adults.
– CAD secondary to infection occurs in younger patients, is a transient and self-limited process, is mediated by polyclonal IgM, lasts a few weeks, and usually does not require more than supportive care [55–57].

25.2.3.2 Pathogenesis of CAD

IgM autoantibodies (cold agglutinins) bind to red cells (commonly are directed against the I antigen) in peripheral parts of the circulation (e.g., fingers, toes, and ears). The classical complement pathway is activated on binding of IgM autoantibodies. The C1 esterase activates C4 and C2, leading to the formation of C3 convertase which cleaves C3 to C3a and C3b. Subsequently, on return to the central portion of circulation (at 37 °C), C3b remains bound to the cell, but IgM autoantibodies dissociate. As a result, intravascular hemolysis is not usually severe in CAD, due to diversity of temperature requirement for IgM antibody fixation and complement activation.

The C3b-coated red cells are then sequestered by macrophages of the reticuloendothelial system (predominantly in liver), causing extravascular hemolysis. C3d remains on the surface, after C3b of the non-sequestered red cells is cleaved. Therefore, patients have positive direct antiglobulin test for C3d but negative for IgG and IgM. However, few exceptions occur in patients with high titers of antibodies (>1:1000) or with moderate titers and activity at 37 °C. Therefore, thermal amplitude is a better predictor of hemolysis then titers.

In around 10% patients with CAD, usually in association with a severe exacerbation (infection, surgery, etc.), intravascular hemolysis resulting from terminal activation may occur. In other CAD cases, the classical pathway activity, due to the expression of CD55 and CD59 on the red cell membrane, does not proceed to activate the terminal pathway of complement [55].

25.2.3.3 Clinical Presentation

Patients usually have symptoms on exposure to cold. There is mild chronic hemolytic anemia in few patients on exposure to cold, with intermittent bursts of hemolysis, associated with hemoglobinemia and hemoglobinuria. Acrocyanosis can occur due to agglutination in the cooler vessels of the hands, ears, nose, and feet, which become cold, stiff, and painful.

On examination, there is pallor and icterus, and in chronic CAD patients, there is mild splenomegaly or hepatomegaly.

CAD secondary to Mycoplasma infections begins during the post-pneumonia recovery period and resolves spontaneously within 1–3 weeks.

CAD after infectious mononucleosis occurs either with the onset of disease or within 3 weeks of onset [55].

25.2.3.4 Laboratory Diagnosis of CAD

Care needs to be taken in collection of blood samples for testing for the thermal amplitude or titer of cold agglutinins. The blood sample is collected and maintained strictly at 37 °C until testing [27, 55].

1. Peripheral blood smear and complete blood counts

    If not obtained from pre-warmed specimen, the peripheral smear shows significant agglutination and RBC clumping. At times, agglutinates may be grossly visible in the specimen tube.

    With automated analyzers, a complete blood count done may show an artifactually low RBC count and a spuriously high MCHC due to red cell agglutination.

    The reticulocyte count is increased, with normal total leucocyte and platelet counts.

2. Direct antiglobulin (Coombs) test

    Red cells characteristically give positive reactions only with anti-complement (anti-C3) sera.

3. Cold antibody specificity

    Most of these cold-type autoantibodies have anti-I specificity, reacting weakly with cord-blood RBC and strongly with the vast majority of adult RBC.

    A minority are anti-I and react strongly with cord-blood cells and weakly with adult red cells.

    Rarely, the antibodies have anti-Pr or anti-M specificity and react with antigens on the red cell surface that are destroyed by enzyme treatment [58].

4. Cold agglutinin titer

    Doubling dilutions of the serum in saline are prepared at 4 °C—ranging from 1 in 1 to 1 in 512 of a 2% suspension of pooled saline-washed adult group O (containing I) cells, cord-blood group O (containing I) cells, and patient's own cells in three separate tubes. If the endpoint has not been reached at a dilution of 1 in 512, then further dilutions should be prepared and tested [27].

5. Determination of thermal range of cold antibody

    Tubes with a drop each of doubling dilutions of serum in saline are kept at 30 °C and at room temperature (20–25 °C), after adding one drop of a 2% saline suspension of pooled normal adult group O (I) red cells, pooled cord-blood group O (I) red cells, and patient's red cells. After incubation for 1 h, the presence or absence of agglutination macroscopically over a light is determined [27].

    Most pathogenic cold agglutinins are of the IgM class, with thermal amplitude exceeding 28–30 °C and titer of 1:256 or greater [54].

25.2.3.5 Treatment

It is very important for patients with CAD to prevent themselves from cold temperatures by protecting their hands, feet, and ears in cold environments.

However, patients who are symptomatic need pharmacologic therapy, and rituximab is the first-line therapy. Around 50% patients achieve remission with rituximab. Rituximab and benda-mustine-and-bortezomib-based therapy have activity in primary CAD, as a combination therapy. Eculizumab therapy has been used in some CAD patients with intravascular hemolysis.

The treatment should target the underlying cause in patients with secondary CAD [55, 59, 60].

Complement-mediated hematologic diseases are not very common. When suspected on the basis of clinical presentation and laboratory findings, should be appropriately worked-up for definitive diagnosis. This is all the more important, as specific therapy for inhibition of complement pathway, eculizumab, is available. We have had a rewarding experience, in diagnosing PNH defect by flow cytometry, using monoclonal antibodies against GPI-AP [61, 62] and FLAER [63, 64].

References

1. Ricklin D, Hajishengallis G, Yang K, et al. Complement: a key system for immune surveillance and homeostasis. Nat Immunol. 2010;11:785–97.
2. Merle NS, Noe R, Halbwachs-Mecarelli L, et al. Complement system part II: role in immunity. Front Immunol. 2015;6:257.
3. Sarma JV, Ward PA. The complement system. Cell Tissue Res. 2011;343:227–35.
4. Merle NS, Church SE, Fremeaux-Bacchi V, et al. Complement system. I. Molecular mechanisms of activation and regulation. Front Immunol. 2015;6:262.

5. Nesargikar PN, Spiller B, Chavez R. The complement system: history, pathways, cascade and inhibitors. Eur J Microbiol Immunol. 2012;2:103–11.
6. Walport MJ. Complement. First of two parts. N Engl J Med. 2001;344:1058–66.
7. Kolev M, Le Friec G, Kemper C. Complement—tapping into new sites and effector systems. Nat Rev Immunol. 2014;14:811–20.
8. Sjöberg AP, Trouw LA, Blom AM. Complement activation and inhibition: a delicate balance. Trends Immunol. 2009;30:83–90.
9. Nilsson B, Nilsson Ekdahl K. The tick-over theory revisited: is C3 a contact-activated protein? Immunobiology. 2012;217:1106–10.
10. Harboe M, Mollnes TE. The alternative complement pathway revisited. J Cell Mol Med. 2008;12:1074–84.
11. Kjaer TR, Thiel S, Andersen GR. Toward a structure-based comprehension of the lectin pathway of complement. Mol Immunol. 2013;56:413–22.
12. Nauta AJ, Castellano G, Xu W, et al. Opsonization with C1q and mannose-binding lectin targets apoptotic cells to dendritic cells. J Immunol. 2004;173:3044–50.
13. Wallis R. Interactions between mannose-binding lectin and MASPs during complement activation by the lectin pathway. Immunobiology. 2007;212:289–99.
14. Davis AE, Mejia P, Lu F. Biological activities of C1 inhibitor. Mol Immunol. 2008;45:4057–63.
15. Blom AM, Villoutreix BO, Dahlback B. Complement inhibitor C4b-binding protein-friend or foe in the innate immune system? Mol Immunol. 2004;40:1333–46.
16. Skerka C, Chen Q, Fremeaux-Bacchi V, et al. Complement factor H related proteins (CFHRs). Mol Immunol. 2013;56:170–80.
17. Medof ME, Kinoshita T, Nussenzweig V. Inhibition of complement activation on the surface of cells after incorporation of decay-accelerating factor (DAF) into their membranes. J Exp Med. 1984;160:1558–78.
18. Rollins SA, Sims PJ. The complement-inhibitory activity of CD59 resides in its capacity to block incorporation of C9 into membrane C5b-9. J Immunol. 1990;144:3478–83.
19. Sahin F, Akay OM, Ayer M, et al. Pesg PNH diagnosis, follow-up and treatment guidelines. Am J Blood Res. 2016;6:19–27.
20. Gulbis B, Eleftheriou A, Angastiniotis M, et al. Epidemiology of rare anaemias in Europe. Adv Exp Med Biol. 2010;686:375.
21. Hillmen P, Lewis SM, Bessler M, et al. Natural history of paroxysmal nocturnal hemoglobinuria. N Engl J Med. 1995;333:1253–8.
22. Bessler M, Mason PJ, Hillmen P, et al. Paroxysmal nocturnal haemoglobinuria (PNH) is caused by somatic mutations in the PIG-A gene. EMBO J. 1994;13:110–7.
23. Miyata T, Takeda J, Iida Y, et al. The cloning of PIG-A, a component in the early step of GPI anchor biosynthesis. Science. 1993;259:1318–20.
24. Nafa K, Mason PJ, Hillmen P, et al. Mutations in the PIG-A gene causing paroxysmal nocturnal hemoglobinuria are mainly of the frameshift type. Blood. 1995;86:4650–5.
25. Takeda J, Miyata T, Kawagoe K, et al. Deficiency of the GPI anchor caused by a somatic mutation of the PIG-A gene in paroxysmal nocturnal hemoglobinuria. Cell. 1993;73:703–11.
26. Kinoshita T, Medof ME, Silber R, et al. Distribution of decay accelerating factor in the peripheral blood of normal individuals and patients with paroxysmal nocturnal hemoglobinuria. J Exp Med. 1985;162:75–92.
27. Bain BJ, Win N. Acquired haemolytic anemias. In: Bain BJ, Bates I, Laffan MA, et al., editors. Dacie and Lewis-practical haematology. 11th ed. China: Churchill Livingstone; 2011. p. 273–300.
28. Parker CJ, Ware RE. Paroxysmal nocturnal hemoglobinuria. In: Greer JP, Arber DA, Glader B, et al., editors. Wintrobes clinical hematology. 13th ed. Philadelphia: Lippincott Williams and Wilkins; 2013. p. 785–808.
29. Parker C, Omine M, Richards S, et al. Diagnosis and management of paroxysmal nocturnal hemoglobinuria. Blood. 2005;106:3699–709.
30. Rosse WF, Dacie JV. Immune lysis of normal human and paroxysmal nocturnal hemoglobinuria (PNH) red blood cells. The sensitivity of PNH red cells to lysis by complement and specific antibody. J Clin Invest. 1966;45:736–48.
31. Rosse WF. Variations in the red cells in paroxysmal nocturnal haemoglobinuria. Br J Haematol. 1973;24:327–42.
32. Dacie JV, Lewis SM. Paroxysmal nocturnal haemoglobinuria: clinical manifestations, haematology, and nature of the disease. Ser Haematol. 1972;5:3–23.
33. Richards SJ, Rawstron AC, Hillmen P. Application of flow cytometry to the diagnosis of paroxysmal nocturnal hemoglobinuria. Cytometry. 2000;42:223–33.
34. Borowitz MJ, Craig FE, DiGiuseppe JA, et al. Guidelines for the diagnosis and monitoring of paroxysmal nocturnal hemoglobinuria and related disorders by flow cytometry. Cytometry B Clin Cytom. 2010;78B:211–30.
35. Savage WJ, Brodsky RA. New insights into paroxysmal nocturnal hemoglobinuria. Hematology. 2007;12:371–6.
36. Nilsson B, Hagstrom U, Englund A, et al. A simplified assay for the specific diagnosis of paroxysmal nocturnal hemoglobinuria: detection of DAF (CD55)- and HRF20 (CD59)-erythrocytes in microtyping cards. Vox Sang. 1993;64:43–6.
37. Telen MJ, Green AM. The Inab phenotype: characterization of the membrane protein and complement regulatory defect. Blood. 1989;74:437–41.
38. Yamashina M, Ueda E, Kinoshita T, et al. Inherited complete deficiency of 20-kilodalton homologous restriction factor (CD59) as a cause of paroxysmal nocturnal hemoglobinuria. N Engl J Med. 1990;323:1184–9.
39. Brodsky RA, Mukhina GL, Li S, et al. Improved detection and characterization of paroxysmal nocturnal hemoglobinuria using fluorescent aerolysin. Am J Clin Pathol. 2000;114:459–66.
40. Galili N, Ravandi F, Palermo G, et al. Prevalence of paroxysmal nocutrnal hemoglobinuria (PNH)

cells in patients with myelodysplastic syndromes (MDS), aplastic anemia (AA) or other bone marrow failure (BMF) syndromes: interim results from the EXPLORE trial. J Clin Oncol. 2009;27:15s.

41. Parker CJ. Management of paroxysmal nocturnal hemoglobinuria in the era of complement inhibitory therapy. Hematology. 2011;2011:21–9.

42. Hillmen P, Hall C, Marsh JC, et al. Effect of eculizumab on hemolysis and transfusion requirements in patients with paroxysmal nocturnal hemoglobinuria. N Engl J Med. 2004;350:552–9.

43. Hillmen P, Young NS, Schubert J, et al. The complement inhibitor eculizumab in paroxysmal nocturnal hemoglobinuria. N Engl J Med. 2006;355:1233–43.

44. Brodsky RA, Young NS, Antonioli E, et al. Multicenter phase 3 study of the complement inhibitor eculizumab for the treatment of patients with paroxysmal nocturnal hemoglobinuria. Blood. 2008;111:1840–7.

45. Kelly RJ, Hill A, Arnold LM, et al. Long term treatment with eculizumab in paroxysmal nocturnal hemoglobinuria: sustained efficacy and improved survival. Blood. 2011;117:6786–92.

46. Hillmen P, Muus P, Duhrsen U, et al. Effect of the complement inhibitor eculizumab on thromboembolism in patients with paroxysmal nocturnal hemoglobinuria. Blood. 2007;110:4123–8.

47. Constantinescu AR, Bitzan M, Weiss LS, et al. Non-enteropathic hemolytic uremic syndrome: causes and short-term course. Am J Kidney Dis. 2004;43:976–82.

48. Noris M, Remuzzi G. Atypical hemolytic-uremic syndrome. N Engl J Med. 2009;361:1676–87.

49. Tsai M. Thrombotic thrombocytopenic purpura, hemolytic-uremic syndrome, and related disorders. In: Greer JP, Arber DA, Glader B, et al., editors. Wintrobes clinical hematology. 13th ed. Philadelphia: Lippincott Williams and Wilkins; 2013. p. 1077–96.

50. Warwicker P, Goodship TH, Donne RL, et al. Genetic studies into inherited and sporadic hemolytic uremic syndrome. Kidney Int. 1998;53:836–44.

51. Caprioli J, Noris M, Brioschi S, et al. Genetics of HUS: the impact of MCP, CFH, and IF mutations on clinical presentation, response to treatment, and outcome. Blood. 2006;108:1267–79.

52. Cataland SR, Wu HM. How I treat: the clinical differentiation and initial treatment of adult patients with atypical hemolytic uremic syndrome. Blood. 2014;123:2478–84.

53. Shih AR, Murali MR. Laboratory tests for disorders of complement and complement regulatory proteins. Am J Hematol. 2015;90:1180–6.

54. Brodsky RA. Complement in hemolytic anemia. Blood. 2015;126:2459–65. https://doi.org/10.1182/blood-2015-06-640995.

55. Friedberg RC, Johari VP. Autoimmune hemolytic anemia. In: Greer JP, Arber DA, Glader B, et al., editors. Wintrobes clinical hematology. 13th ed. Philadelphia: Lippincott Williams and Wilkins; 2013. p. 746–65.

56. Pruzanski W, Shumak KH. Biologic activity of cold reactive autoantibodies. N Engl J Med. 1977;297:538–42.

57. Randen U, Troen G, Tierens A, et al. Primary cold agglutinin associated lymphoprolifertaive disease: a B-cell lymphoma of the bone marrow distinct from lymphoplasmacytic lymphoma. Haematologica. 2014;99:497–504.

58. Roelcke D. Cold agglutination. Transfus Med Rev. 1989;3:140–66.

59. Berentsen S, Ulvestad E, Gjertsen BT, et al. Rituximab for primary chronic cold agglutinin disease: a prospective study of 37 courses of therapy in 27 patients. Blood. 2004;103:2925–8.

60. Shi J, Rose EL, Singh A, et al. TNT003, an inhibitor of the serine protease C1s, prevents complement activation induced by cold agglutinins. Blood. 2014;123:4015–22.

61. Varma V, Garewal G, Varma S, et al. Flow cytometric detection of PNH defect in Indian patients with aplastic anemia and myelodysplastic syndromes. Am J Hematol. 2000;65:264–5.

62. Naseem S, Varma N, Trehan A. Primary/de-novo paroxysmal nocturnal hemoglobinuria in a child from North India: a case report with review of literature. J Pediatr Hematol Oncol. 2009;31:274–6.

63. Sachdeva MU, Varma N, Chandra D, et al. Multiparameter FLAER-based flow cytometry for screening of paroxysmal nocturnal hemoglobinuria enhances detection rates in patients with aplastic anemia. Ann Hematol. 2015;94:721–8.

64. Sreedharanunni S, Sachdeva MU, Bose P, et al. Frequency of paroxysmal nocturnal hemoglobinuria clones by multiparameter flow cytometry in pediatric aplastic anemia patients of Indian ethinic origin. Pediatr Blood Cancer. 2016;63:93–7.

Role of microRNA in Normal and Malignant Hematopoiesis

26

Ruchi Gupta and Khaliqur Rahman

26.1 Introduction

Epigenetic modifications in the recent era have received a lot of attention in a variety of diseases particularly cancer. They are defined as the modulation of gene expression by chromatin modification that does not involve DNA sequence alterations [1]. These modifications act either by altering the chromatin structure to deregulate gene expression or by the post-translational modification. Consequently, epigenetics control cell differentiation and function by "switching on" or "off" certain gene expressions, and a disruption of the normal epigenetic mechanism can lead to uncontrolled gene activation or silencing resulting into an altered homeostasis. Three main types of epigenetic processes which have been identified include DNA methylation, nucleosomal histone modifications, and post-translational alterations by the non-coding RNAs [2]. Prominent among these non-coding RNAs are microRNAs (miRNAs), which have recently emerged as important players in the regulation of normal hematopoietic cell development and differentiation as well as in malignant transformation. In this chapter, we have provided a comprehensive summary of the current knowledge on the role of miRNAs in normal and aberrant hematopoiesis with a focus on the clinical significance of the deranged miRNAs in some of the common hematological neoplasms.

26.1.1 Discovery

Many classes of small RNAs have been identified based on their biological roles and three main categories have been recognized: short interfering RNAs (siRNAs), microRNAs (miRNAs), and piwi-interacting RNAs (piRNAs). miRNA was first discovered in 1993 in nematode *Caenorhabditis elegans*, by genetic screening and later on their role in post translation modification was recognized [3]. miRNAs or "micro-ribonucleoprotein" or "miRNP" are short non-coding RNA molecules, with an approximate length of 15–22 nucleotides. Their genes are distributed non-randomly in human genome and frequently coincide with tumor susceptibility loci. They may be intergenic or intragenic where they share the same promoters of the host genes [4]. The effects of small RNAs on gene expression and control are generally inhibitory, and the corresponding regulatory mechanisms are therefore collectively labeled as RNA silencing. By mid-2013, it had been discovered that the human genome encodes over 2000 different miRNAs that scattered on all human chromosomes except the Y chromosome, though the number of their potential targets validated by experimental studies so far is very small [5].

R. Gupta (✉) · K. Rahman
Department of Hematology, Sanjay Gandhi Post Graduate Institute of Medical Sciences, Lucknow, Uttar Pradesh, India

© Springer Nature Singapore Pte Ltd. 2019
R. Saxena, H. P. Pati (eds.), *Hematopathology*, https://doi.org/10.1007/978-981-13-7713-6_26

435

26.1.2 Genesis and Nomenclature of miRNAs

The generation of mature miRNA is a multistep process involving numerous enzymes [4]. Transcription of miRNA genes is mediated by RNA polymerase II that generates the primary miRNA in the nucleus (Fig. 26.1). The primary miRNA molecule is cleaved by the nuclear microprocessor complex with the help of a member of the RNase II family, Drosha, to yield the precursor miRNA or pre-miRNA. This pre-miRNA is first exported from the nucleus into the cytoplasm by exportin 5 for further processing. In the cytoplasm, another enzyme, Dicer, cleaves the precursor miRNA hairpin loop to yield a double-stranded (duplex) miRNA, a 22 bp miRNA:miRNA* duplex. The double-stranded products of Dicer enter into a RNA-induced silencing complex

(RISC) assembly pathway that involves duplex unwinding and culminating in the stable association of only one of the two strands with the Argonaute (AGO) effector protein (AGO1–4, family member). The "guide strand or the mature miRNA strand" directs target recognition by base pairing, whereas the other strand of the duplex "the passenger strand or the miRNA*" is usually discarded. The mature miRNAs are named as miR- followed by numbers, and the ones with a similar sequence are usually distinguished by an additional letter like a, b, and c following the miRNA number. In addition, since the alternative strands can be differentially expressed in different tissues, the mature miR is also frequently suffixed with "5p" or "3p" to imply the functional miRNA strand. The mature miRNA is designated as miR, while the precursor stem-loop sequence is called a pre-mir [6].

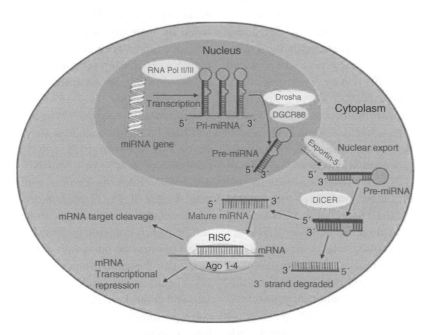

Fig. 26.1 The microRNA (miNA) genes are transcribed by RNA polymerase II (Pol II/III), leading to the production of primary miRNA (pri-miRNA) molecule. The primary processing is carried out by Drosha and DiGeorge syndrome critical region gene-8 (DGCR-S), that produces a pre-miRNA. Exportin 5 mediates the transport of the pre-miRNA to the cytoplasm, where RNase III enzyme Dicer performs the second processing step by cleaving the

stem-loop and generating the miRNA/miRNA* duplex. One of the strands is discarded while the other strand of the duplex, the mature miRNA (miRNA) forms a stable association with the Ago family proteins to form the RISC (RNA-induced silencing complex) assembly. The miRNA in this effector complex guides the RISC to its target mRNA, which is silenced through degradation or translation repression

26.1.3 Mechanism of Action

It is believed that a single miRNA species can regulate hundreds of targets, even if only to a mild degree, and several miRNAs can bind to the target mRNAs and cooperatively fine-tune the signaling of a single miRNA. A key specificity determinant for miRNA target recognition is based on Watson–Crick pairing of 5' proximal "seed" region, i.e., 2–8 nucleotide in the miRNA to the match site in the target mRNA. Besides the target specificity, a number of other factors influence the outcome, namely, the number of target sites for the same miRNA, their relative position, site accessibility, sequences flanking miRNA target site, and RNA secondary structure. Briefly, the gene silencing is carried out by chromatin remodeling, competition with translation initiators or promoting decay of the target mRNAs in the cytoplasmic foci known as processing bodies (P-bodies). Several studies have shown that cell cycle has the potential to determine miRNA-mediated gene regulation direction by promoting or inhibiting special mRNA expressions [7].

26.2 Role of miRNA in Normal Hematopoiesis

Hematopoiesis is initiated by a very small population of pluripotent cells which form the apex of this hierarchical system. A classical model of hematopoiesis describes the well-ordered stepwise lineage restrictions, including the differentiation of multipotent progenitors (MPP) into lymphoid-restricted common lymphoid progenitors (CLPs) or myeloid (CMP) and erythroid-megakaryocytic (MEK) restricted common progenitors. Each of these steps of hematopoiesis is regulated by a highly integrated network of transcription factors and miRNAs [8, 9]. The role of miRNAs was confirmed on the basis of the observation that the loss of key genes required for miRNA processing leads to impaired hematopoiesis. The homozygous Dicer deletion in mice is incompatible with a functional hematopoietic stem cell state, leading to defective hematopoiesis [10, 11]. Similarly, the deletion of AGO2 also leads to severe defects in erythroid and B-cell development. Almost every step in hematopoiesis appears to be finely tuned by specific miRNAs. However, interestingly only five miRNAs have been reported to be highly specific for hematopoietic cells which include miR-142, miR-144, miR-150, miR-155, and miR-223 [12]. Petriv et al. attempted to define the comprehensive profile of miRNA expression patterns of 288 miRNA species in 27 different hematopoietic subsets from all parts of the hematopoietic hierarchy in adult mice. They observed that several miRNAs were generally upregulated in stem cell and progenitor populations as compared to the more differentiated cell types. These miRNAs included miR-125b, miR-196a, miR-196b, miR-130a, let-7d, miR-148b, and miR-351. On the other hand, several miRNAs which were downregulated in these primitive cells were miR-484, miR-200c, miR-331, miR-320, miR-210, miR-324–5p, miR-212, and miR-690, which were expressed widely across differentiated cell types [13]. They further concluded that the analysis of these miRNAs across 27 populations did not reveal any lineage-specific miRNA, rather they displayed a bi- and sometimes trimodal expression patterns in different categories as well as stages of cell maturation [13]. A schematic diagram of the hematopoietic hierarchy and the differentially expressed miRNAs at each step of differentiation is shown in Fig. 26.2. A list of the miRNAs involved in hematopoiesis [12–24], their known targets genes and functions are tabulated in Table 26.1.

26.2.1 miRNA and Hematopoietic Stem Cells (HSC)

A complex epigenetic program safeguards HSCs by maintaining the self-renewal potential, and limiting their over-proliferation; the disruption of which leads to HSC exhaustion. The miRNAs miR-17, miR-24, miR-146, miR-155, miR-128,

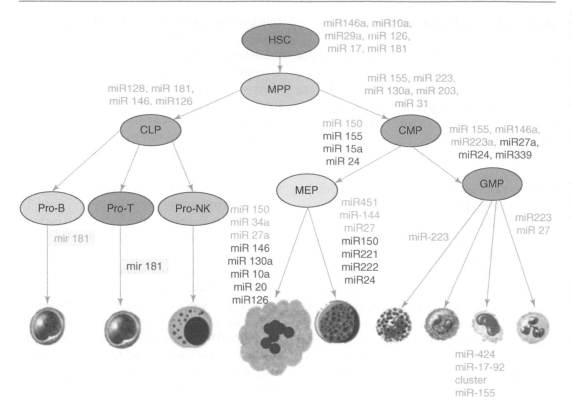

Fig. 26.2 Hematopoietic hierarchy with key regulatory miRNAs. The miRNAs in green color are upregulated while the red color depicts the downregulated miRNAs. *HSC* hematopoietic stem cells, *MPP* multipotent progenitors, *CMP* common myeloid progenitor, *CLP* common lymphoid progenitor, *Pro-B* B lymphocyte progenitor, *Pro-T* T-cell progenitor, *Pro-NK* NK-cell progenitor, *MEP* megakaryocyte/erythroid progenitor, *GMP* granulocyte/macrophage progenitor

and miR-181 were postulated to be involved in sustaining early stem-progenitor cell phenotype and regulating transition of the multipotent progenitor cell to CMP or CLP. On comparing miRNAs isolated from CD133+ long-term and short-term HSC with CD133−/CD34+ HPC, it was observed that miR-10a and miR-146a were higher in CD133+ cells relative to CD34+CD133− and CD34−CD133− cells, indicating their specific roles in hematopoiesis. Further, loss of miR-146a leads to an exhaustion of the HSC pool, due to extensive myeloproliferation. Another study exploring the role of miRNA expression and function in CD34+ progenitors collected from bone marrow and peripheral blood harvest samples revealed the role of 33 miRNAs differentially expressed in these cells which regulated the hematopoietic pool and differentiation [14, 15].

26.2.2 miRNA in Myelopoiesis

miR-16, 103, and 107 have been shown to block commitment of CMPs to granulocyte and macrophage lineage while miRNA 223 enhances granulopoiesis by blocking transcription factor NFI-A a known negative regulator of granulopoiesis and enhancing the expression of transcription factor C/EPB-a, a positive regulator of granulopoiesis. miR-223 is one of the key regulators of granulopoiesis and this was confirmed by studying myeloid differentiation in acute promyelocytic leukemia (APL) cells. Forced expression of miR-223 in APL cell lines enhanced their granulocytic differentiation. Another miRNA whose expression increases during granulocytic maturation is miR-27 expression which acts by negatively regulating the transcription factor AML1.

Table 26.1 Target molecules and regulatory functions of few miRNAs orchestrating normal hematopoiesis

miRNA	Target gene(s)	Known regulatory activities
Hematopoietic stem cells (HSC)		
miR-29a and miR-196b	HBP1, FZD5, TPM1	Both are highly expressed by HSCs; their downregulation leads to differentiation.
miR-125a and miR-125b	Bak1-miR-125a BMF/Klf13– miR-125b	Maintenance of HSC pool by decreasing apoptosis and differentiation *Ectopic expression of miR-125b promotes myelopoiesis*
miR-101	TET 2	HSC expansion
Myelopoiesis		
miR-29a	?	Positively influence myeloid differentiation
miR223	C/EPB-a positive feedback loop, Inhibitor of NFI-A, LMO2	Increases granulocytic maturation
miR-24 and miR-27	RUNX1	Regulates granulocytic differentiation
miR-34a	E2F3	Blocks myeloid cell proliferation
miR-21	NFIB	Monopoiesis
miRNA-17-5p, miR21a, miR106a	AML1	Negatively regulate monocyte differentiation
miRNAs 150/221/222	c-kit	Inhibits early erythroid maturation by downregulation of c-kit receptor
miR-451/144	GATA 2	Promotes erythroid differentiation by suppressing GATA 2 and other transcription factors
miR-24	Activin type I receptor (ALK4)	Highly expressed in HSC, negatively regulates erythroid differentiation
miR-150/miR-105	C-MYB	Promotes megakaryopoiesis
miR-155	Downregulates Ets-1 and Meis1	Blocks megakaryopoiesis
miR-146	CXCR4	Downregulation during megakaryopoiesis
T-cell lymphopoiesis		
miR-181a	PTEN, TCRα, BCL2, and CD69, NLK, inhibitor of Notch signaling	Regulates the metabolic status of thymocytes. Cell proliferation and progression from DN4 stage to the DP stage Mature T-cell activation by increasing TCR pathways NK cell differentiation
miR-150	NOTCH 3	T-cell differentiation Regulation of the differentiation from DP into CD4+ and CD8+ T-cells
miR-155	SOCS1; inhibits IFNγRa expression	Inhibit Th1 differentiation; effects Foxp3 expression and Treg development
miR-29a	?	Inhibit Th1 differentiation
miR-21	Spry1, a negative regulator of the MAP kinase pathway	Promotes Th2 differentiation
miR-17–92a	IKZF4, PTEN, BIM	CD8+ T-cell differentiation and Th17 differentiation
miR-146a	STAT1	Partial loss of Treg function
B-cell lymphopoiesis		
miR181a	AID, BCL2	Promotes B-cell development; *ectopic expression of miR-181 leads to marked B-cell proliferation and impairs somatic hypermutation and class switching*
miR-212/132 cluster	Upregulates SOX4 expression	Suppresses B-cell differentiation at the prepro-B to pro-B transition stage
miR-17–92a	Pro-apoptotic molecule BIM, PTEN, E2F1	B-cell development from pro-B to pre-B stage

(continued)

Table 26.1 (continued)

miR-223	LMO2 and MYBL1	Naive and memory cells development
miR150/miR34a	c-Myb/Foxp1	Expressed at high concentration in mature resting B cells; *ectopic expression of miR-150 impaired B-cell development*
miR-155	PU.1/AID/SHIP or INPP5D and CEBP/β	Key factor in the regulation of germinal center responses, Ig class switching, somatic hypermutation *Overexpression of miR-155 leads to B-cell proliferation*

HBP-1 HMG-box transcription factor, *FZD5* Frizzled class receptor 5, *TPM1* Tropomyosin 1, *BMF* BCL2-modifying factor, *BIM* bcl-2 interacting protein, *Klf13* Kruppel-like factor 13, *TET 2* Ten eleven translocation 2, *C/EBP* CCAAT/ enhancer binding protein, *NF-κB* Nuclear factor kappa-light-chain-enhancer of activated B cells, *LMO2* Lim domain only 2, *NFI-A* Nuclear factor I A, *RUNX1* Runt-related transcription factor 1, *E2F3* E2F transcription factor 3, *AML1* Acute myeloid leukemia 1 protein, *ALK4* Activin type I receptor, *Myb* Myeloblastosis oncogene, *ETS* E26 transformation-specific transcription factor, Meis Homeobox 1, *CXCR4* C-X-C chemokine receptor type 4, *PTEN* Phosphatase and tensin homolog, *TCR* T-cell receptor alpha, *NLK* Nemo-like kinase, *SOCS-1* Suppressor of cytokine signaling, *STAT* Signal transducer and activator of transcription, *AID* Activation induced cytidine deaminase, *SOX4* SRY-related HMG-box gene 4, *INPP5D* Inositol polyphosphate-5-phosphatase D/ Src homology 2 (SH2) domain containing inositol polyphosphate 5-phosphatase 1, *?* Unknown target

Monocyte differentiation is orchestrated by miR-17-5p, 20a, and 106a, which are downregulated leading to the upmodulation of AML1 gene and subsequently M-CSFR, which is essential for monocyte differentiation and proliferation. M-CSFR is also regulated indirectly by miR-424, (targets NFI-A), which in turn induces monocytic/macrophage differentiation [16, 17].

26.2.3 miRNA in Megakaryopoiesis and Erythropoiesis

The earliest progenitor generating megakaryocytic elements are represented by the CMP or colony-forming unit granulocyte–erythrocyte–macrophage–megakaryocyte (CFU-GEMM). At the molecular level, megakaryocytic differentiation is controlled by several transcription factors, including SCL, GATA-1, GATA-2, and NFE2, whose co-ordinated regulation is essential for megakaryopoiesis. One of the miRNAs which have been extensively studied and found to play an essential role in the control of cell fate at the level of megakaryocyte-erythroid progenitors (MEP) is miR-150. It acts on MYB and behaves as a switch for deciding the fate of these EMPs behaves as a switch for deciding the fate of these EMPs; high expression of miR-150 favors megakaryopoiesis while a low expression favors differentiation towards erythroid lineage. [18]. Other miRNAs which are downregulated during

megakaryopoiesis include miR-10a, miR-10b, miR-17, miR-20, miR-106, and miR-126 [17]. Downregulation of miR-221 and miR-222 is essential for erythrocyte differentiation of CD34+ HSCs, and miR-451 is essential for the late stages of erythroid differentiation [19].

26.2.4 miRNA in B-Cell Ontogeny

The first definitive proof that the miRNA pathway is essential for the B-lineage was documented when deletion of Dicer1 gene resulted in a block in the B-cell maturation at the pro-B to pre-B transition and also affected the terminal differentiation of mature B cells into antibody-producing cells [20, 21]. Zhang et al. established the landscape of normal miRNA expression in mature B cells and correlated them with the key transcription factors in B-cell differentiation, namely C-MYB, C-MYC, BCL6, LMO2, and Blimp1 [22]. Early B-cell development is regulated by a number of different miRNAs like miR-17–92a, miR-150, miR-155, miR-30 family. The miR-17–92 cluster and miR-181a positively regulate B-cell development, whereas the others negatively regulate the process. The deficiency of these miRNAs results in a greatly reduced B-cell compartment, with a developmental block at different stages. miR-17-92 targets tumor suppressors or pro-apoptotic proteins and thus has an oncogenic role. It was described as the first

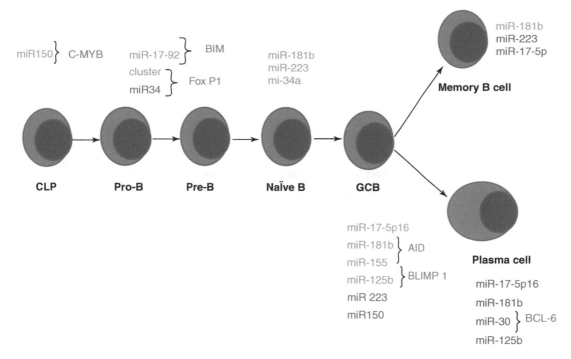

Fig. 26.3 miRNAs involved in B-cell ontogeny. The miRNAs in green color are upregulated while the red color depicts the downregulated miRNAs. The blue color depicts the key interacting transcription factors in each step of maturation. *CLP* common lymphoid progenitors, *GCB* germinal center B cell

"oncomiR" as it was overexpressed in B-cell lymphomas. The key miRNAs and some of their target molecules involved in the B-cell maturation are depicted in Fig. 26.3.

26.2.5 miRNA in T-Cell Ontogeny

T-cell maturation progresses through a series of stages from the double negative (DN, CD4−/CD8−) to the double positive stage (DP CD4+/CD8+), which is followed by differentiation into single positive specific mature T-cell types, based on the TCR rearrangements. Deletion of the genes encoding either Dicer in early T-cell development results in a developmental block at the double negative cells with an increase in gamma-delta T cells and decrease in cell numbers of the mature T cells [21]. The Notch pathway is very important for T-cell development and has been identified as a target for miR-150 [23]. Another key player responsible for T-cell maturation and proliferation of the double positive T cells is the

miRNA-181. It has been shown to modulate TCR signaling by targeting multiple downstream negative regulators of signaling, like *dual-specificity phosphatases* Dusp5, Dusp6 and *SH-2 domain containing phosphotyrosine phosphatase* Shp-2 [24]. Regulation of TCR signaling is critical for T-cell selection and determination of lineage. Differentiation of the mature helper T cells into effector subsets is also modulated by specific miRNAs. The key miRNAs involved in the genesis and differentiation into different T-cell subsets are depicted in Fig. 26.4.

26.3   Role of miRNA in Malignant Hematopoiesis

Given the extensive involvement in normal hematopoiesis, the role of miRNAs in malignant hematopoiesis is tenable. Analysis of the human and mouse genomes revealed that miRNA genes are frequently located at fragile sites and regions of copy number alteration (CNA) associated with

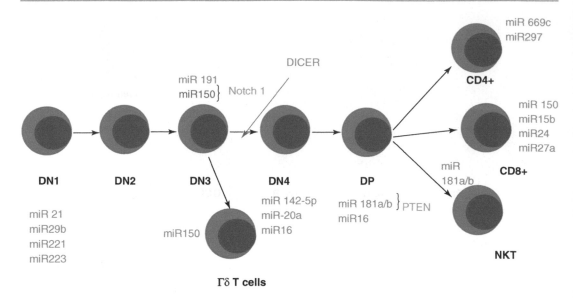

Fig. 26.4 miRNAs involved in T-cell ontogeny. The miRNAs in green color are upregulated while the red color depicts the downregulated miRNAs. The blue color depicts the key interacting transcription factors in each step of maturation. *DN* double negative stage 1, 2, 3, and 4, *DP* double positive, *NKT* Natural killer/T cells

cancer [25]. These findings suggest a very important role of miRNA deregulation in oncogenesis. For cancer research purposes, miRNAs can be divided into two types of groups: those overexpressed, which target tumor suppressor proteins, also known as oncomiRs, and those with decreased expression in cells, which actually target oncogenes. The miRNA genes may be altered either by single nucleotide polymorphism (SNP), epigenetic silencing, or defects in the miRNA biosynthetic pathway. Another interesting observation is that majority of the miRNAs are under the control of the very targets that they regulate by a negative feedback loop [4]. A brief outline of the miRNA profiles and their correlation with known causative genetic abnormalities in few lymphoproliferative disorders and leukemias is discussed below and summarized in Table 26.2.

26.3.1 miRNA in B-Cell Lymphoproliferative Disorders

Chronic lymphocytic leukemia—Among the hematopoietic malignancies, the role of miRNAs was first studied in CLL when Calin et al. found that miR-15a and miR-16-1 located at the 13q14 locus were deleted in the majority of the CLL cases [26]. Both these miRNAs have a tumor suppressor role and act by downregulating the anti-apoptotic molecule Bcl-2. Additionally, it has been shown that miR-15a/miR-16-1 cluster directly targets the TP53 gene, and a positive feedback loop regulates the expression of miR-15a/16-1. Subsequently, other miRNAs like miR-29, miR-181, miR-221/222, miR-106b, miR-155, and miR-34a which regulate the cell cycle were identified [20]. Prognostically, significant among these was a high miR-34a expression, which correlated with chemotherapy-refractory disease, p53 inactivation, and apoptosis resistance [27].

Mantle cell lymphoma and follicular lymphoma harbor a more uniform miRNA signature, which has been confirmed by numerous authors [28, 29]. Several cell cycle genes targeting miRNAs have been detected in mantle cell lymphoma like miR-16-1 and oncomiR-1 targeting cyclin D1, and miR-29, regulating CDK6. The downregulation of miR29a has been shown to be associated with poor prognosis. The follicular lymphoma miRNA signature includes miR-20a/b and miR-194, which target CDKN1A and SOCS2, potentially contributing to tumor cell proliferation and survival.

Table 26.2 Deregulated miRNAs in some of the hematological malignancies

Disease category	miRNAs upregulated	miRNAs downregulated
Chronic lymphocytic leukemia	miR-34a, miR-155	miR-15a and miR-16-1, miR-181, miR-29b
Mantle cell lymphoma	miR-155, miR-17-92,	miR-15a/16-1 cluster gene, miR-29a
Follicular lymphoma	miR-155, let7b, miR-9, miR-20a/b, and miR-194	miR-320, miR-149, miR-139
Diffuse large B cell lymphoma	miR-155, miR-17-92, miR-21, let-7b, miR-199a/b, miR-224	miR30, miR34a, miR-150, miR-222, miR-146b-5p
Multiple myeloma	miR-21, miR-106b~25 cluster, miR-181a/b, miR-17~92, miR-19a	miR-19b and miR-331
Chronic myeloid leukemia	miR-17-92	miR-203, miR-150
B-acute lymphoblastic leukemia	miR-128a and miR-181b, miR-125b, miR-99a	miR-100, miR-196b, and let-7e
T-acute lymphoblastic leukemia	miR-222, 223 and miR19, 17-92 cluster and miR-146a	miR-150, miR-155, miR-200, and miR-193b-3p
Acute myeloid leukemia subtypes		
t(8;21)	miR-27a, miR-126, miR-150, miR-223, miR-29b-3p	miR-126
inv(16) AMLs	miR-126, miR-126*miR-29b-3p	miR-126
t(15;17) AML	miR-224, miR-368, and miR-382	miR-17-5p, miR-20a, miR-126, miR-126*, miRNA-181a-3p, miR-126-5p
Trisomy 8	miR-124a and miR-30d	mir-126
MLL-rearranged AML	miR-17~92 cluster, miR-196b, miR-9 and 9* (miR-9/9*) miR-326, miR-219, miR-194, miR-301, miR-324, miR-339, miR-99b, miR-328	miR-34b, miR-15a, miR-29a, miR-29c, miR-372, miR-30a, miR-29b, miR-30e, miR-196a, let-7f, miR-102, miR-331, miR-299, miR-193 (many are tumor suppressor miRNAs)
Normal karyotype-AML	miR-10a, miR-10b, miR-26a, miR-30c, let-7a-2, miR 16-2, miR-21, miR-181b, miR-368, and miR-192	miR-126, miR-203, miR-200c, miR-182, miR-204, miR-196b, miR-193, miR-191, miR-199a, miR-194, miR-183, miR-299, and miR-145
NPM1 mutations	miR-10, let-7, and miR-29	miR-204 and miR-128a
FLT3-ITD mutations	miR-155	–

In *diffuse large B cell lymphoma (DLBCL)*, gene expression profiles have identified three major subtypes: Germinal center (GC), non-GC or the activated B cell (ABC) type, and primary mediastinal large B-cell lymphoma (PMLBCL). The ABC-type immunophenotypes have been found to express significantly higher levels of miR-155, miR-221, and miR-21 compared with GCB-type immunophenotypes [30]. The miR-NAs, miR-155 and miR-17-72 cluster, target numerous cell cycle regulatory pathways like MYC, SMAD5, BCL-6, BCL-2, and phosphatidylinositol 3-kinase (PI3K)-protein kinase (AKT), thus behaving as important oncomirs for the development of DLBCL. Furthermore, recent studies have shown that low expression of miR21/miR-127/miR-19a/-92a/miR-222 correlated with poor prognosis in DLBCL [20, 31].

26.3.2 miRNA in Multiple Myeloma (MM)

Pichiorri et al. investigated the role of miRNAs in the malignant transformation of plasma cells (PC) in MM-derived cell lines and CD138+ bone marrow PCs from subjects with MM, monoclonal gammopathy of undetermined significance (MGUS), and normal donors. They observed an overexpression of miR-21, miR-106b~25 cluster, miR-181a/b in MM and MGUS and a selective upregulation of miR-32 and miR-17~92 cluster in MM subjects [32]. Similarly, Seckinger et al. explored the role of 559 human miRNAs in myeloma cell lines and observed a differential expression of numerous miRNAs between myeloma cells and healthy controls and a distinct miRNA signature for some cytogenetic subtypes like t(4;14). They identified five miRNAs which were significantly associated with event-free survival: miR-135a/b, miR-200a/b, and miR596 while miR135a and miR596 correlated with high tumor burden [33]. In yet another study, interleukin-6, the key disease mediator in myeloma, is negatively regulated by SOCS-1. The latter is a target for miR-19a/b in MM; hence an upregulation of miR-19a/b leads to the suppression of the SOCS-1 pathway and increased levels of IL-6. Other cell cycle genes which have been found to be negatively regulated by miRNAs include p27Kip1 and p57Kip2, by miR-221/222 and p53 by miR-181a/b, miR-106b-25, and miR-32. Based on these preliminary findings, these miRNAs are being explored as potential targets for the development of novel therapeutic targets [34].

26.3.3 miRNA in Myelodysplastic Syndrome (MDS) and Acute Myeloid Leukemia (AML)

MDS and AML are a consequence of numerous sequential alterations in the genetic cells. A recent genomic analysis of AML and MDS cell lines elicited the role of miRNAs in these malignancies. It was found that about 77% (542 out of 706) of miRNAs were located in regions of leukemia-associated cytogenetic abnormalities, and 18% (99 out of 542) of these miRNAs were relevant in myeloid malignancies [35].

In *MDS*, a differential expression profile of more than 100 miRNAs, spread genome-wide, have been identified between early and advanced stages of MDS. Pons et al. measured the gene expression of 25 mature miRNAs in mononuclear cells (MNCs) isolated from bone marrow and peripheral blood of MDS patients. They revealed an overexpression of miRNA cluster miR-17-92 in MDS and differential expression of miR-15a and miR-16 between low-risk and high-risk subgroups [36]. Similarly, expression levels of miR-422a, miR-617, and four miR-181 family members were found to be associated with progression and their levels were progressively increased in MDS as compared to healthy controls, and also within different risk groups. miR-181a and miR-222 may serve as potential biomarkers for diagnosis and predict progression to secondary AML [37]. Other pathogenetic miRNAs which are significant in MDS include miR-34a, miR-21, and miR22; the target genes being the anti-apoptotic Bcl-2 gene, SMAD7 gene and DNA methylation regulator, TET2 gene [38, 39]. A brief summary of the miRNAs which are deregulated in MDS [35–39] is shown in Fig. 26.5.

In *AML*, known recurrent cytogenetic abnormalities like t(15; 17), t(8;21), inversion 16 have been reported in approximately 24–30% cases, while approximately 50% cases have a normal karyotype (NK-AML). Clinically significant mutations reported in this CN-AML include [40], mutations of the membrane tyrosine kinase FLT3-ITD, mutations of the transcription factor CEBPA (10–15%) and nucleophosmin (NPM1) gene (50–60%). Garzaon et al. reported a distinct miRNA signature profile for each of these subtypes of AML, wherein certain miRNAs are upregulated while others are downregulated (Table 26.2). Of particular interest is the high expression of miR-191 and miR-199a, which were found to be significantly associated with worse overall and event-free survival [41]. In a similar work by Wang et al., expression patterns of four miRNAs, namely, miR-128a, miR-128b, let-7b, and miR-223, were found to be sufficient to discriminate AML from ALL. Further, they observed that a high expression of miR-146a and miR-181a/c and miR-26a, miR-29b, miR-146a, and miR-196b were significantly associated with overall survival in ALL and AML, respectively [42].

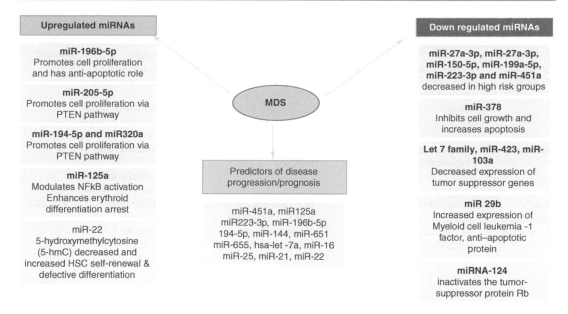

Fig. 26.5 Summary of some of the deregulated miRNAs and their target molecules in myelodysplastic syndrome

26.3.4 miRNA in Acute Lymphoblastic Leukemia (ALL)

B- or T-lineage ALL arise due to arrest in different stages of maturation which have well-defined immunophenotypic profiles and different miRNA signatures. On comparing the miRNA profiles of pediatric B-ALL patient samples with healthy controls, the former showed lower expression levels of miR-100, miR-196b, and let-7e, while miR-128a and miR-181b were increased [43]. Schott et al. evaluated the role of 397 microRNA in 81 cases of pediatric leukemia by the quantitative real-time polymerase chain reaction and concluded that all the major subtypes of ALL, namely, T-lineage, MLL-rearranged, TEL-AML1-positive, E2A-PBX1-positive and hyperdiploid acute lymphoblastic leukemia had a unique microRNA-signatures. Moreover, they observed that the upregulation of miR-125b, miR-99a, and miR-100 in these cases were significantly associated with drug resistance to vincristine and daunorubicin [44]. Similarly, in T-ALL, numerous deregulated miRNAs have been detected which corroborate with specific cytogenetic subgroups. mR221, 222, 223 and 19,

17-92 cluster and 146a are some of the few known tumor oncomirs in T-ALL, while miR-29, miR-31, miR-150, miR-155, and miR-200 behave as tumor suppressors whose inactivation promotes leukemogenesis [45, 46].

26.3.5 miRNA in Chronic Myeloid Leukemia (CML)

One of the initial works on miRNA in CML was performed by Venturiet al., who demonstrated overexpression of the miR-17-92 cluster in CD34+ cells of CML, which later on was seen to be markedly elevated in CML blast crisis [47]. Another pathogenetic miRNA in CML which targets the BCR-ABL1 kinases is miR-203; it was silenced in human leukemic Philadelphia chromosome-positive cell lines. Similarly, the miR-150 expression is decreased in CML, which negatively regulates the Myb oncogene essential for cell survival and proliferation. One of the most important utilities of miRNAs in CML is its applicability as a prognostic marker and prediction of resistance to tyrosine kinase inhibitors. In recent studies [48], several miRNAs, for example, miR-191, miR-29a, miR-422b, miR-100,

Table 26.3 Comparison of the commonly employed techniques for miRNA analysis

Technique	Application	Quantity of input RNA	Advantages	Disadvantages	~Cost/sample
Quantitative RT-PCR	Small-scale experiments, limited no. of targets	500 ng	High sensitivity and specificity	Normalization and identifying a reference miRNA Labor intensive to scale Requires quality miRNA annotation	++
Microarray	Large-scale experiments	100–1000 ng	Identify known miRNAs	Least quantitative and sensitive Requires quality miRNA annotation	++
Next-generation sequencing	Discovery phase research Whole exome analysis	500–5000 ng	Does not require miRNA annotation No problems of background noise and cross-hybridization	Less sensitive than qPCR Good degree of technical and bioinformatics skill necessary	++ - +++

miR-326, miR-26a, and miR-451 have emerged as promising predictors of imatinib resistance in newly diagnosed cases of CML.

A brief summary of the aforementioned deregulated miRNAs and the ones implicated in prognosis [26–48] are depicted in Table 26.2.

26.4 Tools for miRNA Detection

Though there is extensive work on miRNAs by different authors in hematopoietic malignancies, there is very few overlap in the results even in the same disease category. This is possibly due to the differences in the sample types; whole blood, mononuclear cells or plasma and use of separate platforms for miRNA evaluation, which commonly include quantitative real-time-PCR (qRT-PCR), microarrays, and next-generation sequencing. Each of these techniques has its strengths and limitations (Table 26.3).

The clear advantage of high-throughput sequencing is the ability to identify novel miR-NAs. This technology is not affected by differences in the melting temperatures, co-expression of nearly identical miRNA family members, or post-transcriptional modifications. Unlike profiling of miRNAs based on microarray techniques, deep sequencing measures absolute abundance and allows the discovery of novel miRNAs. Therefore deep sequencing methods are emerging

as the best tool for studying miRNA expression, whereas qRT-PCR is often considered a "gold standard" in the detection and quantitation of gene expression. Following detection of the deregulated miRNAs, numerous computational tools like DIANA-microT-CDS, miRanda—mirSVR, and TargetScan are available which aid in the identification and validation of the clinically relevant miRNA: mRNA target interactions, thereby discerning the exact role of miRNAs in the regulatory networks governing the biological processes [49, 50].

26.5 Therapeutic Implications and Future Perspective

Since their discovery way back in early 20th decade researchers have identified more than 2000 miRNAs which regulate the human genome. Extensive work has been performed in delineating the miRNAs in each step of hematopoiesis and identifying their role in diseased states, the entire portrayal of which is beyond the scope of this review. Invariably, it is explicitly clear that microRNAs participate in the regulation of almost every cellular process and are intricately associated with human pathology. However, the information generated by different authors in the same disease is diverse and thus larger studies are required for data reproducibility and generation of universal miRNA signatures. In the recent years, it has been found that "circulating miR-NAs" can also be detected in many extracellular fluids like plasma, serum, and urine, where they are attracting attention as potential noninvasive biomarkers for a range of diseases. Pre-clinical studies [51] are already exploring the utility of miRNA inhibitory molecules, "anti-oncomirs" in various non-hematological and hematological disorders, like anti-miR-155, miR-21, and miR-196b in AML. If successful, they are likely to open up new additional avenues for the management of hematological malignancies.

References

1. Weinhold B. Epigenetics: the science of change. Environ Health Perspect. 2006;114(3):A160–7.
2. Rice KL, Hormaeche I, Licht JD. Epigenetic regulation of normal and malignant hematopoiesis. Oncogene. 2007;26(47):6697–714.
3. Lee RC, Feinbaum RL, Ambros V. The C. elegans heterochronic gene lin-4 encodes small RNAs with antisense complementarity to lin-14. Cell. 1993;75(5):843–54.
4. Carthew RW, Sontheimer EJ. Origins and mechanisms of miRNAs and siRNAs. Cell. 2009;136(4):642–55.
5. Valinezhad Orang A, Safaralizadeh R, Kazemzadeh-Bavili M. Mechanisms of miRNA-mediated gene regulation from common downregulation to mRNA-specific upregulation. Int J Genomics. 2014;2014:970607.
6. Griffiths-Jones S, Grocock RJ, van Dongen S, Bateman A, Enright AJ. miRBase: microRNA sequences, targets and gene nomenclature. Nucleic Acids Res. 2006;34(Database issue):D140–4.
7. Vasudevan S. Posttranscriptional upregulation by microRNAs. Wiley Interdiscip Rev RNA. 2012;3(3):311–30.
8. Hong SH, Kim KS, Oh IH. Concise review: exploring miRNAs—toward a better understanding of hematopoiesis. Stem Cells. 2015;33(1):1–7.
9. Guo S, Lu J, Schlanger R, Zhang H, Wang JY, Fox MC, et al. MicroRNA miR-125a controls hematopoietic stem cell number. Proc Natl Acad Sci U S A. 2010;107:14229–34.
10. Bernstein E, Kim SY, Carmell MA, Murchison EP, Alcorn H, Li MZ, et al. Dicer is essential for mouse development. Nat Genet. 2003;35(3):215–7.
11. Kotaki R, Koyama-Nasu R, Yamakawa N, Kotani A. miRNAs in normal and malignant hematopoiesis. Int J Mol Sci. 2017;18(7):1495.
12. Landgraf P, Rusu M, Sheridan R, Sewer A, Iovino N, Aravin A, et al. A mammalian microRNA expression atlas based on small library sequencing. Cell. 2007;129:1401–14.
13. Petriv OI, Kuchenbauer F, Delaney AD, Lecault V, White A, Kent D, et al. Comprehensive microRNA expression profiling of the hematopoietic hierarchy. Proc Natl Acad Sci U S A. 2010;107(35):15443–8.
14. Georgantas RW III, Hildreth R, Morisot S, Alder J, Liu C-g, Heimfeld S, et al. CD34+ hematopoietic stem progenitor cell microRNA expression and function: a circuit diagram of differentiation control. Proc Natl Acad Sci U S A. 2007;104(8):2750–5.
15. Bissels U, Wild S, Tomiuk S, Hafner M, Scheel H, Mihailovic A, et al. Combined characterization of microRNA and mRNA profiles delineates early differentiation pathways of CD133+ and CD34+ hematopoietic stem and progenitor cells. Stem Cells. 2011;29:847–57.
16. Bhagavathi S, Czader M. MicroRNAs in benign and malignant hematopoiesis. Arch Pathol Lab Med. 2010;134:1276–81.
17. Pelosi E, et al. MicroRNAs in normal and malignant myelopoiesis. Leuk Res. 2009;33:1584–93.
18. Mukai HY, Motohashi H, Ohmeda O, Suzuki N, Nagano M, Yamamoto M. Transgene insertion in proximity to thr c-myb gene disrupts erythroid megakaryocytic lineage bifurcation. Mol Cell Biol. 2006;26:7953–65.
19. Bruchova H, Yoon D, Agarwal AM, Mendell J, Prchal JT. The regulated expression of miRNAs in normal and polycythemia vera erythropoiesis. Exp Hematol. 2007;35(11):1657–67.
20. Lisio LD, Martinez N, Montes-Moreno S, Piris-Villaespesa M, Sanchez-Beato M, Piris MA. The role of miRNAs in the pathogenesis and diagnosis of B-cell lymphomas. Blood. 2012;120(9):1782–90.
21. Johanson TM, Skinner JPJ, Kumar A, et al. The role of microRNAs in lymphopoiesis. Int J Hematol. 2014;100:246.
22. Zhang J, Jima DD, Jacobs C, et al. Patterns of microRNA expression characterize stages of human B-cell differentiation. Blood. 2009;113(19):4586–94.
23. Ghisi M, Corradin A, Basso K, Frasson C, Serafin V, Mukherjee S, et al. Modulation of microRNA expression in human T-cell development: targeting of NOTCH3 by miR-150. Blood. 2011;117:7053–62.
24. Li QJ, Chau J, Ebert PJ, Sylvester G, Min H, Liu G, et al. miR-181a is an intrinsic modulator of T cell sensitivity and selection. Cell. 2007;129:147–61.
25. Lagana A, Russo F, Sismeiro C, Giugno R, Pulvirenti A, Ferro A. Variability in the incidence of miRNAs and genes in fragile sites and the role of repeats and CpG islands in the distribution of genetic material. PLoS One. 2010;5(6):e11166.
26. Calin GA, Dumitru CD, Shimizu M, Bichi R, Zupo S, Noch E, et al. Frequent deletions and down-regulation of micro-RNA genes miR15 and miR16 at 13q14 in chronic lymphocytic leukemia. Proc Natl Acad Sci U S A. 2002;99(24):15524–9.
27. Zenz T, Mohr J, Eldering E, et al. miR-34a as part of the resistance network in chronic lymphocytic leukemia. Blood. 2009;113:3801–8.

28. Deshpande A, Pastore A, Deshpande AJ, Zimmermann Y, Hutter G, Weinkauf M, et al. 3'UTR mediated regulation of the cyclin D1 protooncogene. Cell Cycle. 2009;8(21):3592–600.

29. Wang W, Corrigan-Cummins M, Hudson J, Maric I, Simakova O, Neelapu SS, et al. MicroRNA profiling of follicular lymphoma identifies microRNAs related to cell proliferation and tumor response. Haematologica. 2012;97(4):586–94.

30. Lawrie CH, Soneji S, Marafioti T, Cooper CD, Palazzo S, Paterson JC, et al. Microrna expression distinguishes between germinal center B cell-like and activated B cell-like subtypes of diffuse large B cell lymphoma. Int J Cancer. 2007;121:1156–61.

31. Ni H, Tong R, Zou L, Song G, Cho WC. MicroRNAs in diffuse large B-cell lymphoma. Oncol Lett. 2016;11(2):1271–80.

32. Pichiorri F, Suh SS, Ladetto M, Kuehl M, Palumbo T, Drandi D, et al. MicroRNAs regulate critical genes associated with multiple myeloma pathogenesis. Proc Natl Acad Sci U S A. 2008;105(35):12885–90.

33. Seckinger A, Meißner T, Moreaux J, Benes V, Hillengass J, Castoldi M, et al. miRNAs in multiple myeloma—a survival relevant complex regulator of gene expression. Oncotarget. 2015;6(36):39165–83.

34. Rossi M, Tagliaferri P, Tassone P. MicroRNAs in multiple myeloma and related bone disease. Ann Transl Med. 2015;3(21):334.

35. Starczynowski DT, Morin R, McPherson A, Lam J, Chari R, Wegrzyn J, et al. Genome-wide identification of human microRNAs located in leukemia-associated genomic alterations. Blood. 2011;117(2):595–607.

36. Sokol L, Caceres G, Volinia S, Alder H, Nuovo GJ, Liu CG, et al. Identification of a risk dependent microRNA expression signature in myelodysplastic syndromes. Br J Haematol. 2011;153(1):24–32.

37. Pons A, Nomdedeu B, Navarro A, Gaya A, Gel B, Diaz T, et al. Hematopoiesis-related microRNA expression in myelodysplastic syndromes. Leuk Lymphoma. 2009;50:1854–9.

38. Hussein K, Theophile K, Büsche G, Schlegelberger B, Göhring G, Kreipe H, et al. Aberrant microRNA expression pattern in myelodysplastic bone marrow cells. Leuk Res. 2010;34(9):1169–74.

39. Song SJ, Pandolfi PP. MicroRNAs in the pathogenesis of myelodysplastic syndromes and myeloid leukaemia. Curr Opin Hematol. 2014;21(4):276–82.

40. Scholl S, Fricke HJ, Sayer HG, Hoffken K. Clinical implications of molecular genetic aberrations in acute myeloid leukemia. J Cancer Res Clin Oncol. 2009;135:491–505.

41. Garzon R, Volinia S, Liu CG, Fernandez-Cymering C, Palumbo T, Pichiorri F, et al. MicroRNA signatures associated with cytogenetics and prognosis in acute myeloid leukemia. Blood. 2008;111(6):3183–9.

42. Wang Y, Li Z, He C, Wang D, Yuan X, Chen J, et al. MicroRNAs expression signatures are associated with lineage and survival in acute leukemias. Blood Cells Mol Dis. 2010;44(3):191–7.

43. de Oliveira JC, Scrideli CA, Brassesco MS, Morales AG, Pezuk JA, Queiroz Rde P, et al. Differential miRNA expression in childhood ALL and association with clinical and biological features. Leuk Res. 2012;36(3):293–8.

44. Schotte D, De Menezes RX, Akbari Moqadam F, Khankahdani LM, Lange-Turenhout E, Chen C, et al. MicroRNA characterizes genetic diversity and drug resistance in pediatric acute lymphoblastic leukemia. Haematologica. 2011;96(5):703–11.

45. Sanghvi VR, Mavrakis KJ, Van der Meulen J, Boice M, Wolfe AL, Carty M, et al. Characterization of a set of tumor suppressor microRNAs in T cell acute lymphoblastic leukemia. Sci Signal. 2014;7(352):ra111.

46. Saki N, Abroun S, Solcimani M, Hajizamani S, Shahjahani M, Kast RE, et al. Involvement of microRNA in T-cell differentiation and malignancy. Int J Hematol Oncol Stem Cell Res. 2015;9(1):33–49.

47. Venturini L, Battmer K, Castoldi M, Schultheis B, Hochhaus A, Muckenthaler MU, et al. Expression of the miR-17-92 polycistron in chronic myeloid leukemia (CML) CD34+ cells. Blood. 2007;109(10):4399–405.

48. San José-Enériz E, Román-Gómez J, Jiménez-Velasco A, Garate L, Martin V, Cordeu L, et al. MicroRNA expression profiling in imatinib-resistant chronic myeloid leukemia patients without clinically significant ABL1-mutations. Mol Cancer. 2009;8(1):69.

49. de Planell-Saguer M, Rodicio MC. Detection methods for microRNAs in clinic practice. Clin Biochem. 2013;46(10–11):869–78.

50. Baker M. MicroRNA profiling: separating signal from noise. Nat Methods. 2010;7(9):687–92.

51. Ciccone M, Calin GA. MicroRNAs in myeloid hematological malignancies. Curr Genomics. 2015;16(5):336–48.

Ajit Gorakshakar and Harita Gogri

Immune cytopenia is a reduction in the number of mature blood cells. This can be caused by alloantigens present on the surface of blood cells i.e. red blood cells or erthyrocytes, white blood cells or leucocytes and platelets or thromobocytes. Alloantigens stimulate the immune system of host against foreign antigens causing alloimmunization and subsequent production of alloantibodies which caused decreased survival of blood cells in vivo. This chapter focuses on red blood cell antigens, human platelet antigens, human neutrophil antigens and human leucocyte antigens and their role in immune cytopenias.

27.1 Introduction

Alloantigens present on the blood cells stimulate the immune system of the foreign host causing production of alloantibodies which may ultimately result in an immune cytopenia. Immune cytopenia is a reduction in the number of mature blood cells. This can result in anemia, leukopenia or neutropenia, thrombocytopenia, or pancytopenia. This chapter reviews the immune cytopenias mediated by red cells, white blood cells and platelets, and the alloantigens involved in it.

27.2 Immune Cytopenia Due to Red Blood Cells

27.2.1 Alloantigens

Blood group antigens are sugars or proteins, attached to various components in the red blood cell membrane, whose specificity is controlled by a series of genes. These antigenic determinants decide blood group of an individual. International Society of Blood Transfusion (ISBT) has recognized 346 antigens on human red cells of which 308 are clustered within 36 blood group systems (http://www.isbtweb.org/) [1]. ABO and Rh are the two important blood group systems in transfusion medicine. However, apart from these, there are 34 other blood group systems. Antibodies against these blood group antigens are important in transfusion and prenatal settings.

27.2.1.1 ABO and Rh

ABO blood group system (ISBT No. 1) is the most important system in transfusion medicine and was discovered by Karl Landsteiner in 1900. Based on blood group, individuals are grouped as A, B, AB, and O, depending on the antigens they carry on their red cells. This system consists of two antigens, A and B. Antibodies against these antigens are non-red cell stimulated, naturally occurring antibodies against the ABO antigens that they lack. They are produced during neonatal period (about 3–6 months of age) due to the environmental stimulus.

A. Gorakshakar (✉) · H. Gogri
ICMR-National Institute of Immunohaematology, Mumbai, India

© Springer Nature Singapore Pte Ltd. 2019
R. Saxena, H. P. Pati (eds.), *Hematopathology*, https://doi.org/10.1007/978-981-13-7713-6_27

The ABO antigens are formed due to the interaction of three systems located on different loci (ABO, Hh, and Se). These genes code for specific glycosyltransferases that add specific sugar molecules to a basic precursor substance. The product of H gene is L-fucosyltransferase which catalyzes the addition of L-Fucose to a precursor substance to form H antigen which then acts as a precursor molecule for the formation of ABO antigens. The product of "A" gene is an 1, 3-N-acetylgalactosaminyltransferase, which forms blood group A specific structure by transferring N-acetylagalactosamine residues onto H determinants. The product of the "B" gene is α1, 3-D-galactosyltransferase, which forms B specific structures by transferring α-D-galactose onto H determinants. The silent allele "O" carries no genetic information for a functional glycosyltransferase. Both A- and B-transferases are highly specific towards the blood group H structures as the sugar acceptor. Blood group A is further subgrouped into A1 and A2 which exhibit qualitative and quantitative difference. A1 and A2 can be phenotypically differentiated using anti-A1 extracted from plant lectin, *Dolichos biflorus*. Apart from these, weaker subgroups of A (A_{int}, A_3, A_x, A_m, A_{el}, A_y, A_{end}, and A_{bantu}) and B (B_3, B_x, B_m, and B_{el}) arise due to inheritance of the variant alleles at the ABO locus. The characteristic features of weaker subgroups are their reduced antigenic sites per red cell [2], their reactivity pattern with human anti-A+B, strong reaction with anti-H, and the presence or absence of anti-A1 in the serum.

The ABO gene located on the long arm of chromosome 9 (position 9q34.1-q34.2) which spans over 18–20 kb and consists of 7 exons ranging from 28 to 688 bp and six introns ranging from 554 to 12,982 bp. The 1062 basepair (bp) sequence predicted a 353 amino acid protein. ABO*A101 is considered as a reference sequence. ABO*B101 is distinguishable from ABO*A101 at 7 nt positions: three synonymous mutations at positions 297, 657, and 930 and four nonsynonymous mutations at positions 526, 703, 796, and 803 [3]. The nt sequence of ABO*O01 differs from that of ABO*A101 by a single base deletion at position 261 in exon 6. In contrast, the

ABO*O03 allele lacks the 216delG polymorphism but possesses nonsynonymous mutations that may abolish the protein's enzyme activity by altering the nt sugar binding site. The A2 blood group results from inheritance of ABO*A201, which shows substitution at nucleotide (nt) position 467 and a single deletion (1060delC) in exon 7. This deletion results in disruption of the stop codon and an A-transferase product with an extra 21 amino acid (AA) residue at the C-terminus.

Individuals with the rare Bombay phenotype (Oh) do not express H antigen (also called substance H) (the antigen which is present in blood group O). As a result, they cannot make A antigen (also called substance A) or B antigen (also called "substance B") on their red blood cells, whatever alleles they may have of the A and B blood group genes, because A antigen and B antigen are made from H antigen. Oh individuals can be phenotypically identified using anti-H lectin extracted from *Ulex europeus*. O group has H antigen and hence shows reactivity with anti-H. However, Oh cells do not react with anti-H. Such individuals show the presence of anti-A, anti-B, and anti-H in the serum. Also, they are nonsecretors of A, B, and H soluble substances.

Despite ABO matching, blood transfusions continued to result in morbidity and mortality. In 1939, Levine and Stetson described an antibody in a mother who had recently had a stillborn fetus. The antibody caused hemolytic transfusion reaction (HTR) when she was transfused with ABO compatible blood of her husband [4]. The antibody (now known as anti-D) had been produced in response to D antigen carried by the fetus, which had been inherited from the father and absent in mother. By mid-1940s, several cases of Hemolytic Disease of Newborn (HDN) were than investigated and many could explain on basis of anti-D. Few had specificity similar but not identical to anti-D. They were termed as anti-C, anti-c, anti-E, and anti-e.

Rh system (ISBT No. 4) is the second most important blood group system after ABO. This system consists of more than 60 antigens but five antigens (C, c, D, E, e) and their corresponding antibodies account for 99% of problems related to Rh blood group system. The order of immunogenicity of these antigens is: D > c > E > C > e. Anti-D antibodies are only produced if a patient lacking D antigen is exposed to RhD-positive cells through pregnancy or transfusion. Rh antibodies react at 37 °C, are of the IgG type and capable of causing significant HTR and HDN. RBC destruction by Rh antibodies is mediated almost exclusively via macrophages in the spleen (extravascular hemolysis).

Tippett in 1986 [5] postulated the presence of two homologous RH genes (RHD and RHCE) located on chromosome 1. The RHD and RHCE genes each encode a transmembrane protein over 400 residues in length that traverses the RBC membrane 12 times. RHD determines the production of RhD protein (D antigen), while RHCE gene is responsible for production of RhCE, RhCe, RhcE, and Rhce proteins (C, c, E, e antigens). RhD-positive individuals inherit both RHD and RHCE genes while RhD-negative individuals inherit only the RHCE gene, RHD gene is either deleted or nonfunctional. The C/c polymorphism is due to six nucleotide substitutions resulting in four amino acid changes (Cys 16 trp, Ile 60 Leu, Ser 103 Pro, Ser 68 Asn) and E/e polymorphism is caused by single nucleotide substitution causing the amino acid change Pro 226 Ala.

Variants of RhD include Weak D, Partial D, and Del phenotypes. Very weak D phenotype "DEL" is characterized by low antigenic sites, recognized by only absorption elution method and is produced due to silent mutations in RHD gene [6]. Apart from these variants, rarer phenotypes like Rhnull and D–also exist.

27.2.1.2 Minor Blood Groups

Apart from ABO and Rh, various other minor blood group antigens exist which are not routinely typed during transfusion therapy. These antigens and systems were discovered after the indirect Coomb's test was developed by Robin Coombs in 1945. Antibodies against these antigens do not occur regularly as the corresponding antigens are weak immunogens. Nevertheless, these antibodies are of clinical importance as they can give rise to hemolytic anemias. Different blood groups have characteristic features for serology and clinical relevance; hence, it is important to know them in their due perspective. There are about 34 minor blood group systems, of which Duffy, Kell, Kidd, MNS, P, Lewis, and Lutheran are of major importance as compared to Dombrock, Colton, Indian, Cartwright, etc. blood group systems and the corresponding antibodies are known to cause hemolytic transfusion reactions (HTRs) or hemolytic disease of the newborn (HDFN) (Table 27.1).

The Duffy blood group system (ISBT No. 8): This is named after a hemophiliac multitransfused patient, Mr. Duffy who first showed the presence of anti-Fy^a in 1905. A year later, the antibody defining its antithetical antigen, Fyb, was found in the serum of a woman who had had three pregnancies. Thus, this system consists of two main antigens: Fy^a and Fy^b encoded by FY gene located on chromosome 1q23.2. The three common alleles at the Fy locus include Fya, Fyb, and Fy. The Fya/Fyb polymorphism arises due to single nucleotide alteration 125G>A in the DUFFY gene causing the amino acid change as Gly42Asp. The Fya/Fyb antigens give rise to four phenotypes: Fy(a+b−), Fy(a−b+), Fy(a+b+), and Fy(a−b−) of which phenotype Fy(a−b−) is a rare in general population although it is found with a higher frequency among the Afro-Arab population. This phenotype is caused due to mutations in the promoter region, GATA box of the FY gene. Fyb weak is characterized by a Fy (a−,b+weak) phenotype reacting weakly with anti-Fyb. Fya and Fyb are inherited in a codominant fashion. Antibodies to Duffy antigens are IgG reacting at 37 °C by Indirect Antiglobulin Test (IAT) and have been implicated in hemolytic transfusion reaction and HDFN.

The Kidd blood group system (ISBT No. 9) consists of three antigens which act as urea transporter are encoded by the JK gene found on chromosome 18 (18q11-q12). In 1951, Allen and colleagues reported anti-Jka in the serum of Mrs. Kidd, whose infant had HDFN. Two years later, its antithetical partner, Jkb, was found. The two antigens Jka and Jkb gives rise to four phenotypes, viz. Jk(a+b−), Jk(a−b+), Jk(a+b+), and Jk(a−b−). Jk(a−b−), the null phenotype described in 1959, is rare in most populations but

Table 27.1 Blood group systems and their clinical significance

ISBT no.	System name	Symbol	Epitope or carrier molecule	Chromosome location	Gene names	No. of antigens	Clinical significance
001	ABO	ABO	Carbohydrates	9q34.2	*ABO*	5	Severe AHTRs, rarely HDFN
002	MNS	MNS	CD235a, CD235b; Glycophorins A and B. Main antigens: M, N, S, s	4q31.21	*GYPA, GYPB, and GYPE*	48	AHTRs, DHTRs, HDFN
003	P	P	CD77; Glycolipid with three main antigens: P_1, P, and P^k	22q13.2	*A4GALT*	4	Rarely HTRs
004	Rh	RH	CD240; Protein; Main antigens: C, c, D, E, e antigens	1p36.11	*RHD, RHCE*	61	Severe HTRs and HDFN
005	Lutheran	LU	CD239; Protein (Part of immunoglobulin superfamily)	19q13.32	*LU*	23	Mild DHTRs
006	Kell	KEL	CD238; Glycoprotein	7q34	*KEL*	14	Severe AHTRs, DHTRs
007	Lewis	LE	Carbohydrate; Main antigens: Le^a and Le^b	19p13.3	*FUT3*	6	Not clinically significant generally
008	Duffy	FY	CD234: Chemokine receptor/Receptor for malarial parasite binding	1q23.2	*DARC*	6	AHTRs, DHTRs, and HDFN
009	Kidd	JK	Urea transporter	18q12.3	*SLC14A1*	3	DHTRs
010	Diego	DI	CD233; Glycoprotein, an anion exchanger	17q21.31	*SLC4A1*	22	Sometimes HTRs, severe HDFN
011	Yt	YT	Protein: (AChE, acetylcholinesterase)	7q22.1	*ACHE*	2	Very rarely HTR
012	XG	XG	CD99 (MIC2 product); Glycoprotein	Xp22.33	*XG,MIC2*	2	None
013	Scianna	SC	Glycoprotein	1p34.2	*ERMAP*	7	None
014	Dombrock	DO	CD297; Glycoprotein	12p12.3	*ART4*	8	AHTRs, DHTRs
015	Colton	CO	Aquaporin 1; main antigens Co^a and Co^b	7p14.3	*AQP1*	4	AHTRs, DHTRs, HDFN
016	Landsteiner-Wiener	LW	CD242; member of the immunoglobulin superfamily	19p13.2	*ICAM4*	7	None
017	Chido	CH	Complement fractions C4A C4B	6p21.3	*C4A,C4B*	9	None
018	Hh	H	CD173; Carbohydrate	19q13.33	*FUT1*	1	Can cause HTRs/HDFN
019	XK	XK	Glycoprotein	Xp21.1	*XK*	1	Severe HTRs
020	Gerbich	GE	CD236; Glycophorins C and D	2q14.3	*GYPC*	12	HDFN
021	Cromer	CROM	CD55; Glycoprotein (DAF)	1q32.2	*CD55*	18	None
022	Knops	KN	CD35; Glycoprotein (CR1)	1q32.2	*CR1*	9	None
023	Indian	IN	CD44 Glycoprotein	11p13	*CD44*	4	HTR

024	Ok	OK	CD147; Glycoprotein	19p13.3	*BSG*	3	None
025	Raph	RAPH	CD151; Transmembrane glycoprotein	11p15.5	*CD151*	1	None
026	JMH (John Milton Hagen)	JMH	CD108; Semaphorin 7A	15q24.1	*SEMA7A*	6	AHTR
027	Ii	I	Polysaccharide	6p24.2	*GCNT2*	1	–
028	Globoside	GLOB	Glycolipid. Antigen P	3q26.1	*B3GALT3*	2	Intravascular HTRs
029	GILL	GIL	Aquaporin 3	9p13.3	*AQP3*	1	None
030	Rh-associated glycoprotein	RHAg	CD241; Rh-associated glycoprotein	6p21-qter	*RHAG*	4	
1031	Forssman	FORS	Globoside alpha-1,3-*N*-acetylgalactosaminyltransferase 1 (GBGT1)	9q34.13	*GBGT1*	1	
0132	Langereis	LAN	ABCB6, human ATP-binding cassette (ABC) transporter	2q36	*ABCB6*	1	
033	Junior	JR	CD338: Multi-drug transporter protein	4q22	*ABCG2*	1	
034	Vel	Vel	Human red cell antigens	1p36.32	*SMIM1*	1	HTRs
035	CD59	CD59	CD59: GPI linked glycoprotein	11p13	*CD59*	1	
036	Augustine	AUG	Glycoprotein: equilibrative nucleoside transporter 1 (ENT1)	6p21.1	*SLC29A1*	2	

less uncommon among the Polynesians. The Jk locus (SLC12A1 gene; for solute carrier family 14, member 1) is located on chromosome 18 at position 18q12.3 and consists of 11 exons. The Jka/Jkb polymorphism is caused due to SNP 838G>A associated with an amino acid substitution Asp280Asn, predicted to be located on the fourth extracellular loop of the glycoprotein. JK3 antigen is present in all but Jk(a−b−) individuals who can produce anti-Jk3. Individuals with the null Jk(a−b−) phenotype lack Jka, Jkb, and Jk3. Red cells of these individuals are resistant to 2M urea. The antibodies are red cell immune, produced through incompatible transfusion or pregnancy and majority of them are IgG, reacting at 37 °C. Rarely, the antibodies show a great degree of dosage effect and being a short live entity, they remain obscure in pretransfusion test causing delayed HTR. The antibodies are associated with mild HDFN.

The Kell blood group system (ISBT No. 6) is highly polymorphic and the antigens are encoded by the KEL locus on chromosome 7q34. It has three sub-loci: K/k, Kpa/Kpb, and Jsa/Jsb. The polymorphisms associated with common Kell antigens include: K>k− 578T>C; Met193Thr, Kpa>Kpb− 841T>C; Trp281Arg and Jsa>Jsb- 1790C>T; Pro597Leu. The absence of all Kell antigens on red cells of individual results in Ko, a rare null phenotype characterized with anti-Ku in serum. Lack of XK protein results in weak expression of Kell antigens (The McLeod syndrome). The term "Kmod" is used to describe phenotypes with very weak Kell expression, often requiring adsorption-elution tests for detection. Some Kmod individuals make an antibody that resembles anti-Ku but does not react with other Kmod RBCs. Antibodies of this system are immune IgG, non-complement binding, react at 37 °C by IAT and have been implicated in HTR and HDFN.

The MNS system (ISBT No. 2) was discovered by Landsteiner and Levine in the year 1927 and the antigens are carried on glycophorin A(GYPA) and B(GYPB). The GYPA has three allelic forms M, N, and Mg that correspond to the M, N, and Mg antigens, respectively, while GYPB has two co-dominant alleles viz. S and s, encode the S

and s antigens. GYPE, the third glycophorin gene is responsible for production of variant antigens of this system. The genes GYPA and GYPB, encoding GPA and GPB, respectively, are located at chromosome 4q28–q31. The known alleles for GYPA (M/N) and GYPB (S/s) are co-dominant. The MNS antigens arise due to: M>N change is due to nucleotide changes 59C>T; 71G>A; 72T>G causing Ser20Leu, Gly24Glu changes in the protein. S/s polymorphism is caused due to Thr48Met because of single nucleotide change 143T>C. Gene rearrangements due to unequal crossing over between GYPA and GYPB give rise to GP(A-B) and GP(B-A) hybrid glycophorins.

Antibodies of the MNSs blood groups are red cell non-immune (i.e. naturally occurring) IgM agglutinins reacting at lower temperatures, e.g. anti-M, anti-N, and anti-Mg or are the red cell immune, IgG immunoglobulins reacting at 37 °C by the indirect antiglobulin test (IAT), e.g., anti-S and anti-s. The immune antibodies are susceptible to proteolytic enzymes and have been reported to cause HTR and HDFN.

Other systems of lesser clinical significance include P, Colton, Dombrock, Diego, Catwright, Indian, Lutheran, Lewis, etc. Common and clinically significant antigens of most of these blood systems are encoded by single nucleotide polymorphisms (SNPs) which give rise to change in amino acid resulting in change in antigen specificity (Table 27.2). Other molecular mechanisms encoding these antigens include deletions, insertions, missense mutations, frame shift mutations, and gene rearrangements [7].

27.2.2 Immune Anemias

The milestone for blood transfusion was in 1900 when Karl Landsteiner discovered the human ABO blood group system in Vienna. This fast forwarded the understanding for blood group incompatibility.

Alloimmunization is sensitization of the host immune system against foreign antigens and subsequent development of alloantibodies. Alloimmunization may occur due to blood

Table 27.2 Single nucleotide polymorphisms responsible for blood group antigens

Blood group system	Antigen specificity	Nucleotide	Amino change	Antigen specificity	Nucleotide	Amino change
MNS	M	59C; 71G; 72T	Ser20, Gly24	N	59T; 71A; 72G	Leu20, Glu24
	S	143T	Thr48	s	143C	Met48
Lutheran	Lu^a	230A	His77	Lu^b	230G	Arg77
Kell	K	578T	Met193	k	578C	Thr193
	Kp^a	841T	Trp281	Kp^b	841C	Arg281
	Js^a	1790C	Pro597	Js^b	1790T	Leu597
Duffy	Fy^a	125G	Gly42	Fy^b	125A	Asp42
Kidd	Jk^a	838G	Asp280	Jk^b	838A	Asn280
Diego	Di^a	2561T	Leu854	Di^b	2561C	Pro854
Cartwright	Yt^a	1057C	His353	Yt^b	1057A	Asn353
Scianna	Sc1	169G	Gly57	Sc2	169A	Arg57
Dombrock	Do^a	793A	Asn256	Do^b	793G	Asp256
Colton	Co^a	134C	Ala45	Co^b	134T	Val45
Indian	In^a	137C	Pro	In^b	137G	Arg

transfusion or via feto-maternal hemorrhage. Even very small amounts of donor antigenic RBCs can elicit an alloimmune response [8]. With the first exposure to foreign antigen, lymphocyte memory is invoked which results in moderate production of IgM and IgG antibodies. Secondary exposure elicits rapid production of large amounts of IgG-class antibody, rising rapidly in the first 2 days after exposure to the antigen. The antibody produced attaches to the antigenic surface and may interact with the complement system or reticuloendothelial system (RES) or monocyte phagocytic system [9]. Alloimmunization against multiple blood group antigens may lead to production of multiple antibodies which may cause difficulty in finding compatible RBC units, cause transfusion reactions, or platelet refractoriness. Retrospective studies in the general population reported antibody frequencies after transfusion of less than 1–3%. However, in multitransfused patients alloimmunization occurs from 10–38% and up to 60–70% of patients [10–12]. About 25% of such patients receive unsatisfactory transfusion support and it may even be impossible to find suitable units in some cases [13]. Blood transfusion also predisposes patient to formation of autoantibodies, which may result in development of autoimmune hemolytic anemia (AIHA), which can lead to increased hemolysis of transfused RBCs. Thus, the presence of RBC

alloantibodies creates the potential for serologic incompatibility, makes selection of appropriate units for future transfusion more difficult, delays blood transfusion, and presents risk of HDN. Non-hematooncologic alloimmunized patients are high antibody responders, with a more than 20 times increased risk to form antibodies compared to first-time alloimmunization risk [14].

In a Transfusion setting, an immediate HTR occurs very soon after the transfusion of incompatible RBCs. The RBCs are rapidly destroyed, releasing hemoglobin and RBC stomata into the circulation. In an anesthetized patient, hemoglobinuria, abnormal bleeding at the surgical wound site, and hypotension may be the only warning signs of IHTR. The reaction period varies from within few minutes to 1–2 h [15]. ABO-incompatible transfusions may be life-threatening, causing shock, acute renal failure, and disseminated intravascular coagulation (DIC).

Delayed HTR (DHTR) is most often the result of an anamnestic response in a patient who has been previously sensitized by transfusion, pregnancy, or transplant and in whom antibody is not detectable by standard pretransfusion methods. It is of two types: 1/primary alloimmunization wherein the patient has no past history of pregnancy, transfusion, or transplant and 2/secondary (anamnestic) response to transfused RBCs which occurs about 3–5 days later from the transfusion during which time enough antibody is produced by the patient to cause an immune reaction. Clinical signs and symptoms are usually mild; severe DHTR cases and fatalities are uncommon. Unexpected or unexplained decreases in hemoglobin or hematocrit values following transfusion should be investigated as a possible DHTR.

Hemolytic disease of the fetus and newborn (HDFN) or HDN or erythroblastosis fetalis is an alloimmune condition in the fetus when maternally produced IgG molecules against the paternal antigens present on the fetuses RBCs cross the placenta and cause in vivo destruction of fetal RBCs. The two common types of HDN are the ABO-HDN and the Rh-HDN. ABO-HDN is caused due to maternal anti-A or anti-B, but it is generally mild. Rh-HDN is caused when the maternal anti-D crosses the placental barrier and binds to fetal RhD-positive red cells. However, HND due to other blood group antigens has also been reported. Severe reaction may cause death of the fetus and hence the name erythroblastosis fetalis. The antibody binds to alloantigens of the fetus and these Ab coated cells are then removed from the circulation by spleen macrophages. The degree of destruction of fetal cells depends on the amount and functional characteristics of antibody [16]. Hemolysis of the sensitized cells releases hemoglobin, which is metabolized to bilirubin. Since fetal liver is immature, the bilirubin remains unconjugated and transported across the placenta to the mother. Therefore, during intrauterine life, there is no risk of jaundice to the fetus. The process of RBC destruction goes on even after the infant is delivered and the bilirubin accumulates in the fetal circulation causing jaundice.

27.2.3 Diagnosis and Management

Various laboratory tests are used to evaluate transfusion reactions and HDN. Biochemical tests for jaundice, testing for the presence of increased reticulocytes and positive direct and indirect antiglobulin tests are carried out. To further evaluate the severity, semi-quantitative estimation of the IgG antibody in mother's serum is carried out. Screening of all antenatal women in their early pregnancy and subsequent follow-ups for the presence of Rh and other antibodies will help in the management and prevention of HDFN. In case of RhD incompatibility, IVIG is prophylactically given postpartum to prevent alloimmunization in RhD-negative mother. Also, HDN cases are managed through intrauterine transfusions, postpartum-phototherapy, exchange transfusion, and plasma exchange.

In case of HTR, pretransfusion and posttransfusion sample should be tested for the presence of alloantibodies. Preliminary tests include blood grouping, direct and indirect antiglobulin tests and antigen profiling of donor and patient. In case of DHTR, additional tests may include testing for hemoglobin, hematocrit, coagulation studies, and renal function tests. Sometimes, it may not be possible to determine the clinical significance of an RBC antibody, or there may be evidence of an HTR in the absence of serologic evidence. RBC survival studies may be carried out to evaluate the clinical significance of the antibody involved.

It has been shown that extended phenotyping of minor blood group antigens and provision of antigen-matched blood reduces the incidence of alloimmunization and post-transfusion reactions. It also reduces iron overload and subsequent iron-chelation. In already alloimmunized patients, antigen-matched blood can reduce chances of producing antibodies against other antigens present on recipients' RBCs. In a 12.5-year study, patients with sickle cell anemia were divided into two groups. Group I which had no history of transfusion and was given antigen matched blood (C, c, E, e, K, S, Fya, and Fyb) did not show development of clinically significant alloantibodies. However, group II who received a mixture of antigen-matched and non-antigen-matched RBCs, 34.8% patients presented with clinically significant alloantibodies or developed them upon follow-up. Within Group II, 75% patients who presented with alloantibodies developed further new antibodies and only 22.2% of those patients who had not formed any alloantibodies at presentation developed alloantibodies [17]. Among

Table 27.3   Human platelet alloantigens

System	Glycoprotein	Antigen	Nucleotide substitution	Amino acid change
HPA-1	Integrin β3	HPA-1a	196T	Leu33
		HPA-1b	196C	Pro33
HPA-2	GPIbα	HPA-2a	524C	Thr145
		HPA-2b	524T	Met145
HPA-3	Integrin αIIb	HPA-3a	2622T	Ile843
		HPA-3b	2622G	Ser843
HPA-4	Integrin β3	HPA-4a	526G	Arg143
		HPA-4b	526A	Gln143
HPA-5	Integrin α2	HPA-5a	1648G	Glu505
		HPA-5b	1648A	Lys505
HPA-15	CD109	HPA-15a	2108C	Ser703
		HPA-15b	2108A	Tyr703

thalassemics, transfusion of phenotypically matched blood for the Rh and Kell systems reduced alloimmunization from 33 to 2.9% as compared to ABO-RhD-matched blood ($P = .0005$) [18]. Pujani et al. [19] reported no alloimmunization in thalassemics who were received partially better matched (PBM) blood (matched for ABO, Rh cDE, and Kell antigens). Castro et al. [20] observed that partial antigen matching of C, c, E, e, and K, along with ABO and D would have prevented alloimmunization in 53.3% of Caucasian patients and in 70.8% if S, Fya, and Jkb were further matched. Transfusion management is problematic is patients with autoantibodies. In these cases, the presence of an underlying alloantibody complicates transfusion therapy. Shirey et al. [21] adopted an algorithm for providing prophylactic antigen-matched RBCs to 20 consecutive patients with warm autoantibodies requiring chronic RBC transfusions. In 60% of these patients, adsorption studies could be precluded.

27.3   Immune Cytopenia Due to Human Platelet Antigens (HPA)

27.3.1   Alloantigens

Platelet-specific antigens are immunogenic glycoprotein structures present on the surface of platelets. These antigenic determinants are expressed as complex proteins, namely GPIIb/

IIIa (integrin alpha IIbbeta3), GPIa/GPIIa (integrin alpha2beta1), GPIb/IX/V, and CD109 which serve as binding receptors for ligands during platelet adhesion and aggregation. Currently, there are 33 different antigens grouped into six systems [22, 23]. Of the two biallelic antigens of the systems HPA-1, 2, 3, 4, 5 and 15, the designated "a" antigen is typically a high frequency antigen whereas the "b" is a low frequency antigen (Table 27.3). The remaining HPAs are low frequency antigens and thus designated as "b". HPAs are important in transfusion and prenatal settings have antibodies against these antigens have been known to cause refractoriness for platelet antigens, fetal neonatal alloimmune thrombocytopenia (FNAIT), and post-transfusion purpura (PTP) [24].

27.3.2   Immune Thrombocytopenias

In Neonatal Alloimmune Thrombocytopenia (NAIT), fetal/neonatal thrombocytopenia occurs due to transplacental transmission of maternal HPA alloantibodies that react with platelets of the fetus/neonate. It is characterized by a platelet count less than 150×10^9/L. It is hypothesized that, like maternal red cell antigen alloimmunization, a mother is exposed to paternal HPA produces an alloantibody which binds to and causes the rapid clearance/destruction of fetal/neonate platelets. NAIT can cause thrombocytopenia without overt bleeding or utero fetal demise secondary to intracranial hemorrhage or other severe bleeding complications. Alloantibodies against HPA-1a have been implicated in the majority of cases of NAIT (80–85%), with HPA-5b being the second most frequent target [25, 26].

Post-Transfusion Purpura (PTP) is a thrombocytopenic condition which occurs 2–14 days after an uneventful red blood cell (RBC) transfusion. RBC units containing contaminant platelets expressing HPA foreign to the patient have been implicated in this disease process. The generation of alloantibodies against a specific HPA not only affects platelets with said HPA, but a bystander effect is observed where the patient's native platelets are also cleared/destroyed.

Immune Platelet Refractoriness: Immune refractoriness to allogeneic platelets is most frequently associated with human leukocyte antigen class I alloimmunization; however, there are cases which have been documented as due to alloantibodies against HPAs lacking on the patient's platelets. As in NAIT, HPA-1a and HPA-5b have been implicated in this immune refractoriness. In patients congenitally lacking GPIb (Bernard Soulier) and GPIIb/IIIa (Glanzmann thrombasthenia), a wide range of alloimmune HPA antibodies can result from allogeneic platelet exposure.

27.3.3 Diagnosis and Management

NAIT is generally suspected if neonatal thrombocytopenia is seen in newborn especially to a mother with a previously affected child. The symptoms include bleeding into the skin or major organs like lungs or gastrointestinal tract. The management involves transfusion of washed and irradiated platelets from mother or plateletpheresis on a pregnant or peripartum mothers who are hospitalized. However, the cost of these procedures is the main limitations. Therefore, other alternative management involves platelet transfusion from a donor. If we get antigen-negative platelets, then they are more helpful.

In case of PTP, instead of providing antigen-negative platelet transfusion, immunosuppressive strategies are more useful. Intravenous immuno-globulin (IVIG) is more useful as compared to corticosteroid treatment which is sometimes not effective. The main purpose of this treatment is to increase the platelet count. Once it is increased, then PTP is usually a self-limited disease. The knowledge of both the patient's HPA phenotype and the specificity of the alloantibody can be very useful when attempting to provide platelets to patients with platelet alloantibodies.

A variety of laboratory techniques now exist to determine the HPA phenotype and genotype of the patient and potential platelet donors. Originally, typing was performed with patient-derived antisera, but was often contained contaminating anti-HLA antibodies. Since the discovery of the molecular determinants for HPA viz. single nucleotide polymorphisms leading to amino acid substitutions at specific points, the application of molecular methods to perform typing using DNA-based techniques became the "gold standard." Polymerase chain reaction (PCR) can be used to differentially amplify specific SNPs to determine type. For detection of HPA antibodies, Flow cytometry-based and Solid Phase Techniques methods have been used for antibody detection. Two common methods in wide use are the mixed passive hemagglutination assay (MPHA) and the monoclonal antibody-specific immobilization of platelet antigen (MAIPA) assay.

27.4 Immune Cytopenia Due to Human Neutrophil Antigens (HNA)

27.4.1 Alloantigens

Human neutrophil antigens (HNAs) are polymorphic structures located on several glycoproteins in the neutrophil membrane. The first granulocyte antigen was discovered by Lalezari and colleagues during their investigation of a neonate with transient alloimune neonatal neutropenia and since the antigens were neutrophil specific they designated it as the N system consisting of seven antigens (NA1, NA2, NB1, NB2, NC1, ND1, and NE1) [27–34]. Subsequently, several different granulocyte antigens were identified at the same time with sera from patients with auto-antibodies or alloantibodies directed against granulocytes. Currently, eight well characterized antigens are assigned to five HNA systems (Table 27.4).

27.4.2 HNA-1

HNA-1 is expressed exclusively on neutrophils and is located on the FCγRIIIb receptor (CD16b) which belongs to the Fc receptor family and is anchored to the membrane by glycosyl-phosphatidylinositol (GPI) [35, 36]. Consequently, whenCD16b binds to IgG, it interacts with other transmembrane proteins such as FcRII to generate an intracellular signal to activate neutrophil phago-cytosis, degranulation, or the respiratory burst [37, 38]. The FcγRIIIb possesses two IgG-like domains of which the membrane proximal domain contains residues critical for ligand binding. About 30% of granulocyte autoantibodies recognize epitopes on the Fcγ RIIIb with a preferential binding to the HNA-1a receptor [39].

Initially, HNA-1 was thought to be a biallelic system consisting of two main antigens: NA1 (HNA-1a) and NA2 (HNA-1b) [40]. However in 1997, a new alloantigen SH (HNA-1c) was char-acterized when the antibodies against this anti-gen was found in maternal sera of four neonatal alloimmune neutropenia cases. The antigens of HNA-1 are encoded by FCGR3B gene, a part of which is highly homologous FCγ-encoding genes on chromosome 1q22 and consists of five exons [41].

The FCGR3B*01 and FCGR3B*02 alleles differ in five nucleotide positions within exon 3 including one synonymous mutation, resulting in two isoforms HNA-1a (NA1; 50–65 kDa) and HNA-1b (NA2; 65–80 kDa), respectively [42–44]. The five nucleotide polymorphisms (nt 141, 147, 227, 277, and 349) result in four amino acid substitutions (positions 36, 65, 82, and 106) and two additional N-linked glycosilation sites. Individuals having zero expression of all the three antigens (HNA-1 null) have also been described [45]. This is due unequal crossing lead-ing to loss of FcγRIIIb. Homozygous individuals do not express FcγRIIIb on their neutrophils and are resistant to suffer from repeated infections, autoimmune or immune complex diseases. However, pregnant women with HNA-1 null phe-notype can form FcγRIIIB-specific isoantibodies which can cause alloimmune neutropenia in the neonates [46].

Recently, in a study by Reil et al. [47], it was observed that in two cases of neonatal alloim-mune neutropenia, both mothers were typed as FCGR3B*1+, *02−, and *03+. However, they produced antibodies reactive with FcγRIIIb encoded by FCGR3B*02 but not by FCGR3B*03. The antibodies detected the antithetical epitope to HNA-1c covering Ala78 and Asn82 which resides on the same glycoprotein as the HNA-1b epitope and is now proposed to be assigned as HNA-1d [47].

Antibodies to HNA-1 are involved in autoim-mune neutropenia, alloimmune neonatal neutro-penia and TRALI [27, 48–52]. The differing population frequencies for HNA-1a and HNA-1b, which both appear to be highly anti-genic, should be borne in mind when investigat-ing a potential ANN in a neutropenic newborn from a cross-cultural family. The binding of cog-nate antibodies to these antigens in vivo can result in severe functional impairment as well as neutropenia [53].

27.4.3 HNA-2

The second most clinically significant neutrophil specific antigen was described as "NB1" in 1971. It is located on a 58–64 kDa glycoprotein, CD177. It is not only found on the membrane but also attached intracellularly on the membranes of small vesicles and specific granules [54].

A unique characteristic of HNA-2a is its het-erogenous expression, i.e., a single individual has two or three subpopulations of expression: one negative reacting population and one or two pop-ulations that express the antigen with different intensities. HNA-2 is a high frequency antigen.

The gene encoding HNA-2a, i.e., CD177 is mapped on chromosome 19q13.2. The HNA-2a

Table 27.4 Summary of human neutrophil alloantigens systems

Antigen system	Carrier glycoprotein	Anchor/link	Antigen	Former name	Alleles	Expression	Nucleotide polymorphisms	Clinical significance
HNA-1	Fcγ Receptor IIIb (CD16b)	Glycosyl-phosphatidylinositol link (GPI)	HNA-1a	NA1	FCGR3B*01	Neutrophils	141G,147C,227A,266C,277G,349G	ANN, AIN, TRALI
			HNA-1b	NA2	FCGR3B*02		141C,147T,227G,266C,277A,349A	
			HNA-1c	SH	FCGR3B*03		141C,147T,227G,266A,277A,349A	
HNA-2	NB1 glycoprotein (CD177)	GPI	HNA-2	NB1	CD177*01	Neutrophils (monocytes of pregnant women)	Post-transcriptional modification/splicing defects	ANN, AIN, TRALI, drug-induced neutropenia, febrile transfusion reactions
HNA-3	Choline transporter-like protein 2 (CTL2)	Transmembrane	HNA-3a	5b	SLC44A2*1	Neutrophils, granulocytes, monocytes, lymphocytes, platelets, kidney, placental tissue, spleen, lymph node tissue, endothelial cells	461G	ANN, TRALI, febrile transfusion reactions
			HNA-3b	5a	SLC44A2*2		461A	
HNA-4	MAC-1; CR3; αMβ2-integrin (CD11b)	Transmembrane	HNA-4a	MART	ITGAM*01	Granulocytes, monocytes, T-lymphocytes	302G	ANN
HNA-5	LFA-1; αLβ2-integrin (CD11a)	Transmembrane	HNA-5a	OND	ITGAL*01	Granulocytes, monocytes, lymphocytes	2466G	AIN

AIN Autoimmune neutropenia, *ANN* Alloimmune neonatal neutropenia, *TRALI* Transfusion related acute lung injury cDNA consist of 1311 bp encoding 437 amino acids and a signal peptide of 21 amino acids. Apart from this, there a pseudogene that is located adjacent to the HNA-2 gene, but oriented in the opposite direction. Exons 4–9 are homologous. The HNA null allele is the result of different off-frame insertions at RNA level resulting in deficiency of the antigen on neutrophils [55].

The alloantibodies formed by HNA-2a-negative individuals are important in neonatal alloimmune neutropenia, TRALI, autoimmune drug-induced neutropenia, and graft failure following bone marrow transplantation [56–60].

27.4.4 HNA-3

Antibodies to the human neutrophil antigen 5b (now known as HNA-3a) was first described in 1964 by van Leeuwen and his co-workers from sera of alloimmunized pregnant women which agglutinated leucocytes of normal individuals [61]. It was suggested that the antigen is located on a 70–95 kDa protein, which is not linked to the plasma membrane via a GPI anchor as the HNA-1 and -2 antigens [62]. It was later characterized by Curtis B et al. in 2010. HNA-3a is carried on choline transporter-like protein 2 (CTL2), a member of the choline transporter-like family of membrane glycoproteins [63]. HNA-3 is a bialleleic system consisting of two antigens-3a and 3b (formerly 5a). The antigens arise due to a nonsynonymous single nucleotide polymorphism 461G>A in exon seven of the CTL2 gene (*SLC44A2*) located on chromosome 19p13.1 resulting in amino acid change arginine at position 154 (HNA-3a) to glutamine (HNA-3b) in the first extracellular loop of the mature protein.

The HNA-3 alloantigens reside on neutrophils, lymphocytes, platelets, and various tissues such as lung, liver, colon, and the inner ear. An additional 457C>T exchange (SLC44A2*03; rs147820753) constituting the amino acid change Leu151Phe in close proximity to the HNA-3a epitope alters HNA-3a antibody binding and also influences PCR-SSP typing when the SLC44A2*01 allele-specific primer covers this polymorphic position

[64, 65]. Occasional cases of febrile transfusion reactions and alloimmune neonatal neutropenia caused by anti-HNA-3 have been reported. HNA-3a alloantibodies have been increasingly reported in conjunction with TRALI, particularly with severe cases, in which patients required artificial ventilation, or with fatal reactions [66]. Alloantibodies to HNA-3a in donor plasma have been reported cause two fatalities [67]. This is possibly the result of the neutrophil priming capacity for reactive oxygen species production, and probably the marked capability of the HNA-3a antibodies to agglutinate neutrophils.

27.4.5 HNA-4

HNA-4a antigen (originally known as "Mart") and identification of HNA-4a-negative individuals were first reported in 1986. HNA-4 system is located on the CD11b/αM subunit of the αMβ2-integrin, a member of the Leu-CAM family and integrin superfamily, which shares a common β subunit (β2 or CD18) noncovalently associated with four different α subunits. HNA-4a is expressed on monocytes and NK cells along with neutrophils [68] and plays an important role in the leukocyte adhesion to endothelial cells and platelets, as well as in phagocytosis. The HNA-4a antigen is a polymorphic variant of αM (CR3; CD11b) subunit which is the result of a single nucleotide change G230A, substituting histidine by arginine at position 61 which is essential for HNA-4a alloantibody binding. HNA-4a has been reported to be present in more than 90% of population studied so far.

27.4.6 HNA-5

HNA-5a antigen—originally known as "Ond[a]," is located on the αL (CD11a) subunits of the lymphocyte function-associated (LFA)-1 complex and functions as a leucocyte adhesion molecule. It is the result of G2466C substitution in the coding sequence leading to the amino acid change Arg776Thr [68]. Antibodies to both

HNA-4a and HNA-5a were originally identified in sera from a multiparous blood donor and a multitransfused male patient respectively, indicating that the antigens are immunogenic. NAN cases have been associated with HNA-4a and HNA-5a antigens [69, 70].

27.4.7 Immune Neutropenias

Investigators have observed since the beginning of the twentieth century that sera of some patients caused agglutination of leucocytes from other individuals. These granulocyte reacting antibodies are involved in the pathophysiology of various clinical conditions, mainly associated with neutropenia, i.e., decrease in neutrophil count. Cases of alloimmune neutropenia (caused due anti-neutrophil antibodies to non-self-neutrophil-specific antigens) and autoimmune neutropenia (caused due to anti-neutrophil antibodies against self-specific neutrophil antigens) triggered scientists in the 1960s to late 1970s to develop reliable serological techniques for detecting antibodies against neutrophil antigens. Granulocyte antibodies have been detected in sera of multitransfused persons, women after pregnancy, patients with neutropenia, patients with febrile transfusion reactions, and in blood of donors that caused pulmonary transfusion reactions in the transfusion recipient.

Neutrophil antibodies have been shown to play a key role in the pathophysiology of several clinical conditions. One of the major conditions includes transfusion-related acute lung injury (TRALI). TRALI occurs during or within 6 h of transfusion with one or more units of blood products and represents similar to acute lung injury. The pathogenesis of TRALI is explained by identifying of anti-human leukocyte antigen (anti-HLA) or anti-HNA antibodies in blood products which react with cognate antigen present on neutrophils of the transfusion recipient. Patient with TRALI shows dyspnea, tachypnea, hypoxemia, bilateral pulmonary opacities on chest radiograph, edema fluid in the endotracheal tube of intubated patients (severe TRALI), and the absence of evidence of volume overload or car-

diac dysfunction as the principal cause of pulmonary edema. HNA-3a antibodies have known to be the major causative agent of TRALI. Other clinical conditions where HNA play a key role include: neonatal alloimmune neutropenia in neonates (NAN), autoimmune neutropenia during childhood, febrile non-hemolytic transfusion reactions, immune neutropenia post bone marrow transplantation, drug-induced neutropenia, and refractoriness to granulocyte transfusion. The identification of neutrophil antigens and antibodies is relevant for the diagnosis of these disorders [71, 72].

The prevalence of granulocyte antibodies among previously pregnant and never allo-exposed donors was 3% and 2%, respectively, in the Dutch population. The type of pregnancy outcome could influence both the degree of exposure of the mother to paternal granulocyte antigens and the extent of tissue damage and related inflammation involved in this exposure, which together influence the probability of developing antibodies [73]. Lucas et al. [74] reported 4.9% of granulocyte reacting antibodies in a study of female donors in the UK [74]. However, Gottschall et al. reported a much lower frequency of 0.7% in US donors with different specificities of HNA antibodies 23 [75] and Reil et al. [76] reported 0.45% rate of alloimmunization among female donors in Germany [76].

The presence of granulocyte antibodies have also been reported among multitransfused and multiparous women. In Japanese multitransfused patients who were transfused with filtered leucocytes and unfiltered leucocytes, it was found that the rate of alloimmunization was 0.44% against granulocyte antibodies among patients who received unfiltered leucodepleted blood products [77] and where transfused frequently. It has been reported that as the number of pregnancies increase the incidence of granulocyte reacting antibodies increased up to 26.3% in women with three or more parity indicating that plasma products from these donors cause highest risk for inducing TRALI [78]. Sachs et al. [79] studied sera of multiparous women and found 11.2% of granulocyte reacting antibodies in women with three or more parity [79].

27.4.8 Diagnosis and Management

There are no specific tests to detect TRALI. However, analyzing echocardiogram, measuring brain natriuretic peptide (BNP) levels, performing pulmonary edema fluid protein analysis and estimating white blood cell count (WBC) can be done to eliminate other clinical conditions. In addition to these tests, confirmatory laboratory tests which involve testing for the presence/absence of granulocyte/HLA antibodies can provide definitive evidence for the diagnosis of TRALI. The ultimate detection of TRALI depends on the clinical conditions and laboratory test results. As with other forms of ALI/ARDS, there is no specific treatment for TRALI. In most cases, prompt diagnosis allows immediate supportive care. In case if the patient is still being transfused after suspecting TRALI, the transfusion should be immediately stopped. In mild cases, supplemental oxygen may be sufficient while in severe cases, mechanical ventilation, intravenous fluids, invasive hemodynamic monitoring, and vasopressors are required. In rare cases, extracorporeal oxygenation may be required to treat hypoxemia resulting from TRALI. As a preventive measure, donors who have granulocyte/HLA reactive antibodies should be deferred from donating. Female blood donors with only two previous pregnancies can form clinically important granulocyte-reactive alloantibodies leading to fatal TRALI reactions in recipients and also should be deferred from blood donation.

Traditionally, the neutrophil antigen phenotyping has been performed using human alloantibodies in the granulocyte agglutination test (GAT), or the granulocyte immunofluorescence test (GIFT). HNA phenotyping by serological techniques requires granulocyte isolation, which is a time-consuming process and may affect test results due to low viability and also alloantisera specific to neutrophil antigens are not always available. Hence, genotyping methods are more commonly used for detection of antigens of HNA-1, 3, 4, and 5 systems as they are easy and cost-effective. However, HNA-2 is studied by flow cytometry because even though it has been characterized at the molecular level, genotyping methods are yet to be developed. It may be pos-

sible to distinguish HNA-2-positive phenotypes from HNA-2a-negative phenotypes by analyzing neutrophil *CD177* mRNA for accessory sequences, but working with mRNA is much more difficult than working with DNA.

Human neutrophil antibodies have been studied using GAT, GIFT, and monoclonal antibody immobilization of granulocyte antigens (MAIGA). GAT method is based on the principle of agglutination in which the antibodies actively cause agglutination of neutrophils. GIFT uses fluorescently labeled antibody to detect the antigens. Microscopic GIFT and FLOW-GIFT are both based on the same principle; however, FLOW-GIFT uses flow cytometer to analyze antigen antibody reactions and microscopic GIFT uses fluorescent microscope. MAIGA assay allows the detection of antibodies to specific neutrophil membrane glycoproteins even when antibodies to human leucocyte antigen (HLA) antigens are present.

27.4.9 Immune Cytopenia Due to Leucocytes

In 1947, Jean Dausset provided the first evidence for human leukocyte blood groups. He observed that patients receiving a large number of transfusions contained leukoagglutinins in their sera which were produced by the infusion of cells bearing alloantigens not present in the recipient [80]. Based on the reactivity of the alloantibodies, HLA-A2 was the first human leucocyte antigen (HLA) to be identified [81]. HLA are surface receptors responsible for the antigen recognition and represent them on the external surface of the is recognized by the T cells eventually resulting in the elimination of foreign tissues. In humans, HLA are also referred to as the major histocompatibility complex (MHC). Apart from the recognition of foreign agents, MHC also participates in correlating the cell mediated and the humoral immunity and also plays a role in a successful solid organ transplantation [82]. HLA testing supports a number of clinical specialties in transplantation, transfusion, and immunogenetics. Though HLA system has a primary clinical importance in transplantation, it has recently become of great interest due to its association with certain diseases than any other known genetic marker in humans. Also, the HLA system has huge applicability in resolving cases of disputed paternity.

27.4.10 Alloantigens

The HLA gene complex encodes for the human leukocyte antigen (HLA) complex. This gene complex consists of more than 200 genes located closely together on chromosome 6. HLA gene products are globular glycoproteins, composed of chains which are noncovalently linked. In humans, the MHC complex is categorized into three classes: MHC class I, II, and III.

The three main MHC class I genes are HLA-A, HLA-B, and HLA-C; the proteins of which are present on the surface of almost all cells. HLA-A, HLA-B, and HLA-C are made up of a heavy chain (molecular weight: 45,000 Da) which is associated noncovalently with β 2-microglobulin, a nonpolymorphic protein (12,000 Da). The heavy chain folds into three domains and is inserted through the cell membrane via a hydrophobic sequence [83]. Viral protein compartments, peptides derived from tumor cells and also self-antigens are represented by this type of MHC. MHC class I also encodes for additional nonclassic genes such as HLA-E, HLA-F, and HLA-G.

MHC class II contains six main genes: HLA-DPA1, HLA-DPB1, HLA-DQA1, HLA-DQB1, HLA-DRA, and HLA-DRB1. These molecules are made up of two chains of a molecular weight of 33,000 (α) and 28,000 (β) daltons which are noncovalently associated with each other via their extracellular regions. Both the α and β chains are inserted into through the cell membrane via hydrophobic regions. The extracellular portions of these chains fold into two domains [84]. The DP molecules are the product of DPA1 and DPB1 alleles while DPB2 and DPA2 are pseudogenes. DQ molecules are the product of DQA1 and DQB1 alleles. DR molecules use DRA but can use alleles coded by DRB1 (the classic DR specificities), DRB3 (DR52 molecules), and DRB4 (DR53). MHC class II genes provide instructions for making proteins that are present almost exclusively on the surface of certain immune system cells. These proteins display peptides to the immune system.

MHC class III gene located between Class I and II produces proteins such as complement proteins (C2, C4, Bf), 21-hydroxylase, and tumor necrosis factor. These gene products are involved in inflammation and other immune system activities. The functions of some MHC genes are unknown.

The antigenic specificities, defined by serologic reactivity, are designated by numbers following the locus symbol (e.g., HLA-A1, HLA-A2, HLA-B5, and HLA-B7). Several HLA alleles demonstrate serologic cross-reactivity due to structural similarity. For example, HLA-A9, HLA-A23, and HLA-A24 all react with antibodies specific for HLA-A9, but HLA-A23 and HLA-A24 can be "split" from A9 by unique reactivity with antibodies specific for each. Two exceptions to HLA nomenclature are the Bw4 and Bw6 epitopes, where the "w" is present to distinguish them as significant serologic epitopes found on multiple HLA-A and HLA-B alleles, rather than independent HLA specificities.

Class I molecules are present on all nucleated cells, dendritic cells, and platelets, whereas class II molecules are found only on B lymphocytes, activated T-lymphocytes, macrophages, monocytes, and endothelial cells.

The majority of HLA alloantibodies are IgG. Antibodies to HLA molecules can be divided into two groups: (1) Those that detect a single HLA gene product ("private" antibodies binding to an epitope unique to one HLA gene product) (2) those that detect more than one HLA gene product. These may be "public" (binding to epitopes shared by more than one HLA gene product) or cross-reactive (binding to structurally similar HLA epitopes).

27.4.11 Immune Cytopenias Due to HLA

HLA class I antigens are expressed variably on platelets [85–89]. Alloimmunization against HLA results in refractoriness to random donor platelet transfusions. This is manifested by the failure to achieve a rise in the circulating platelet count 1 h after infusion of adequate numbers of platelets. Lymphocytotoxic HLA antibodies are often associated with the refractory state.

Antibodies against HLA class I and class II molecules have been found in 50–89% of products associated with TRALI along with anti-HNA antibodies [90–92].

HLA antibodies are also involved in clinical transplantation such as hematopoietic stem cell transplantation, kidney transplantation, liver transplantation, lung transplantation, pancreas, and islet cell transplantation.

27.4.12 Detection of HLA and Associated Antibodies

HLA class I (HLA-A, HLA-B, HLA-C) and class II (HLA-DR, HLA-DQ, HLA-DP) are genotyped using DNA-based analysis techniques [93]. The three most common molecular assays currently employed in the clinical laboratory are sequence-specific oligonucleotides (SSO), sequence-specific primers (SSP), and sequence-based typing (SBT). SSO has been traditionally used and most of the SNPs can be detected, depending on the extent of resolution required. Although it is a very reliable and accurate technology, it has been superseded by the more rapid technique of PCR-SSP. Sequence-based typing of HLA genes is utilized for high-resolution typing and is required in the definition of a new allele.

Screening for and determining the specificity of anti-HLA class I and II antibodies has been reported for the clinical management of patients, pre- and post-transplant and useful in excluded antibody containing donor blood products that can cause TRALI in blood recipients. Microcytotoxicity testing, enzyme-linked immunosorbent crossmatch assays and Luminex based assays are being carried out.

References

1. Storry JR, Castilho L, Chen Q, Daniels G, Denomme G, Flegel WA, Gassner C, Haas M, Hyland C, Keller M, Lomas-Francis C. International Society of Blood Transfusion Working Party on red cell immunogenet-ics and terminology: report of the Seoul and London meetings. ISBT Sci Ser. 2016;11(2):118–22.
2. Cartron JP. Elute quantitative et thermo dynamique des phenotypes erythrocytaires "Afaible". Rev franc Transfus Immunohaemat. 1976;19:35.
3. Yamamoto F, Clausen H, White T, Marken J, Hakomori S. Molecular genetic basis of the histo-blood group system. Nature. 1990;345:229–33.
4. Levine P, Stetson RE. An unusual case of intragroup agglutination. JAMA. 1939;13:126–7.
5. Tippett P. A speculative model for Rh blood groups. Ann Hum Genet. 1986;50:241–7.
6. Shao CP, Maas JH, Su YQ, Köhler M, Legler TJ. Molecular background of Rh Dpositive, D-negative, D(el) and weak D phenotypes in Chinese. Vox Sang. 2002;83:156–61.
7. Patnaik SK, Helmberg W, Blumenfeld OO. BGMUT database of allelic variants of genes encoding human blood group antigens. Transfus Med Hemother. 2014;41(5):346–51.
8. Silberstein LE, Naryshkin S, Haddad JJ, Strauss JF. Calcium homeostasis during therapeutic plasma exchange. Transfusion. 1986;26:151.
9. Cox JV, Steane E, Cunningham G, Frenkel EP. Risk of alloimmunization and delayed hemolytic transfusion reactions in patients with sickle cell disease. Arch Intern Med. 1988;148:2488.
10. Singerb ST, Wu V, Mignacca R, et al. Alloimmunisation and erythrocyte autoimmunisation in transfusion-dependent thalassemia patients of predominant Asian descent. Blood. 2000;96:3369–73.
11. Hoeltge GA, Domen RE, Rybicki LA, Schaffer PA. Multiple red cell transfusions and alloimmunization. Experiences with 6996 antibodies detected in a total of 159,262 patients from 1985-1993. Arch Pathol Lab Med. 1995;119:42–5.
12. Makarovska-Bojadzieva T, Blagoevska M, Kolevski P, Kostovska S. Optimal blood gouping and antibody screening for safe transfusion. Contrib Sec Biol Med Sci MASA. 2009;30:119–28.
13. Seltsam A, Wagner FF, Salama A, et al. Antibodies to high-frequency antigens may decrease the quality of transfusion support: an observational study. Transfusion. 2003;43:1563–6.
14. Schonewille H, Van De Watering LM, Brand A. Additional red blood cell alloantibodies after blood transfusions in a nonhematologic alloimmunized patient cohort: is it time to take precautionary measures? Transfusion. 2006;46:630–5.
15. Holland PV. The diagnosis and management of transfusion reactions and other adverse effects of transfusion. In: Petz LD, Swisher SN, editors. Clinical practice of transfusion medicine. 2nd ed. New York: Churchill Livingstone; 1989. p. 714.
16. Zupanska B, Thomson EE, Merry AH. Fc receptors for IgG1 and IgG3 on human mononuclear cells and evaluation with known levels of erythrocyte bound IgG. Vox Sang. 1986;50:97–103.
17. Tahhan HR, Holbrook CT, Braddy LR, et al. Antigen matched donor blood in the transfusion management

of patients with sickle-cell disease. Transfusion. 1994;34:562–9.

18. Singer ST, Wu V, Mignacca R, Kuypers FA, Morel P, Vichinsky EP. Alloimmunization and erythrocyte autoimmunization in transfusion-dependent thalassemia patients of predominantly Asian descent. Blood. 2000;96:3369–73.

19. Pujani M, Pahuja S, Dhingra B, Chandra J, Jain M. Alloimmunisation in thalassaemics: a comparison between recipients of usual matched and partial better matched blood. An evaluation at a tertiary care centre in India. Blood Transfus. 2014;12:s100.

20. Castro O, Sandler SG, Houston-Yu P, Rana S. Predicting the effect of transfusing only phenotype-matched RBCs to patients with sickle cell disease: Theoretical and practical implications. Transfusion. 2002;42:684–90.

21. Shirey RS, Boyd JS, Parwani AV, Tanz WS, Ness PM, King KE. Prophylactic antigen-matched donor blood for patients with warm autoantibodies: an algorithm for transfusion management. Transfusion. 2002;42:1435–41.

22. Novotny VM. Prevention and management of platelet transfusion refractoriness. Vox Sang. 1999;76:1–13.

23. Peterson JA, Gitter ML, Kanack A, et al. New low-frequency platelet glycoprotein polymorphisms associated with neonatal alloimmune thrombocytopenia. Transfusion. 2010;50:324–33.

24. Kroll H, Kiefel V, Santoso S. Clinical aspects and typing of platelet alloantigens. Vox Sang. 1998;74:s345–54.

25. Davoren A, Curtis BR, Aster RH, McFarland JG. Human platelet antigen-specific alloantibodies implicated in 1162 cases of neonatal alloimmune thrombocytopenia. Transfusion. 2004;44:1220–5.

26. Knight M, Pierce M, Allen D, Kurinczuk JJ, Spark P, Roberts DJ, Murphy MF. The incidence and outcomes of fetomaternal alloimmune thrombocytopenia: a UK national study using three data sources. Br J Haematol. 2011;152:460–8.

27. Lalezari P, Bernard GE. An isologous antigen-antibody reaction with human neutrophils, related to neonatal neutropenia. J Clin Invest. 1966;45:1741–50.

28. Lalezari P, Radel E. Neutrophil-specific antigens: immunology and clinical significance. Semin Hematol. 1974;11:281–90.

29. Lalezari P, Murphy GB, Allen FH. NB1, a new neutrophil antigen involved in the pathogenesis of neonatal neutropenia. J Clin Invest. 1971;50:1108–15.

30. Huang ST, Lin J, McGowan EL, et al. NB2, a new allele of NB1 antigen involved in febrile transfusion reaction (abstract). Transfusion. 1982;22:426.

31. Lalezari P, Petrosova M, Jiang AF. NB2, an allele of NB1 neutrophil specific antigen: relationship to 9a (abstract). Transfusion. 1982;22:433.

32. Lalezari P, Thelenfeld B, Weinstein WJ. The third neutrophil antigen. In: Terasaki PI, editor. Histocompatibility testing. Baltimore: Williams & Wilkins; 1970. p. 319–22.

33. Verheugt FWA, von dem Borne AE, van Noord-Bokhorst JC, et al. ND1, a new neutrophil granulocyte antigen. Vox Sang. 1978;35:13–7.

34. Claas FHJ, Langerak J, Sabbe LJM, et al. NE1, a new neutrophil specific antigen. Tissue Antigens. 1979;13:129–34.

35. Bux J, Sohn M, Hachmann R, et al. Quantitation of granulocyte antibodies in sera and determination of their binding sites. Br J Haematol. 1992;82:20–5.

36. Huizinga TW, van der Schoot CE, Jost C, et al. The PI-linked receptor FcRIII is released on stimulation of neutrophils. Nature. 1988;333:667–9.

37. Huizinga TW, van Kemenade F, Koenderman L, et al. The 40-kDa Fc gamma receptor (FcRII) on human neutrophils is essential for the IgG-induced respiratory burst and IgG-induced phagocytosis. J Immunol. 1989;142:2365–9.

38. Unkeless JC, Shen Z, Lin CW, et al. Function of human Fc gamma RIIA and Fc gamma RIIIB. Semin Immunol. 1995;7:37–44.

39. Bux J, Behrens G, Jäger G, Welte K. Diagnosis and clinical course of autoimmune neutropenia in infancy: analysis 240 cases. Blood. 1997;89:1027–34.

40. Huizinga TW, Kleijer M, Tetteroo PA, et al. Biallelic neutrophil Na-antigen system is associated with a polymorphism on the phospho-inositol-linked Fcc Receptor III (CD16). Blood. 1990;75:213–7.

41. Qiu WQ, de Bruin D, Brownstein BH, Pearse R, Ravetch JV. Organization of the human and mouse low-affinity FcgR genes: Duplication and recombination. Science. 1990;248:732.

42. Ravetch JV, Perussia B. Alternative membrane forms of FcRIII (CD16) on human natural killer cells and neutrophils. J Exp Med. 1989;170:481–97.

43. Ory PA, Clark MR, Kwoh EE, Clarkson SB, Goldstein IM. Sequences of complementary DNAs that encode the NA1 and NA2 forms of Fc receptor III on human neutrophils. J Clin Invest. 1989;84:1688–91.

44. Ory PA, Goldstein IM, Kwoh EE, Clarkson SB. Characterization of polymorphic forms of Fc receptor III on human neutrophils. J Clin Invest. 1989;83:1676–81.

45. De Haas M, Kleijer M, Van Zwieten R, Roos D, Von Dem Borne AE. Neutrophil Fcγ RIIIb deficiency, nature and clinical consequences: a study of 21 individuals from 14 families. Blood. 1995;86:2403–13.

46. Huizinga TW, Kuijpers RWA, Kleijer M, Schulpen TW, Cuypers HTM, Roos D, Von Dem Borne AE. Maternal genomic FcRIII deficiency leading to neonatal isoimmune neutropenia. Blood. 1990;76:1927–32.

47. Reil A, Sachs UJ, Siahanidou T, Flesch BK, Bux J. HNA-1d: a new human neutrophil antigen located on Fcγ receptor IIIb associated with neonatal immune neutropenia. Transfusion. 2013;53:2145–51.

48. Bux J, Hartmann C, Mueller-Eckhart C. Alloimmune neonatal neutropenia resulting from immunization to a high-frequency antigen on the granulocyte Fc g receptor III. Transfusion. 1994;34:608–11.

49. Bux J, Kissel K, Nowak K, et al. Autoimmune neutropenia: clinical and laboratory studies in 143 patients. Ann Hematol. 1991;63:249–52.

50. Stroncek DF, Skubitz KM, Plachta LB, et al. Alloimmune neonatal neutropenia due to an antibody to the neutrophil Fc-greceptor III with maternal deficiency of CD16 antigen. Blood. 1991;77:1572–80.

51. Fung YL, Goodison KA, Wong JK, et al. Investigating transfusion-related acute lung injury (TRALI). Intern Med J. 2003;33:286–90.

52. Lucas GF, Rogers S, Evans R, et al. Transfusion-related acute lung injury associated with interdonor incompatibility for the neutrophil-specific antigen HNA-1a. Vox Sang. 2000;79:112–5.

53. Bux J, Dickmann JO, Stockert U, et al. Influence of granulocyte antibodies on granulocyte function. Vox Sang. 1993;64:220–5.

54. Goldschmeding R, van Dalen CM, Faber N, Calafat J, Huizinga TWJ, van der Schoot CE, et al. Further characterization of the NB1 antigen as a variably expressed 56–62 kD GPI-linked glycoprotein of plasma membranes and specific granules of neutrophils. Br J Haematol. 1992;81:336–45.

55. Kissel K, Scheffler S, Kerowgan M, et al. Molecular basis of NB1 (HNA-2a, CD177) deficiency. Blood. 2002;99:4231–3.

56. Stroncek D. Granulocyte antigens and antibody detection. Vox Sang. 2004;87(S1):91–4.

57. Bux J, Jung KD, Kauth T, et al. Serological and clinical aspects of granulocyte antibodies leading to alloimmune neonatal neutropenia. Transfus Med. 1992;2:143–9.

58. Bux J. Granulocyte antibody mediated neutropenias and transfusion reactions. Infus Ther Transfus Med. 1999;26:152–7.

59. Bux J, Becker F, Seeger W, et al. Transfusion-related acute lung injury due to HLR-A2-specific antibodies in recipient and NB1-specific antibodies in donor blood. Br J Haematol. 1996;93:707–13.

60. Stroncek DF, Shankar RH, Herr GP. Quininedependent antibodies to neutrophils react with a 60kD glycoprotein on which neutrophil-specific antigenNB1 is located and an 85 kD glycosylphosphatidylinositol–linked N-glycosylated plasma membrane protein. Blood. 1993;81:2758–66.

61. van Leeuwen A, Eernisse JG, van Rood JJ. A new leucocyte group with two alleles: leucocyte group five. Vox Sang. 1964;9:431–46.

62. De Haas M, Muniz-Dias E, Alonso LG, Van Der Kolk K, Kos M, Buddelmeijer L, Porcelijn L, Von Dem Borne AE. Neutrophil antigen 5b is carried by a protein, migrating from 70 to 95 kDa, and may be involved in neonatal alloimmune neutropenias. Transfusion. 2000;40:222–7.

63. Curtis BR, Cox NJ, Sullivan MJ, Konkashbaev A, Bowens K, Hansen K, Aster RH. The neutrophil alloantigen HNA-3a (5b) is located on choline transporter-like protein 2 and appears to be encoded by an R> Q154 amino acid substitution. Blood. 2010;115(10):2073–6.

64. Huvard MJ, Schmid P, Stroncek DF, et al. Frequencies of SLC44A2 alleles encoding human neutrophil antigen-3 variants in the African American population. Transfusion. 2011;52:1106–11.

65. Flesch BK, Reil A, Bux J. Genetic variation of the HNA-3a encoding gene. Transfusion. 2011;51:2391–7.

66. Lalezari P, Bernard GE. Identification of a specific leukocyte antigen: another presumed example of 5b. Transfusion. 1965;5(2):135–42.

67. Davoren A, Curtis BR, Shukman IA, Mohrbacher AF, Bux J, Kwiatkowska BJ, Mcfarland JG, Aster RH. TRALI due to granulocyte-agglutinating human neutrophil antigen-3a (5b) alloantibodies in dnor plasma: a report of 2 fatalities. Transfusion. 2003;43:641–5.

68. Simsek S, van der Schoot CE, Daams M, et al. Molecular characterization of antigenic polymorphisms (Ond(a) and Mart(a)) of the beta 2 family recognized by human leukocyte alloantisera. Blood. 1996;88:1350–8.

69. Fung YL, Pitcher LA, Willett JE, et al. Alloimmune neonatal neutropenia linked to anti-HNA-4a. Transfus Med. 2003;13:49–52.

70. Porcelijn L, Abbink F, Terraneo L, Onderwater-vd Hoogen L, Huiskes E, de Hass M. Neonatal alloimmune neutropenia due to immunoglobulin G antibodies against human neutrophil antigen-5a. Transfusion. 2011;51:574–7.

71. Moritz E, Norcia AM, Cardone JD, et al. Human neutrophil alloantigens systems. An Acad Bras Cienc. 2009;81:559–69.

72. Fung YL, Minchinton RM. The fundamentals of neutrophil antigen and antibody investigations. ISBT Sci Ser. 2011;6:381–6.

73. Middelburg RA, Porcelijn L, Lardy N, Briët E, Vrielink H. Prevalence of leucocyte antibodies in the Dutch donor population. Vox Sang. 2011;100:327–35.

74. Lucas G, Win N, Calvert A, et al. Reducing the incidence of TRALI in the UK: the results of screening for donor leucocyte antibodies and the development of national guidelines. Vox Sang. 2012;103:10–7.

75. Gottschall JL, Triulzi DJ, Curtis B, et al. The frequency and specificity of human neutrophil antigen antibodies in a blood donor population. Transfusion. 2011;51:820–7.

76. Reil A, Keller-Stanislawski B, Günay S, Bux J. Specificities of leukocyte alloantibodies in transfusion-related acute lung injury and results of leucocyte antibody screening of blood donors. Vox Sang. 2008;95:313–7.

77. Zhang X, Araki N, Ito K. Post-transfusion alloimmunization to granulocytes and platelets in Japanese patients as determined by the MPHA method. Transfus Apher Sci. 2001;25:163–72.

78. Densmore TL, Goodnough LT, Ali S, Dynis M, Chaplin H. Prevalence of HLA sensitization in female apheresis donors. Transfusion. 1999;39:103–6.

79. Sachs UJ, Link E, Hofmann C, Wasel W, Bein G. Screening of multiparous women to avoid transfusion-related acute lung injury: a single centre experience. Transfus Med. 2008;18(6):348–54.

80. Dausset H. Leukoagglutinins: leukoagglutinins and blood transfusion. J Vox Sang. 1954;4:190.

81. Dausset J. Iso-leuco-anticorps. Acta Haematol. 1958;20:156.

82. Horton R, Wilming L, Rand V, Lovering RC, Bruford EA, Khodiyar VK, et al. Gene map of the extended human MHC. Nat Rev Genet. 2004;5:889–99.

83. Bjorkman PJ, et al. Structure of the HLA class I histocompatibility antigen, HLA-A2. Nature. 1987;329:506.

84. Brown JH, et al. Three-dimensional structure of the human class II histocompatibility antigen HLA DR1. Nature. 1993;364:33.

85. Colombani J. Blood platelets in HL-A serology. Transplant Proc. 1971;3:1078.

86. Svejgaard A, Kissemeyer-Nielson F, Thorsby E. HL-A typing of platelets. In: Terasaki PI, editor. Histocompatibility testing 1970. Copenhagen: Munksgaard; 1970. p. 160.

87. Leibert M, Aster RH. Expression of HLA-B12 on platelets, on lymphocytes, and in serum: a quantitative study. Tissue Antigens. 1977;9:199.

88. Aster RH, Szatkowski N, Liebert M. Expression of HLAB12, HLA-B8, W4, and W6 on platelets. Transplant Proc. 1977;9:1965.

89. Duquesnoy RJ, Testin J, Aster RH. Variable expression of W4 and W6 on platelets: Possible relevance to platelet transfusion therapy of alloimmunized thrombocytopenic patients. Transplant Proc. 1977;9:1827.

90. Popovski MA, Moore SB. Diagnostic and pathogenic considerations in transfusion-related acute lung injury. Transfusion. 1985;25:573.

91. Kopko PM, et al. HLA class II antibodies in transfusion-related acute lung injury. Transfusion. 2001;41:1244.

92. Eder AF, et al. Transfusion-related acute lung injury surveillance (2003–2005) and the potential impact of the selective use of plasma from male donors in the American Red Cross. Transfusion. 2007;47:599.

93. Tiercy JM, Jannet M, Mach B. A new approach for the analysis of HLA class II polymorphism: HLA oligo typing. Blood Rev. 1990;4:9.

Molecular Techniques for Prenatal Diagnosis

28

Anita Nadkarni and Priya Hariharan

28.1 Inherited Haematological Disorders

28.1.1 Introduction

A disease that is caused by an abnormality in an individual's genome and which is transmitted from one generation to another is known as an inherited disease. Based on the type of anomalies present, a genetic disorder can be classified into chromosomal aberrations, monogenetic diseases which are caused by single gene mutation, polygenetic/multifactorial diseases, which are caused by mutations in several genes as well as exogenous factors [1]. These diseases are generally inherited in a recognizable pattern of autosomal dominant, autosomal recessive or X-linked disorders of which inherited haematological diseases are the disorders that primarily affect the fundamental process of haematopoiesis and blood components (red blood cells, white blood cells, and platelets) [1]. The common inherited haematological disorders can be broadly classified as cellular and non-cellular.

28.1.1.1 Cellular Disorders

Bone Marrow
These include disorders of bone marrow failure, which act as the primary site of new blood cell production and cellular components of the blood. The inherited bone marrow failure syndromes are heterogeneous group of disorders that generally lead to aplastic anaemias associated with pancytopenias [2].

Fanconi Anaemia
One of the common forms of inherited bone marrow failure is Fanconi anaemia that is an autosomal recessive disorder characterized by defects in DNA repair mechanism and a predisposition to leukaemia and solid tumours [3]. Fanconi anaemia is usually inherited as an autosomal recessive trait but in a small subset of patients it can be an X-linked recessive disorder. Over the last two decades, about 33 genes have been found to be associated with this disorder. Majority of the patients show their clinical presentation towards the end of the first decade of life. The proteins encoded by the Fanconi anaemia genes mainly (*FANCA, FANCB, FANCC, FANCE, FANCF, FANCG, FANCL and FANCM*) participate in a complicated network important in DNA repair. Approximately 30% of patients with Fanconi anaemia have no overt somatic abnormalities [4].

A. Nadkarni (✉) · P. Hariharan
National Institute of Immunohematology (ICMR), Mumbai, India

© Springer Nature Singapore Pte Ltd. 2019
R. Saxena, H. P. Pati (eds.), *Hematopathology*, https://doi.org/10.1007/978-981-13-7713-6_28

Dyskeratosis Congenita

Classical dyskeratosis congenita is an inherited bone marrow failure syndrome characterized by the muco-cutaneous triad of abnormal skin pigmentation, nail dystrophy and mucosal leucoplakia. Bone marrow failure is the major cause of mortality with patients having an additional predisposition to malignancy and fatal pulmonary complications. X-linked recessive, autosomal dominant and autosomal recessive subtypes of dyskeratosis congenita are recognized. Six dyskeratosis congenita genes (*DKC1, TERC, TERT, NOP10, NHP2, TINF2*) have been identified to date. Heterozygous mutations in *TERC* and *TERT* (telomerase reverse transcriptase) have been found in patients with autosomal dominant dyskeratosis congenita. X-linked DC (*DKC1*) encodes a highly conserved nucleolar protein called dyskerin [5].

Diamond–Blackfan Anaemia

Diamond–Blackfan anaemia (DBA) usually presents in early infancy, with features of anaemia. The hallmark of classical Diamond–Blackfan anaemia is a selective decrease in erythroid precursors and normochromic microcytic anaemia associated with a variable number of somatic abnormalities such as craniofacial, thumb, cardiac and urogenital malformations. The heterozygous mutations in the genes encoding for ribosomal proteins of the small (*RPS24, RPS17, RPS7, RPS10, RPS26*) and large (*RPL5, RPL11, RPL35A*) subunits have been reported; collectively the genetic basis of approximately 50–60% of cases of DBA can now be established [5].

Other congenital anomalies include maturational arrest in the myeloid lineage (leucopenia) and isolated thrombocytopenia, reduction or absence of megakaryocytes in the bone marrow (congenital amegakaryocytic thrombocytopenia) [5].

Inherited Disorders of Red Blood Cells (RBCs)

RBCs may lead to an enormous degree of genetic variability that may generate a disease condition. The main three components of RBCs are haemoglobin, membrane and its enzymes.

Haemoglobinopathies

The most common is genetic disorders of haemoglobin, the quantitative defect (thalassaemia) or the qualitative defect (variant structural haemoglobin) of the globin genes [6]. Thalassaemias can mainly be classified into two groups α-thalassaemia and β-thalassaemia, which is based on the globin gene that is affected. In α-thalassaemia, α-globin gene cluster located in chromosome 16 has one or more deletions affecting the output of one, two, three, or four of the α-globin gene. Clinically there are four α-thalassaemia syndromes based on the deletion of the α-globin gene: silent carrier ($-\alpha/\alpha\alpha$), α-thalassaemia trait ($-\alpha/-\alpha$ or $--/\alpha\alpha$), HbH disease ($--/-\alpha$) and hydrops fetalis syndrome ($--/--$). The more severe life-threatening thalassaemia syndrome is β-thalassaemia, where in the β-globin gene is affected. Depending on the degree of quantitative reduction in the β-globin chain output, the mutations that result in no β-globin production cause β-thalassaemia and those that allow production of some β-globin chain are classified as β+ or β++ ("silent") thalassaemia. The second class of haemoglobinopathies comprises of synthesis of structural variant or abnormal haemoglobin due to missense mutation in the globin genes. These abnormal haemoglobins have altered physio-chemical properties as compared to the normal adult haemoglobin. The most common variant haemoglobins prevalent in the Indian subcontinent are: HbS, HbE, HbD[Punjab] that form the β-variants and HbQ India forming the most common α-variant. Both types of haemoglobinopathies are inherited as autosomal recessive condition [7].

Red Cell Membrane Disorders

The proteins of the red cell membrane skeleton are responsible for the deformability, flexibility and durability of the red blood cell, enabling it to squeeze through capillaries less and recovering the discoid shape as soon as these cells stop receiving compressive forces. A deficiency or dysfunction of the membrane proteins weakens or destabilizes the cytoskeleton and distorts the RBC shape that leads to membrane disability giving rise to haemolytic anaemia [8]. Disorders of the erythrocyte membrane, including hereditary spherocytosis (HS), hereditary elliptocytosis (HE), hereditary pyropoikilocytosis (HPP), and hereditary stomatocytosis (HSt), are autosomal recessive disorders that comprise an important group of inherited haemolytic anaemias [9]. These syndromes are characterized by marked clinical and laboratory heterogeneity. Recent molecular studies have revealed that there is also significant genetic heterogeneity in these disorders. The mutations in the gene for band 3, spectrin {α and β}, ankyrin and protein 4.1 have been reported leading to membrane disorders [8].

Enzymopathy

Hereditary red blood cell enzymopathies are genetic disorders affecting genes encoding red blood cell enzymes. They cause a specific type of anaemia designated as hereditary nonspherocytic haemolytic anaemia (HNSHA). Enzymopathies affect cellular metabolism, of the red cell, mainly the enzymes involved in anaerobic glycolysis, hexose monophosphate (HMP) shunt, glutathione metabolism and nucleotide metabolism. Enzymopathies are commonly associated with normocytic normochromic haemolytic anaemia. The morphology of the red blood cell shows no specific abnormalities. Diagnosis is based on the detection of reduced specific enzyme activity and molecular characterization of the defect on the DNA level. The most common enzyme disorders are deficiencies of glucose-6-phosphate dehydrogenase (G6PD) [X-linked disorder] and pyruvate kinase (PK) [autosomal recessive disorder]. However, there are a number of other enzyme disorders, often much less known, causing HNSHA. These disorders are rare and often underdiagnosed [10].

Inherited Disorders of White Blood Cells

White blood cells (leucocytes) help defend the body against infection and foreign substances. Disorders of white blood cell can affect immune response.

Primary Immunodeficiency (PID)

Congenital immunity defects leading to primary immunodeficiency (PID) is a heterogeneous group of inheritable genetic disorders that affects the immune system development and/or function [11]. They are broadly classified as disorders of adaptive immunity (i.e. T-cell, B-cell or combined immune deficiencies) or of innate immunity (e.g. phagocyte and complement disorders) [11]. Severe combined immunodeficiency is a heterogeneous group of disorders characterized by profound deficiency of both T and B lymphocytes, causing secondary susceptibility to infections, autoimmunity, uncontrolled inflammation and malignancy [11].

Malignant or Benign Leucocytosis

Leucocytosis is defined as an elevation of the WBC count for the patient's age. Acute myeloid leukaemia (AML) is a heterogeneous group of neoplastic disorders with great variability in clinical course, genetic and molecular basis of the pathology. In AML, somatic genetic changes are often thought to contribute to leukaemogenesis through two types of mutations: (1) a mutation that improves haematopoietic cell's ability to proliferate (*FLT3* and *KIT*) and (2) a mutation that prevents the cells from maturing (class II, including *CBFB-MYH11, CEBPA, DEK-NUP214, MLL-MLLT3, NPM1, PML RARA, RUNX1-RUNX1T1*) and depends on the mutational pathway that is activated [12]. Chronic myeloid leukaemia is a slow-growing cancer, wherein the bone marrow produces too many white blood cells called myeloblasts (or blasts) accumulated in the blood and bone marrow. Chronic myeloid leukaemia is caused by a rearrangement (translocation) of genetic material between chromosome 9 and 22. This translocation, written as t (9;22), fuses part of the ABL1 gene from chromosome 9 with part of the BCR gene from chromosome 22, creating an abnormal fusion gene called *BCR-ABL1*. The abnormal chromosome 22 containing a piece of chromosome 9 and the fusion gene is often referred to as the Philadelphia chromosome. The abnormal protein produced from the fusion gene, called BCR-ABL1, promotes cell proliferation and is insensitive to apoptosis signals [13].

Inherited Disorders of Platelets

Blood platelets are the first responders to the injury. They gather at the site of the injury, creating a temporary plug to stop blood loss. Bleeding disorders can be classified as thromocytopenias or thrombocytopathies. Inherited thrombocyto-penias (ITs) are a heterogeneous group of disorders characterized by a sustained reduction in platelet count manifested as a bleeding diathesis and defects in the size of the platelets [14].

Glanzmann's Thrombasthenia

Glanzmann's thrombasthenia is an autosomal recessive disorder of platelet function caused by deficiency or abnormality of platelet glycoproteins (IIb, III A) which are the fibrinogen receptors. Due to defective receptors, platelets do not aggregate with each other at the site of injury, and there is difficulty for the formation of normal blood clot [15].

Bernard–Soulier Syndrome

Bernard–Soulier syndrome (BSS) is an inherited, usually autosomal recessive, platelet bleeding abnormality, characterized by a prolonged bleeding time, large platelets and thrombocytopenia. This disorder of platelet function is caused due to abnormality of platelet glycoproteins (Ib, IX) [15].

28.1.1.2 Non-Cellular Disorders

Thrombocytopathies are induced by different platelet defects based on the aberrations in the fundamental function of platelet adhesion, activation, aggregation, secretion and signal transduction. Inherited coagulopathies causing prolonged bleeding time arise from the mutations within the genes responsible for the synthesis or processing of the active coagulation factors. Haemophilia A and B, sex-linked inherited single gene disorders that occur due to mutation in factor VIII or factor IX gene leading to repeated haemorrhagic episodes in joints and soft tissues are one of the most common bleeding disorder with X-linked inheritance [16]. Table 28.1 enlists the details of the inherited haematological disorders.

After birth an individual inheriting the malfunctional genes from the parents can only be managed for the disease; however, it cannot be cured completely. Hence a potentially applicable approach to any congenital inherited disease is to conduct prenatal diagnosis for detecting the presence or absence of the mutated gene in the growing foetus. In the following section, we have discussed various foetal tissue sampling procedures and methodology for the diagnosis of the mutation in the foetal sample.

28.2 Prenatal Diagnosis of Inherited Disorders

Prenatal examination is an important medical technique that helps in the diagnosis of hereditary disorders in the foetus. To date, various methodologies are being used to determine the foetal health. Owing to the advances in the research technology, two pivotal domains of the prenatal diagnosis have been emerging steadily—the foetal sampling and the mutation diagnosis techniques. The prenatal sampling techniques have been headed from traditional sampling methods like invasive chorionic villi sampling, amniocentesis, cordocentesis to non-invasive cell-free DNA from maternal plasma and pre-implantation genetic diagnosis. Similarly there has been a gradual advancement in molecular diagnosis of the mutation from southern blotting, restriction fragment length polymorphism, automated DNA sequencing to the newer multiple ligation probe amplification, next-gen sequencing and DNA arrays.

28.2.1 Foetal Sampling

The diagnosis of the foetal health is dependent on gestational age of foetus, ease of carrying the procedure and varied techniques that mainly aims in accurate detection of the presence of mutation [17]. The sampling of the foetal tissue forms the first part of prenatal diagnosis: This includes the conventional invasive procedures which require direct removal of foetal sample from the growing foetus in the womb and the future non-invasive techniques where in the foetal genetic material is assessed without directly affecting the foetus.

Table 28.1 Genetics of inherited haematological disorders

Disease	Common gene affected	Mutational effects	Pattern of inheritance
Bone marrow malfunction			
Fanconi anaemia	FANCA[a], FANCB, FANCC, FANCD2, FANCE, FANCF, FANCG, BRCA2, BRIP1	Impaired DNA repair mechanism, increased chromosome breakage and radial forms when exposed to DNA cross-linking agents: diepoxybutane or mitomycin C	Autosomal and X-linked recessive disorder
Diamond–Blackfan anaemia	RPS19	Pure red cell aplasia	Autosomal dominant
Severe congenital neutropenia	ELA2[a], GFI1	Profound peripheral neutropenia, maturation arrest in the myeloid lineage	Autosomal dominant
Congenital amegakaryocytic thrombocytopenia	c-MPL	Reduction or absence of megakaryocytes in the bone marrow	Autosomal recessive
Red blood cells disorders			
Haemoglobinopathies	Alpha (α)/beta (β)-globin gene	Decreased synthesis of haemoglobin/variant haemoglobin production	Autosomal recessive
Membrane defects	Ankyrin[a], spectrin, band 3, protein 4.1, protein 4.2, glycophorin	Heterogeneous RBC shapes, unstable RBC membrane leading to haemolytic anaemia	Autosomal dominant[a], autosomal recessive
Enzymopathies	G6PD[a]	Profound decrease in the red cell metabolic enzymes	X-linked recessive
	Pyruvate kinase[a], glucose phosphate isomerase, pyrimidine 5′ nucleotidase		Autosomal recessive
Immunodeficiency syndromes			
T−B+ Severe combined immunodeficiency (SCID)	γc deficiency	Defect in γ chain of receptors for IL-2, -4, -7, -9, -15, -21	X-linked recessive
	JAK3 deficiency CD45 deficiency	Defect in Janus activating kinase 3, CD 45 deficiency	Autosomal recessive
T−B− SCID	RAG 1/2 deficiency Adenosine deaminase (ADA) deficiency	Defective VDJ recombination Absent ADA activity, deficiency of T-cells and B-cells from birth	Autosomal recessive
ZAP-70 deficiency	ZAP70 mutation	Defects in ZAP-70 signalling kinase, decreased CD8	Autosomal recessive
Acute myeloid leukaemia	FLT3, KIT, CEBPA, DEK-NUP214, MLL-MLLT3, NPM1, PML RARA, RUNX1-RUNX1T1	Infinite proliferation of haematopoietic stem cells with their maturational arrest	Mostly non-hereditary, certain conditions CEBPA gene mutations: autosomal dominant
Chronic myeloid leukaemia	Translocation between chromosome 9 and 22	Increased and unregulated growth of predominantly myeloid cells	Somatic mutation

(continued)

Table 28.1 (continued)

Bleeding disorders			
X-linked thrombocytopenia Wiskott–Aldrich syndrome (WAS)	Defects in the WAS gene	Mild haemorrhagic condition severe thrombocytopenia and smaller sized platelets	X-linked recessive
Thrombocytopenia-absent radius (TAR) syndrome	HOXA10, HOXA11, HOXD11, (homeobox genes)	Bilateral absence of the radii and hypomegakaryocytic thrombocytopenia	Autosomal recessive
von Willebrand's disease-platelet type	GPIb/GPIX/V	Platelet adhesion	Autosomal recessive
Glanzmann's thrombasthenia	GPIIb/GPIIIa	Platelet aggregation	Autosomal recessive
Haemophilia A[a] Haemophilia B	Factor VIII deficiency[a] Factor IX deficiency	Reduced levels or lack of clotting factors	X-linked recessive

[a]Common mutations

28.2.1.1 Conventional Invasive Procedures

Although conventional invasive prenatal diagnosis is associated with potential risk factors, still there is no effective replacement for these techniques.

Chorionic Villus Sampling (CVS)

Sampling of the chorionic villi in the field of antenatal genetic diagnosis is carried out in the first trimester of the pregnancy. The method was first carried out in China for foetal sex determination and later on for diagnosis of genetic disorders; however, the continuous clinical implementation of CVS was started in 1983, by Denis Fairweather and Humphrey Ward in London for the diagnosis of the haemoglobinopathies [18]. The method involves the biopsy of foetal tissue from the chorionic plate at its site of attachment to the uterine wall transcervically or transabdominally at 10–12 weeks of gestation in coordination with real-time guided ultrasound, without anaesthesia (Fig. 28.1). The CVS tissue obtained is further cleaned by careful microscopic dissection to remove any maternal contamination. Figure 28.2 is a comparative image of uncleaned and cleaned CVS tissue viewed under the inverted microscope. The main advantage of this method is early termination of affected foetuses. However, there are potential risks as well. The disruption of the chorionic plate and amniotic sac, together with possible direct trauma to the foetus, might have unknown long-term effects. Foetal growth retardation following CVS, antepartum haemorrhage, infection, premature rupture of the amniotic sac, lowered birth weight and premature delivery have all been postulated as possible consequences [19, 20]. The method also has 0.5–2.0% risk of miscarriage. The phenomenon confined to placental mosaicism which leads to misdiagnosis is also reported in 0.8–2.0% of the pregnancies [21].

Amniocentesis

This method was first carried out by an American physician Steele and Breg in 1966 for chromosome analysis by culturing of amniotic cells. Over the years, amniocentesis has become the method of choice for mid-trimester prenatal diagnosis. The method is carried out during 14–16 weeks of gestation [22]. It involves aspiration of 20–30 mL of amniotic fluid that contains cells derived from the foetal membranes and the foetus (Fig. 28.1). The main challenge involves difficulty to aspirate amniotic fluid commonly due to membrane "tenting". This occurs more frequently with amniocentesis performed before 14 weeks gestation because amnion and chorion are usually not fused early in gestation [23]. The biggest advantage of this technique is that the risk of miscarriage is only 0.6–0.68% as compared to other invasive techniques, less chances of maternal contamination and overall reduced risk to the growing foetus, thus making this technique the most widely used invasive method [21].

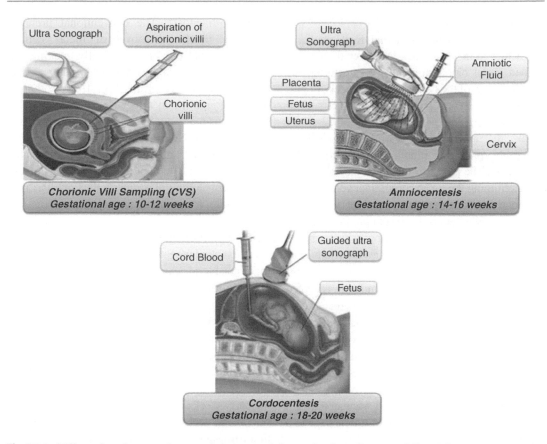

Fig. 28.1 Different invasive procedures carried out at varied gestational age for prenatal diagnosis

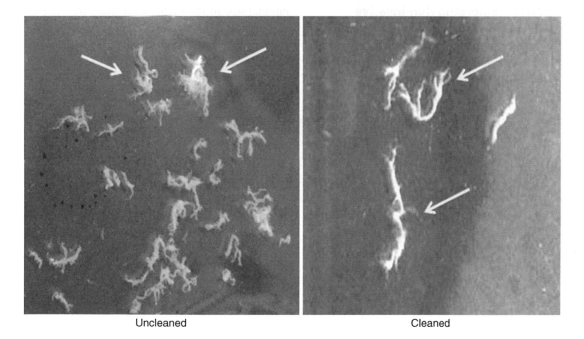

Uncleaned   Cleaned

Fig. 28.2 First trimester prenatal diagnosis: view of chorionic Villi sample (CVS) under inverted microscope

Cordocentesis

A major advancement in maternal–foetal medicine was achieved in 1983 when Daffos et al. first performed foetal blood sampling by puncturing the umbilical vein of the foetus on 18–20 weeks of gestation [24]. The procedure involves ultrasonography guided aseptic insertion of 22 gauge needle, that aspirates 0.5–2.0 mL of blood from preferably placental umbilical cord vein [25] (Fig. 28.1). The purity of the foetal blood is tested by determining the mean corpuscular volume (foetal blood MCV > maternal blood MCV) and by performing Kleihauer–Betke staining for detecting the maternal blood contamination in foetal blood sample [26]. Figure 28.3 illustrates the Kleihauer–Betke staining of the foetal sample obtained after cordocentesis. Though this technique is accepted worldwide due to its rapid and simple procedure, it is generally performed when chorionic villi sampling or amniocentesis results are inconclusive or when couple is referred late for prenatal diagnosis as it is associated with numerous risks. The procedure involves 2% risk of foetal bradycardia, foetal–maternal haemorrhage and cord haematoma [27, 28]. There is 2.5–3.0% chance of miscarriage and premature delivery [29].

28.2.1.2   Emerging Non-invasive Techniques

To obtain complete foetal genetic information and to avoid endangering the foetus, non-invasive prenatal diagnosis has become the vital goal of prenatal diagnosis. The conventional prenatal sampling involves removal of foetal sample transabdominally or transcervically, making the entire procedure unpleasant for mothers. Also these procedures carry a risk of 1–2.5% chance of miscarriage or may affect the growth of healthy foetus, thus many not opting for invasive prenatal diagnosis [30]. Non-invasive prenatal testing primarily involves isolation of foetal genetic material either from the maternal blood or from the in vitro developing blastomere, thus not harming the growing foetus in the womb directly.

Cell-Free Foetal Nucleic Acids

The first evidence of foetal cells circulating in maternal blood was shown by Bianchi et al., in 1997, followed by the discovery of male free circulating foetal DNA in the plasma of pregnant women by Dennis Lo et al. in the same year [31]. These circulating cell-free DNA originates from the trophoblasts that make up the placenta and comprise 3–13% of the total cell-free DNA in most of the maternal blood samples [32]. During the early weeks of pregnancy (4 weeks), the cell-free foetal DNA is highly diluted (16 fl/mL in first trimester); however, their concentration positively increases with the progression of the gestational age of the foetus with sharp increase in its concentration beyond 28 weeks of pregnancy (80 fl/mL in the third trimester) [31, 33]. Postdelivery the cell-free foetal DNA is rapidly cleared from the maternal circulation with a

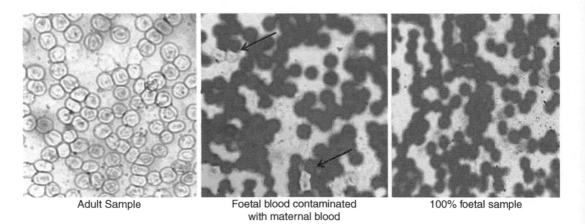

Adult Sample   Foetal blood contaminated   100% foetal sample
                                  with maternal blood

Fig. 28.3 Purity of foetal blood sample checked by Kleihauer–Betke staining

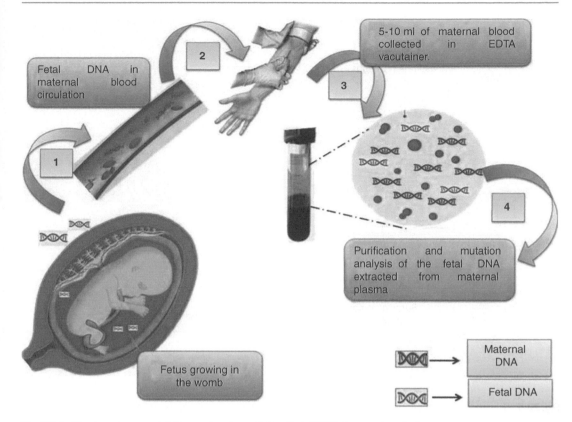

Fig. 28.4 Non-invasive prenatal diagnosis using cell-free foetal DNA from maternal plasma

half-life of 16 min and is undetectable by 2 h after delivery [34]. Figure 28.4 shows a schematic representation of the steps involved in cell-free foetal DNA procedure. The main challenge of this technique is to selectively amplify the foetal cell-free DNA from the maternal plasma. These include detection and enrichment of foetal DNA based on the length of the foetal DNA fragment [foetal DNA < 200 bp and maternal DNA > 500 bp] and carefully excising the foetal DNA fragment followed by gel extraction [35]. The maternal DNA release from the sample is also suppressed by addition of formaldehyde such that there is only relative increase in the foetal DNA. Another recent advancement is identification of universal markers, the epigenetic regulators of the gene. The promoter region of two tumour suppressor genes Maspin and RASSF1A are differentially methylated in placenta and maternal cell-free foetal DNA, thus aiding in selection of foetal DNA from maternal DNA [36].

Clinical application includes identification of any sex-linked disorders like haemophilia, X-linked immunodeficiency in foetus. In haemoglobinopathies, paternally inherited mutations that cause β-thalassemia can be detected in cell-free foetal DNA. However, in case of two identical copies of single point mutation [same mutation in both the parents], one cannot make use of this technique, thus leading to a major drawback [36].

Pre-implantation Genetic Diagnosis

Pre-implantation genetic diagnosis or PGD is the most recent technology that allows genetic testing of an embryo under in vitro conditions, prior to implantation. This technology is used in conjunction with in vitro fertilization (IVF) and allows only embryos diagnosed free of a specific genetic disease to be transferred into the womb, thus leading to an unaffected pregnancy (Fig. 28.5). Pre-implantation genetic diagnosis was first successfully performed by Edwards and

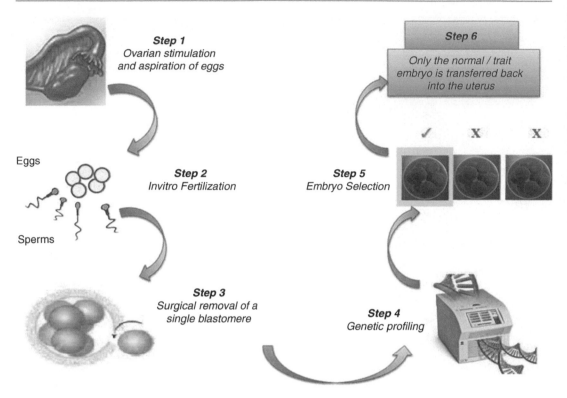

Fig. 28.5 Schematic representation of steps involved in pre-implantation genetic diagnosis (PGD)

Gardner way back in 1968 to determine the sex of the rabbit embryos. Further in humans, with the advent of IVF, this method was primarily performed for an X-linked disorder by Kontogianni et al., in 1989 to selectively amplify Y chromosome-specific repeat sequences [37]. The first clinical application by Handyside et al. in 1990 that lead to the first unaffected child born following PGD performed for an X-linked disorder which marked a progress in reproductive medicine, genetic and molecular biology [38]. The basic methodology involves in vitro fertilization of the oocyte with intracytoplasmic sperm injection. The embryos are biopsied at 6–8 cell stage to remove a 1–2 blastomere which is followed by fluorescent in situ hybridization (FISH) for cytogenetic diagnosis, or polymerase chain reaction (PCR) for molecular diagnosis [39].

Advantages and Challenges

Pre-implantation diagnosis surpasses the most difficult and traumatic decision of the expecting parents of pregnancy termination when the foetus

is revealed having a genetic disease. Also in hundreds of infants born following PGD worldwide, there are no reports of increased foetal malformation rates or any other identifiable problems. However, this technique has more challenges over advantages. The diagnosis from a single cell remains a technically challenging procedure and hence the risk of misdiagnosis cannot be eliminated. The causes of misdiagnosis include confusion of embryo and cell number, transfer of the wrong embryo, maternal or paternal contamination and chromosomal mosaicism [40, 41]. The technology requires extremely skilled personnel for careful removal of a single cell without breaking it or causing serious damage to the growing embryo. A relatively large number of eggs or embryos may be found to be abnormal, thus leaving only a few or no healthy embryos for transfer. The limitation of single cell analysis is development of mosaic embryo. During mitosis, if nondisjunction occurs after fertilization, then two or more cell lines may be present in the embryo. Thus, a mosaic embryo with normal and abnormal cells may be misdiagnosed with the present single cell biopsy technique. The diagnostic methodology is relatively expensive and time consuming as compared to the conventional invasive techniques and for diagnosing a new disease mutation it is a time-consuming and expensive process [41].

Detection of Maternal Contamination

An additional precaution should be taken when the foetal genotype is the same as the maternal genotype. To rule out maternal DNA contamination, the polymorphic DNA markers including the variable tandem repeats (VNTRs) such as ApoB, D1S80 and other short tandem repeats or micro satellites should be checked by PCR amplification of the parents and CVS sample and should provide an informative result or else there would be chances of misdiagnosis [42].

28.3 Molecular Diagnosis of the Disease (Characterization of the Mutation)

Accurate diagnosis of the disease is essential for appropriate treatment of patients, genetic counselling and prevention strategies. Thus the second important diagnostic tier involves accurate detection for the presence or absence of genetic mutation in the foetal DNA sample. The advent of polymerase chain reaction (PCR) has revolutionized the molecular diagnostic field which helps in the detection of wide range of DNA variations in the form of point mutations, gene deletion, insertion or inversion on much smaller quantities of DNA by a simple and cheap PCR-based technique that allows the detection of the common mutations simultaneously. The detection of these variations also depends on the variability and specificity of the techniques used. Mutation detection techniques can be divided into techniques that test for known mutations (genotyping) and those that scan for any mutation in a particular target region (mutation scanning) [43].

The strategy for the identification of the known mutation depends on the frequency of occurrence of the specific mutation in the given population and is carried out by various PCR-based screening techniques. The conventional methods to identify mutation include allele-specific oligonucleotide (ASO) hybridization or dot-blot analysis which is based on the binding of allele-specific oligonucleotide probe (15–21 nucleotides) to the complementary DNA present in the patient's sample and its detection using the colorimetric principle [44], allele-specific priming or amplification refractory mutation system (ARMS) that discriminates between normal and mutant alleles by 3′ nucleotide of the primers [45], restriction fragment length polymorphism that exploits the ability of *restriction enzymes* to cleave the DNA at specific sites in the genome and gap PCRs [46]. Conventional PCR-based approaches for scanning or screening for unknown mutations involve techniques like Denaturing Gradient Gel Electrophoresis (DGGE) and Single-Strand Conformation Polymorphism (SSCP) which are based on the principle that a mutation changes the melting behaviour of the single stranded DNA under increasing denaturing conditions or may show different migration patterns due to altered conformation of the DNA strand [47, 48].

In case of X-linked recessive disorders, sex determination of the foetus becomes an important application because carrier mothers have 25% chance to give birth to a baby with related abnormalities. Hence the first step during prenatal diagnosis for X-linked recessive disorders involves determination of the sex of the foetus, by polymerase chain reaction (PCR), which specifically detects the presence of Y chromosome in the foetal sample. Also couples at risk of having an affected child can have embryo diagnosis before implantation, thereby avoiding the termination of an affected pregnancy [49].

With the recent development, lot of new upcoming techniques like multiple ligation probe amplification, next-gen gene sequencing and array CGH are used to detect and characterize unknown deletions or gene duplications.

28.3.1 Multiplex Ligation-Dependent Probe Amplification (MLPA)

This is a recent molecular technique developed that is used to characterize, screen and map large deletions or duplications in the genomic DNA, thus helps in detecting the copy number variations in the genome. MLPA is a multiplex PCR assay that utilizes up to 40–42 probes, each specific for a different region of the genome [50]. Although well-characterized deletions and amplifications can be detected by PCR, the exact breakpoint site of most deletions is unknown. This technique is widely used for characterized large deletions in the β-globin cluster, leading to hereditary persistence of foetal haemoglobin (HPFH) [51].

28.3.2 Microarray Analysis for Point Mutations

A slight variation to allele-specific oligonucleotides technique has led to the development of microarray procedure which can be used potentially for rapid genotyping, for screening a large number of samples and varied number of mutations simultaneously. The Arrayed Primer Extension (APEX) method is based upon the attachment of oligonucleotides, on a glass surface by the 5' end which terminates one nucleotide before the mutation site. The amplified patient DNA anneals to the 3' of the oligonucleotide and is extended by DNA polymerase which adds fluorescently labelled dideoxynucleotide complementary to the mutant base. Thus the presence of a mutation is detected by a colour change in the primer site [46].

28.3.3 Next Generation Sequencing (NGS)

For monogenic disorders, automated DNA sequencing is still the method of choice to screening for the mutation; however, its basic drawback is analysis limited to only one amplified fragment and the read length is maximum of 1000 base pairs. NGS systems provide several sequencing options which include sequencing of the entire genome, exome or a transcript such that the multigenic factors leading to a disease syndrome could be identified rapidly [52]. Sequencing of the complete exome will thus reveal the mutations causing rare genetic disorders [53, 54].

28.3.4 Summary

A change in the DNA sequence is considered to be deleterious if it has a pathogenic effect on the normal biological pathway. Thus the molecular characterization of the disease is required for an accurate diagnosis. In the last few decades, the genetic basis of numerous diseases has been identified, and safe, efficacious, foetal diagnostic techniques have been developed. An expansive progress in the field of prenatal diagnosis is thus likely to continue into the future, and the advances in molecular genetics will continue to accelerate and expand the accuracy of prenatal diagnosis.

References

1. Wieacker P, Steinhard J. The prenatal diagnosis of genetic diseases. Dtsch Arztebl Int. 2010;107:857–62.
2. Brodsky R, Jones R. Aplastic anaemia. Lancet. 2005;365:1647–56.
3. Wang W. Emergence of a DNA-damage response network consisting of Fanconi anaemia and BRCA proteins. Nat Rev Genet. 2007;8:735–48.
4. Chirnomas S, Kupfer G. The inherited bone marrow failure syndromes. Pediatr Clin North Am. 2013;60:1–21.
5. Dokal I, Vulliamy T. Inherited bone marrow failure syndromes. Haematologica. 2010;95:1236–40.
6. Kohne E. Haemoglobinopathies clinical manifestations, diagnosis, and treatment. Dtsch Arztebl Int. 2011;108:532–40.
7. Clarke G, Higgins T. Laboratory investigation of haemoglobinopathies and thalassaemias: review and update. Clin Chem. 2000;46:1284–90.
8. Gallagher P. Abnormalities of the erythrocyte membrane. Pediatr Clin North Am. 2013;60:1349–62.
9. Bianchi P, Fermo E, Imperiali F, et al. Hereditary red cell membrane defects: diagnostic and clinical aspects. Blood Transfus. 2011;9:274–7.
10. Koralkova P, Solinge W, Wijk R. Rare hereditary red blood cell enzymopathies associated with

haemolytic anaemia—pathophysiology, clinical aspects, and laboratory diagnosis. Int J Lab Hematol. 2014;36:388–97.

11. McCusker C, Warrington R. Primary immunodeficiency. Allergy Asthma Clin Immunol. 2011;7:1–8.

12. Renneville A, Roumier C, Biggio V, et al. Cooperating gene mutations in acute myeloid leukemia: a review of the literature. Leukemia. 2008;22:915–31.

13. Buyukasik Y, Haznedaroglu I, Ilhan O. Chronic myeloid leukemia: practical issues in diagnosis, treatment and follow-up. Int J Hematol Oncol. 2010;20:1–12.

14. Johnson B, Fletcher S, Morgan N. Inherited thrombocytopenia: novel insights into megakaryocyte maturation, proplatelet formation and platelet lifespan. Platelets. 2016;27:519–25.

15. D'Andrea G, Chetta M, Margaglione M. Inherited platelet disorders: thrombocytopenias and thrombocytopathies. Blood Transfus. 2009;7:278–92.

16. Bowen J. Haemophilia A and haemophilia B: molecular insights. Mol Pathol. 2002;55:1–18.

17. Cheng W, Hsiao C, Tseng H, et al. Non invasive prenatal diagnosis. Taiwan J Obstet Gynecol. 2015;54:343–9.

18. Old J, Ward R, Petrou M, et al. First-trimester fetal diagnosis for haemoglobinopathies: three cases. Lancet. 1982;2:1413–6.

19. Stott P. Sampling of the chorionic villi: a technique to complement amniocentesis. J R Coll Gen Pract. 1985;35:316–7.

20. Kazy Z, Rozofsky I, Bakharev V. Chorion biopsy in early pregnancy: a method of early prenatal diagnosis for inherited disorders. Prenat Diagn. 1982;2:39–45.

21. South S, Chen W, Brothman A. Genomic medicine in prenatal diagnosis. Clin Obstet Gynecol. 2008;51:62–73.

22. Simoni G, Colognato R. The amniotic fluid-derived cells: the biomedical challenge for the third millennium. J Prenat Med. 2009;3:34–6.

23. Shulman L, Elias S. Amniocentesis and chorionic villus sampling. West J Med. 1993;159:260–8.

24. Daffos F, Capella-Pavlovsky M, Forestier F. Fetal blood sampling via the umbilical cord using a needle guided by ultrasound. Report of 66 cases. Prenat Diagn. 1983;3:271–7.

25. Henderson J, Weiner C. Cordocentesis. Glob Libr Womens Med. 2008. https://doi.org/10.3843/GLOWM.10212. Accessed 25/12/2017.

26. Kleihauer E, Braun H, Betke K. Demonstration of fetal hemoglobin in erythrocytes of a blood smear. Klin Wochenschr. 1957;35:637–8.

27. Budau G, Anastasiu D, Muresan C, et al. Cordocentesis in prenatal diagnosis case report. J Exp Med Surg Res. 2008;3:100–4.

28. Liao C, Wei J, Li Q, et al. Efficacy and safety of cordocentesis for prenatal diagnosis. Int J Gynaecol Obstet. 2006;93:13–7.

29. Orlandi F, Damiani G, Jakil C, et al. The risks of early cordocentesis (12-21 weeks): analysis of 500 procedures. Prenat Diagn. 1990;10:425–8.

30. Wright C, Burton H. The use of cell-free fetal nucleic acids in maternal blood for non-invasive prenatal diagnosis. Hum Reprod Update. 2009;15:139–51.

31. Lo Y, Tein M, Lau T, et al. Quantitative analysis of fetal DNA in maternal plasma and serum: implications for non-invasive prenatal diagnosis. Am J Hum Genet. 1998;62:768–75.

32. Alberry M, Maddocks D, Jones M, et al. Free fetal DNA in maternal plasma in an embryonic pregnancies: confirmation that the origin is the trophoblast. Prenat Diagn. 2007;27:415–8.

33. Birch L, English A, O'Donoghue K, et al. Accurate and robust quantification of circulating fetal and total DNA in maternal plasma from 5 to 41 weeks of gestation. Clin Chem. 2005;51:312–20.

34. Lo D, Zhang J, Leung N, et al. Rapid clearance of fetal DNA from maternal plasma. Am J Hum Genet. 1999;64:218–24.

35. D'Souza E, Sawant P, Nadkarni A, et al. Detection of fetal mutations causing hemoglobinopathies by non-invasive prenatal diagnosis from maternal plasma. J Postgrad Med. 2013;59:15–20.

36. Https://emedicine.medscape.com/article/273415-overview. Accessed 25/12/2017.

37. Harper C. Introduction. Preimplantation genetic diagnosis. London: Wiley; 2001. p. 3–12.

38. Handyside A, Kontogianni E, Hardy K, et al. Pregnancies from biopsied human preimplantation embryos sexed by Y-specific DNA amplification. Nature. 1990;344:768–70.

39. Basille C, Frydman R, El Aly A, et al. Preimplantation genetic diagnosis: state of the art. Eur J Obstet Gynecol Reprod Biol. 2009;145:9–13.

40. Http://www.ivf-worldwide.com/cogen/oep/pgd-pgs/history-of-pgd-and-pgs.html. Accessed 26/12/2017.

41. Geraedts J, De Wert G. Preimplantation genetic diagnosis. Clin Genet. 2009;76:315–25.

42. Decorte R, Cuppens H, Marynen P, et al. Rapid detection of hypervariable regions by the polymerase chain reaction technique. DNA Cell Biol. 1990;9:461–9.

43. Fakher R, Bijan K, Taghi A. Application of diagnostic methods and molecular diagnosis of hemoglobin disorders in Khuzestan province of Iran. Indian J Hum Genet. 2007;13:5–15.

44. Colah R, Gorakshakar A, Lu C, et al. Application of covalent reverse dot-blot hybridization for rapid prenatal diagnosis of the common Indian thalassemia syndromes. Indian J Hematol Blood Transfus. 1997;15:10–3.

45. Newton R, Graham A, Heptinstall E, et al. Analysis of any point mutation in DNA. The amplification refractory mutation system (ARMS). Nucleic Acids Res. 1989;17:2503–16.

46. Old J, Harteveld C, Traeger-Synodinos J, et al. Prevention of thalassaemias and other haemoglobin disorders. Vol. 2. Laboratory protocols [Internet]. 2nd ed. 2012. Thalassemia International Federation, Nicosia, Cyprus.

47. Gorakshakar A, Lulla C, Nadkarni A, et al. Prenatal diagnosis of beta-thalassemia among Indians using denaturing gradient gel electrophoresis. Haemoglobin. 1997;21:421–35.

48. Nataraj A, Olivos-Glander I, Kusukawa N, et al. Single-strand conformation polymorphism and heteroduplex analysis for gel-based mutation detection. Electrophoresis. 1999;20:1177–85.

49. Rahimi A, Shahhosseiny H, Ahangari G, et al. Prenatal sex determination in suspicious cases of X-linked recessive diseases by the amelogenin gene. Iran J Basic Med Sci. 2014;17:134–7.

50. Stuppia L, Antonucci I, Palka G, et al. Use of the MLPA assay in the molecular diagnosis of gene copy number alterations in human genetic diseases. Int J Mol Sci. 2012;13:3245–76.

51. Gallienne A, Dréau H, McCarthy J, et al. Multiplex ligation-dependent probe amplification identification of 17 different β-globin gene deletions (including four novel mutations) in the UK population. Hemoglobin. 2009;33:406–16.

52. Ku C, Cooper D, Polychronakos C, et al. Exome sequencing: dual role as a discovery and diagnostic tool. Ann Neurol. 2012;71:5–14.

53. Bamshad M, Ng S, Bigham A, et al. Exome sequencing as a tool for Mendelian disease gene discovery. Nat Rev Genet. 2011;12:745–55.

54. Schuster S. Next-generation sequencing transforms today's biology. Nat Methods. 2008;5:16–8.

Autoimmune Myelofibrosis: A Diagnosis by Exclusion

Preeti Tripathi, Shivangi J. Harankhedkar, and Hara Prasad Pati

29.1 Background

Myelofibrosis or bone marrow (BM) fibrosis is a common phenomenon occurring with various benign and malignant disorders. Neoplastic causes of BM fibrosis include various myeloproliferative neoplasms (MPNs), acute megakaryocytic leukemia, lymphoid malignancies, and metastasis of various solid malignancies. Nonneoplastic causes of BM fibrosis include chronic infections (e.g., tuberculosis, kala azar), metabolic causes, storage disorders, drug reactions, and autoimmune disorders [1]. Despite varied etiology and pathogencsis, it is the aberrant production of the fibrogenic cytokines, which is the main cause mediating the fibrosis of BM through stimulation of BM fibroblasts [1].

Autoimmune myelofibrosis (AIMF) is a benign disorder that was first described in 1994 by Paquette et al. as a distinct clinicopathological entity associated with diffuse bone marrow fibrosis and autoimmune phenomenon [2]. However, it has been recently found to be present even in the absence of a well-defined autoimmune disorder (Primary AIMF) [3]. The disease is characterized by isolated or combined cytopenia,

autoimmune phenomenon, and bone marrow fibrosis. However, due to the rarity of the disease, patients are frequently misdiagnosed as primary myelofibrosis (PMF) which is otherwise a common neoplastic cause of BM fibrosis. Given the significant therapeutic and prognostic differences between the two disorders, it is essential to correctly identify patients with autoimmune myelofibrosis, which has a favorable course as compared to primary myelofibrosis [3].

29.2 Classification and Diagnostic Criteria

Autoimmune myelofibrosis can be classified as follows:

- Primary autoimmune myelofibrosis (primary AIMF)
- Secondary autoimmune myelofibrosis (secondary AIMF)

Primary autoimmune myelofibrosis refers to AIMF cases in which patients have the presence of autoantibodies but do not have a well-characterized autoimmune disorder. It has been recently recognized as a distinct entity as described by Pullarkat et al. (2003).

Secondary autoimmune myelofibrosis refers to AIMF secondary to an autoimmune disorder. It is well recognized in context of various autoimmune disorders, e.g., systemic lupus erythromatosus

P. Tripathi · S. J. Harankhedkar
D.M. Hematopathology, All India Institute of Medical Sciences, New Delhi, India

H. P. Pati (✉)
Department of Hematology, All India Institute of Medical Sciences, New Delhi, India

© Springer Nature Singapore Pte Ltd. 2019
R. Saxena, H. P. Pati (eds.), *Hematopathology*, https://doi.org/10.1007/978-981-13-7713-6_29

Table 29.1 Autoimmune disorders found to be associated with secondary AIMF

Systemic lupus erythromatosus
Rheumatoid arthritis
Autoimmune hemolytic anemia
Evans syndrome
Autoimmune hepatitis
Antiphospholipid syndrome
Autoimmune demyelinating polymyositis
Diabetes mellitus type 1
Hashimotos thyroiditis
Primary sclerosing cholangitis
Psoriasis
Vitiligo

Table 29.2 Diagnostic criteria for primary AIMF

(a) Grade 3 or 4 reticulin fibrosis of bone marrow (WHO grading)
(b) Lack of clustered or atypical megakaryocytes
(c) Lack of myeloid or erythroid dysplasia, eosinophilia, or basophilia
(d) Lymphocytic infiltration of bone marrow
(e) Lack of osteosclerosis
(f) Absent or mild splenomegaly
(g) Presence of autoantibodies
(h) Absence of a disorder known to cause MF

(SLE), rheumatoid arthritis, and autoimmune hemolytic anemia. [4]. Table 29.1 provides list of autoimmune disorders found to be associated with AIMF.

Primary and secondary autoimmune myelofibrosis are pathologically indistinguishable from each other and can be differentiated only clinically by the presence of a well-defined autoimmune disorder in cases of secondary AIMF. To diagnose primary AIMF and to differentiate it from other causes of myelofibrosis, Pullarkat et al. described following criteria as shown below. Only cases satisfying *all* the eight criteria mentioned in Table 29.2 *and not meeting* the WHO criteria of any myeloproliferative disorders can be diagnosed as primary AIMF [3].

29.3 Epidemiology

In addition to being a rare entity, AIMF is also an underecognized disorder due to general unawareness, incomplete work up of cases, and lack of definite diagnostic criteria. Presently, there is no available data regarding prevalence of the disease and the current knowledge about the entity mainly stems from the case reports and series. Larger series like Vergara-Lluri et al. and Pullarkat et.al. describe a prominence of female patients in their series with mean age of 40–45 years [4, 5]. In series described by Pullarkat et al. (2003), 69% patients had established diagnosis of an autoimmune disorder (secondary AIMF) while 31% patients had only elevated levels of autoantibodies in the absence of any well-established autoimmune disorder [3].

29.4 Pathogenesis

Although the pathophysiology of autoimmune myelofibrosis remains poorly understood, aberrant cytokine production by monocytes and T cells has been found to play pivotal role. Harrison and colleagues reported significantly higher levels of fibrogenic cytokines (e.g., TGF-β, FGF-β, peptide substance P) in an AIMF patient as compared to healthy controls and showed dramatic reduction in their serum levels with treatment, indicating the role of immune dysregulation, including T cell dysfunction, in the development of AIMF [6].

29.5 Clinical Features

The clinical spectrum of patients with AIMF is broad, with patients presenting either with classical features of autoimmune disorders first or with just cytopenias initially. Common signs and symptoms of underlying autoimmune disorder include arthralgias, oral ulcers, pain abdomen, gingival bleedings, pleuritis, pericarditis, lymphadenopathy, and malar rash. Patients usually do not have hepatosplenomegaly, spleen if present, may be mildly enlarged but massive splenomegaly (as described in PMF) is rare in AIMF [7]. Patients with primary AIMF may be missed altogether if BM examination and autoimmune work up is not taken up in these cases due to lack of any other definitive features. The various antibodies found

Table 29.3 Approach to a suspected case of autoimmune myelofibrosis

(a) *History*
Duration of illness
Any underlying disorder
Low grade fever of long duration
Unexplained fatigue
Joint pains
Skin rash or any history of photosensitivity
Pain abdomen/altered bowel movements
Xerostomia/dry conjunctiva
Numbness and tingling of extremities
Neuropsychiatric symptoms
(b) *Clinical examination*
Oral ulcers
Malar rash
Pleuritis/pericarditis
Lymphadenopathy
Hepatosplenomegaly
Deformities in hand/spine
Neuromuscular system
(c) *Investigations*
Complete blood count
Peripheral smear examination
Liver function tests
Renal function tests
Autoimmune work up
Antinuclear antibody
Direct coombs test
Anti-double-stranded DNA (dsDNA)
Rheumatoid factor
Anti-cyclic citrullinated peptide Ab (Anti-CCP)
Lupus anticoagulant
Anticardiolipin antibody
pANCA and cANCA
Anti-smooth muscle antibody (ASMA)
Anti-SSA
Anti-SSB
Bone marrow examination with reticulin staining
BM cytogenetics
Mutation study; JAK2 V617F, CAL-R, and MPL mutations

in association of AIMF are: ANA, dsDNA, RF, anti-CCP, DAT, lupus anticoagulant, anticardiolipin AB, pANCA, anti-MPO, anti-SMA, anti-SSA, and anti-SSB [8]. Table 29.3 provides the list of suggested work up in a suspected case of autoimmune myelofibrosis.

Nearly all patients of autoimmune myelofibrosis have cytopenias during the course of evolution and almost 50% cases present with it.

Hence, autoimmune myelofibrosis should be kept as a differential in patients presenting with idiopathic long standing cytopenias [7]. Vergara-Lluri et al. described pancytopenia (28%) as the most common manifestation followed by anemia and thrombocytopenia (24%), isolated anemia (21%), and lastly combined anemia and leucopenia (14%) [5]. The cytopenia is generally mild to moderate and clinical symptoms due to cytopenias per se is rare [9, 10]. However, if compounded with other causative variables may lead to symptoms.

29.5.1 Peripheral Smear Morphology

Peripheral smear in AIMF patients may show bi- or pancytopenia. Cases with underlying AIHA or ITP may show classical blood picture. No evidence of eosinophilia/basophilia/dysplasia is noted. Few cases may show mild tear drop poikilocytosis and occasional nucleated red cells but frank leukoerythroblastic picture with immature myeloid forms is rare [3, 7].

29.5.2 Bone Marrow Morphology

BM aspirates are cellular with preserved myeloid to erythroid ratio and normal morphology. No evidence of dysplasia is noted. Cases with associated AIHA/Evans syndrome may show erythroid hyperplasia. BM biopsy usually shows hypercellularity; however, occasional cases of normocellular/hypocellular BM are also described (Fig. 29.1) [3]. Reticulin stain shows mild to moderate increase in fibrosis (MF grade 1–3) (Figs. 29.2 and 29.3). Even grade 3 fibrosis has also been described in cases of AIMF; however, osteosclerosis is not common [3, 5]. Megakaryocytes may be increased or normal in number. However, their distribution and morphology remains normal. Clustering is not a feature of AIMF and increases suspicion for underlying MPNs.

Increased lymphoid aggregates/interstitial lymphocytes (Figs. 29.4 and 29.5) are a common finding which are non-paratrabecular generally

Fig. 29.1 Bone marrow biopsy showing presence of diffuse fibrosis, and presence of hypocellular areas (arrow) (10×, Hematoxylin and Eosin)

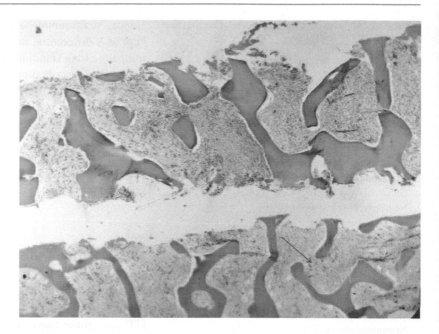

Fig. 29.2 Bone marrow biopsy showing hypercellular area in a case of AIMF. Presence of lymphocytes and background fibrosis is also seen (40×, Hematoxylin and Eosin)

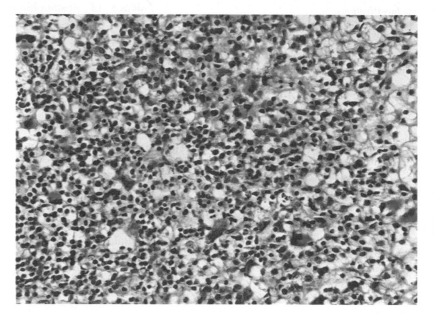

and on immunohistochemistry show benign pattern (mixture of B and T lymphocytes) [3, 5]. Prominent plasma cells infiltration which is a feature of all autoimmune disorders are common in AIMF too and should not show any Kappa/lambda restriction. Intrasinusoidal hematopoiesis may be noted [7].

29.6 Differential Diagnosis

Clinically, patients of autoimmune myelofibrosis present with cytopenias hence need to be differentiated from aplastic anemia/BM failure syndrome. Presence of increased reticulin fibers in bone marrow biopsy should exclude aplastic anemia.

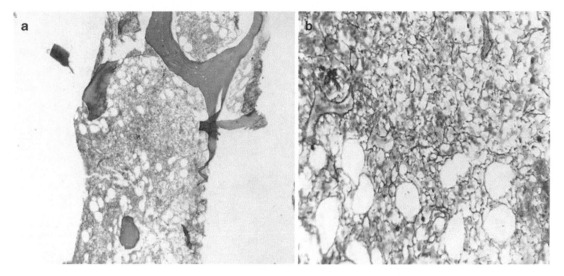

Fig. 29.3 Bone marrow biopsy showing Grade 1 fibrosis (10× (**a**), 40× (**b**), Reticulin stain)

Fig. 29.4 Presence of marrow fibrosis along with lymphoid aggregates (20×, Hematoxylin and Eosin)

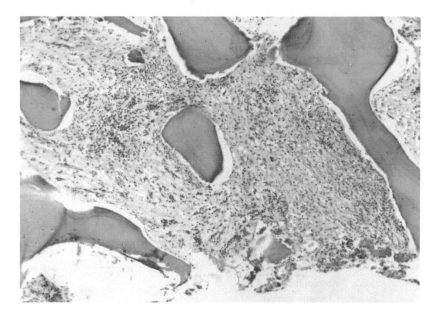

On morphology, the close differentials of autoimmune myelofibrosis include myelodysplastic syndrome with fibrosis, acute panmyelosis with myelofibrosis, lymphoproliferative disorders, and primary myelofibrosis. Patients with myelodysplastic syndrome with fibrosis and acute myelofibrosis may have similar clinical presentation as AIMF (pancytopenia with lack of organomegaly and significant leukoerythroblastosis). Presence of dysplasia and increase in blast count and cytogenetic study may help to exclude these two conditions, respectively.

Lymphoproliferative disorders may be suspected due to increased lymphoid cell infiltrate. Any lymphadenopathy or hepatosplenomegaly along with atypical lymphocytes on peripheral smear or bone marrow would point towards a diagnosis of lymphoid malignancy. In suspected cases, the lymphoid aggregates should be subjected to immunohistochemistry to exclude any clonal disease [5].

Fig. 29.5 Collection of lymphocytes and plasma cells in a background of fibrosis and stromal edema (40×, Hematoxylin and Eosin)

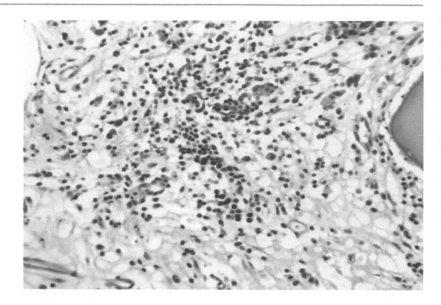

Table 29.4 Distinguishing features of AIMF and PMF

	Features	AIMF	PMF
Clinical	Underlying autoimmune disorder	May be present/absent	Absent
	Spleen	Absent/mild	Moderate/massive
Peripheral smear	Cytopenia	Bi/pancytopenia	May have increase TLC/platelet count
	Leukoerthyroblastic picture	Rare	Common
	Eosinophilia/basophilia	Absent	May be present
Bone marrow	Cellularity	Mostly hypercellular	Variable (hypocellular)
	Megakaryocytes	Increased with normal morphology	Increased and dysplastic morphology
	Megakaryocytic clustering	Absent	Present
	Intrasinusoidal hematopoiesis	Rare	Prominent
	Lymphoid infiltrates	Frequent	Rare
	Plasma cells	Prominent	Absent
	Reticulin fibrosis	MF gd 1–2 (rare3)	MF gd 2–3 with osteosclerosis
Investigations	Autoimmune Abs	Positive	Negative
	Clonality marker	Negative	Positive (e.g., JAK V 617F, CAL-R or MPL)
Management	Treatment	Steroids	Supportive/HS CT/JAK2 inhibitors
	Prognosis	Favorable	Unfavorable

It is a difficult task to distinguish primary AIMF from primary myelofibrosis and close observation of morphological details are required in the absence of mutation positivity (Jak2/CAL R/MPL) and other evidence of clonality. Usually, patients with PMF have appreciable to significantly palpable spleen, leukoerythroblastic picture, megakaryocytic clustering, and atypia on bone marrow.

Table 29.4 provides the list of distinguishing features between AIMF and PMF.

29.7 Management

Steroids are the mainstay in the treatment of autoimmune myelofibrosis with patients showing rapid improvements in cytopenias[1, 11]. Those who fail to respond to corticosteroids can benefit from other immunosuppressive therapies [11]. Definition of complete response includes normalization of hemoglobin level and platelet count in the absence of transfusion requirements[7]. Count recovery generally precedes resolution of BM fibrosis with 50% patients showing residual fibrosis even with complete response [3]. Overall, AIMF patients have a significant better overall survival as compared to primary myelofibrosis.

29.8 Conclusion

Autoimmune myelofibrosis is an underrecognized cause of myelofibrosis in patients presenting with cytopenias that responds to steroids and has a good clinical outcome in majority of patients. The spectrum of clinical presentation of primary and secondary AIMF may be broad but the BM findings are usually similar. It is imperative to differentiate AIMF from PMF due to drastic prognostic and therapeutic differences between these entities.

Points to Remember
1. Autoimmune myelofibrosis (AIMF) is a distinct clinicopathological entity.
2. Two types: primary AIMF and secondary AIMF.
3. Usual presentation includes—cytopenias with or without preexisting autoimmune disorder.
4. Splenomegaly is rare.
5. Immunosuppressive therapy leads to complete or partial response of cytopenias (independent of resolution of fibrosis).
6. Good morphological assessment of BM biopsy features clinches the diagnosis.

Conflicts of Interest Nil.

References

1. Kuter DJ, Bain B, Mufti G, Bagg A, Hasserjian RP. Bone marrow fibrosis: pathophysiology and clinical significance of increased bone marrow stromal fibres. Br J Haematol. 2007;139:351–62. https://doi.org/10.1111/j.1365-2141.2007.06807.x.
2. Paquette RL, Meshkinpour A, Rosen PJ. Autoimmune myelofibrosis. A steroid-responsive cause of bone marrow fibrosis associated with systemic lupus erythematosus. Medicine (Baltimore). 1994;73(3):145–52.
3. Pullarkat V, Bass RD, Gong JZ, Feinstein DI, Brynes RK. Primary autoimmune myelofibrosis: definition of a distinct clinicopathologic syndrome. Am J Hematol. 2003;72(1):8–12.
4. Chalayer E, Ffrench M, Cathebras P. Bone marrow fibrosis as a feature of systemic lupus erythematosus: a case report and literature review. Springerplus. 2014;3:349. https://doi.org/10.1186/2193-1801-3-349.
5. Vergara-Lluri ME, Piatek CI, Pullarkat V, Siddiqi IN, O'Connell C, Feinstein DI, Brynes RK. Autoimmune myelofibrosis: an update on morphologic features in 29 cases and review of the literature. Hum Pathol. 2014;45(11):2183–91. https://doi.org/10.1016/j.humpath.2014.07.017.
6. Agarwal A, Morrone K, Bartenstein M, Zhao ZJ, Verma A, Goel S. Bone marrow fibrosis in primary myelofibrosis: pathogenic mechanisms and the role of TGF-β. Stem Cell Investig. 2016;3:5. https://doi.org/10.3978/j.issn.2306-9759.2016.02.03.
7. Piatek CI, Vergara-Lluri ME, Pullarkat V, Siddiqi IN, O'Connell C, Brynes RK, Feinstein DI. Autoimmune myelofibrosis: clinical features, course, and outcome. Acta Haematol. 2017;138:129–37.
8. Piatek CI, Vergara-Lluri ME, Pullarkat V, Siddiqi IN, O'Connell C, Brynes RK, Feinstein DI. Autoimmune myelofibrosis (AIMF)—clinical features, course and outcome. Blood. 2013;122(21):3714.
9. Hua J, Matayoshi S, Uchida T, Inoue M, Hagihara M. Primary autoimmune myelofibrosis with severe thrombocytopenia mimicking immune thrombocytopenia: a case report. Mol Clin Oncol. 2016;5(6):789–91. https://doi.org/10.3892/mco.2016.1064.
10. Santos FPS, Konoplev SN, Lu H, Verstovsek S. Primary autoimmune myelofibrosis in a 36-year old patient presenting with isolated extreme anemia. Leuk Res. 2010;34(1):e35–7. https://doi.org/10.1016/j.leukres.2009.08.026.
11. Abaza Y, Yin CC, Bueso-Ramos CE, et al. Int J Hematol. 2017;105:536–7. https://doi.org/10.1007/s12185-016-2129-5.

Role of Next Generation Sequencing (NGS) in Hematological Disorders

Sanjeev Kumar Gupta

30.1 Introduction

Sequencing techniques are at the forefront of medical diagnostics in the current era of personalized medicine and targeted therapy. These techniques can identify the exact genetic change at the nucleotide level which aids in delineating the molecular pathogenesis and may also help in development of tailored therapy. Different sequencing approaches can be used for either the discovery of new genetic aberrations or checking the known genetic change for diagnostic purposes, depending on the requirement. *Next generation sequencing (NGS)* refers to the post-Sanger technologies, i.e., sequencing technologies developed after Sanger sequencing. So, NGS includes a group of technologies having the capacity to sequence large segments of genome or entire genome in high-throughput experiments to detect genetic aberrations in a much faster and reliable way [1]. The current high-throughput NGS techniques, which are also being made available at affordable costs, are gradually replacing the conventional or first generation sequencing techniques in the clinical settings. In this chapter, the basic workflow of next generation sequencing (NGS) and its application in hematological disorders has been briefly discussed.

Whole-genome sequencing (WGS) is the study of entire genome (complete set of DNA including all of its genes). It provides a comprehensive analysis of all genetic changes in the genome. However, the limitation of this assay is that a very large data output is generated resulting in difficulties in data analysis. Another problem encountered in genome sequencing is that certain portions of the genome, particularly from centromeric, telomeric, and other repetitive regions have ambiguous sequences and thus create difficulties in analysis.

A more specialized approach is to do *"targeted sequencing,"* i.e., focus on specific parts of the genome like gene mutation hotspots or recurrent gene fusions using PCR or hybrid capture methods [2]. If we target the recurrent or known mutations, it is known as *"targeted resequencing."* The number of targeted gene can be single or many genes. If it covers only the protein-coding regions (exons) and leaves out non-coding areas (introns), then it is termed as *exome sequencing* and if it covers entire set of exons, then it would be labelled as *whole-exome sequencing (WES)*. WES focuses on the exons which are functionally the most relevant portion of the genome and only 1–2% of genome. This results in achievement of much higher sequence

S. K. Gupta (✉)
Lab Oncology Unit, IRCH, All India Institute of
Medical Sciences (AIIMS), New Delhi, India
e-mail: drskgupta@aiims.ac.in

© Springer Nature Singapore Pte Ltd. 2019
R. Saxena, H. P. Pati (eds.), *Hematopathology*, https://doi.org/10.1007/978-981-13-7713-6_30

coverage (or depth)[1] compared with WGS and thus lowers the detection limit of mutations. The higher depth allows analysis of specimens with lower purity, and particularly useful for cancer specimens.

Another approach could be to do *whole transcriptome sequencing (WTS)* or RNA sequencing (RNA-seq) including coding as well as noncoding RNAs. The coding RNA (mRNA) accounts for 1–4% of the whole transcriptome and can be studied using *mRNA-sequencing (mRNA-seq)*. RNA-seq helps to study alternative gene splicing, gene fusions, post-transcriptional modifications, mutations, single nucleotide polymorphisms, and gene expression in different groups.

30.2   Advantages of NGS

There are three main advantages of NGS over the classical sequencing platforms. Firstly, it allows sequencing of multiple markers, in multiple samples in single run. Secondly, a variety of genetic aberrations like insertions and deletions, single and multi-nucleotide variants, copy number alterations, and gene fusions can be screened simultaneously. Lastly, sequencing of genomic regions multiple times or at high sequencing coverage increases the detection sensitivity (lowers the limit of detection). The correlation of number of fragments carrying the mutation with the background can also give an estimation of clonality in the sample. It also provides an opportunity to detect molecular mutations accurately in heterogeneous tumor samples [1].

The ultimate goal of genomic analysis is to detect and interpret acquired somatic mutations to reveal clinically useful information. These efforts have led to a better understanding of the molecular landscape in various diseases including hematological disorders, often uncovering new molecular pathogenetic mechanisms and resulting in changes in classification systems and prognostic models [3]. The NGS is providing

new insights into hematology, oncology, clinical genetics, and other areas of research. It has the potential to enable more precision in medical research and practice [4].

30.3   Evolution of Sequencing Techniques

The field of DNA sequencing technology has a rich history. In brief, the early DNA sequencing introduced by Sanger and Gilbert was done by chain termination followed by gel electrophoresis. The basic requirements of the classical chain termination method included a DNA primer (fluorescently or radioactively labelled), a singlestranded template, DNA polymerase, deoxyribonucleotide triphosphates (dNTPs) (dATP, dTTP, dGTP, and dCTP), and dideoxynucleotide triphosphates (ddNTPs) (ddATP, ddTTP, ddGTP, or ddCTP). The ddNTPs act as DNA chain terminators, resulting in DNA fragments of various lengths. The procedure was cumbersome as four different PCR reactions needed to be set up with one of the four ddNTPs added in each. The DNA bands could be seen either by UV light or autoradiography after denaturing polyacrylamide gel electrophoresis and the sequence was manually interpreted based on the four parallel runs (lanes A, T, G, C). Later, development of fluorescently labelled ddNTPs allowed the use of four ddNTP chain terminators, tagged with fluorochromes having different emission spectrum, in same sequencing reaction. Subsequently, the advent of capillary electrophoresis and computerized data analysis provided automation to gel electrophoresis which was much faster and provided a higher resolution. This led to the development of capillary-based DNA sequencing, initially using single and later multi-capillary sequencers.

30.4   Next Generation Sequencing (NGS) and Its Workflow

The next generation of sequencing technologies like 454 pyrosequencing (Roche) and Solexa (Illumina) have their origin in the cyclic-array

---

[1] *Coverage*: The average number of times each base pair in the target genome is covered by reads. For example, 30× coverage implies that each base in the genome was covered by 30 reads on an average.

sequencing which was first employed by Shendure et al. (2005) [5]. The process involved library preparation by DNA fragmentation and adaptor sequence ligation. The clustered fragments gathered on a plane surface or on microbeads. The DNA polymerase incorporates fluorescently labelled dNTPs into a DNA template during sequential cycles of DNA synthesis and the nucleotides are identified by excitation of fluorophore during each cycle. The critical difference from capillary electrophoresis-based sequencing is that, instead of sequencing a single DNA fragment, NGS extends this process across millions of fragments in a massively parallel fashion. In short, alternative cycles of enzyme-catalyzed elongation and spectral imaging create the sequence, using the "*sequencing by synthesis*" principle. This facilitates screening of multiple genes in multiple samples at one time. The four basic steps in the NGS workflow, as done in Illumina platform, are given below. Although the sequencing chemistries may vary in other commercially available platforms, the basic sample preparation steps and analysis steps are quite similar.

1. *Library Preparation*—The library preparation for sequencing involves random fragmentation of DNA/cDNA sample, followed by ligation of adapter sequence at both ends (Fig. 30.1). PCR amplification and gel purification is done for adapter-ligated fragments. Other platforms may use different methods of amplification of the genomic areas of interest, e.g., hybrid capture.

2. *Cluster Generation*—After library preparation, library is loaded in a flow cell for cluster generation. The adaptors on the fragments then bind complimentary oligos bound to the surface of flow cell. The clonal clusters are generated from each fragment after "bridge amplification" process (Fig. 30.2). The templates are ready for sequencing after cluster generation.

3. *Sequencing*—Illumina *sequencing by synthesis* (SBS) technology uses reversible chain termination method. It detects single bases in the sequence as they are incorporated in the

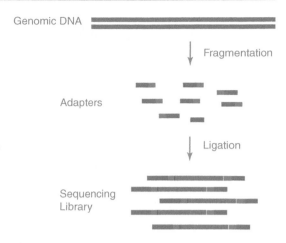

Fig. 30.1 NGS library preparation by fragmentation and adaptor ligation to both fragment ends

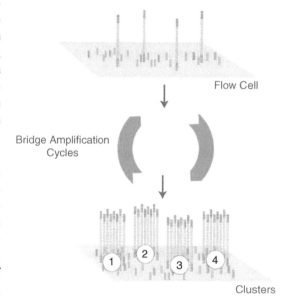

Fig. 30.2 Cluster amplification of fragments bound on flow cell surface

DNA template strands (Fig. 30.3). The readout could be optical like in Illumina and Pacific Biosciences (PacBio) platforms or non-optical, e.g., by pH measurement in Ion Torrent (Thermo Fisher) platform which uses unlabelled and unmodified nucleotides.

4. *Data Analysis*—Multiple steps of NGS data analysis can be divided into primary, secondary, and tertiary analysis steps. This analysis helps to convert the raw data into clinically relevant knowledge. Primary analysis includes

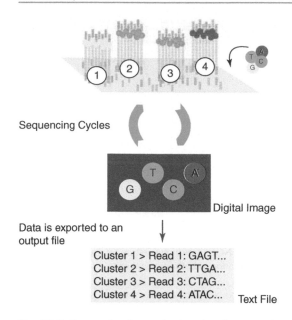

Sequencing Cycles

Digital Image

Data is exported to an output file

Cluster 1 > Read 1: GAGT...
Cluster 2 > Read 2: TTGA...
Cluster 3 > Read 3: CTAG...
Cluster 4 > Read 4: ATAC...   Text File

Fig. 30.3 Sequencing by synthesis using fluorescently labelled nucleotides and imaging of flow cell

Reads

ATGGCATTGCAATTTGACAT
TGGCATTGCAATTTG
AGATGGTATTG
GATGGCATTGCAA
GCATTGCAATTTGAC
ATGGCATTGCAATT
AGATGGCATTGCAATTTG

Reference Genome   AGATGGTATTGCAATTTGACAT

Fig. 30.4 Alignment of sample read with the reference genome revealing a T to C change

signal processing and base-calling with assessment of quality scores ("Phred score"[2]). Secondary analysis involves sequence alignment and variant calling. Tertiary level analysis includes annotation and filtering of variants.

At these multiple steps of NGS data analysis, different file formats are generated, including base-calling (FASTA files), base with quality score (FASTQ files), files after alignment to a reference genome—SAM (Sequence Alignment/Map format) followed by BAM files (Binary Alignment/Map format) and sequence variations files (VCF files) (Variant Calling Format). The main steps during data analysis are:

(a) *Alignment*: The sequence read generated after base-calling is aligned to a reference genome in order to compare it with reference and identify variations. This is known as sequence alignment (Fig. 30.4). This can be done using several alignment algorithms, e.g., MiSeq Reporter software (Illumina) preferentially uses the Burrows–Wheeler Aligner; Ion Torrent prefers the Torrent Mapping Alignment Program; and PacBio uses the Basic Local Alignment with Successive Refinement aligner.

(b) *Variant calling*: After alignment, the next step is identification of aberrations in the sequence, known as "variant calling." These structural variations or genetic aberrations can be of various sizes and types, including single nucleotide polymorphism (SNP) or insertion-deletion (indel), copy number alterations, and gene fusions. Several variant calling algorithms are available to analyze the NGS data from different platforms and purposes. These algorithms take into consideration the quality of base-calling and level of coverage to assess any nucleotide change with respect to the reference.

(c) *Variant annotation*: Annotation of the variant calls should be done according to nomenclature guidelines from Human Genome Variation Society. The obtained variants should also be compared against reference data like public SNP databases to correctly identify somatic alterations and rule out germline variants. On analysis of matched normal sample, the germline variant will be observed in both test sample and normal reads, whereas somatic variants will be seen only in test sample. Other variants can be incidental and/or of unknown significance (variants of unknown significance—VUS). An example given below shows both an SNP and a deletion (Fig. 30.5).

[2] Phred Quality score (Q) indicates base call accuracy and is logarithmically related to the probability of error (p) in base-calling. If Q is 10, then p is 1 in 10 and base call accuracy is 90%. If Q is 40, then p is 1 in 10^4, i.e., 1 in 10,000 and base call accuracy is 99.99%.

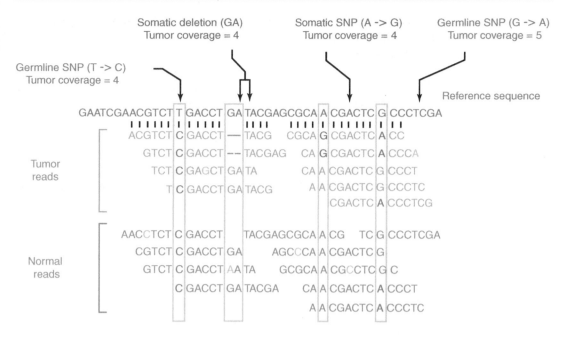

Fig. 30.5 Example showing somatic single nucleotide polymorphism (SNP), germline SNP, and somatic deletion with coverage

30.5   Next Generation Sequencing (NGS) in Hematological Disorders

The application of NGS to hematologic disorders has provided new insights into disease initiation, progression, and therapy outcome. The rapid progress in the sequencing techniques and data analysis methods as well as better integration of the NGS data with clinical information will further help in fine-tuning the therapy of patients with hematologic disorders. Although the usage of NGS has penetrated more in the field of cancer including hematological malignancies, other applications in non-malignant hematological disorders have also been documented. Some of the examples of application of NGS in malignant and non-malignant hematological disorders are listed below.

30.6   Acute Myeloid Leukemia (AML)

The first complete cancer genome was obtained from an acute myeloid leukemia (AML) patient using whole-genome sequencing (WGS). The

acquired (or somatic) mutations were identified using paired germline DNA from a normal skin biopsy of the same patient [6]. A paired non-neoplastic sample like peripheral blood, saliva, skin biopsy, buccal swabs, from the same patient, or adjacent normal tissue in an FFPE (formalin fixed paraffin embedded) sample, helps to accurately identify somatic mutations and filter the germline polymorphisms. It is also important to note that additional relevant variants may emerge on later analysis, subsequent to improvement of sequencing techniques and bioinformatics analytical tools. Two years later, a novel recurrent mutation in the DNA methyltransferase gene *DNMT3A* was reported in the same AML patient on re-examination with improved sequencing techniques, better coverage, and newer data analysis methods [7]. It was later shown that *DNMT3A* mutations were predictive of improved survival, in patients less than 60 years of age, in response to high-dose induction chemotherapy [8]. This is an example of how clinical outcome data can complement the results from the sequencing and improve patient care. NGS has been utilized to describe tumor evolution and patterns of clonal architecture in AML recently, which has the potential to guide therapeutic options [9, 10].

Recently, there has been an increased interest in the field of hematolymphoid genomes, exomes, etc., and a lot of mutations have been identified by large-scale NGS. However, it is still a challenge to be able to differentiate *"driver" mutations* that confer growth or survival advantages and contribute to pathogenesis and *"passenger" mutations,* the acquired mutations that have been carried along during the course of disease but are neutral. Further functional studies are required on candidate variants to further elucidate their clinical and biological significance.

The comprehensive characterization of the AML-associated variants was done by "The Cancer Genome Atlas Research Network" (2013). The genomes of 200 clinically annotated adult de novo AML cases were analyzed using either whole-genome or whole-exome sequencing, along with DNA methylation analysis, RNA and microRNA sequencing. AML genomes were found to have an average of 13 mutations in genes and having at least one nonsynonymous mutation in one of nine categories of genes listed in Table 30.1, in nearly all samples. These potentially "driver" mutations are very likely to be relevant for pathogenesis, and a complex network of genetic events may contribute to AML pathogenesis. A strong biologic relationship among several of the genes and classes was suggested by various patterns of involvement [11, 12].

30.7 Myelodysplastic Syndrome (MDS)

The use of NGS approaches has led to the identification of around 40 recurrent gene mutations in MDS, with many of them having prognostic implication or related to specific disease biology. Integration of sequencing data into existing international prognostic scoring system (IPSS) or revised IPSS (IPSS-R) may be challenging, but this additional information may help in selecting patients for allogeneic hematopoietic stem cell transplantation or for clinical trials of novel targeted agents. The spliceosome subunit gene *SF3B1* is commonly mutated in patients with ring sideroblasts (RS) (80–90% of MDS-RS-SLD (single lineage dysplasia) and 30–70% of MDS-RS-MLD (multilineage dysplasia)) and is associated with a relatively indolent disease course. Mutations of genes involved in DNA methylation, splicing factors other than *SF3B1*, *RAS* pathway genes and cohesin complex genes have been found to be independently associated with multilineage dysplasia. Co-mutation of *TET2* and *SRSF2* was found to be predictive of a myeloid neoplasm with myelodysplasia and monocytosis including chronic myelomonocytic leukemia. MDS patients with *TET2* mutations are more likely to respond to the DNA hypomethylating agents, e.g., azacytidine, compared to patients with wild-type *TET2*. This is in contrast to *ASXL1* mutations which is less likely to respond to hypo-

Table 30.1 Functional complementation groups of genetic alterations in AML

	Type	Examples
Class 1	Transcription-factor fusions	t(8;21), t(15;17), inv(16)
Class 2	Nucleophosmin 1	*NPM1* mutations
Class 3	Tumor-suppressor genes	*TP53* and *PHF6* mutations
Class 4	DNA methylation-related genes	DNA hydroxymethylation, e.g., *TET2*, *IDH1*, *IDH2* DNA methyltransferases, e.g., *DNMT3A*
Class 5	Activated signalling genes	*FLT3*, *KIT*, *RAS* mutations
Class 6	Chromatin-modifying genes	*ASXL1* and *EZH2* mutations, *KMT2A* fusions, *KMT2A-PTD*
Class 7	Myeloid transcription-factor genes	*CEBPA*, *RUNX1* mutations
Class 8	Cohesion complex genes	*STAG2*, *RAD21*, *SMC1*, *SMC2* mutations
Class 9	Spliceosome-complex genes	*SRSF2*, *U2AF1*, *ZRSR2* mutations

methylating agents in MDS. *TP53* mutations may identify patients with less chances of progression to higher-risk MDS or AML, when treated with lenalidomide. The patients with targetable mutation like *IDH1* or *IDH2* may be taken up for clinical trial of targeted therapy [13, 14].

The detection of a clonal genetic change in patients with "idiopathic cytopenias of undetermined significance" (ICUS) can help in the diagnosis and may also indicate a higher chance of progression to overt neoplasm, and a negative result on NGS assay has a high negative predictive value for a clonal myeloid neoplasm including MDS. However, one should not over-interpret the presence of clonal change alone in the absence of other clinical features because nearly 10% healthy persons over 70 years of age have clonal mutations in putative leukemia driver genes, known as clonal hematopoiesis of indeterminate potential (CHIP). Another fact to consider is that many variants detected by genomic studies may be germline polymorphisms, and other variants may be non-specific, e.g., *SF3B1* mutation can also be detected in a CLL clone, the *KRAS* mutations detected in MDS, and AML may also be present in other non-myeloid malignancies and lymphoproliferative disease. So, it is more likely that NGS results will not be able to replace the existing risk stratification schemes like IPSS and IPSS-R in MDS but may augment these existing clinic-pathological prognostic tools [13].

30.8   Chronic Lymphocytic Leukemia (CLL)

Quesada et al. did exome sequencing of matched CLL and normal cells from 105 patients to identify genes involved in CLL pathogenesis. Recurrent somatic mutations in 78 genes resulted in protein-coding changes. Majority of the mutations occurred in only a small fraction of cases and only *NOTCH1* and the splicing factor *SF3B1* were mutated in around 10% patients [15]. Wang et al. independently sequenced exomes of CLL

and matched normal cells in 88 CLL patients and performed WGS of another three CLL cases. They found an average of 20 (range 2–76) nonsynonymous somatic mutations per CLL patient. They identified nine genes, with a possible causative relationship, to be mutated at a significantly higher rate. Four of these genes were *TP53, ATM, MYD88,* and *NOTCH1,* known to be implicated in CLL biology. The other five included splicing factor gene *SF3B1* and four novel genes—*FBXW7, DDX3X, MAPK1,* and *ZMYM3.* These nine genes are involved in five pathways: DNA damage repair and cell-cycle control, Notch signalling, Wnt signalling, inflammatory pathways, and RNA processing. Many other genes involved in these pathways were mutated at a low rate in these CLL exomes. These observations suggest that even though a large number of genes may be mutated, only a common set of pathways gets affected in CLL [16].

30.9   Hairy Cell Leukemia (HCL)

Recently, whole-exome sequencing analysis of leukemic and matched normal cells in a hairy cell leukemia (HCL) patient led to the identification of recurrent *BRAF V600E* mutation in HCL. The *BRAF V600E* mutation were found in all patients with HCL and absent in other B-cell lymphomas like HCL variant and splenic marginal zone lymphoma, thus helping in their differential diagnosis. Moreover, a possibility of targeting mutated *BRAF V600E* (using PLX-4720) was also shown [17]. This is a good example to show how NGS techniques may have implications for explaining the pathogenesis, in differential diagnosis, and also targeted therapy.

30.10   Waldenstrom's Macroglobulinemia

NGS studies have detected that about 90% of lymphoplasmacytic lymphoma (LPL) or Waldenstrom's macroglobulinemia (LPL plus an immunoglobulin M [IgM] paraprotein) have *MYD88 L265P* mutations [18]. This mutation is also found in IgM monoclonal gammopathy of undetermined significance (MGUS) cases, few other small B-cell lymphomas but not in IgG or IgA MGUS or plasma cell myeloma. Review of cases with and without the *MYD88 L265P* mutation has led to revised criteria for LPL.

30.11 Multiple Myeloma

WGS and WES in multiple myeloma patients revealed mutations in genes involved in protein translation, genes involved in histone methylation, and NF-kB signalling pathway. In addition, few patients also showed mutations of the *BRAF*, suggesting a role of *BRAF* inhibitors in multiple myeloma [19].

30.12 T-Cell Large Granular Lymphocytic Leukemia (T-LGL)

Koskela et al. performed targeted re-sequencing in a cohort of 76 patients with T-LGL, after finding the candidate gene, signal transducer and activator of transcription 3 (*STAT3*) in the whole-exome sequencing of an index patient. They found *STAT3* mutations in 40% patients of T-LGL, suggesting a role of aberrant *STAT3* signalling in its pathogenesis [20].

30.13 Acute lymphoblastic leukemia (ALL)

Roberts et al. reported targetable kinase activating lesions in a cohort of 154 patients with Ph-like B-ALL, taking help of NGS techniques—predominantly using transcriptome sequencing and also whole-genome and whole-exome sequencing in few patients. Using various methods, rearrangements with activation of kinase signalling were seen in 62% (96/154) patients [21].

30.14 Thalassemia and Other Hemoglobinopathies

Some recent studies have shown the use of NGS for population screening for carriers of thalassemia and other hemoglobinopathies and prenatal testing. Shang et al. (2017) recently developed and validated a single target-based NGS assay for molecular screening and genotyping in hemoglobinopathies [22]. Their target regions included all eight globin genes (*HBZ, HBA1, HBA2, HBE1, HBG1, HBG2, HBD,* and *HBB*) and validated genetic modifiers (*KLF1, BCL11A,* and *MYB*) with an aim to detect variants in known genes related to hemoglobinopathies. The assay was designed to capture key regions, such as α- and β-globin gene clusters, associated with hemoglobinopathies to ensure the detection of any disease-associated aberrations. Unlike traditional carrier screening assays, which are designed to search for only the most common mutations within a gene, the NGS-based approach identified both common and rare, annotated and novel variants in carriers, significantly improving the detection of carrier status and at-risk couples. The NGS assay additionally identified few at-risk couples which were missed by traditional screening or molecular testing methods. Although the cost of instruments and reagents usually appear as limiting factors, this study with NGS had a high throughput of 3000 samples per run and showed NGS to be a feasible and effective methodology for preconception screening and diagnosis of hemoglobinopathies in large populations. He et al. (2017) also found NGS to be a competitive thalassemia screening method for population screening among populations with a high prevalence of disease [23]. The re-sequencing approach targeting the common point mutations and deletions was found to be useful and could be successfully validated. NGS-based screening was found to be better for screening of α-thalassemia carriers and composite α- and β-thalassemia carriers.

Carlberg et al. investigated NGS for non-invasive prenatal testing for beta thalassemia, using cell-free fetal DNA (cfFDNA) in maternal plasma [24]. This can potentially eliminate risks associated with invasive procedures like chorionic villus sampling and amniocentesis. They developed an NGS assay using probe capture enrichment, with short oligonucleotide probes complementary to the target region. Their assay was applicable to short, fragmented DNA, like cell-free DNA and could identify informative single nucleotide polymorphisms (SNPs) (i.e., an allele in the fetus which is absent in the mother) to estimate the fraction of cfDNA from the fetus.

30.15 Aplastic Anemia

Up to a third of adult aplastic anemia (AA) patients have shown somatic mutations in MDS-associated genes using targeted NGS for genes mutated in hematological malignancies. The most commonly mutated malignancy-associated genes in AA are *ASXL1, BCOR/BCORL1,* and *DNMT3A.* The mutations in *BCOR* and *BCORL1* may predict an improved response to immunosuppressive therapy and have favorable prognosis along with *PIGA* mutations. Several genes (*DNMT3A, ASXL1, TP53, RUNX1,* and *CSMD1*) were associated with worse overall survival, when analyzed in aggregate, but not individually in a study by Yoshizato et al. It is noted that majority of pediatric and adult AA patients develop clonal hematopoiesis, with many adult AA patients having somatic mutations in genes, usually affected in MDS and aging. However, long-term prospective studies are required to decode the prognostic implications of somatic mutations in MDS-associated genes [25, 26].

30.16 Hereditary Hemolytic Anemias

NGS has helped in study of RBC membrane disorders, e.g., exome sequencing in anemias due to altered permeability of RBC membrane led to identification of *PIEZO1* (encoding a mechanoreceptor) as the affected gene in both isolated and syndromic forms of dehydrated hereditary stomatocytosis (DHS1), which can be clinically confused with Hereditary Spherocytosis (HS) [27]. Other disorders in heterogeneous group of hereditary hemolytic anemias have also been studied with various NGS panels, including RBC membrane disorders like HS, elliptocytosis/pyropoikilocytosis; enzymopathies like Glucose 6 phosphate dehydrogenase deficiency, pyruvate kinase deficiency; disorders of erythropoiesis like congenital dyserythropoietic anemia, etc. These complex genetic disorders are difficult to diagnose due to their clinical and molecular heterogeneity. Targeted NGS panels incorporating genes coding for cytoskeletal proteins and enzymes, and covering complete coding region, splice site junctions, some deep intronic or regulatory regions have been tested and found useful. Many pathogenic variants, likely pathogenic variants, and complex combinations of known and novel mutations could be detected on NGS [28]. Russo et al. tested RedPlex panel composed of 34 loci causative or candidates of hereditary hemolytic anemias and found high sensitivity and specificity in patients with ambiguous phenotypes. It also allowed the identification of "polygenic" conditions, i.e., patients in which the phenotypic variability was possibly by modifier variants associated with causative mutations [29]. However, extensive clinical and hematologic information is needed to support the interpretation of molecular data.

30.17 Venous Thromboembolism (VTE)

The possibility of using NGS techniques has also been explored for VTE patients. Lee et al. reported the use of whole-exome sequencing in VTE to find out lesser known genetic causes of thrombophilia. Their analysis focused on 55 novel genes associated with thrombophilia, based on literature or correlation with protein modelling studies. Their analysis could detect probable disease causing variants in around 60% of patients compared to only around 25% using conventional thrombophilia testing for heritable thrombophilia in their cohort [30]. So, with easy availability of NGS at affordable price, it may be an alternative strategy to screen the whole genome/exome rather than the limited thrombophilia screening done currently.

30.18 Iron Metabolism Disorders

McDonald et al. reported the use of NGS to sequence 39 iron regulatory genes in parallel at a cost comparable to that of sequencing each gene sequentially using the Sanger approach. This approach can be particularly useful in detecting the patients with atypical iron disorders including iron-refractory iron-deficiency anemia (IRIDA) and hereditary hemochromatosis without HFE mutations which are difficult to diagnose genetically and have overlapping clinical presentation with the more common iron overload conditions [31].

30.19 Major Challenges of Using NGS

1. *Volume of data*: The major challenges are regarding the volume and complexity of the data generated due to the large size of genome tested in multiple samples. It is not practical to store all the files generated as NGS assay output. As a policy, the laboratory may store files which have adequate data to repeat the analysis. In general, a storage period of 2 years is recommended for these files as per the Clinical Laboratory Improvement Amendment policies [1].
2. *Choice of markers*: With an extensive ability of NGS to screen multiple targets simultaneously, the selection of appropriate genes to be included in a panel becomes important. For specific needs and better sample throughput, custom panels with mutational hotspot regions are a better choice rather than screening the entire coding region of genes.
3. *Clinical implications of the data generated*: It is a challenging task to translate the wealth of data generated by the NGS experiments into clinically actionable information. Determination of the pathogenicity of the numerous identified genomic variants is difficult and requires correlation with clinical information from a large number of patients. The general approach to characterize the impact of mutation on prognosis is to sequence the "index patients" or the "discovery cohorts" first and then verify the findings in larger and independent patient cohorts. The functional characterization of mutation and biochemical analyses may help to assess the pathogenicity of identified genetic variants. Another way of better interpretation of the data in inherited genetic disorders is the simultaneous evaluation of parents and other family members, to establish the inheritance pattern of the variants and to understand its role. Moreover, it is better to focus on key pathways or genes to generate data on clinically relevant genetic changes.
4. *Ethical and medico-legal issues*: During the NGS studies, particularly WGS and WES, there is a chance of encountering clinically relevant germline mutations unrelated to the disease being studied. An informed consent should be taken for both research and clinical genomic testing, particularly for reporting the unrelated or secondary findings. The current American College of Medical Genetics and Genomics (ACMG) policy recommends 59 medically actionable genes, for return in clinical genomic sequencing [32].

30.20 Future of NGS

Sequencing technologies and analysis methods have shown continued improvement over time. This trend is likely to continue and further speed up in near future, providing more comprehensive characterization of genomic variants and their biological function. Initial efforts have focused on target identification and further efforts are likely in the areas of prognostication, resistance detection, disease monitoring, and early detection with the help of integration of RNA sequencing and epigenetic analysis. The addition of genomic findings into classification and prognostic scoring systems as well as prospective clinical trials will allow further fine-tuning of clinical care. Over time, these efforts will ultimately facilitate precision medicine, with therapy being guided by the genetic makeup of the individual.

References

1. Singh RR, Luthra R, Routbort MJ, Patel KP, Medeiros LJ. Implementation of next generation sequencing in clinical molecular diagnostic laboratories: advantages, challenges and potential. Expert Rev Precis Med Drug Dev. 2016;1(1):109–20.
2. Sulonen A, Ellonen P, Almusa H, Lepisto M, Eldfors S, Hannula S, et al. Comparison of solution-based exome capture methods for next generation sequencing. Genome Biol. 2011;12(9):R94.
3. Kohlmann A, Grossmann V, Nadarahjah N, Haferlach T. Next generation sequencing—feasibility and practicality in hematology. Br J Haematol. 2013;160(6):736–53.
4. Merker JD, Valouev A, Gotlib J. Next-generation sequencing in hematologic malignancies: what will be the dividends? Ther Adv Hematol. 2012;3(6):333–9.
5. Shendure J, Porreca GJ, Reppas NB, Lin X, McCutcheon JP, Rosenbaum AM, et al. Accurate multiplex polony sequencing of an evolved bacterial genome. Science. 2005;309:1728–32.
6. Ley TJ, Mardis ER, Ding L, Fulton B, McLellan MD, Chen K, et al. DNA sequencing of a cytogenetically normal acute myeloid leukemia genome. Nature. 2008;456:66–72.
7. Ley TJ, Ding L, Walter MJ, McLellan MD, Lamprecht T, Larson DE, et al. DNMT3A mutations in acute myeloid leukemia. N Engl J Med. 2010;363: 2424–33.
8. Patel JP, Gonen M, Figueroa ME, Fernandez H, Sun Z, Racevskis J, et al. Prognostic relevance of integrated genetic profiling in acute myeloid leukemia. N Engl J Med. 2012;366:1079–89.
9. Ding L, Ley TJ, Larson DE, Miller CA, Koboldt DC, Welch JS, et al. Clonal evolution in relapsed acute myeloid leukaemia revealed by whole-genome sequencing. Nature. 2012;481:506–10.
10. Walter MJ, Shen D, Ding L, Shao J, Koboldt DC, Chen K, et al. Clonal architecture of secondary acute myeloid leukemia. N Engl J Med. 2012;366: 1090–8.
11. Cancer Genome Atlas Research Network. Genomic and epigenomic landscapes of adult de novo acute myeloid leukemia. N Engl J Med. 2013;368:2059–74.
12. Arber DA, Orazi A, Hasserjian RP, Brunning RD, Le Beau MM, Porwit A, et al. Introduction and overview of the classification of myeloid neoplasms. In: Swerdlow SH, Campo E, Harris NL, et al., editors. WHO classification of tumours of haematopoietic and lymphoid tissues. Revised 4th ed. Lyon: IARC; 2017. p. 16–27.
13. Steensma DP. The evolving role of genomic testing in assessing prognosis of patients with myelodysplastic syndromes. Best Pract Res Clin Haematol. 2017;30(4):295–300.
14. Malcovati L, Papaemmanuil E, Ambaglio I, Elena C, Galli A, Della Porta MG, et al. Driver somatic mutations identify distinct disease entities within myeloid neoplasms with myelodysplasia. Blood. 2014;124(9):1513–21.
15. Quesada V, Conde L, Villamor N, Ordonez GR, Jares P, Bassaganyas L, et al. Exome sequencing identifies recurrent mutations of the splicing factor SF3B1 gene in chronic lymphocytic leukemia. Nat Genet. 2012;44:47–52.
16. Wang L, Lawrence MS, Wan Y, Stojanov P, Sougnez C, Stevenson K, et al. SF3B1 and other novel cancer genes in chronic lymphocytic leukemia. N Engl J Med. 2011;365:2497–506.
17. Tiacci E, Trifonov V, Schiavoni G, Holmes A, Kern W, Martelli MP, et al. BRAF mutations in hairy-cell leukemia. N Engl J Med. 2011;364:2305–15.
18. Treon SP, Xu L, Yang G, et al. MYD88 L265P somatic mutation in Waldenstrom's macroglobulinemia. N Engl J Med. 2012;367(9):826–33.
19. Chapman MA, Lawrence MS, Keats JJ, Cibulskis K, Sougnez C, Schinzel AC, et al. Initial genome sequencing and analysis of multiple myeloma. Nature. 2011;471:467–72.
20. Koskella HL, Eldfors S, Ellonen P, van Adrichem AJ, Kuusanmaki H, Andersson EI, et al. Somatic STAT3 mutations in large granular lymphocytic leukemia. N Engl J Med. 2012;366:1905–13.
21. Roberts KG, Li Y, Payne-Turner D, Harvey RC, Yang Y-L, Pei D, et al. Targetable kinase-activating lesions in Ph-like acute lymphoblastic leukemia. N Engl J Med. 2014;371(11):1005–15.
22. Shang X, Peng Z, Ye Y, Asan, Zhang X, Chen Y, et al. Rapid targeted next-generation sequencing platform for molecular screening and clinical genotyping in subjects with hemoglobinopathies. EBioMedicine. 2017;23:150–9.
23. He J, Song W, Yang J, Lu S, Yuan Y, Guo J. Next-generation sequencing improves thalassemia carrier screening among premarital adults in a high prevalence population: the Dai nationality, China. Genet Med. 2017;19(9):1022–31.
24. Carlberg K, Bose N, Deng J, Lal A, Erlich H, Calloway C. Towards the development of a noninvasive prenatal test for beta-thalassemia: utilization of probe capture enrichment and next generation sequencing. Blood. 2016;128(22):3622.
25. Yoshizato T, Dumitriu B, Hosokawa K, Makishima H, Yoshida K, Townsley D, et al. Somatic mutations and clonal hematopoiesis in aplastic anemia. N Engl J Med. 2015;373(1):35–47.
26. Kulasekararaj AG, Jiang J, Smith AE, Mohamedali AM, Mian S, Gandhi S, et al. Somatic mutations identify a subgroup of aplastic anemia patients who progress to myelodysplastic syndrome. Blood. 2014;124(17):2698–704.
27. Andolfo I, Russo R, Gambale A, Iolascon A. New insights on hereditary erythrocyte membrane defects. Haematologica. 2016;101(11):1284–94.
28. Agarwal AM, Reading NS, Frizzell K, Shen W, Sorrells S, Salama ME, et al. Using a next generation sequencing panel to discover the obscure causes of hereditary hemolytic anemias. Blood. 2016;128(22):2433.

29. Russo RAI, Manna F, Gambale A, Pignataro P, De Rosa G, Iolascon A. RedPlex: a targeted next generation sequencing-based diagnosis for patients with hereditary hemolytic anemias. Haematologica. 2016;101(s1):1.

30. Lee E, Dykas DJ, Leavitt AD, Camire RM, Ebberink E, García de Frutos P, et al. Whole-exome sequencing in evaluation of patients with venous thromboembolism. Blood Adv. 2017;1:1224–37.

31. McDonald CJ, Ostini L, Wallace DF, Lyons A, Crawford DH, Subramaniam VN. Next-generation sequencing: application of a novel platform to analyze atypical iron disorders. J Hepatol. 2015;63(5):1288–93.

32. Kalia SS, Adelman K, Bale SJ, Chung WK, Eng C, Evans JP, et al. Recommendations for reporting of secondary findings in clinical exome and genome sequencing, 2016 update (ACMG SF v2.0): a policy statement of the American College of Medical Genetics and Genomics. Genet Med. 2017;19(2):249–55.

Printed by Printforce, the Netherlands